AF743839

Current Cancer Research

Series Editor
Wafik El-Deiry

For further volumes:
http://www.springer.com/series/7892

Joseph D. Rosenblatt • Eckhard R. Podack
Glen N. Barber • Augusto Ochoa
Editors

Advances in Tumor Immunology and Immunotherapy

Springer

Editors
Joseph D. Rosenblatt
Sylvester Comprehensive Cancer Center (SCCC)
School of Medicine
University of Miami
Miami, FL, USA

Glen N. Barber
Sylvester Comprehensive Cancer Center
University of Miami
Miami, FL, USA

Eckhard R. Podack
Department of Microbiology and Immunology
University of Miami
Miami, FL, USA

Augusto Ochoa
Department of Pediatrics
Louisiana State University Health Sciences Center
New Orleans, LA, USA

ISBN 978-1-4614-8808-8 ISBN 978-1-4614-8809-5 (eBook)
DOI 10.1007/978-1-4614-8809-5
Springer New York Heidelberg Dordrecht London

Library of Congress Control Number: 2013951429

© Springer Science+Business Media New York 2014
This work is subject to copyright. All rights are reserved by the Publisher, whether the whole or part of the material is concerned, specifically the rights of translation, reprinting, reuse of illustrations, recitation, broadcasting, reproduction on microfilms or in any other physical way, and transmission or information storage and retrieval, electronic adaptation, computer software, or by similar or dissimilar methodology now known or hereafter developed. Exempted from this legal reservation are brief excerpts in connection with reviews or scholarly analysis or material supplied specifically for the purpose of being entered and executed on a computer system, for exclusive use by the purchaser of the work. Duplication of this publication or parts thereof is permitted only under the provisions of the Copyright Law of the Publisher's location, in its current version, and permission for use must always be obtained from Springer. Permissions for use may be obtained through RightsLink at the Copyright Clearance Center. Violations are liable to prosecution under the respective Copyright Law.
The use of general descriptive names, registered names, trademarks, service marks, etc. in this publication does not imply, even in the absence of a specific statement, that such names are exempt from the relevant protective laws and regulations and therefore free for general use.
While the advice and information in this book are believed to be true and accurate at the date of publication, neither the authors nor the editors nor the publisher can accept any legal responsibility for any errors or omissions that may be made. The publisher makes no warranty, express or implied, with respect to the material contained herein.

Printed on acid-free paper

Springer is part of Springer Science+Business Media (www.springer.com)

Contents

Introduction

The first decades of immunotherapy applied to cancer yielded modest and sporadic successes, largely confined to the treatment of a handful of solid tumors such as melanoma, renal cell carcinoma, and bladder cancer, either through the installation of local adjuvants such as BCG or through systemic administration of cytokines such as interferon-alpha and interleukin-2 in pharmacologic doses. Despite a dearth of mechanistic underpinning and immunologic insight, these successes demonstrated the potential power inherent in harnessing the immune system to combat malignant disease, as well as the durability of the responses in the handful of patients in which such responses were observed. Early therapeutic success derived from serendipitous application of newly discovered immune-effector molecules such as high-dose interleukin-2, and insight into underlying mechanisms was lacking. Recent advances have allowed for the application of our evolving understanding of immunologic principles and provided new avenues by which both innate and adaptive immune responses can be harnessed to augment antitumor therapies. There is growing appreciation that the cytolytic CD8+ T-cell, while necessary is but one actor in a complex environment in which tolerance and effector function may coexist and may facilitate or alternatively inhibit tumor growth. Immune response and/or tolerance is shaped from the inception of tumorigenesis by complex interaction between the tumor, its microenvironment, the innate and adaptive immune systems, and immune editing. Antigen processing and presentation, chemokines, cytokines, costimulatory ligands and their receptors, including members of the TNF receptor family, toll-like receptors and their ligands, NK-cells and activating and repressive signals, and a variety of cells with immune regulatory function act in coordinate fashion to shape the ultimate outcome of the encounter between the immune system and tumor. Such immune regulatory function has been ascribed to plasmacytoid dendritic cells, tumor-associated macrophages, myeloid suppressor cells, and T- and B-regulatory cells as well as the tumor cells themselves which may usurp normal cellular mechanisms conferring immune tolerance such as elaboration of TGF-β, and interleukin 10 (IL-10), expression of tolerogenic costimulatory ligands such as PDL-1 and ICOS-ligand, and soluble forms of NKG2D ligand which may serve to tolerize the host.

Despite manifest complexity, recent therapeutic successes leading to the approval of anti CTLA-4 antibody (ipilimumab), and successful targeting of the PD1 pathway in lung cancer, demonstrate the potential inherent in selective manipulation of even a single important pathway in altering the balance between immune tolerance and rejection. While a host of autoimmune phenomena have been encountered as a result of such manipulations, ultimately the increasingly frequently observed therapeutic successes offer real promise that manipulation of such key pathways is feasible and may be used to augment response in a variety of solid and hematologic malignancies.

In this volume leaders in the immune therapy field as well as clinically engaged investigators have summarized selected advances in our understanding of immune suppression and anti-tumor immunity and highlighted promising new approaches which may foretell the next generation of immune interventions. The volume is not meant to be all encompassing; this would not have been possible within the context of a volume of this size. Rather, it seeks to highlight new and evolving approaches and insights which may shape a new generation of immune therapies. The editors have elected to survey territory somewhat less well explored in an effort to take a fresh look at new trends in this rapidly evolving field. These include for example, the role of myeloid suppressor cells in human malignancies and the evolving body of knowledge relevant to the potential role of B-regulatory cells in addition to the better appreciated T-regulatory cell. While most human data regarding B reg function has been amassed in the setting of autoimmune disease, extensive murine studies point to a likely role for B cells in shaping of the human anti-tumor response, an area of emerging study surveyed by Zhang and Rosenblatt in this volume. Novel approaches harnessing potent innate pathways such as those involving biology of heat shock proteins which have already advanced into the clinic are reviewed by Schreiber and Podack who have pioneered the use of gp96 in secreted form now being tested in Phase I/II trials alone, and which will shortly be tested in combination with therapeutic manipulation of adenosinergic tolerizing pathways. Biology and manipulation of natural killer cells is summarized by George Weiner, who has pioneered the manipulation of NK cell biology in relation to therapeutic antibody administration. Drs. Paul Sondel and Lou Weiner extensively review developments in antibody engineering, and early experiences and challenges using bifunctional molecules incorporating both antibody targeting sequences as well as immune effector molecules such as cytokines. These approaches while still in their infancy have been unusually successful in murine models, yet have proven quite difficult to apply in the human setting. Nevertheless, they offer considerable promise and versatility and perspective is provided by leading researchers in the field.

Dr. Eli Gilboa, highlights an unusual new approach to altering the inherent immunogenicity of tumors through manipulation of nonsense RNA editing functions within the cell, an innovative approach which has garnered significant recent attention. The creation of "space" for homeostatic T cell expansion and its utility is summarized by Bernie Fox who has pioneered understanding of this mechanism in relation to clinical immunotherapy. Perhaps nowhere is the complex interplay between tolerance, NK, B, and T cell repopulation more routinely and effectively manipulated than in the setting of allogeneic stem cell transplantation and lessons learned from decades of preclinical and clinical investigation are summarized in a comprehensive chapter by Lazaros Lekakis and Krishna Komanduri.

The recent successes in the genetic manipulation of T-cell specificities as well as intracellular signaling within T-cells following encounter with tumor cells are highlighted in the two chapters by Zelig Esshar and Aaron Rapoport, pioneers in the development of T cell engineering and redirection of T cell specificity, and their application to hematologic malignancies, respectively. The striking results recently reported to great acclaim by Carl June and colleagues observed in a small number of patients with ALL and CLL following introduction of the CAR-T technology, highlight the considerable promise of the approach.

Renal cell carcinoma and melanoma continue to serve as principal examples of success of immunotherapeutic approaches. The current status of tumor immunotherapeutic approaches in renal cell carcinoma is reviewed by Jaime Merchan, providing perspective in an area in which immune and non-immune approaches are rapidly coalescing to alter prognosis.

Finally, the recent successes using anti CTLA4 antibody and other targets in the TNF receptor family in solid tumors are reviewed from a clinical vantage point as the underlying immunology has been extensively addressed elsewhere. These and other new approaches in the clinic have increased our need for improved means of assessing immune response, and correlation of such response with clinical outcomes are comprehensively reviewed by Theresa Whiteside, a leading authority in clinical immune assessment.

The strong association between the human papilloma virus infection and a subset of human head and neck squamous cell carcinoma suggests that head and neck cancer may be particularly susceptible to immune intervention, and also may afford unique accessibility of tumor for correlative study. Rationale and opportunities for manipulation of the immune response in head and neck cancer are carefully reviewed by Dr. Paolo Serafini and Donald Weed.

This volume could not have been expansive but rather is meant to highlight evolving new areas and critical recent advances in the field. The authors, recognized as leaders in an exciting field have been given free reign of thought and have been encouraged to raise critical questions for future investigation. The editors certainly hope that this volume will be of substantial interest to clinicians as well as basic and translational scientists working in the rapidly moving and exciting field of antitumor immunity.

We owe a special debt of gratitude to my coeditors and our accomplished colleagues who have contributed to this volume. Special thanks to Fiona Sarne, Cancer Research Editor at Springer for her tireless and enthusiastic encouragement and persistence in seeing this volume to completion and to my editorial assistants Zulema Rivero and Angie Monnar for their dedicated efforts. We truly hope you enjoy the volume.

Part I
Immune Activation, Suppression and Manipulation of the Immune Antitumor Response

Myeloid-Derived Suppressor Cells in Cancer

Christos E. Kyriakopoulos, Alberto J. Montero, and Claudia Marcela Diaz-Montero

Abstract Immune evasion is an emerging hallmark of cancer. Many cancers evade the immune system through the overproduction of a wide array of immunosuppressive cells and cytokines, which not only inhibit the host's antitumor immune response, but also hinder the clinical efficacy of immune-based therapies. Myeloid-derived suppressor cells (MDSCs) represent a heterogeneous collection of immature myeloid cells that play an important role in cancer immune evasion. Their presence has been extensively investigated in preclinical models. MDSCs arise from myeloid progenitor cells that have failed to terminally differentiate into mature granulocytes and macrophages and are recruited from the marrow to the tumor microenvironment through production of various cytokines. One of the major obstacles in developing clinical strategies targeting MDSCs in cancer patients has been their heterogeneity in humans, which thus far has prevented determination of an unambiguous phenotype, shared between mice and humans, that has clinical relevance and correlates with their suppressive function. In this chapter we review the current clinical literature on MDSCs in cancer patients, showing that there appear to be two major subsets of MDSCs which are present under different situations. We also discuss the potential use of MDSC as prognostic and predictive markers in cancer patients. Finally, we examine current strategies designed to modulate MDSCs in cancer patients, which represents an innovative and promising approach to enhance the effectiveness of immune-based therapies.

Keywords Myeloid derived suppressor cells • Cancer • Tumor immunology • Cancer immune evasion

---

C.E. Kyriakopoulos
Department of Medicine, Sylvester Comprehensive Cancer Center,
University of Miami, Miami, FL, USA

A.J. Montero (✉) • C.M. Diaz-Montero
Taussig Cancer Institute Cleveland Clinic, Cleveland, OH 44195, USA
e-mail: montero2@ccf.org

J.D. Rosenblatt et al. (eds.), *Advances in Tumor Immunology and Immunotherapy*,
Current Cancer Research, DOI 10.1007/978-1-4614-8809-5_1,
© Springer Science+Business Media New York 2014

1 Introduction

Myeloid-derived suppressor cells (MDSCs), first described over 30 years ago in patients with cancer, are a heterogeneous population of myeloid cells with the ability to suppress the immune system. The biology of MDSCs in malignant disease has now been more thoroughly characterized as a result of work in preclinical models as well as a more refined understanding of the varied mechanisms by which tumor cells utilize them to evade the immune system. However, advances in clinical research have been hindered by their heterogeneous phenotype in humans, and thus far there is no uniform consensus regarding which is the most clinically relevant phenotype to study. In this chapter we provide an overview of what has been learned about the biology of MDSCs in the setting of cancer from preclinical models, review what has been learned from clinical studies, and discuss pharmacologic strategies to directly modulate MDSCs, as a novel therapeutic approach in oncology.

2 Preclinical Data

2.1 Phenotype

MDSCs constitute a diverse population of cells derived from bone marrow progenitor cells that are at varying stages of differentiation from early myeloid to more granulocytic or monocytic in phenotype. In murine tumor models, MDSCs have been isolated from peripheral blood, spleen, lymph nodes, and tumor sites and are known to have the ability to block both innate and adaptive immunity. MDSC recruitment to the tumor microenvironment is currently thought to be one of the central mechanisms by which tumor cells evade the immune system [1]. Our current understanding from the published literature is that there are two main subtypes of MDSCs with either polymorphonuclear or monocytic characteristics, termed granulocytic and monocytic MDSCs, respectively, each of which employs slightly different mechanisms to suppress antitumor immunity (Fig. 1).

The distinction between the two different phenotypes was initially based on the expression of Ly6G and Ly6C. Granulocytic MDSCs were described as $Ly6G^{+}Ly6C^{low}$, whereas the monocytic subpopulation was described as $Ly6G^{-}Ly6C^{high}$. In terms of their function, the granulocytic MDSCs are known to express high levels of arginase, but not inducible nitric oxide synthetase (iNOS), and have been shown to produce higher levels of reactive oxygen species (ROS). Monocytic MDSCs are known to express both arginase and iNOS but do not produce high levels of ROS [2]. The production of ROS is believed to be important, as this is one mechanism by which granulocytic MDSCs are able to suppress T-cells that are in close proximity through production of high levels of ROS, such as hydrogen peroxide and peroxynitrite, that can induce T-cell apoptosis. The production of ROS could also lead to nitration of tyrosine residues in the T-cell receptor (TCR)

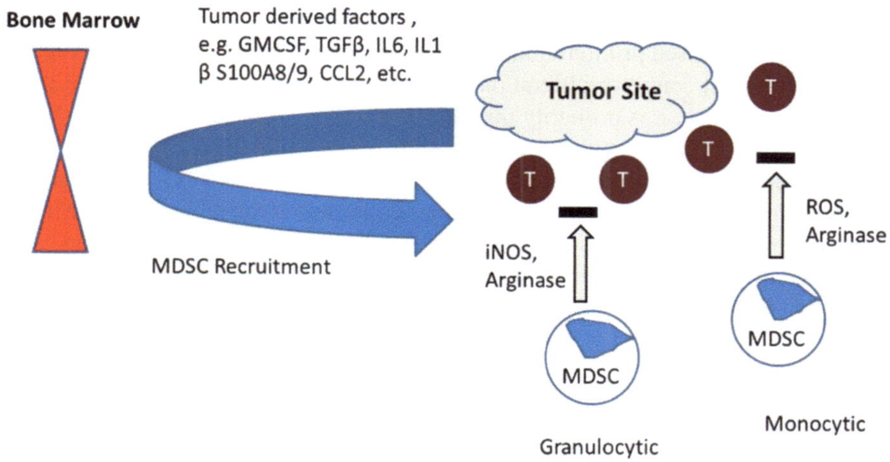

Fig. 1 Schematic of tumor-induced mobilization of MDSCs

during direct cell–cell contact which renders it unable to bind to antigen, thus blocking their activation [3].

Further classification of those cells in mice was based on the intensity of Gr-1 expression [4] which is associated with specific functional traits [5]. Monocytic MDSCs have been described as $CD11b^{+}/Gr\text{-}1^{int/low}$ and are capable of constantly suppressing the $CD8^{+}$ T-cell activation in tumor-bearing mice [6]. These cells show high expression of IL-4Rα when compared to granulocytic MDSCs, and their activity appears to be driven by tumor-secreted GM-CSF [6] and by IFN-γ released from T lymphocytes [7]. Granulocytic MDSCs have been described phenotypically as $CD11b^{+}/Gr\text{-}1^{high}$ and exert limited immune suppression in some tumor models and only when present in high numbers [6]. Although they require GM-CSF secretion in order to expand, they do not appear to respond when GM-CSF is given externally [6] since GM-CSF is a required but not a sufficient factor for their maturation [8].

2.2 *Expansion and Activation of MDSCs in Tumor Models*

In tumor-bearing mice, expansion and activation of MDSCs are controlled by several factors released by tumor cells, the surrounding stroma, and/or the immune system. Factors released from the tumors mostly induce MDSC proliferation through the stimulation of myelopoiesis and inhibition of their differentiation, whereas factors released from the tumor stroma or the immune system directly impact on their activation.

The majority of these tumor-derived factors are growth factors, cytokines, or chemokines and trigger different signaling pathways on MDSCs that are mainly mediated through the signal transducer and activator of transcription (STAT) family of transcriptional factors [9]. The activation of STAT3 is known to lead to prolonged survival and increased proliferation of MDSCs through the induction and upregulation of genes that control proliferation and apoptosis, such as MYC, BCL-XL, and cyclin D1 [9]. Also, it is primarily through both STAT 3 and NADPH that ROS are overproduced in granulocytic MDSCs as well.

There are also more complex and interrelated chemokine and cytokine networks between tumor cells, stroma, and immune cells that ultimately lead to MDSC recruitment and activation, a process that is required before the MDSCs can exert their immunosuppressive activity. Those factors include IFNγ, ligands for Toll-like receptors, IL-4, IL-3, and TGFβ, among others [9].

2.3 Mechanisms of Immunosuppression of MDSCs in Cancer

MDSCs mediate immune suppression through various metabolic pathways and direct cell-to-cell contact. Even though most of the functional studies have been conducted in the preclinical setting, there is an increasing body of evidence supporting the notion that similar mechanisms are also involved in humans.

2.3.1 Metabolism of L-Arginine

While both granulocytic and monocytic MDSCs utilize a variety of mechanisms to suppress tumor immunity, both are known to utilize a strategy that involves depletion of an amino acid in the tumor microenvironment that is important for proper T-cell function. MDSCs produce high intracellular levels of arginase, the enzyme that catabolizes L-arginine. L-arginine is a semi-essential amino acid, and is fundamental for proper T-cell function. L-arginine serves as a substrate for two different enzymes implicated in MDSC-induced immunosuppression, arginase 1 and iNOS. Like most cells, both MDSCs and T-cells need L-arginine for protein synthesis, but as a direct consequence of MDSCs having high intracellular arginase levels, they need to import excess arginine through their CAT-2B transporter. This results in L-arginine depletion from the microenvironment which leads T-cells to cell cycle arrest [10].

Arginase 1 secretion by murine MDSCs is modulated by several cytokines such as IL-4, IL-13, TGF-β, and GM-CSF [11]. Arginase 1 metabolizes L-arginine to L-ornithine and urea, thus depleting L-arginine from the tumor microenvironment. The exact mechanism of inhibition of T-cell proliferation through L-arginine depletion is still unclear; however different potential mechanisms have been postulated. One possible mechanism that has also been observed in humans is that depletion of L-arginine may lead to decreased expression of CD3 ζ-chain of the T-cell receptor, thereby interfering with their function [12]. Furthermore L-arginine depletion prevents T-cell upregulation by cyclin D3- and cyclin-dependent kinase 4 [13]. In addition, increased expression of arginase 1 by MDSCs in a lymphoma mouse model has been shown to induce antigen-specific tolerance through recruitment and expansion of regulatory T-cells (T_{reg}) [14].

2.3.2 ROS and Peroxynitrite

ROS are another important mechanism by which MDSCs can directly suppress T-cells. High levels of ROS, mainly H_2O_2, have been found at sites heavily infiltrated by MDSCS in both cancer patients and animal models [4, 15–18]. ROS production is mainly regulated by NADPH oxidase (NOX2) whose expression is regulated by STAT3 [15]. The exact mechanism of immunosuppression triggered by ROS is not fully elucidated; however, it has been shown that high levels of ROS correlate with either impaired dendritic cell maturation [19] or decreased CD3ζ-chain expression of the T-cell receptor and thus diminished T-cell proliferation and cytokine production [20]. These immunosuppressive properties have only been observed in granulocytic MDSCs [4, 15], and they were abrogated by eliminating ROS [15, 17].

In addition to ROS, peroxynitrite, which in vivo has been ascribed to the reaction of the free radical superoxide with the free radical nitric oxide (NO), is a powerful prooxidant that has emerged as a crucial mediator of MDSC-related suppression of T-cell function. In both cancer patients and tumor models increased levels of peroxynitrite accumulate in areas of tumor progression [21–25]. Even though the immunosuppressive properties of peroxynitrite are not fully understood, it has been shown that it promotes apoptosis of T-cells [26] and alteration of their function [3]. In the latter, nitration of tyrosine residues in the T-cell receptor–CD8 complex by MDSCs, through ROS and peroxynitrite production, resulted in marked decrease in the binding of specific peptide-major histocompatibility complex (pMHC) to the $CD8^+$ T-cells and thus resulted in T-cell tolerance.

3 Clinical Data

Since the initial identification and description of MDSCs, in the preclinical literature, there have been many studies in cancer patients with solid and hematologic malignancies that have evaluated the presence and clinical significance of MDSCs (Table 1). One of the main challenges has been the absence of a universally accepted clinical definition of MDSCs. This is due to their highly heterogeneous nature and also in part due to the absence of the cognate Gr-1 molecule in humans [1].

One of the first published clinical studies that evaluated the presence of MDSCs in cancer patients was in the tumor of patients with head and neck cancer, mostly squamous histology ($n=18$) [51]. This study reported the presence of intra-tumoral $CD34^+$ myeloid cells that were significantly correlated ($r^2=0.65$) with levels of secreted GM-CSF in tumor fragments. Moreover, depletion of $CD34^+$ cells by immunomagnetic separation was associated with a reversal of T-cell suppression, evidenced by increased IL-2 production from intra-tumoral lymphocytes. A subsequent study [27] analyzed peripheral blood samples from patients with HNSCC, NSCLC, and breast cancer of unknown clinical stages ($n=44$) that identified a population of immature myeloid cells (ImC). These cells were described as lineage negative (Lin^-), defined here as $CD3^-$, $CD14^-$, $CD19^-$, and $CD57^-$. The immunosuppressive properties of

Table 1 Heterogeneity of MDSC phenotypes utilized in clinical studies

Phenotype	Cancer type	References
Lin^{-a}/$HLA\text{-}DR^{-}$	Breast	[27]
	HNSCC	
	NSCLC	
$CD15^{+}$ granulocytes	Breast	[20]
	Colon	
	Pancreatic	
$CD11b^{+}/CD14^{-}/CD15^{+}$	Renal cell	[28]
$CD14^{+}$/arginase^{+}	HNSCC	[29]
	MM	
$CD14^{+}/HLA\text{-}DR^{-/low}$	Melanoma	[30]
$CD11b^{+}/CD33^{+}$	NSCLC	[31]
$Lin1^{-/low\ b}/HLA\text{-}DR^{-}/CD33^{+}/CD11b^{+}$	Multiple solid tumors (breast, esophageal, gastric, colorectal, and other solid malignancies)	[32–34]
$Lin^{-c}/HLA\text{-}DR^{-}/CD33^{+}$	Melanoma	[35]
$CD11b^{+}/CD14^{-}/CD33^{+}/CD15^{+}$	NSCLC	[36, 37]
$CD14^{+}/IL\text{-}4Ra^{+}$	Colon	[38]
	Melanoma	
$CD11b^{+}/CD13^{+}/CD34^{+}/CD14^{-}/CD45^{+}$	Hodgkin lymphoma	[39]
$CD14^{+}/HLA\text{-}DR^{-/low}$	Melanoma	[40]
$DC\text{-}Sign^{+}/CD80^{+}/CD83^{+}$		
$CD14^{+}/CD15^{+}/CD33^{+}/HLA\text{-}DR^{-}$	Bladder	[41]
$CD14^{+}/HLA\text{-}DR^{-/low}$	MM	[42]
	MGUS	[43]
	NHL	[44, 45]
	HCC	
$SSC^{high}/CD66b^{+}/CD125^{-}/CD33^{+}/HLA\text{-}DR^{-}$	Urothelial tract	[46]
	HNSCC	
	NSCLC	
$CD34^{+}/CD45^{+}/CD116^{+}/CD13^{+}/CD14^{-}$	NHL	[47]
$CD11b^{+}/CD15^{high}/CD33^{low}$	Bladder	[48]
$Lin^{-b}/HLA\text{-}DR^{-}/CD33^{+}$	Multiple solid tumors	[49]
$CD14^{+}/HLA\text{-}DR^{low/-}$	Prostate	[50]

[a]Lineage defined as -CD3, -CD14, -CD19, and -CD57

[b]Lineage-1 defined as-CD3, -CD14, -CD16, -CD19, -CD20, and -CD56; HNSCC: head and neck squamous cell carcinoma; NSCLC: non-small-cell lung cancer; MDS: myelodysplastic syndrome; MGUS: monoclonal gammopathy of undetermined significance; MM: multiple myeloma; NHL: non-Hodgkin lymphoma

[c]Lineage defined as -CD3, -CD14, -CD19, and -CD56

those cells were confirmed by restoration of the ability of the dendritic cells to stimulate allogeneic T-cells in vitro when the ImC were depleted.

The next major study of MDSCs in cancer patients described a more mature granulocytic population of circulating cells with T-cell immunosuppressive properties in metastatic renal cell carcinoma (RCC) patients [28]. In this study, peripheral blood levels of granulocytic cells ($CD11b^{+}$, $CD14^{+}$, and $CD15^{+}$) in patients without previous treatment ($n=123$) were found to be significantly higher ($p=0.037$) than in healthy controls ($n=33$). Additional phenotypic characterization of this population revealed negative expression of CD11a, CD80, CD83, CD86, and HLA-DR and increased arginase activity. A subsequent study in patients with metastatic RCC ($n=27$) confirmed the presence of a granulocytic population of MDSCs that were $CD11b^+/CD15^+/CD66b^+$ and $CD14^-/CD16^{low}/CD62L^{low}$ [52].

To address the question of whether MDSCs aberrantly accumulate in cancer patients with a variety of different malignancies and whether levels in circulation were proportional to clinical stage, a subsequent study [33] by Diaz-Montero et al. prospectively evaluated MDSC levels in patients ($n=106$) with newly diagnosed solid tumors of various clinical stages. Approximately 50 % of patients had breast cancer, followed by 30 % of patients with gastrointestinal cancers and 20 % of various other types of cancer. In that study MDSCs were defined as a population of cells that were $Lin1^{-/low}/HLA\text{-}DR^-/CD33^+/CD11b^+$. Lineage-1 here was a cocktail of antibodies against CD3, CD14, CD16, CD19, CD20, and CD56. Overall circulating levels of MDSCs were significantly higher in patients with cancer ($P<0.0001$) compared to a cohort of matched healthy individuals ($n=21$). Furthermore, levels of circulating MDSCs were directly proportional to clinical stage of disease, with the highest overall numbers in patients with stage IV disease compared to patients with stage I/II disease ($P<0.0001$). Levels in patients with advanced metastatic disease also appeared to be highest among patients experiencing extensive metastatic burden.

Another study [48] examined the presence of two distinct populations of MDSCs in patients with superficial noninvasive and invasive bladder cancer. Both peripheral blood and fresh tumor samples were collected and analyzed by flow cytometry. Two different circulating MDSC populations were described: (1) $CD11b^+/CD15^{high}/CD33^{low}$ with co-expression of the neutrophil markers CD114 and CD117; and (2) $CD11b^+/CD15^{low}/CD33^{high}$ with co-expression of the monocyte–macrophage markers CD14, CD115, CD116, and CCR2. When circulating levels were compared, only the population of $CD11b^+/CD15^{high}/CD33^{low}$ cells were found to be present in higher levels in bladder cancer patients, whereas the $CD11b^+/CD15^{low}/CD33^{high}$ population was also found to be present in significant amounts in healthy individuals. Only the $CD11b^+/CD15^{high}/CD33^{low}$ population was noted to have immunosuppressive activity. Additionally, two distinct MDSC populations were found to infiltrate the tumors: 60–70 % of those cells were described as $CD11b^+/HLA\text{-}DR^+$ with the remaining 30–40 % described as $CD11b^+$ and $CD15^+$. The clinical significance of those cells though was not fully explored.

In summary, MDSCs in cancer patients consist of (1) a monocytic population characterized by the presence of CD14 and absence of CD15, which could also comprise a cell subset expressing CD15 at low levels, possibly representing a more immature stage of monocyte development, likely less differentiated than monocytic $CD15^-$ MDSCs, and (2) a more differentiated granulocytic population having the opposite pattern of expression, i.e., $CD15^+$ and $CD14^-$.

Despite the fact that immune evasion is an emerging hallmark of cancer, there is a clear paucity of validated immune related biomarkers that are known to correlate with prognosis and clinical outcome. In the setting of breast cancer, the most established and validated prognostic markers are tumor related, for example HER-2/neu gene amplification, hormone receptor status, tumor histologic grade, and circulating tumor cells [53]. However, recent comprehensive microarray analyses have validated immune gene signatures as valuable prognostic indicators in localized breast cancer and other solid tumors [54, 55]. MDSCs are clearly an important mechanism of tumor-mediated immune evasion, but thus far there are few published studies that have explored in detail the overall prognostic or predictive significance of MDSCs in cancer patients. Even if we put aside the issue of how to best define MDSCs, very few studies have fully addressed the clinical implications of circulating MDSCs. To the best of our knowledge, only three published studies have shown that overall levels of a monocytic population of MDSCs ($Lin1^{-/low}/HLADR^{-}/CD33^{+}/CD11b^{+}$) in the peripheral blood correlate with clinical stage [32–34]. Another study reported MDSC levels in NHL patients correlated with clinical cancer stage and aggressiveness of disease; however a different phenotype was utilized ($CD14^{+}/HLA\text{-}DR^{-/low}$) [43]. Moreover, two studies [32, 34] have independently shown that in patients with advanced breast cancer and gastrointestinal malignancies, higher MDSC levels were associated with poorer overall survival times. In the study by Solito et al. patients with stage IV breast cancer ($n=25$) with circulating MDSC levels >3.17 % (median) at baseline had significantly shorter median OS times than patients with circulating MDSCs less than the median at 5.5 months [95 % confidence interval (CI), 0.5–11.3] and 19.32 months (95 % CI, 8.7–infinity), respectively ($P<0.048$) [32]. Similarly, in the study by Gabitass et al., levels of circulating MDSCs >2.0 % were found to be an independent prognostic factor in patients with pancreatic, esophageal, and gastric cancers in a multivariate analysis [34]. Patients with elevated MDSCs (>2 %) were found to have an overall poorer prognosis, with a median OS of only 4.6 months (95 % CI, 2.2–6.0), relative to a median OS of 9.3 months (95 % CI, 6.3–12.1) ($P<0.001$), in patients with circulating MDSCs <2 %. Although these studies were retrospective in nature and involved relatively small number of patients, they provided important initial data using a similar MDSC phenotype, i.e., $Lin1^{-/low}/HLA\text{-}DR^{-}/CD33^{+}/CD11b^{+}$, on the prognostic significance of MDSCs. It is presently unknown whether blood MDSC levels are an independent prognostic factor in different cancers; future appropriately powered prospective studies are needed to address this.

4 Pharmacologic Modulation of MDSCs

The myriad strategies utilized by MDSCs to promote evasion of the immune system represent major hurdles for the clinical success of any type of cancer immunotherapy. Moreover, recruitment of MDSCs to pre-metastatic niches appears to be an early event in the development of metastatic disease. Several drugs known to pharmacologically modulate MDSCs have been tested clinically and can be classified into at least three different categories: (1) drugs that decrease MDSCs through

Table 2 Drugs known to modulate MDSCs

Agent	Cancer type	References
25-Hydroxyvitamin D3	HNSCC	[56]
ATRA	Renal cell carcinoma	[57, 58]
	Breast cancer	[59]
	Sarcoma	
Nitroaspirin	Colon cancer	[60]
Sildenafil	HNSCC	[29]
	Multiple myeloma	
Sunitinib	Renal cell carcinoma	[61]
	Transitional cell bladder cancer	[41]
Taxane	Melanoma	[62]
Gemcitabine	Pancreatic and esophageal cancer	[63]
Fluropyrimidine		
Gemcitabine	Breast cancer	[64]
5-Fluorouracil	Thymoma	[65]
Triterpenoid	Multiple solid tumors (colon, lung, thymoma, renal cell, sarcoma)	[66]
Celecoxib	Mesothelioma	[67]

promotion of cell differentiation; (2) drugs that modulate one or more different immunosuppressive mechanisms of MDSCs, without affecting overall levels; and (3) non-differentiating agents that decrease MDSCs levels, through decreasing their recruitment or production in the bone marrow (Table 2).

Two agents that have been shown to promote the differentiation of MDSCs include 25-hydrooxyvitamin D3 and all-trans-retinoic acid (ATRA). Treatment of locally advanced or metastatic head and neck squamous cell carcinoma (HNSCC) patients with 25-hydrooxyvitamin D3 resulted in a decrease of $CD34^+$ suppressive cells and an increase in the frequency of HLA-DR^+ cells, increased plasma levels of IL-12 and IFN-γ, and improved T-cell proliferation [56]. However, the small nature of this study prevented the determination of any clinical correlates.

ATRA was initially found to promote the in vivo differentiation of Gr-1^+CD11b^+ MDSCs into mature dendritic cells, macrophages, and granulocytes, thereby improving T-cell-mediated immune response in fibrosarcoma and mammary adenocarcinoma mouse models [59]. Further vaccination of the pretreated animals with two different types of cancer vaccines resulted in a prolonged antitumor effect through immune-mediated mechanisms.

Subsequent testing of ATRA in metastatic renal cell carcinoma patients with subcutaneous IL-2 revealed decreased number of Lin^-/HLA-DR^-/$CD33^+$ MDSCs, improved myeloid/lymphoid dendritic cell ratios, and was associated with an improvement in antigen-specific T-cell responses as measured by stimulation with tetanus-toxoid [57]. Similar results were observed when ATRA was used in patients with stage III–IV renal cell carcinoma [58].

Several drugs have been shown to modulate the immunosuppressive properties of MDSCs both in vivo and in vitro without affecting their overall accumulation.

Nitroaspirin was one of the first drugs that was shown to decrease the immunosuppressive properties of splenic MDSCs in animal models [60]. Elevated levels of NO lead to feedback inhibition of NOS and arginase (AGR) with subsequent decreased production of ROS. Furthermore, the addition of nitroaspirin to a tumor vaccine in a preclinical model increased the number and improved the function of tumor-specific T-cells. Similar effects were also observed with the phosphodiesterase-5 (PDE-5) inhibitor sildenafil [29]. Sildenafil was shown to down regulate ARG1 and NOS2 in vivo in murine models for colon carcinoma, mammary adenocarcinoma, and fibrosarcoma and in vitro in peripheral blood from multiple myeloma and HNSCC patients. Another promising approach in the same direction has been the use of anti-inflammatory agents, with two studies showing evidence of the ability to modulate MDSC function [66, 67]. The first study [66] examined the effect of triterpenoid in various tumor models and also in blood samples from patients with renal cell cancer, soft tissue sarcomas, and pancreatic cancer and showed that only the function but not the number of MDSCs was impaired through a decrease in the levels of ROS. The second study [67] showed that the COX-2 inhibitor celecoxib, when used in a mesothelioma mouse model, affected both the number and the function of MDSCs by inhibiting prostaglandin E2 synthesis and decreasing ROS and NO production.

Even though there is extensive literature on the effect of chemotherapy on MDSCs in mice, only two studies have shown a direct effect in humans. The first study [62] examined the effect of taxane-based chemotherapy on circulating MDSCs in stage I–IV melanoma patients ($n=77$). In this study, pretreatment MDSC levels were found to correlate with clinical cancer stage, with levels decreasing after taxane-based chemotherapy. A second study [63] evaluated changes in MDSC levels after chemotherapy in patients with pancreatic cancer ($n=16$) treated with gemcitabine-based chemotherapy and in patients with esophago-gastric cancer ($n=23$) treated with 5-FU-based chemotherapy. A significant decrease in circulating MDSC levels after chemotherapy was observed ($p<0.0001$); however, this decrease did not correlate with response to treatment and was also observed in patients with progressive disease.

5 Conclusions

The literature provides substantial evidence that MDSCs are important in the biology of tumor progression and immune evasion. However, one of the major obstacles in the study of MDSCs in cancer patients is the considerable heterogeneity of their phenotype. The most extensive clinical data demonstrating an inverse correlation between MDSC levels and prognosis and cancer clinical stage has involved an early and immature myeloid population (Lin1$^{-/low}$ HLADR^{-} CD33^{+} CD11b^{+}). Early clinical data suggests that levels circulating MDSCs may potentially serve as a predictive marker in cancer patients receiving immunotherapy. Although these initial studies are interesting and suggest that MDSCs could be a potential marker correlating clinical outcome and response to therapy, they need to be validated by larger prospective trials. Another important aspect related to the biology of MDSCs in cancer patients that requires further elucidation is the driving tumor-derived factors produced that control both recruitment of MDSCs from the bone marrow to the tumor site and activation of MDSCs. Finally, MDSCs represent a novel and attractive therapeutic target in oncology. A greater understanding of the biology of MDSCs would certainly help to accelerate the clinical development of novel strategies for the prevention of metastases, and may also potentially enhance the effectiveness of immune-based therapies.

References

1. Montero AJ, Diaz-Montero CM, Kyriakopoulos CE, Bronte V, Mandruzzato S. Myeloid-derived suppressor cells in cancer patients: a clinical perspective. J Immunother. 2012;35(2):107–15.
2. Youn JI, Nagaraj S, Collazo M, Gabrilovich DI. Subsets of myeloid-derived suppressor cells in tumor-bearing mice. J Immunol. 2008;181(8):5791–802.
3. Nagaraj S, Gupta K, Pisarev V, Kinarsky L, Sherman S, Kang L, Herber DL, Schneck J, Gabrilovich DI. Altered recognition of antigen is a mechanism of CD8+ T cell tolerance in cancer. Nat Med. 2007;13(7):828–35.
4. Kusmartsev S, Nefedova Y, Yoder D, Gabrilovich DI. Antigen-specific inhibition of CD8+ T cell response by immature myeloid cells in cancer is mediated by reactive oxygen species. J Immunol. 2004;172(2):989–99.
5. Movahedi K, Guilliams M, Van den Bossche J, Van den Bergh R, Gysemans C, Beschin A, De Baetselier P, Van Ginderachter JA. Identification of discrete tumor-induced myeloid-derived suppressor cell subpopulations with distinct T cell-suppressive activity. Blood. 2008; 111(8):4233–44.
6. Dolcetti L, Peranzoni E, Ugel S, Marigo I, Fernandez Gomez A, Mesa C, Geilich M, Winkels G, Traggiai E, Casati A, Grassi F, Bronte V. Hierarchy of immunosuppressive strength among myeloid-derived suppressor cell subsets is determined by GM-CSF. Eur J Immunol. 2010;40(1):22–35.
7. Gallina G, Dolcetti L, Serafini P, De Santo C, Marigo I, Colombo MP, Basso G, Brombacher F, Borrello I, Zanovello P, Bicciato S, Bronte V. Tumors induce a subset of inflammatory monocytes with immunosuppressive activity on CD8+ T cells. J Clin Invest. 2006;116(10):2777–90.
8. Marigo I, Bosio E, Solito S, Mesa C, Fernandez A, Dolcetti L, Ugel S, Sonda N, Bicciato S, Falisi E, Calabrese F, Basso G, Zanovello P, Cozzi E, Mandruzzato S, Bronte V. Tumor-induced tolerance and immune suppression depend on the C/EBPbeta transcription factor. Immunity. 2010;32(6):790–802.
9. Gabrilovich DI, Nagaraj S. Myeloid-derived suppressor cells as regulators of the immune system. Nat Rev Immunol. 2009;9(3):162–74.
10. Ostrand-Rosenberg S. Myeloid-derived suppressor cells: more mechanisms for inhibiting antitumor immunity. Cancer Immunol Immunother. 2010;59(10):1593–600.
11. Rodríguez PC, Ochoa AC. Arginine regulation by myeloid derived suppressor cells and tolerance in cancer: mechanisms and therapeutic perspectives. Immunol Rev. 2008;222:180–91.
12. Rodriguez PC, Zea AH, Culotta KS, Zabaleta J, Ochoa JB, Ochoa AC. Regulation of T cell receptor CD3zeta chain expression by L-arginine. J Biol Chem. 2002;277(24):21123–9.
13. Rodriguez PC, Quiceno DG, Ochoa AC. L-Arginine availability regulates T-lymphocyte cell-cycle progression. Blood. 2007;109(4):1568–73.
14. Serafini P, Mgebroff S, Noonan K, Borrello I. Myeloid-derived suppressor cells promote cross-tolerance in B-cell lymphoma by expanding regulatory T cells. Cancer Res. 2008; 68(13):5439–49.

15. Corzo CA, Cotter MJ, Cheng P, Cheng F, Kusmartsev S, Sotomayor E, Padhya T, McCaffrey TV, McCaffrey JC, Gabrilovich DI. Mechanism regulating reactive oxygen species in tumor-induced myeloid-derived suppressor cells. J Immunol. 2009;182(9):5693–701.
16. Szuster-Ciesielska A, Hryciuk-Umer E, Stepulak A, Kupisz K, Kandefer-Szerszeń M. Reactive oxygen species production by blood neutrophils of patients with laryngeal carcinoma and anti-oxidative enzyme activity in their blood. Acta Oncol. 2004;43(3):252–8.
17. Hamilton MJ, Banáth JP, Lam V, Lepard NE, Krystal G, Bennewith KL. Serum inhibits the immunosuppressive function of myeloid-derived suppressor cells isolated from 4T1 tumor-bearing mice. Cancer Immunol Immunother. 2012;61(5):643–54.
18. Mantovani G, Macciò A, Madeddu C, Mura L, Gramignano G, Lusso MR, Massa E, Mocci M, Serpe R. Antioxidant agents are effective in inducing lymphocyte progression through cell cycle in advanced cancer patients: assessment of the most important laboratory indexes of cachexia and oxidative stress. J Mol Med (Berl). 2003;81(10):664–73.
19. Nefedova Y, Huang M, Kusmartsev S, Bhattacharya R, Cheng P, Salup R, Jove R, Gabrilovich D. Hyperactivation of STAT3 is involved in abnormal differentiation of dendritic cells in cancer. J Immunol. 2004;172(1):464–74.
20. Schmielau J, Finn OJ. Activated granulocytes and granulocyte-derived hydrogen peroxide are the underlying mechanism of suppression of t-cell function in advanced cancer patients. Cancer Res. 2001;61(12):4756–60.
21. Cobbs CS, Whisenhunt TR, Wesemann DR, Harkins LE, Van Meir EG, Samanta M. Inactivation of wild-type p53 protein function by reactive oxygen and nitrogen species in malignant glioma cells. Cancer Res. 2003;63(24):8670–3.
22. Bentz BG, Haines GK, Radosevich JA. Increased protein nitrosylation in head and neck squamous cell carcinogenesis. Head Neck. 2000;22(1):64–70.
23. Ekmekcioglu S, Ellerhorst J, Smid CM, Prieto VG, Munsell M, Buzaid AC, Grimm EA. Inducible nitric oxide synthase and nitrotyrosine in human metastatic melanoma tumors correlate with poor survival. Clin Cancer Res. 2000;6(12):4768–75.
24. Nakamura Y, Yasuoka H, Tsujimoto M, Yoshidome K, Nakahara M, Nakao K, Nakamura M, Kakudo K. Nitric oxide in breast cancer: induction of vascular endothelial growth factor-C and correlation with metastasis and poor prognosis. Clin Cancer Res. 2006;12(4):1201–7.
25. Bronte V, Kasic T, Gri G, Gallana K, Borsellino G, Marigo I, Battistini L, Iafrate M, Prayer-Galetti T, Pagano F, Viola A. Boosting antitumor responses of T lymphocytes infiltrating human prostate cancers. J Exp Med. 2005;201(8):1257–68.
26. Brito C, Naviliat M, Tiscornia AC, Vuillier F, Gualco G, Dighiero G, Radi R, Cayota AM. Peroxynitrite inhibits T lymphocyte activation and proliferation by promoting impairment of tyrosine phosphorylation and peroxynitrite-driven apoptotic death. J Immunol. 1999; 162(6):3356–66.
27. Almand B, Clark JI, Nikitina E, van Beynen J, English NR, Knight SC, Carbone DP, Gabrilovich DI. Increased production of immature myeloid cells in cancer patients: a mechanism of immunosuppression in cancer. J Immunol. 2001;166(1):678–89.
28. Zea AH, Rodriguez PC, Atkins MB, Hernandez C, Signoretti S, Zabaleta J, McDermott D, Quiceno D, Youmans A, O'Neill A, Mier J, Ochoa AC. Arginase-producing myeloid suppressor cells in renal cell carcinoma patients: a mechanism of tumor evasion. Cancer Res. 2005;65(8):3044–8.
29. Serafini P, Meckel K, Kelso M, Noonan K, Califano J, Koch W, Dolcetti L, Bronte V, Borrello I. Phosphodiesterase-5 inhibition augments endogenous antitumor immunity by reducing myeloid-derived suppressor cell function. J Exp Med. 2006;203(12):2691–702.
30. Filipazzi P, Valenti R, Huber V, et al. (2007) Identification of a new subset of myeloid suppressor cells in peripheral blood of melanoma patients and modulation by GM-CSF-based antitumor vaccine. American Society Clinical Oncology Annual Meeting, Chicago; J Clin Oncol, ASCO Annual Meeting Proceedings Part I. Vol 25, No. 18S (June 20 Supplement), 2007: 21082
31. Srivastava MK, Bosch JJ, Thompson JA, Ksander BR, Edelman MJ, Ostrand-Rosenberg S. Lung cancer patients' CD4(+) T cells are activated in vitro by MHC II cell-based vaccines

despite the presence of myeloid-derived suppressor cells. Cancer Immunol Immunother. 2008;57(10):1493–504.

32. Solito S, Falisi E, Diaz-Montero CM, Doni A, Pinton L, Rosato A, Francescato S, Basso G, Zanovello P, Onicescu G, Garrett-Mayer E, Montero AJ, Bronte V, Mandruzzato S. A human promyelocytic-like population is responsible for the immune suppression mediated by myeloid-derived suppressor cells. Blood. 2011;118(8):2254–65.
33. Diaz-Montero CM, Salem ML, Nishimura MI, Garrett-Mayer E, Cole DJ, Montero AJ. Increased circulating myeloid-derived suppressor cells correlate with clinical cancer stage, metastatic tumor burden, and doxorubicin-cyclophosphamide chemotherapy. Cancer Immunol Immunother. 2009;58(1):49–59.
34. Gabitass RF, Annels NE, Stocken DD, Pandha HA, Middleton GW. Elevated myeloid-derived suppressor cells in pancreatic, esophageal and gastric cancer are an independent prognostic factor and are associated with significant elevation of the Th2 cytokine interleukin-13. Cancer Immunol Immunother. 2011;60(10):1419–30.
35. Daud AI, Mirza N, Lenox B, Andrews S, Urbas P, Gao GX, Lee JH, Sondak VK, Riker AI, Deconti RC, Gabrilovich D. Phenotypic and functional analysis of dendritic cells and clinical outcome in patients with high-risk melanoma treated with adjuvant granulocyte macrophage colony-stimulating factor. J Clin Oncol. 2008;26(19):3235–41.
36. Wang Y, Chung F, Wang C, et al. (2008) The population alteration of CD11b+/CD14− myeloid-derived suppressor cells in patients with advanced stage, non-small cell lung cancer and the clinical relevance to the responsiveness to epidermal growth factor receptor (EGFR). American Society Clinical Oncology Annual Meeting; Chicago: J Clin Oncol. 2008;26:(Suppl.):Abstract 19082.
37. Liu CY, Wang YM, Wang CL, Feng PH, Ko HW, Liu YH, Wu YC, Chu Y, Chung FT, Kuo CH, Lee KY, Lin SM, Lin HC, Wang CH, Yu CT, Kuo HP. Population alterations of L-arginase- and inducible nitric oxide synthase-expressed CD11b+/CD14^{-}/CD15+/CD33+ myeloid-derived suppressor cells and CD8+ T lymphocytes in patients with advanced-stage non-small cell lung cancer. J Cancer Res Clin Oncol. 2010;136(1):35–45.
38. Mandruzzato S, Solito S, Falisi E, Francescato S, Chiarion-Sileni V, Mocellin S, Zanon A, Rossi CR, Nitti D, Bronte V, Zanovello P. IL4Ralpha+ myeloid-derived suppressor cell expansion in cancer patients. J Immunol. 2009;182(10):6562–8.
39. Parrinello N, La Cava P, Tibullo D, et al. (2009) Myeloid-derived suppressor cells in patients with Hodgkin lymphoma. American Society Hematology Annual Meeting Abstracts, New Orleans. Blood. 2009;114:3662.
40. Poschke I, Mougiakakos D, Hansson J, Masucci GV, Kiessling R. Immature immunosuppressive CD14+HLA-DR-/low cells in melanoma patients are Stat3hi and overexpress CD80, CD83, and DC-sign. Cancer Res. 2010;70(11):4335–45.
41. Shepard DR, Ireland J, Stephenson AJ, et al. (2010) Effects of sunitinib on immune dysfunction in patients with transitional cell carcinoma (TCC) of the bladder. American Society of Clinical Oncology Genitourinary Cancers Symposium, Orlando, 2010. Abstract-295.
42. Brimnes MK, Vangsted AJ, Knudsen LM, Gimsing P, Gang AO, Johnsen HE, Svane IM. Increased level of both CD4+FOXP3+ regulatory T cells and CD14+HLA-DR^{-}/low myeloid-derived suppressor cells and decreased level of dendritic cells in patients with multiple myeloma. Scand J Immunol. 2010;72(6):540–7.
43. Lin Y, Gustafson MP, Bulur PA, Gastineau DA, Witzig TE, Dietz AB. Immunosuppressive CD14+HLA-DR(low)/- monocytes in B-cell non-Hodgkin lymphoma. Blood. 2011; 117(3):872–81.
44. Hoechst B, Ormandy LA, Ballmaier M, Lehner F, Krüger C, Manns MP, Greten TF, Korangy F. A new population of myeloid-derived suppressor cells in hepatocellular carcinoma patients induces CD4(+)CD25(+)Foxp3(+) T cells. Gastroenterology. 2008;135(1):234–43.
45. Hoechst B, Voigtlaender T, Ormandy L, Gamrekelashvili J, Zhao F, Wedemeyer H, Lehner F, Manns MP, Greten TF, Korangy F. Myeloid derived suppressor cells inhibit natural killer cells in patients with hepatocellular carcinoma via the NKp30 receptor. Hepatology. 2009;50(3):799–807.

46. Brandau S, Trellakis S, Bruderek K, Schmaltz D, Steller G, Elian M, Suttmann H, Schenck M, Welling J, Zabel P, Lang S. Myeloid-derived suppressor cells in the peripheral blood of cancer patients contain a subset of immature neutrophils with impaired migratory properties. J Leukoc Biol. 2011;89(2):311–7.
47. Pitini V, Santarpia M, Tomasello C, et al. (2011) Myeloid-derived suppressor cells absolute counts in predicting durable response to R-CHOP in patients with follicular lymphoma. American Society Clinical Oncology Annual Meeting, Chicago, 2011. J Clin Oncol. 2011;29:(Suppl):Abstract e18504.
48. Eruslanov E, Neuberger M, Daurkin I, Perrin GQ, Algood C, Dahm P, Rosser C, Vieweg J, Gilbert SM, Kusmartsev S. Circulating and tumor-infiltrating myeloid cell subsets in patients with bladder cancer. Int J Cancer. 2012;130(5):1109–19.
49. Fricke I, Mirza N, Dupont J, Lockhart C, Jackson A, Lee JH, Sosman JA, Gabrilovich DI. Vascular endothelial growth factor-trap overcomes defects in dendritic cell differentiation but does not improve antigen-specific immune responses. Clin Cancer Res. 2007;13(16):4840–8.
50. Vuk-Pavlović S, Bulur PA, Lin Y, Qin R, Szumlanski CL, Zhao X, Dietz AB. Immunosuppressive CD14+HLA-DRlow/- monocytes in prostate cancer. Prostate. 2010;70(4):443–55.
51. Pak AS, Wright MA, Matthews JP, Collins SL, Petruzzelli GJ, Young MR. Mechanisms of immune suppression in patients with head and neck cancer: presence of CD34(+) cells which suppress immune functions within cancers that secrete granulocyte-macrophage colony-stimulating factor. Clin Cancer Res. 1995;1(1):95–103.
52. Rodriguez PC, Ernstoff MS, Hernandez C, Atkins M, Zabaleta J, Sierra R, Ochoa AC. Arginase I-producing myeloid-derived suppressor cells in renal cell carcinoma are a subpopulation of activated granulocytes. Cancer Res. 2009;69(4):1553–60.
53. Carey LA, Perou CM, Livasy CA, Dressler LG, Cowan D, Conway K, Karaca G, Troester MA, Tse CK, Edmiston S, Deming SL, Geradts J, Cheang MC, Nielsen TO, Moorman PG, Earp HS, Millikan RC. Race, breast cancer subtypes, and survival in the Carolina Breast Cancer Study. JAMA. 2006;295(21):2492–502.
54. Kuo WH, Chang YY, Lai LC, Tsai MH, Hsiao CK, Chang KJ, Chuang EY. Molecular characteristics and metastasis predictor genes of triple-negative breast cancer: a clinical study of triple-negative breast carcinomas. PLoS One. 2012;7(9):e45831.
55. Yoshihara K, Tsunoda T, Shigemizu D, Fujiwara H, Hatae M, Masuzaki H, Katabuchi H, Kawakami Y, Okamoto A, Nogawa T, Matsumura N, Udagawa Y, Saito T, Itamochi H, Takano M, Miyagi E, Sudo T, Ushijima K, Iwase H, Seki H, Terao Y, Enomoto T, Mikami M, Akazawa K, Tsuda H, Moriya T, Tajima A, Inoue I, Tanaka K, J. S. O. C. S. Group. High-risk ovarian cancer based on 126-gene expression signature is uniquely characterized by downregulation of antigen presentation pathway. Clin Cancer Res. 2012;18(5):1374–85.
56. Lathers DM, Clark JI, Achille NJ, Young MR. Phase 1B study to improve immune responses in head and neck cancer patients using escalating doses of 25-hydroxyvitamin D3. Cancer Immunol Immunother. 2004;53(5):422–30.
57. Mirza N, Fishman M, Fricke I, Dunn M, Neuger AM, Frost TJ, Lush RM, Antonia S, Gabrilovich DI. All-trans-retinoic acid improves differentiation of myeloid cells and immune response in cancer patients. Cancer Res. 2006;66(18):9299–307.
58. Kusmartsev S, Su Z, Heiser A, Dannull J, Eruslanov E, Kübler H, Yancey D, Dahm P, Vieweg J. Reversal of myeloid cell-mediated immunosuppression in patients with metastatic renal cell carcinoma. Clin Cancer Res. 2008;14(24):8270–8.
59. Kusmartsev S, Cheng F, Yu B, Nefedova Y, Sotomayor E, Lush R, Gabrilovich D. All-trans-retinoic acid eliminates immature myeloid cells from tumor-bearing mice and improves the effect of vaccination. Cancer Res. 2003;63(15):4441–9.
60. De Santo C, Serafini P, Marigo I, Dolcetti L, Bolla M, Del Soldato P, Melani C, Guiducci C, Colombo MP, Iezzi M, Musiani P, Zanovello P, Bronte V. Nitroaspirin corrects immune dysfunction in tumor-bearing hosts and promotes tumor eradication by cancer vaccination.". Proc Natl Acad Sci U S A. 2005;102(11):4185–90.
61. Ko JS, Zea AH, Rini BI, Ireland JL, Elson P, Cohen P, Golshayan A, Rayman PA, Wood L, Garcia J, Dreicer R, Bukowski R, Finke JH. Sunitinib mediates reversal of myeloid-derived

suppressor cell accumulation in renal cell carcinoma patients. Clin Cancer Res. 2009; 15(6):2148–57.

62. Wilcox RA, Nevala WK, Thompson MA, et al. (2009) CD14+hla-DR-/lo myeloid-derived suppressor cells express immunosuppressive B7-H family members and are depleted following taxane-based chemotherapy in melanoma. American Society Hematology Annual Meeting Abstracts, New Orleans. Blood. 2009;114:464.
63. Gabitass RF et al. (2011) Use of gemcitabine- (Gem) and fluropyrimidine (FP)-based chemotherapy to reduce myeloid-derived suppressor cells (MDSCs) in pancreatic (PC) and esophagogastric cancer (EGC). American Society of Clinical Oncology Annual Meeting, Chicago. J Clin Oncol. 2011;29(Suppl):Abstract 2588.
64. Le HK, Graham L, Cha E, Morales JK, Manjili MH, Bear HD. Gemcitabine directly inhibits myeloid derived suppressor cells in BALB/c mice bearing 4T1 mammary carcinoma and augments expansion of T cells from tumor-bearing mice. Int Immunopharmacol. 2009; 9(7–8):900–9.
65. Vincent J, Mignot G, Chalmin F, Ladoire S, Bruchard M, Chevriaux A, Martin F, Apetoh L, Rébé C, Ghiringhelli F. 5-Fluorouracil selectively kills tumor-associated myeloid-derived suppressor cells resulting in enhanced T cell-dependent antitumor immunity. Cancer Res. 2010;70(8):3052–61.
66. Nagaraj S, Youn JI, Weber H, Iclozan C, Lu L, Cotter MJ, Meyer C, Becerra CR, Fishman M, Antonia S, Sporn MB, Liby KT, Rawal B, Lee JH, Gabrilovich DI. Anti-inflammatory triterpenoid blocks immune suppressive function of MDSCs and improves immune response in cancer. Clin Cancer Res. 2010;16(6):1812–23.
67. Veltman JD, Lambers ME, van Nimwegen M, Hendriks RW, Hoogsteden HC, Aerts JG, Hegmans JP. COX-2 inhibition improves immunotherapy and is associated with decreased numbers of myeloid-derived suppressor cells in mesothelioma. Celecoxib influences MDSC function. BMC Cancer. 2010;10:464.

The Role of B Cells in Shaping the Antitumor Immune Response

Yu Zhang, Taylor H. Schreiber, and Joseph D. Rosenblatt

Abstract Although many experimental tumor models have demonstrated the importance of CTL, Th1 response, and NK cells in antitumor immunity, relatively little is known about the role of B cells in tumor immunity. The ability and mechanism of B cell-mediated regulation of cellular immune responses and inflammation have only recently been described and remain incompletely understood. Although B cells are recognized as a significant proportion of tumor-infiltrating lymphocytes in both mouse models and human tumors, relatively little mechanistic information is available describing how these cells influence antitumor immunity and immunosurveillance. Recently, studies in several murine models have found an association indicating that reduced number of tumor-infiltrating B cells is associated with improved CD8+ T cell and NK cell infiltration into the tumor bed and decreased tumor growth. Multiple mechanisms have been implicated in B cell-mediated suppression of antitumor immunity including (1) preferential polarization of immune responses to Th2; (2) direct suppression of tumor immunity by immunosuppressive regulatory B cells (Breg), and (3) coordination of regulatory T cell (Treg) recruitment and suppression within the tumor microenvironment. Because B cells are readily targeted in the clinic with monoclonal antibodies, understanding of how these cells influence tumor immunity may lead to rapidly translatable approaches to enhancing therapeutic immunity for both solid and hematological malignancy.

Keywords B regulatory cell (Breg) • B cell-deficient mice (BCDM) • T regulatory cells (Treg) • B lymphocyte • IL-10 • TGF-β • CD5 • GITR • GITR-L • Antitumor immunity

---

Y. Zhang • J.D. Rosenblatt (✉)
Division of Hematology/Oncology, Department of Medicine, Sylvester Comprehensive Cancer Center; University of Miami Miller School of Medicine, Miami, FL 33136, USA
e-mail: jrosenblatt@med.miami.edu

T.H. Schreiber
Department of Microbiology and Immunology, University of Miami Miller School of Medicine, Miami, FL 33136, USA

J.D. Rosenblatt et al. (eds.), *Advances in Tumor Immunology and Immunotherapy*, Current Cancer Research, DOI 10.1007/978-1-4614-8809-5_2,
© Springer Science+Business Media New York 2014

1 Introduction

A variety of animal models suggest that B cells can play a role in shaping antitumor immune responses [1–5]. While the role of Tregs and myeloid suppressor cells has been extensively investigated, the role of B cells in shaping antitumor immunity has been less well characterized. It is increasingly appreciated that B cell subsets may participate in the shaping of Th1 and Th2 responses through the so-called Be1 and Be2 B cell subsets [6–10]. A variety of B cell subsets have also been reported to mediate immunosuppressive activity in experimental systems, although a formal definition of a Breg subset similar to the widely appreciated CD25+FoxP3+ Treg has yet to be agreed upon. This review focuses on the potential role and proposed mechanisms of B cells in modulating therapeutic antitumor immunity.

2 B Cells and Antitumor Immunity

Although many human tumors are heavily infiltrated with B cells [11, 12], relatively little is known about the role of B cells in tumor immunity. Cancer patients often develop antibodies to tumor-associated antigens such as HER2/neu, p53, ras, myc, and myb; however, these antibodies do not confer protection, and often antibodies correlate with poor prognosis [13]. In some murine models, antibody-secreting B cells were reported to inhibit antitumor CTL responses [5, 14].

We and others have demonstrated decreased growth of several histologically distinct murine tumors in B cell-deficient mice (BCDM) relative to wild-type (WT) mice [2, 3, 15]. EMT-6 mammary carcinoma, EL-4 thymoma, and MC38 colon carcinoma grew progressively in WT mice but regressed spontaneously in BCDM. In addition, growth of B16 melanoma was slowed significantly in BCDM compared to the WT mice [1, 3]. Reduced tumor growth in BCDM was associated with increased T cell infiltration of tumors, increased Th1 cytokine response, and, in the case of EMT-6, EL-4, and MC38, a significantly higher CTL response [1, 3, 15]. Adoptive transfer of WT splenic B cells to BCDM abrogated tumor rejection and resulted in diminished antitumor Th1 responses, providing evidence that B cells were causal in dampening antitumor immunity in vivo [15]. Similar results were reported for other murine tumor models, such as Friend murine leukemia virus gag-expressing mouse EL-4 (EL-4 gag) and the D5 mouse melanoma [4]. Thus, in multiple murine tumor models the evidence suggests that despite production of antibodies to tumor-specific antigens, B cells may be detrimental to therapeutic antitumor immunity. A variety of mechanisms may be involved in B cell-mediated suppression of the antitumor response.

B cells also affect T cell responses to vaccination and to chemotherapy in several murine tumor models. Single immunization with melanoma-associated antigens (Ad2/gp100, Ad2/mTRP-2) inhibited established B16 tumor growth in BCDM but not in wild-type C57BL/6 mice [16]. Using a secreted gp96-Ig-based vaccine and the LLC-OVA tumor model, the rejection of established tumors required frequent vaccination in the presence of B cells, while in the absence of B cells, a single vaccine administration was sufficient to elicit rejection [17]. In a lung metastasis model, BCDM showed complete recovery in response to a combination of cyclophosphamide and IL-15, whereas WT C57BL/6 mice showed only a partial response [18]. B cells may also directly promote tumorigenesis through indirect effects on T cell immunity. In a DMBA/TPA (7,12-dimethylbenz(α)anthracene/terephthalic acid) induced skin carcinoma mouse model, Schioppa et al. [19] found that both B cells and TNF-α were critical for the development of DMBA/TPA-induced papilloma. Transfer of B cells from DMBA/TPA-treated wild-type mice to TNF(−/−) mice rescued papilloma development to levels seen in wild-type mice, but when B cells from TNF(−/−) mice were transferred to Rag2(−/−) mice or when TNF-α was selectively eliminated in the transferred B cells, this did not occur. Increased IFN-γ and CD8+ T cells in skin and a significant reduction in IL-10-producing B regulatory cells were associated with resistance to papilloma development in TNF (−/−) mice. Thus, in this model B cell-derived TNF-α appears to directly foster tumorigenesis in response to a chemical carcinogen.

Collectively these results suggest that B cells are important in shaping the antitumor immune response and that cancer vaccination strategies designed to elicit a Th1-type response might in theory be augmented by B cell depletion.

3 Mechanisms of B Cell Modulation of Immune Response

3.1 Be1 and Be2 Differentiation and Skewing of T Cell Response

In addition to their well-defined role in antibody production, B cells may regulate immune responses to infectious pathogens through their production of cytokines. Activated B cells produce a variety of cytokines including: proinflammatory molecules (IL-1, IL-6, TNF, and lymphotoxin-α), hematopoietic growth factors (CSF, GM-CSE, M-CSF, and IL-7), and immunosuppressive cytokines (TGF-β1 and IL-10) [20–22]. Harris et al. identified two populations of "effector" B cells that produce distinct patterns of cytokines depending on the cytokine environment present during their primary encounter with antigen and T cells [8]. These effector B cells can differentiate into two functionally polarized effectors, one (*Be1*) producing a Th1-like cytokine pattern and the other (*Be2*) producing a Th2-like pattern. Depending on the profile of cytokines they produce, these effector B cell subsets subsequently regulate the differentiation of naïve CD4+ T cells to Th1 and Th2 cells through production of polarizing cytokines such as IL-4 or IFN-γ.

Type-I interferons are produced early in the immune response and directly stimulate B cells. Specifically, IFN-α triggers a signaling cascade in resting human naïve B cells, involving STAT4 and T-bet, two key IFN-γ gene imprinting factors. Subsequent production of IFN-α in naïve B cells facilitates their differentiation toward Be1-type B cells and is further reinforced by exogenous IL-12 [8]. IFN-α and

IFN-γ therefore condition B and T cell response to IL-12, resulting in coordinated Be1 polarization of naive B cells [23]. IFN-γ-producing Be1 cells may further amplify Th1 responses and potentially imprint a type 1 phenotype on additional B cells. This B cell-driven autocrine loop is likely to be beneficial in response to bacterial or viral pathogens, while in relation to autoantigens, it may result in increased autoimmune pathology. Be2 B cell differentiation, in contrast, is dependent on the expression of IL-4Rα, IL-4, and Th2 CD4+ T cells in the microenvironment [6]. Be2 cells predominantly secrete cytokines which augment Th2 responses. Be1 and Be2 cells can be readily identified in animals following infection with pathogens that preferentially induce a type 1 and type 2 immune response, respectively [9]. Whether tumor-infiltrating B cells are imprinted or differentiated along Be1or Be2 pathways is unknown, but the theoretical implication is that such imprinting might further amplify Th1- and/or Th2-type responses.

3.2 B Cells and Antigen Presentation

B cells are also capable to function as abundant antigen-presenting cells (APC). Presentation of antigens by B cells has been observed to skew T cell responses to the Th2 type [21, 24]. Conversely, T cell responses may be skewed to Th1 in the absence of B cells. Because Th1 and Th2 responses are mutually suppressive, B cells may be deleterious for Th1-dependent antitumor immunity if they function as the dominant source of APC in the tumor microenvironment. Adoptively transferred B cells, but not serum from either tumor-immunized or naive WT mice, abolished the increased response of BCDM to tumor vaccination, perhaps indicating that B cells themselves, and not B cell-derived soluble factors, are responsible for immune suppression [2]. Our studies using the MC38 model and transfer of B cells from BCR-transgenic anti-HEL mice into BCDM indicated that B cells may inhibit antitumor T cell responses by antigen-nonspecific mechanisms since neither tumor-specific antibodies nor cognate T:B interactions were necessary for inhibition of tumor immunity by B cells [3]. IFN-γ secretion in vitro in co-cultures of tumor-challenged BCDM splenocytes with tumor cells was inhibited by addition of wild-type but not $CD40^{-/-}$ B cells suggesting that B cells may inhibit antitumor Th1cytokine responses in a CD40-dependent manner. However, adoptive transfer of $CD40^{-/-}$ B cells into BCDM also restored growth of MC38 implicating factors other than CD40 [3]. Together, these data indicate that the molecular mechanism of immune suppression provided by B cells is dependent upon a B cell-derived ligand(s) that functions in an antigen-nonspecific fashion.

3.3 B Cells and Expansion of Tregs

CD4+Foxp3+ Tregs have been increasingly implicated in the suppression of antitumor immune response. Increasing evidence suggests that B cells may support the expansion of CD4+Foxp3+ Treg in vitro and in vivo [1, 25–29]. Induction of oral tolerance is B cell dependent and is associated with Treg cell expansion, suppression, and/or deletion of effector T cells [28]. Antigens such as ovalbumin, coupled to cholera toxin B subunit (CTB), enhanced antigen uptake by B cells and induced expression of latency-associated polypeptide (LAP)/TGF-β on the B cell surface and production of IL-10 by B cells [25, 28]. Provision of TGF-β by these B regulatory cells may promote the induction of Tregs, particularly in the mucosal environment, and has been shown to stimulate antigen-specific Treg proliferation in vivo and in vitro [25, 28]. In a similar model using myelin oligodendrocyte glycoprotein peptide (MOGp) as antigen coupled to CTB, similarly expanded Tregs are markedly suppressive and protective against development of experimental autoimmune encephalomyelitis [25].

GITR and GITR-L are co-stimulatory molecules belonging to the TNF superfamily that play an important role in Treg and T effector cell proliferation, activation, and differentiation [30]. In mice, B cells, NK cells, NK-T cells, CD4+ T cells, CD8+ T cells, Treg cells, granulocytes, and macrophages express GITR, particularly upon activation. In humans, only activated macrophages and NK cells express GITR. The cognate ligand of GITR (GITR-L) is expressed on endothelial cells, dendritic cells, and macrophages in humans and on B cells, dendritic cells, monocytes, macrophages, dendritic cells, and endothelial cells in the mouse. In an EAE mouse model, Ray et al. have shown that B cells appear to regulate the number of CD4+Foxp3+ Treg in the CNS through interactions with B cell-expressed GITR-L but that they do so independently of IL-10 secretion by B cells. In an adoptive transfer experiment, WT, $CD80^{-/-}$, $CD86^{-/-}$, and $MHC\text{-}II^{-/-}$ B cell transfer into μMT mice restored both Treg numbers and enhanced their ability to recover from EAE, while B cells deficient in GITR-L failed to protect against EAE. These studies showed that B cells play a major role in immune tolerance through maintenance of the Treg subpopulation via their expression of GITR-L [26]. Whether GITR-L-expressing B cells are also implicated in the suppression of antitumor immunity is not yet known.

In naïve BCDM, Treg number in peripheral blood, spleen, and lymph nodes are lower than wild-type mice while similar numbers of Treg are seen in the thymus [1]. In EMT-6 tumor-bearing mice, although Treg number increased following tumor inoculation in both BCDM and wild-type mice, much higher Treg numbers were detected in wild-type mice compared to BCDM [15]. When adoptive transfer of B cells into BCDM is followed by EMT-6 tumor implantation, a dramatic increase in CD4+Foxp3+ Treg was observed in B cell-reconstituted BCDM, compared to BCDM. Increased Treg number correlated with increased tumor growth in B cell-reconstituted BCDM as compared to BCDM (Fig. 1). The observed increase in tumor growth was associated with decreased CD8+ T cell and NK+ cell infiltration into tumor tissue and increased infiltration of Treg and B cells into the tumor bed. CTL activity was significantly decreased in B cell-reconstituted BCDM compared to BCDM. Depletion of Treg by anti-CD25 antibody resulted in tumor rejection, despite adoptive transfer of B cells, implicating CD4+ CD25+ Treg as mediators of the B cell effects on tumor growth (Fig. 1). IL-10 secretion by Breg cells has been

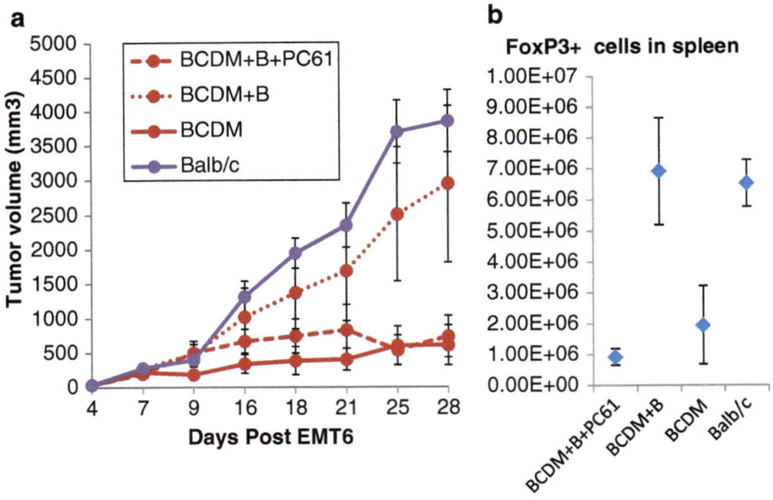

Fig. 1 Tumor growth in BCDM and B cell-reconstituted BCDM and wild-type (WT) mice and Treg number in spleen. 10^6 EMT-6 tumor cells were implanted subcutaneously at day 0; purified splenic B cells from wild-type mice were adoptively transferred at days -7, 0, and 7. Anti-CD25 antibody (PC61) and isotype control rat IgG1was administered at days -7 and 0 at 150 μg/mouse, i.v. Thirty days post EMT-6 implantation, spleens were harvested and processed for flow cytometry analysis. (**a**). Tumor growth in indicated groups, mean ± SEM, 8 mice/group. (**b**). CD4+Foxp3+ Treg number in spleen at day 30, 3 mice/group, mean ± S.D

implicated in immune suppression [31]. However in the EMT-6 model mentioned above, IL-$10^{-/-}$ B cell reconstitution of BCDM facilitated EMT-6 growth and Treg expansion similarly to reconstitution with wild-type B cells [15].

3.4 B10 Cells and Immune Suppression

Studies using murine disease models have demonstrated that regulatory B cells play a significant role in autoimmune connective tissue diseases, such as rheumatoid arthritis and systemic lupus erythematosus, as well as organ-specific autoimmune diseases including experimental autoimmune encephalomyelitis and inflammatory bowel disease [3, 22, 32–35]. In several murine disease models the function of regulatory B cells is dependent on IL-10 [20, 32, 36]. IL-10-producing B cells (B10) were the first B regulatory cell that has been recognized and are well described in the mouse and human setting [36]. This B regulatory cell has the distinct phenotypic marker characterized as CD1d^{hi}CD5+CD19^{hi} and upon activation secretes IL-10. B10 cells are potent negative regulators of inflammation and autoimmunity in mouse models of disease in vivo. Adoptive transfer of this B subset into BCDM ameliorated EAE development and prevented the onset of disease [32]. An IL-10-competent Breg subset that parallels the mouse B10 Breg has been identified in humans [37]. CD19+CD24^{high}CD38^{high} B cells are another phenotypic subset that have been linked to protection against SLE in man [38]. Such B cells can suppress Th1 differentiation by CD4+ cells, and this activity appears to be impaired in SLE patients. Diminished IL-10 secretion by these B cells appears to play an important role in the immune dysregulation observed in SLE patients.

In a murine model for neonatal infectious disease, Zhang et al. have demonstrated that IL-10 production by neonatal B cells suppressed proinflammatory cytokine secretion by dendritic cells in response to CpG stimulation of TLR9 response, and this effect was mediated through type 1 IFN and its receptor on B cells [39]. In these studies the suppressive phenotype was linked to IFNα signaling in B cells, because IFN-$\alpha^{-/-}$R knockout B cells did not suppress as well [39]. In this mouse model, BCR engagement and/or TLR signals induced B10 cells to produce and secrete IL-10 that negatively influenced the activation of T cells, macrophages, and dendritic cells (DCs) and thereby dampened both cellular and humoral immunity. As in autoimmunity and infection, B10 cells are likely to be involved in regulating antitumor immunity.

To investigate the role of B cell-secreted IL-10 in antitumor response, we adoptively transferred B cells obtained from IL-10$^{-/-}$ mice or wild-type mice into BCDM and compared Treg number, EMT-6 tumor growth, immune cell infiltration into tumor tissue, and cytolytic CD8+ T cell generation. EMT-6 growth was inhibited in BCDM but was restored in IL-10$^{-/-}$ B or WT B cell-reconstituted BCDM. Treg expansion was seen in IL-10$^{-/-}$ B or wild-type B cell-reconstituted BCDM to a level similar to that seen in WT mice. NK and CD8+ T cell infiltration and cytolytic activity of CD8+ T cells were suppressed in the presence of both WT and IL10$^{-/-}$ B cells [15]. This indicates that B cell suppression of antitumor response may be mediated in whole or partly by expansion of Treg and that Treg expansion could proceed independently of IL-10 production by B cells.

Phenotypically distinct B cell populations that may be involved in the suppression of antitumor immunity including the so-called B10 cells, B1b cells, B2-like cells, and/or T2 MZP-like B cells. Different phenotypic and functional characteristics have been ascribed to various Breg populations in mice including CD19+CD43^{-}CD 21^{high}CD23+CD24^{high}IgD+IgM+ CD1d^{high} (production of IL-10; inhibition of TH1 response) [40, 41]; CD19+CD1d+CD21+CD23IgM+CD24+CD62L+ (production of IL-10, TGF-β; Treg induction) [42–45]; CD19+CD43+CD5+ Breg (production of IL-10; IFN-α [39, 46, 47]; and CD19+CD43-CD80+CD86+CD40+ (production of IL-10; Treg induction; inhibition of TH1 response; costimulation via B7) [48–51]. Emerging evidence implicates the B10-cell in regulation of tumor immunity [20]. However, in adoptive transfer experiments using the EMT-6 model in BCDM both wild-type and IL-10$^{-/-}$ B cell successfully suppressed antitumor response, suggesting that the predominant immunosuppressive effect of B cells is not IL10 dependent in that model and that other B cell subsets may suppress response independently of IL-10 [15].

3.5 Other Breg Subsets and Role of TGF-β

Other B cell subsets have been described with regulatory function, such as CD5+B-1a cells [52, 53], CD1d+ marginal zone B cells, and transitional-2-marginal zone precursor B cells [54]. Finally a novel GM-CSF–IL-15 fusokine was found to induce a regulatory B cell subset which could attenuate EAE in the murine setting [55].

Emerging evidence also indicates that specific subsets of Bregs evolve under inflammatory conditions that may promote tolerance. In a recent model of allergic airway disease TGF-β-expressing CD5+ B cells expanded locally in hillar lymph nodes of tolerant mice, and inhalational tolerance could be induced by adoptive transfer of CD5+ B cells [56].

CD5+ B cells from tolerant mice induced expression of FoxP3 in CD4+CD25− B cells in vitro and appeared to co-localize with CD4+ FoxP3+ Treg in vivo. In contrast to TGF-β, IL-10 levels did not differ between CD5+ B cells of inhalationally tolerant vs. allergic mice. Whether similar CD5+ TGF-β-expressing B cells are implicated in tumor tolerance is not known.

Another mechanism of B cell inhibition of Th1 response is secretion of IgG linked to latent transforming growth factor-beta (IgG/TGF-β) which prevents CTL response in the presence of macrophage and Fc receptor. If CTL responses in man are similarly regulated by B lymphocytes, ongoing B cell response in patients with chronic viral infections or patients with potentially immunogenic cancers may prevent effective therapeutic vaccination [5].

Recently Olkhanud et al. demonstrated that lung metastasis of 4T1 mammary carcinoma cells in mice following orthotopic implantation required active Treg participation. In that model Foxp3+ Treg population conversion appeared to be dependent upon Breg-induced TGF-β. These tumor-evoked Bregs phenotypically resembled the so-called "B2" cells (CD19+CD25+CD69^{high}), expressed Stat3, B7-H1^{high}CD81^{high} CD86^{high}CD62^{low}IgM^{int} markers and also appeared to inhibit NK-mediated function, thereby facilitating metastasis [57]. The primary role of tumor-evoked Bregs (tBregs) in lung metastases was to induce TGF-β-dependent conversion of FoxP3+ Tregs from resting CD4+ T cells. In the absence of tBregs, 4T1 tumors did not metastasize into the lungs efficiently due to poor Treg conversion. In contrast to the results reported in 4T1, in the EMT-6 model, a very low percentage of tumor-infiltrating B cells expressed CD25, suggesting that an alternate subset of B cells may have been involved in attenuating the immune response. Whether or not there is a common surface phenotype, suppressive cytokine or transcription factor that delineates Breg cells from non-immunosuppressive B cells currently remains unknown.

3.6 B Cells and Chronic Inflammation

B cells may also play a role in modulating levels of inflammation associated with tumor development. In addition to the role of B cell-derived TNF-α previously

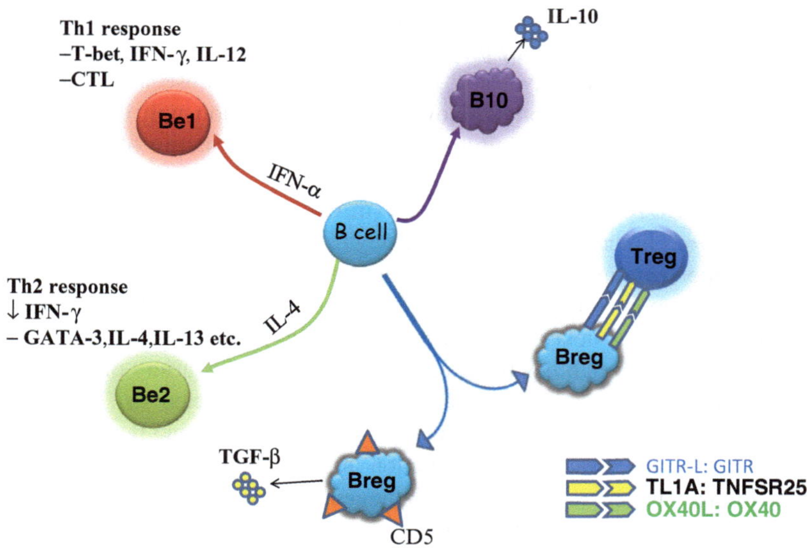

Fig. 2 Hypothetical scheme for B regulatory cell development. B cell precursors can differentiate into subsets with Th1-like cytokine pattern (Be1) or Th2-like cytokine pattern (Be2). Be2 cells may depress Th1 response. B cell may also differentiate into IL-10-secreting B10 cells, GITR-L+ B cell, TL1A, and/or OX40L and/or differentiate into Bregs that co-express CD5 and TGF-β. Details in text

mentioned, B cells have been implicated in the recruitment of inflammatory cells leading to development of neoplasia. De Visser et al. [58] reported that the elimination of mature T and B lymphocytes in K14-HPV16 mice, a transgenic model of inflammation-associated epithelial carcinogenesis, limits neoplastic progression due to the failure to recruit innate immune cells. Adoptive transfer of B lymphocytes or of serum from HPV16 mice into T and B cell-deficient/HPV16 mice restored innate immune cell infiltration into premalignant tissue leading to chronic inflammation, enhanced angiogenesis, and a hyperproliferative epidermis. In this model, B lymphocytes participate in the generation of a chronic inflammatory state that is required for carcinogenesis.

Potential regulatory B cell subsets that can affect antitumor immunity and suppress T cell response are illustrated in Fig. 2.

4 Effects of B Cell Depletion on Antitumor Immunity

Since B cells appear to modulate immune response in the context of mouse models genetically deficient in B cells, it would follow that therapeutic B cell depletion may be useful in the context of antitumor immune therapies. However the effects of B cell depletion may vary substantially according to the disease context. In some diseases, B cells may play a direct pathogenic role due to elaboration of pathogenic antibodies. In others B cells may play a supportive role leading to augmented T cell responses or alternatively may lead to attenuated T cell response, as we have shown in several murine tumor models. However, this regulation will be significantly influenced by the immunogenicity of the tumor and the nature of the antitumor immune response.

A chimeric CD20 monoclonal antibody (mAb), rituximab, was the first mAb to be approved for clinical use in cancer therapy [59]. Rituximab effects appear to be primarily dependent upon antibody-dependent cellular cytotoxicity (ADCC) and to a lesser degree upon complement-mediated cytotoxicity (CDC), but evidence also supports induction of delayed T cell anti-idiotypic tumor responses [60]. B cell depletion using rituximab has reported to be effective in a variety of autoimmune settings including SLE, rheumatoid arthritis, and multiple sclerosis. The effects of rituximab may involve direct depletion of autoantibody-producing B cells, decreased autoreactive T cell activation, or a reduction in pathogenic cytokine production by B cells. In many instances depletion of pathogenic B cell populations also results in an observed increase in Treg. These results are interesting and puzzling in view of the observed decrease in both Treg function and number seen in response to EMT-6 tumor implantation in BCDM and the rise in Treg seen following B cell reconstitution. We have also observed a paradoxical rise in CD4+Foxp3+ Treg following B cell depletion in wild-type mice [15]. Different B cell subsets may be disproportionately affected by CD20 B cell depletion leading to variable effects. Selective elimination of carefully identified Breg subsets might still be feasible and may be required in order to produce desired results in relation to T cell immunity.

Several investigators have tested the effects of B cell depletion on antitumor vaccination. Injection of anti-mouse CD20 antibody was effective in depleting circulating B cells from blood and lymph nodes, although depletion was less complete in the spleen [61]. In the TC1 murine lung cancer model (murine lung cancer cells expressing human papilloma virus-E7 and transformed with c-Ha-ras), B cell depletion slowed primary tumor growth and retarded the growth of established tumors but did not induce tumor regression. However, when the antibody was combined with an active immunotherapy approach using an adenovirus vaccine expressing the human papilloma virus-E7 gene (Ad.E7) in mice bearing TC1 tumors, Kim et al. noted increased number of tetramer+/CD8+ T cells within the spleens, increased activated CD8+ T cells within tumors, and enhanced antitumor immunity [61]. B cell depletion using an anti-CD20 antibody was thus effective in augmenting immunotherapy in a tumor vaccine model. These studies raise the possibility that B cell depletion may be a useful adjunct in human immunotherapy trials [61].

The effects of B cell depletion vary depending on the tumor model being examined. In B16 melanoma, mature B cell depletion using CD20 mAb dramatically exacerbates tumor progression and metastasis, arguing that B cells, or a depletion-resistant subset of B cells, may support antitumor immune responses in this model [62]. Following anti-CD20 treatment of BL3750, a CD20-expressing primary Burkitt-like lymphoma cell line, "B10" cells, suppressed the effects of CD20 mAb-mediated lymphoma depletion by inhibiting mAb-mediated monocyte activation and effector function through IL-10-dependent mechanisms. This suppression could be overcome by using a TLR3 agonist that did not activate B10 cells but rather activated monocytes and enhanced effector cell-mediated ADCC [63]. Although neither MC38 nor EL-4 grow well in BCDM and growth is restored by adoptive B cell transfer, we have observed little or no effect of B cell depletion using anti-murine CD20 antibody on the growth of either MC38 or EL-4 in normal mice. One possible explanation is that B cell depletion may deplete both suppressive as well as stimulatory subsets, with effects varying depending on the balance between these elements. Put simply B cell depletion may be a blunt instrument, similar to CD3 depletion of T cells. For example there are numerous animal tumor models in which CD3 and/or CD8 depletion will abrogate response, while CD25 or CD4 depletion might augment response through more selective elimination of Treg. Alternatively, CD20-based therapeutic B cell depletion may spare depletion of immunosuppressive Breg or Be2 B cell subsets. Since a clear phenotypic characterization of Breg is still not available, anti-CD20 antibody depletion of B cells may eliminate multiple B cell subsets that are involved in immune suppression and/or alternatively in promotion of antitumor response.

Whether B cell depletion using CD20 antibodies can be used to augment human antitumor immune response following vaccination or tumor treatment remains to be seen, and effects may be context dependent. Better phenotypic characterization of Breg "subsets" may allow more selective depletion of regulatory B cells and afford more predictable effects on immune response.

5 B Cell Infiltration in Human Tumors

Treg infiltration into solid tumors is associated with local immune suppression and carries a negative relationship to prognosis [64–72]. Similar to Tregs, infiltration with myeloid suppressor cells (MDSC) also appears to inhibit antitumor responses [73]. In contrast to Treg and MDSC however, the extent and prevalence of B cell infiltration in human tumors and the nature and phenotypic characteristics of infiltrating B cells that may be involved in tumor growth or tumor rejection are poorly characterized.

In humans, B cell infiltration in ovarian carcinoma and oral cancers predicts poor prognosis [11, 12], and combined NK and B cell infiltration in metastatic ovarian cancer also correlates with poor outcome [11]. Progression of oral epithelium from hyperkeratosis to dysplasia and carcinoma is accompanied by increased B cell infiltration into tongue lesions that appears to parallel the degree of transformation [12]. In patients with advanced melanoma, plasma cell infiltration in primary melanomas has been reported to carry negative prognostic significance [74, 75]. In advanced renal carcinoma, B cells infiltrate tumor tissue out of proportion to circulating peripheral blood B lymphocyte levels, while fewer T cells infiltrate compared to circulating T lymphocytes. In addition, the infiltrative T lymphocytic population was represented predominantly by CD4+ T cells [76]. In these patients Th2 response appears to predominate vs. Th1 response [77]. Thus in human ovarian, oral, melanoma, and renal cell carcinomas, B cell infiltration of the tumor microenvironment carries a negative prognostic value. Whether B cell depletion could be used to augment immune therapy of melanoma or renal cell carcinoma in the setting of either IL-2 or anti-CTLA-4 immune-directed therapy remains to be prospectively tested.

Although some studies in human infiltrating ductal and medullary breast carcinomas suggest that B cell infiltration may be associated with a favorable prognosis [78], this does not preclude a supportive role for B cells in facilitating tumor growth, since the B cell infiltration may simply be a marker for a more favorable type of breast cancer. Medullary carcinomas are reported to carry an improved prognosis compared to the so-called atypical medullary carcinomas, in which increased B cell infiltration and decreased CD8+ T cell infiltration are seen [79]. The reasons for B cell recruitment in medullary breast cancer are poorly understood. Whether B cell infiltration in medullary and/or atypical medullary carcinomas affects immune response is not known. Whether B cell depletion would impact tumor growth is also unknown.

6 Conclusions

In recent years investigators have identified an important role for a variety of immune-suppressive cells in human tumors. Examples include myeloid suppressor cells, tumor -ssociated macrophages, and CD4+CD25+FoxP3+ Tregs. Increasing evidence now points to the presence of B cell subsets with similar immune-modulating properties. The role of such Breg in suppression of antitumor immunity remains poorly understood. Abundant evidence in mouse models suggests that B cells may modulate innate and Th1 response in a manner conducive to tumor growth. A variety of B cell subsets have been implicated in suppression of both autoimmune disease and antitumor response. Much remains to be learned about the phenotypic characteristics of Breg cells, underlying mechanisms of action, and the prevalence of Breg in human tumors of both lymphoid and non-lymphoid origin. Breg may conceivably suppress immunity in certain breast, renal, or ovarian cancers in which significant B cell infiltrates have been described.

Understanding mechanisms of B cell-mediated suppression of antitumor response and the identification of human tumors with evidence of B cell-mediated immune suppression may allow rational design of clinical trials incorporating B cell depletion to augment antitumor immune responses.

References

1. Tadmor T, Zhang Y, Cho HM, Podack ER, Rosenblatt JD. The absence of B lymphocytes reduces the number and function of T-regulatory cells and enhances the anti-tumor response in a murine tumor model. Cancer Immunol Immunother. 2011;60(5):609–19.
2. Qin Z, Richter G, Schuler T, Ibe S, Cao X, Blankenstein T. B cells inhibit induction of T cell-dependent tumor immunity. Nat Med. 1998;4(5):627–30.

3. Shah S, Divekar AA, Hilchey SP, Cho HM, Newman CL, Shin SU, Nechustan H, Challita-Eid PM, Segal BM, Yi KH, Rosenblatt JD. Increased rejection of primary tumors in mice lacking B cells: inhibition of anti-tumor CTL and TH1 cytokine responses by B cells. Int J Cancer. 2005;117(4):574–86.
4. Inoue S, Leitner WW, Golding B, Scott D. Inhibitory effects of B cells on antitumor immunity. Cancer Res. 2006;66(15):7741–7.
5. Rowley DA, Stach RM. B lymphocytes secreting IgG linked to latent transforming growth factor-beta prevent primary cytolytic T lymphocyte responses. Int Immunol. 1998;10(3): 355–63.
6. Harris DP, Goodrich S, Mohrs K, Mohrs M, Lund FE. Cutting edge: the development of IL-4-producing B cells (B effector 2 cells) is controlled by IL-4, IL-4 receptor alpha, and Th2 cells. J Immunol. 2005;175(11):7103–7.
7. Wojciechowski W, Harris DP, Sprague F, Mousseau B, Makris M, Kusser K, Honjo T, Mohrs K, Mohrs M, Randall T, Lund FE. Cytokine-producing effector B cells regulate type 2 immunity to H. polygyrus. Immunity. 2009;30(3):421–33. doi:10.1016/j.immuni.2009.01.006.
8. Harris DP, Haynes L, Sayles PC, Duso DK, Eaton SM, Lepak NM, Johnson LL, Swain SL, Lund FE. Reciprocal regulation of polarized cytokine production by effector B and T cells. Nat Immunol. 2000;1(6):475–82. doi:10.1038/82717.
9. Gjertsson I, Foster S, Tarkowski A. Polarization of cytokine responses in B- and T-lymphocytes during Staphylococcus aureus infection. Microb Pathog. 2003;35(3):119–24.
10. Lund FE, Garvy BA, Randall TD, Harris DP. Regulatory roles for cytokine-producing B cells in infection and autoimmune disease. Curr Dir Autoimmun. 2005;8:25–54. doi:10.1159/000082086.
11. Dong HP, Elstrand MB, Holth A, Silins I, Berner A, Trope CG, Davidson B, Risberg B. NK- and B-cell infiltration correlates with worse outcome in metastatic ovarian carcinoma. Am J Clin Pathol. 2006;125(3):451–8.
12. Gannot G, Gannot I, Vered H, Buchner A, Keisari Y. Increase in immune cell infiltration with progression of oral epithelium from hyperkeratosis to dysplasia and carcinoma. Br J Cancer. 2002;86(9):1444–8.
13. Disis ML, Pupa SM, Gralow JR, Dittadi R, Menard S, Cheever MA. High-titer HER-2/neu protein-specific antibody can be detected in patients with early-stage breast cancer. J Clin Oncol. 1997;15(11):3363–7.
14. Houbiers JG, van der Burg SH, van de Watering LM, Tollenaar RA, Brand A, van de Velde CJ, Melief CJ. Antibodies against p53 are associated with poor prognosis of colorectal cancer. Br J Cancer. 1995;72(3):637–41.
15. Zhang Y, Eliav Y, Shin SU, Schreiber TH, Podack ER, Tadmor T, Rosenblatt JD. B lymphocyte inhibition of anti-tumor response depends on expansion of Treg but is independent of B-cell IL-10 secretion. Cancer Immunol Immunother. 2012;62(1):87–99. doi:10.1007/s00262-012-1313-6.
16. Perricone MA, Smith KA, Claussen KA, Plog MS, Hempel DM, Roberts BL, St George JA, Kaplan JM. Enhanced efficacy of melanoma vaccines in the absence of B lymphocytes. J Immunother. 2004;27(4):273–81.
17. Oizumi S, Deyev V, Yamazaki K, Schreiber T, Strbo N, Rosenblatt J, Podack ER. Surmounting tumor-induced immune suppression by frequent vaccination or immunization in the absence of B cells. J Immunother. 2008;31(4):394–401. doi:10.1097/CJI.0b013e31816bc74d 00002371-200805000-00008 [pii].
18. Chapoval AI, Fuller JA, Kremlev SG, Kamdar SJ, Evans R. Combination chemotherapy and IL-15 administration induce permanent tumor regression in a mouse lung tumor model: NK and T cell-mediated effects antagonized by B cells. J Immunol. 1998;161(12):6977–84.
19. Schioppa T, Moore R, Thompson RG, Rosser EC, Kulbe H, Nedospasov S, Mauri C, Coussens LM, Balkwill FR. B regulatory cells and the tumor-promoting actions of TNF-alpha during squamous carcinogenesis. Proc Natl Acad Sci U S A. 2011;108(26):10662–7. doi:10.1073/pnas.1100994108.
20. DiLillo DJ, Matsushita T, Tedder TF. B10 cells and regulatory B cells balance immune responses during inflammation, autoimmunity, and cancer. Ann N Y Acad Sci. 2010; 1183:38–57.

21. Stockinger B, Zal T, Zal A, Gray D. B cells solicit their own help from T cells. J Exp Med. 1996;183(3):891–9.
22. Bouaziz JD, Yanaba K, Tedder TF. Regulatory B cells as inhibitors of immune responses and inflammation. Immunol Rev. 2008;224:201–14.
23. de Goer de Herve MG, Durali D, Dembele B, Giuliani M, Tran TA, Azzarone B, Eid P, Tardieu M, Delfraissy JF, Taoufik Y. Interferon-alpha triggers B cell effector 1 (Be1) commitment. PloS one. 2011;6(4):e19366. doi:doi:10.1371/journal.pone.0019366.
24. Macaulay AE, DeKruyff RH, Goodnow CC, Umetsu DT. Antigen-specific B cells preferentially induce CD4+ T cells to produce IL-4. J Immunol. 1997;158(9):4171–9.
25. Sun JB, Czerkinsky C, Holmgren J. B lymphocytes treated in vitro with antigen coupled to cholera toxin B subunit induce antigen-specific Foxp3(+) regulatory T cells and protect against experimental autoimmune encephalomyelitis. J Immunol. 2012;188(4):1686–97. doi:10.4049/jimmunol.1101771.
26. Ray A, Basu S, Williams CB, Salzman NH, Dittel BN. A novel IL-10-independent regulatory role for B cells in suppressing autoimmunity by maintenance of regulatory T cells via GITR ligand. J Immunol. 2012;188(7):3188–98. doi:10.4049/jimmunol.1103354.
27. Reichardt P, Dornbach B, Rong S, Beissert S, Gueler F, Loser K, Gunzer M. Naive B cells generate regulatory T cells in the presence of a mature immunologic synapse. Blood. 2007;110(5):1519–29. doi:doi:blood-2006-10-053793 [pii] 10.1182/blood-2006-10-053793.
28. Sun JB, Flach CF, Czerkinsky C, Holmgren J. B lymphocytes promote expansion of regulatory T cells in oral tolerance: powerful induction by antigen coupled to cholera toxin B subunit. J Immunol (Baltimore, Md : 1950). 2008;181(12):8278–87.
29. Chen X, Jensen PE. Cutting edge: primary B lymphocytes preferentially expand allogeneic FoxP3+ CD4 T cells. J Immunol (Baltimore, Md : 1950). 2007;179(4):2046–50.
30. Placke T, Kopp HG, Salih HR. Glucocorticoid-induced TNFR-related (GITR) protein and its ligand in antitumor immunity: functional role and therapeutic modulation. Clinical & developmental immunology 2010:239083. doi:10.1155/2010/239083
31. Matsushita T, Tedder TF. Identifying regulatory B cells (B10 cells) that produce IL-10 in mice. Methods Mol Biol. 2011;677:99–111.
32. Matsushita T, Horikawa M, Iwata Y, Tedder TF. Regulatory B cells (B10 cells) and regulatory T cells have independent roles in controlling experimental autoimmune encephalomyelitis initiation and late-phase immunopathogenesis. J Immunol. 2010;185(4):2240–52.
33. Lemoine S, Morva A, Youinou P, Jamin C. Regulatory B cells in autoimmune diseases: how do they work? Ann N Y Acad Sci. 2009;1173:260–7.
34. Mauri C, Blair PA. Regulatory B cells in autoimmunity: developments and controversies. Nat Rev Rheumatol. 2010;6(11):636–43.
35. Fujimoto M. Regulatory B cells in skin and connective tissue diseases. J Dermatol Sci. 2010;60(1):1–7.
36. Yanaba K, Bouaziz JD, Haas KM, Poe JC, Fujimoto M, Tedder TF. A regulatory B cell subset with a unique CD1dhiCD5+ phenotype controls T cell-dependent inflammatory responses. Immunity. 2008;28(5):639–50.
37. Iwata Y, Matsushita T, Horikawa M, Dilillo DJ, Yanaba K, Venturi GM, Szabolcs PM, Bernstein SH, Magro CM, Williams AD, Hall RP, St Clair EW, Tedder TF. Characterization of a rare IL-10-competent B-cell subset in humans that parallels mouse regulatory B10 cells. Blood. 2011;117(2):530–41.
38. Blair PA, Norena LY, Flores-Borja F, Rawlings DJ, Isenberg DA, Ehrenstein MR, Mauri C. CD19(+)CD24(hi)CD38(hi) B cells exhibit regulatory capacity in healthy individuals but are functionally impaired in systemic Lupus Erythematosus patients. Immunity. 2010;32(1):129–40.
39. Zhang X, Deriaud E, Jiao X, Braun D, Leclerc C, Lo-Man R. Type I interferons protect neonates from acute inflammation through interleukin 10-producing B cells. J Exp Med. 2007;204(5):1107–18.
40. Evans JG, Chavez-Rueda KA, Eddaoudi A, Meyer-Bahlburg A, Rawlings DJ, Ehrenstein MR, Mauri C. Novel suppressive function of transitional 2 B cells in experimental arthritis. J Immunol. 2007;178(12):7868–78.

41. Naqvi SA, Khan MS, Vohora SB. Antibacterial, antifungal and anthelmintic studies on Ochrocarpus longifolius. Planta Med. 1976;29(1):98–100.
42. Brummel R, Lenert P. Activation of marginal zone B cells from lupus mice with type A(D) CpG-oligodeoxynucleotides. J Immunol. 2005;174(4):2429–34.
43. Wei B, Velazquez P, Turovskaya O, Spricher K, Aranda R, Kronenberg M, Birnbaumer L, Braun J. Mesenteric B cells centrally inhibit CD4+ T cell colitis through interaction with regulatory T cell subsets. Proc Natl Acad Sci U S A. 2005;102(6):2010–5.
44. Sonoda KH, Stein-Streilein J. CD1d on antigen-transporting APC and splenic marginal zone B cells promotes NKT cell-dependent tolerance. Eur J Immunol. 2002;32(3):848–57.
45. Mizoguchi A, Mizoguchi E, Takedatsu H, Blumberg RS, Bhan AK. Chronic intestinal inflammatory condition generates IL-10-producing regulatory B cell subset characterized by CD1d upregulation. Immunity. 2002;16(2):219–30.
46. Paciorkowski N, Shultz LD, Rajan TV. Primed peritoneal B lymphocytes are sufficient to transfer protection against Brugia pahangi infection in mice. Infect Immun. 2003;71(3):1370–8.
47. O'Garra A, Chang R, Go N, Hastings R, Haughton G, Howard M. Ly-1 B (B-1) cells are the main source of B cell-derived interleukin 10. Eur J Immunol. 1992;22(3):711–7.
48. Mann MK, Maresz K, Shriver LP, Tan Y, Dittel BN. B cell regulation of CD4+CD25+ T regulatory cells and IL-10 via B7 is essential for recovery from experimental autoimmune encephalomyelitis. J Immunol. 2007;178(6):3447–56.
49. Mauri C, Gray D, Mushtaq N, Londei M. Prevention of arthritis by interleukin 10-producing B cells. J Exp Med. 2003;197(4):489–501.
50. Fillatreau S, Sweenie CH, McGeachy MJ, Gray D, Anderton SM. B cells regulate autoimmunity by provision of IL-10. Nat Immunol. 2002;3(10):944–50.
51. Hernandez HJ, Wang Y, Stadecker MJ. In infection with Schistosoma mansoni, B cells are required for T helper type 2 cell responses but not for granuloma formation. J Immunol. 1997;158(10):4832–7.
52. Silverman GJ, Srikrishnan R, Germar K, Goodyear CS, Andrews KA, Ginzler EM, Tsao BP. Genetic imprinting of autoantibody repertoires in systemic lupus erythematosus patients. Clin Exp Immunol. 2008;153(1):102–16.
53. Carroll MC, Prodeus AP. Linkages of innate and adaptive immunity. Curr Opin Immunol. 1998;10(1):36–40.
54. Alam MS, Kurtz CC, Rowlett RM, Reuter BK, Wiznerowicz E, Das S, Linden J, Crowe SE, Ernst PB. CD73 is expressed by human regulatory T helper cells and suppresses proinflammatory cytokine production and Helicobacter felis-induced gastritis in mice. J Infect Dis. 2009;199(4):494–504.
55. Rafei M, Hsieh J, Zehntner S, Li M, Forner K, Birman E, Boivin MN, Young YK, Perreault C, Galipeau J. A granulocyte-macrophage colony-stimulating factor and interleukin-15 fusokine induces a regulatory B cell population with immune suppressive properties. Nat Med. 2009;15(9):1038–45.
56. Natarajan P, Singh A, McNamara JT, Secor Jr ER, Guernsey LA, Thrall RS, Schramm CM. Regulatory B cells from hilar lymph nodes of tolerant mice in a murine model of allergic airway disease are CD5(+), express TGF-beta, and co-localize with CD4(+)Foxp3(+) T cells. Mucosal Immunol. 2012. doi:10.1038/mi.2012.42.
57. Olkhanud PB, Damdinsuren B, Bodogai M, Gress RE, Sen R, Wejksza K, Malchinkhuu E, Wersto RP, Biragyn A. Tumor-Evoked Regulatory B Cells Promote Breast Cancer Metastasis by Converting Resting CD4+ T Cells to T-Regulatory Cells. Cancer Res. 2011;71(10): 3505–15.
58. de Visser KE, Korets LV, Coussens LM. De novo carcinogenesis promoted by chronic inflammation is B lymphocyte dependent. Cancer cell. 2005;7(5):411–23. doi:10.1016/j.ccr.2005.04.014.
59. Maloney DG, Grillo-Lopez AJ, Bodkin DJ, White CA, Liles TM, Royston I, Varns C, Rosenberg J, Levy R. IDEC-C2B8: results of a phase I multiple-dose trial in patients with relapsed non-Hodgkin's lymphoma. J Clin Oncol. 1997;15(10):3266–74.
60. Hilchey SP, Hyrien O, Mosmann TR, Livingstone AM, Friedberg JW, Young F, Fisher RI, Kelleher Jr RJ, Bankert RB, Bernstein SH. Rituximab immunotherapy results in the induction

of a lymphoma idiotype-specific T-cell response in patients with follicular lymphoma: support for a "vaccinal effect" of rituximab. Blood. 2009;113(16):3809–12. doi:10.1182/blood-2008-10-185280.
61. Kim S, Fridlender ZG, Dunn R, Kehry MR, Kapoor V, Blouin A, Kaiser LR, Albelda SM. B-cell depletion using an anti-CD20 antibody augments antitumor immune responses and immunotherapy in nonhematopoetic murine tumor models. J Immunother. 2008;31(5):446–57. doi:10.1097/CJI.0b013e31816d1d6a.
62. DiLillo DJ, Yanaba K, Tedder TF. B cells are required for optimal CD4+ and CD8+ T cell tumor immunity: therapeutic B cell depletion enhances B16 melanoma growth in mice. J Immunol. 2010;184(7):4006–16. doi:10.4049/jimmunol.0903009.
63. Horikawa M, Minard-Colin V, Matsushita T, Tedder TF. Regulatory B cell production of IL-10 inhibits lymphoma depletion during CD20 immunotherapy in mice. J Clin Invest. 2011;121(11):4268–80. doi:10.1172/JCI59266.
64. El Andaloussi A, Lesniak MS. CD4+ CD25+ FoxP3+ T-cell infiltration and heme oxygenase-1 expression correlate with tumor grade in human gliomas. J Neurooncol. 2007;83(2):145–52. doi:10.1007/s11060-006-9314-y.
65. Yamagami W, Susumu N, Tanaka H, Hirasawa A, Banno K, Suzuki N, Tsuda H, Tsukazaki K, Aoki D. Immunofluorescence-detected infiltration of CD4+FOXP3+ regulatory T cells is relevant to the prognosis of patients with endometrial cancer. Int J Gynecol Cancer. 2011; 21(9):1628–34. doi:10.1097/IGC.0b013e31822c271f.
66. Heimberger AB, Abou-Ghazal M, Reina-Ortiz C, Yang DS, Sun W, Qiao W, Hiraoka N, Fuller GN. Incidence and prognostic impact of FoxP3+ regulatory T cells in human gliomas. Clin Cancer Res. 2008;14(16):5166–72. doi:10.1158/1078-0432.CCR-08-0320.
67. Schwarz S, Butz M, Morsczeck C, Reichert TE, Driemel O. Increased number of CD25 FoxP3 regulatory T cells in oral squamous cell carcinomas detected by chromogenic immunohistochemical double staining. J Oral Pathol Med. 2008;37(8):485–9. doi:10.1111/j.1600-0714.2008.00641.x.
68. Fu J, Xu D, Liu Z, Shi M, Zhao P, Fu B, Zhang Z, Yang H, Zhang H, Zhou C, Yao J, Jin L, Wang H, Yang Y, Fu YX, Wang FS. Increased regulatory T cells correlate with CD8 T-cell impairment and poor survival in hepatocellular carcinoma patients. Gastroenterology. 2007;132(7):2328–39. doi:10.1053/j.gastro.2007.03.102.
69. Yan M, Jene N, Byrne D, Millar EK, O'Toole SA, McNeil CM, Bates GJ, Harris AL, Banham AH, Sutherland RL, Fox SB. Recruitment of regulatory T cells is correlated with hypoxia-induced CXCR4 expression, and is associated with poor prognosis in basal-like breast cancers. Breast Cancer Res. 2011;13(2):R47. doi:10.1186/bcr2869.
70. Sugihara AQ, Rolle CE, Lesniak MS. Regulatory T cells actively infiltrate metastatic brain tumors. Int J Oncol. 2009;34(6):1533–40.
71. Chaput N, Darrasse-Jeze G, Bergot AS, Cordier C, Ngo-Abdalla S, Klatzmann D, Azogui O. Regulatory T cells prevent CD8 T cell maturation by inhibiting CD4 Th cells at tumor sites. J Immunol. 2007;179(8):4969–78.
72. Wang W, Hodkinson P, McLaren F, Mackinnon A, Wallace W, Howie S, Sethi T. Small cell lung cancer tumour cells induce regulatory T lymphocytes, and patient survival correlates negatively with FOXP3(+) cells in tumour infiltrate. Int J Cancer. 2012. doi:10.1002/ijc.27613.
73. Lesokhin AM, Hohl TM, Kitano S, Cortez C, Hirschhorn-Cymerman D, Avogadri F, Rizzuto GA, Lazarus JJ, Pamer EG, Houghton AN, Merghoub T, Wolchok JD. Monocytic CCR2(+) myeloid-derived suppressor cells promote immune escape by limiting activated CD8 T-cell infiltration into the tumor microenvironment. Cancer Res. 2012;72(4):876–86. doi:10.1158/0008-5472.CAN-11-1792.
74. Mascaro JM, Molgo M, Castel T, Castro J. Plasma cells within the infiltrate of primary cutaneous malignant melanoma of the skin. A confirmation of its histoprognostic value. A J Dermatopathol. 1987;9(6):497–9.
75. Weissmann A, Roses DF, Harris MN, Dubin N. Prediction of lymph node metastases from the histologic features of primary cutaneous malignant melanomas. Am J Dermatopathol. 1984;6(Suppl):35–41.

76. Shabtai M, Ye H, Frischer Z, Martin J, Waltzer WC, Malinowski K. Increased expression of activation markers in renal cell carcinoma infiltrating lymphocytes. J Urol. 2002;168(5):2216–9. doi:10.1097/01.ju.0000031960.09503.89.
77. Elsasser-Beile U, Grussenmeyer T, Gierschner D, Schmoll B, Schultze-Seemann W, Wetterauer U, Schulte Monting J. Semiquantitative analysis of Th1 and Th2 cytokine expression in CD3+, CD4+, and CD8+ renal-cell-carcinoma-infiltrating lymphocytes. Cancer Immunol Immunother. 1999;48(4):204–8.
78. Nzula S, Going JJ, Stott DI. Antigen-driven clonal proliferation, somatic hypermutation, and selection of B lymphocytes infiltrating human ductal breast carcinomas. Cancer Res. 2003;63(12):3275–80.
79. Lim KH, Telisinghe PU, Abdullah MS, Ramasamy R. Possible significance of differences in proportions of cytotoxic T cells and B-lineage cells in the tumour-infiltrating lymphocytes of typical and atypical medullary carcinomas of the breast. Cancer Immun. 2010;10:3.

Heat-Shock Protein-Based Cancer Immunotherapy

Taylor H. Schreiber

Abstract Despite the registration of over 1,000 clinical trials assessing the activity of therapeutic cancer vaccines in human patients with multiple cancer types, only a single vaccine has received FDA approval for clinical use. Nonetheless, the therapeutic potential of immune modulation for treating cancer has continued to be validated with both preclinical and clinical studies, most recently in studies investigating so-called checkpoint inhibitory antibodies targeting CTLA-4 and PD-1. One important class of therapeutic cancer vaccines seeks to generate therapeutic immunity based on the combined adjuvant and antigen delivery characteristics of heat-shock proteins. Heat-shock protein-based vaccines are unique among other approaches due to the unique ability of certain heat-shock proteins to dually activate antigen-presenting cells and specifically deliver tumor antigens to cytotoxic CD8+ T cells via the antigen cross-presentation pathway. The enclosed chapter provides a comprehensive overview of heat-shock protein-based cancer vaccines assessed in human clinical trials within the context of parallel progress in understanding the interactions between a developing tumor and the human immune system.

1 Heat-Shock Proteins, Sterile Inflammation, and Immunosurveillance

Molecular alarm systems are an essential component of vertebrate immunity and function to signify the occurrence of an event which threatens the survival of the host. One such system operates through the family of receptors known as "Toll-like" receptors (TLRs), which evolved to recognize common pathogen-associated

T.H. Schreiber (✉)
Department of Microbiology and Immunology, University of Miami Miller School of Medicine, Miami, FL, USA
e-mail: TSchreiber@med.miami.edu

J.D. Rosenblatt et al. (eds.), *Advances in Tumor Immunology and Immunotherapy*, Current Cancer Research, DOI 10.1007/978-1-4614-8809-5_3,

© Springer Science+Business Media New York 2014

molecular patterns (PAMPs) such as bacterial cell wall sugars, single-stranded viral DNA, and flagella [1, 2]. Other pattern recognition molecules include C-type lectin receptors (CLRs), caspase-recruitment domain (CARD), and nucleotide-binding domain (NOD) family members [3]. There are currently 13 known TLRs that recognize PAMPs derived from many of the most common human pathogens [4, 5]. The predetermined specificity of the TLR/PAMP warning system provides a very efficient mechanism for host notification of an invading pathogen but performs this function principally by promoting inflammation and is incapable of directly stimulating antigen-specific immunity. Instead, TLR ligation signals the maturation of antigen-presenting cells (APCs) via upregulation of costimulatory molecules including CD80 and CD86, production of inflammatory cytokines including interleukins-12 and -18, and migration of activated APCs to local lymphoid organs [6–8].

The limitation inherent to screening for PAMPs is that such a system requires a unique receptor for each PAMP. Likely as a mechanism to increase efficiency in this process, the immune system evolved an antigen-specific presentation system to screen not just for pathogen-specific patterns but also for individual peptide sequences that are specific to the pathogen in question. Such a candidate system would ideally have at least several of the following properties: (1) abundant expression in all cell types, (2) ability to bind a diverse array of proteins, (3) ability for specific detection by immune cells, and (4) ability to inform immune cells as to the identity of the pathogen in question. These requirements describe precisely the role of the major histocompatibility complex (MHC) in the evolution of adaptive immunity. Reviewed extensively elsewhere, the MHC consists of two complexes (MHC I and MHC II) which provide a division of labor for defense against intracellular (MHC I) and extracellular (MHC II) pathogens [9–11]. The expression patterns of these receptors follow the behavioral patterns of the pathogens to which they provide defense, with the MHC I molecules being ubiquitously expressed by all cells (save erythrocytes) and the MHC II molecules being restricted to cells capable of engulfing or directly binding extracellular pathogens such as dendritic cells, macrophages, and B cells. Together, the MHC molecules and TLR system provide an integrated, but parallel, system of antigen presentation and expression of costimulatory molecules which lead to the antigen-specific activation of adaptive immunity (exerted by T and B cells) in response to the dual presence of both "danger signals" and specific antigens presented by MHC I and/or MHC II.

Survival to reproductive age is threatened by not only invasion from foreign pathogens but also maladaptive mutations throughout development. Adaptation itself is a process afforded by the acquisition of individual mutations in the human genome which may lead to cellular progeny with differential fitness from the parental cell. For this to occur DNA replication must, *by necessity*, be an imperfect process. Taking into account all DNA proofreading mechanisms, the fidelity of eukaryotic DNA replication is estimated to be on the order of 10^{-10}, which predicts that a cell will progressively and randomly acquire a single mutation every 1–2 cell divisions (in a human genome containing approximately 6.6 billion nucleotides) even in the absence of genotoxic stress and in proportion to the overall rate of cell division throughout development. Thus, the evolutionary trade-off for adaptation is the acquisition of mutations during development that may lead to the dysregulated growth and potentially transformation of otherwise normal cells into cancer cells. This is a process against which both cell-intrinsic and -extrinsic defense systems have developed; the extrinsic defense system is known today as cancer immunosurveillance [12, 13].

An immunological defense against transformed cells is fundamentally distinct from defense against exogenous pathogens in that the immune response must be initiated under the so-called sterile conditions for non-virus-associated malignancies. Sterile inflammation is detected through a distinct group of molecules known collectively as "damage-associated molecular patterns" (DAMPs) and their receptors [14, 15]. DAMPs include a range of endogenous molecules including heat-shock proteins, HMGB1, S100 proteins, as well as nucleic acids and extracellular matrix components [16]. In general, DAMPs are molecules that are released as a result of cell necrosis as occurs during conditions of extreme cellular stress or trauma. Many DAMPs are also recognized by the TLR system and are important for mediating inflammatory cytokine production in response to tissue damage that may contribute to recruitment of innate immune cells and wound healing [17–19]. Certain DAMPs, including HMGB1, may play critical roles in the efficacy of cancer chemotherapy and radiotherapy by generating inflammation within the tumor microenvironment via TLR and RAGE interactions [20]. Dysregulation of DAMP-mediated immune activation is also associated with a variety of pathological conditions including atherosclerosis, pseudogout, type 1 diabetes, and Alzheimer's disease, which may represent the evolutionary trade-off for a DAMP-mediated sensor system to detect necrotic cell death.

In addition to TLRs, DAMPs can also interact with several other receptors, of which CD91 and CLEC9 are unique in bridging sterile inflammation to antigen cross-presentation [21–25]. CD91 and CLEC9 are both expressed by CD11c+ dendritic cells and in particular by the CD8α+ subset of dendritic cells that play a critical role in antigen cross-presentation [22, 25–27]. The ligand for CLEC9 was recently identified as F-actin [28, 29], and the ligands for CD91 include well-described members of the heat-shock protein family, which constitutes the oldest and most abundant class of protein in all mammalian cells [25, 30, 31]. Because the adaptive immune response is developmentally programmed to recognize foreign antigens [32], the existence of a linkage between sterile inflammation and adaptive immunity implies that certain antigens may arise in metabolically stressed "self" cells that are sufficiently nonself to engage the adaptive immune response and that such a pathway provides a survival advantage to the host at large. It has been suggested in the "neo-ligand" hypothesis that such a linkage is purely maladaptive and contributes only to autoimmunity [33]; however, the possibility that this pathway provides a survival advantage via tumor immunosurveillance must also be considered. This linkage may also be important for defense against the introduction of exogenous antigens during traumatic tissue damage; however, it is clear that a role of HSP/CD91 in this situation would be redundant with the PAMP/MHC system. Such redundancy may provide benefit in response to infection with pathogens that have developed mechanisms to evade (low-frequency CpG DNA by adenoviruses for example) or thwart (V-proteins by paramyxoviruses for example) innate immune activation by TLRs; however, this may not be the only benefit. The recent identification of antigen cross-presentation as a critical mechanism for tumor immunosurveillance supports a specialized role of the HSP/CD91 system in this process [26, 34].

Heat-shock proteins are an abundant family of intracellular proteins that collectively facilitate protein folding, trafficking, localization, and degradation [35–37]. The classification of this family of proteins as being related to "heat shock" dates to their accidental discovery as molecular mediators of cell stress, and the name has persisted despite the knowledge that their primary role is to chaperone protein folding and trafficking [38]. The ability of a relatively small number of HSP to function as protein chaperones for a large number of unique proteins expressed across all cell types requires that these HSP have unusual promiscuity in peptide binding specificity. This property has been confirmed by several groups, all seeking to identify the source of immunogenicity of different HSP. Most comprehensively shown for HSP gp96, efforts to identify specific HSP peptide-binding motifs have failed to elucidate a defined peptide profile based on amino acid content or peptide length that defines HSP binding capacity. In the specific case of gp96, nearly every peptide analyzed has been found in association with gp96 and the binding of these peptides has surprisingly high affinity, surviving SDS-PAGE and only weakly released by high temperature or high salt conditions in vitro [39]. The peptide binding promiscuity of HSP70 is slightly more limited than for gp96, being specific for aliphatic amino acid motifs and extremely sensitive to peptide release in the presence of ATP [31, 40]. This promiscuity in peptide binding is likely the source of evolutionary efficiency in APC adaptation to screen for extracellular HSP via CD91 as a sensor for necrotic cell death. CD91 is the endocytic receptor for all known heat-shock proteins, including HSP70, HSP90, gp96, and calreticulin [5, 9]. Among DAMP receptors, CD91 is also the primary endocytic receptor, which indicates that among DAMPs, HSPs are highly specialized adjuvants that can provide APCs with both a maturation signal (via TLRs) and a source of antigen via endocytosis of HSP/antigen complexes. The remarkable efficiency of HSP/peptide complex uptake by CD91 facilitates the induction of antigen-specific immunity at femto-molar concentrations of antigen, which represent physiologic concentrations [37, 41]. The evolution of HSP proteins as dual-purpose adjuvants may have taken place as a specific immunosurveillance mechanism in cancer, because linkage of adaptive immunity to sterile inflammation in diseases other than cancer is usually maladaptive.

The combined adjuvant properties of APC activation via TLRs and antigen delivery via CD91 are what make HSP ideal candidates for vaccine development. The hypothesis that the dual adjuvant role of HSP evolved specifically as an antigen-cross-presenting mechanism for immunosurveillance against cancer arising under conditions of sterile inflammation remains to be experimentally confirmed; however, this evidence would heighten the validity of utilizing HSP as cancer immunotherapy. Such findings would provide an elegant circularity to the original description of HSP as the critical tumor rejection "antigens" (now understood to be HSP/antigen complexes) for sarcoma tumors in mice [42]. To date, 20 clinical trials have been conducted in the United States with HSP-based oncology vaccines. Of these, 13

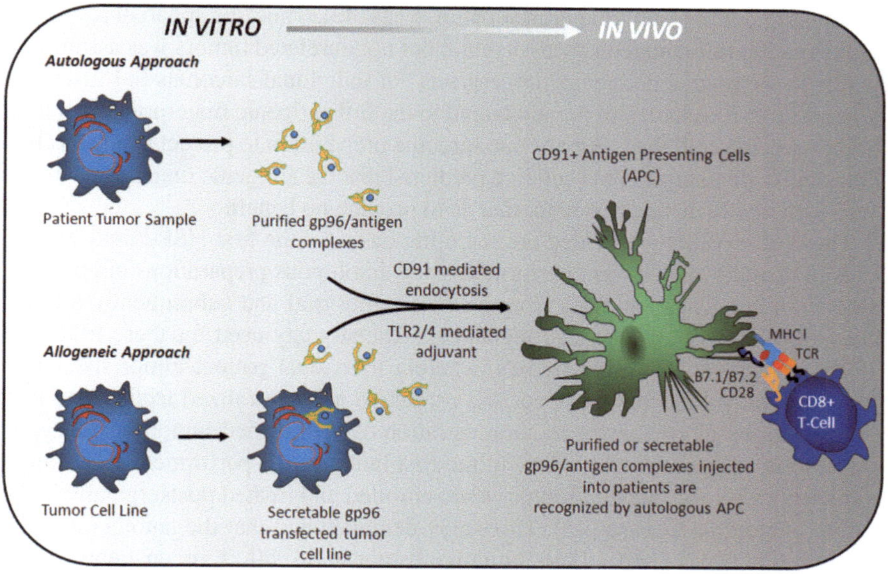

Fig. 1 Schematic overview of the key characteristics of autologous and allogeneic HSP based vaccines in clinical development

utilized gp96-based approaches and 7 HSP70-based approaches. There are not yet any immunotherapy trials testing calreticulin, HSP90, or grp170 listed on clinicaltrials.gov. The major focus of the following sections is geared toward those approaches that have been studied in human patients. A schematic overview of the core attributes of autologous and allogeneic HSP vaccines is illustrated in Fig. 1, using gp96 as the archetypal HSP.

2 Autologous Purified HSP Vaccines

The initial discovery of HSP gp96 as a "tumor rejection antigen" demonstrated that purified preparations of gp96 provided T cell-mediated protection against parental, but not unrelated, sarcoma tumors [42]. In these experiments, the immunogenic component within individual chemically induced murine sarcoma cell lysates was meticulously chased using several fractionation strategies into a fraction of glycoproteins of approximately 96 kDa molecular weight. Subsequent immunization of mice with these 96 kDa molecular weight proteins was protective against a subsequent challenge with the parental, but not unrelated, sarcoma cell lines. The proposed explanation for the immunogenicity of gp96 and the limited protection it provided only to parental tumor cells was that gp96 itself must be uniquely mutated in various sarcoma tumor cell lines. This hypothesis was quickly proven false, and the specific immunogenicity of gp96 was unequivocally demonstrated to be due to the client tumor peptides chaperoned by gp96 [24, 43]. Thus, the apparent restriction of therapeutic immunogenicity to parental but not unrelated tumors was assumed to be due to the unique antigenic "fingerprints" of individual sarcomas [44]. Because purified gp96 is assumed to remain bound to the full antigenic fingerprint of an individual sarcoma cell, the failure of one sarcoma preparation to protect against a challenge with a distinct sarcoma cell line predicted that the antigenic fingerprints of one were sufficiently distinct from another as to provide no benefit.

These observations provided the scientific basis for the first HSP-based vaccine trials in humans, which were performed using autologous preparations of gp96 isolated from surgical specimens from a small safety trial and subsequently a larger study in patients with advanced melanoma. The strategy used for these trials was similar to the initial murine studies, wherein individual patient tumor specimens were surgically collected, shipped, and processed at a centralized facility and then returned to the physician for re-administration of the purified tumor-derived gp96 preparation to the original patient. In the first human trial, performed in Germany, 16 patients with various tumor types were enrolled and treated postsurgically in the setting of residual disease [45]. This study demonstrated that the autologous gp96 vaccine was safe, induced an immune response in 50 % of patients tested (as measured by tumor antigen-specific CD8+ T cells), and produced interesting, albeit anecdotal, tumor responses in at least one patient with coincident hepatocellular and breast carcinoma.

This safety study set the stage for the next human trial, performed in Italy: 39 patients with stage IV melanoma were treated with at least one cycle (four vaccinations) of autologous gp96 starting 5–8 weeks after surgical resection of at least one lesion by intradermal or subcutaneous injection [46]. Patients who did not progress were eligible to continue on a second cycle of vaccinations and continue with monthly injections thereafter until progression or exhaustion of the autologous gp96 preparation. The vaccine was observed to be safe in all patients tested, and 10/21 evaluable patients demonstrated a positive and specific immune response to melanoma antigens by the ELISPOT assay [47]. Of the 28 patients with residual disease post surgery, there were 2 complete responses (CR) and another 3 patients with stable disease (SD) for varying intervals. Of the two patients with CRs, one responded extremely quickly to the vaccine, with resolution of lung metastasis after only the first cycle, and remained disease free for 24 months after vaccination. In the second patient the immune response took over a year to resolve the metastatic lesions, which extended well beyond the period of vaccination and led to a CR in excess of 38 months in duration. These two patients in the very early studies serve to highlight the variability in the time required for an immune response to manifest in patients, which is a phenomenon that is only now becoming accepted by clinicians and well highlighted by recent data with anti-CTLA-4 antibodies [48, 49]. In total, this initial trial demonstrated that autologous gp96 was safe, feasible in at least 60 % of patients enrolled, and warranted further testing in humans [46]. A separate phase I/II study performed in the United States on a similar population of patients with advanced melanoma obtained similar findings, including the intriguing, but unconfirmed, suggestion that patients fared better following treatment in the adjuvant setting [50].

In a subsequent phase II clinical trial, also conducted in Italy, autologous gp96 preparations were prepared from a similar population of patients with stage IV melanoma; however, the trial design was significantly modified. A total of 20 patients completed the first cycle of vaccinations and were evaluable in the study for immune response and survival. Once again, no safety issues were observed in any patients and only minor injection-site reactions including erythema and induration were common. In this study each weekly vaccination was performed together with GM-CSF injection and patients received two injections of interferon-alpha (IFNα) between vaccinations [51]. A greater number of patients achieved SD (11/20) than in the phase I study, and a single patient had a CR after the first cycle of vaccination. It remains unclear whether these responses were related to an increased immune response or to the combination therapy with GM-CSF and IFNα because as in the phase I study, approximately half of the patients (7/13) had a positive ELISPOT result. Interestingly, the patient achieving a CR had the lowest expression of the melanoma antigens MART1 and gp100, perhaps indicating that other antigens not highly expressed by the ELISPOT target cells contributed to the clinical response [51]. These data served to extend the safety database, immunological activity, and potential clinical benefit of autologous gp96 for the treatment of melanoma and facilitated testing in a controlled phase III clinical trial.

An international phase III trial of 322 patients with stage IV melanoma was subsequently conducted with autologous gp96 to determine overall survival compared to physicians' choice [52]. Once again, the study design was revised significantly from the phase II study. In both prior studies, patients were pretreated with a combination of surgery + chemotherapy or radiotherapy and in some patients with IFNα or IL-2. In contrast to the phase II study, patients did not receive peri-vaccination treatment with GM-CSF or intermittent IFNα; however, the patient population was otherwise similar to the two prior studies. As was observed in the phase I and II studies, vaccination was feasible in just over 60 % of patients enrolled, with a significant number of patients not receiving treatment due to quality control failures in manufacturing. Unfortunately, this trial failed to demonstrate a benefit in overall survival for patients treated with autologous gp96 as compared to physicians' choice. In a subset analysis, a trend toward increased overall survival was observed in all patient subsets depending on the number of vaccine doses administered to each patient. In this analysis, it was reported that patients with stage M1a and M1b disease who received at least ten doses of the vaccine demonstrated a survival benefit as compared to physicians' choice [52]. Whether or not the failure of this trial was due to feasibility questions related to vaccine production and adequate supply of product to reach a therapeutic dose in a majority of patients remains unclear; however, such a conclusion is supported both by preclinical studies and the overall trends observed in this randomized phase III trial [44, 53]. In addition, it is worth noting that the trend toward increased survival also correlated with earlier stage disease, suggesting that vaccine therapy may be more effective early in the course of disease.

At the same time the first trials in melanoma were running, phase II and III trials were also conducted in patients with metastatic renal cell carcinoma. Renal cell carcinoma was chosen because, similar to melanoma, it was believed to be a relatively immunogenic tumor type that demonstrated intermittent responses to cytokine-based therapy and immunotherapy [54]. In the phase II study, 60 out of 84 enrolled patients were treated and evaluable, demonstrating an improvement in feasibility in this tumor type as compared to melanoma patients, potentially due to increased access to tumor tissue following nephrectomy. Out of these 60 patients, 2 CRs, 2 PRs, and 7 SDs were observed. This trial also included a single patient who developed severe complications that were potentially related to the vaccination. The remaining 59 patients experienced similar injection-site reactions to what was observed in the melanoma trials.

Despite the fact that this study concluded that autologous gp96 was "… relatively ineffective …" a large phase III study was subsequently performed in patients with metastatic renal cell carcinoma. As in melanoma, the design of this phase III trial was a significant departure from the phase II trial and was tested as adjuvant therapy to prevent disease recurrence in non-metastatic patients following nephrectomy [55]. A total of 318 patients were treated with autologous gp96, and both PFS and OS were compared to 367 patients in the observation-only control group. This trial was therefore the first of its kind to examine the efficacy of HSP vaccine therapy in a minimal-residual disease setting but unfortunately also missed its primary endpoint of reducing recurrence-free survival. A post hoc analysis suggested that patients with the earliest stage disease (AJCC stage I and II) may have enjoyed a delayed rate of recurrence; however, this conclusion requires further validation. As in the phase II in renal cell carcinoma, nearly 90 % of the patients randomized to autologous gp96 were able to receive the vaccine, demonstrating that feasibility was significantly improved as compared to melanoma.

In addition to melanoma and renal cell carcinoma, autologous preparations of gp96 have been tested in patients with colorectal and pancreatic cancer as well as non-Hodgkin's lymphoma. A study including 29 patients with metastatic colorectal cancer treated with autologous gp96 in the adjuvant setting reported impressive increases in MHC I-restricted immune responses in the majority of patients treated [56]. The presence of a positive immune response detected by interferon-γ enzyme-linked immunospot (ELISPOT) assay was significantly correlated with both increased overall survival and increased progression-free survival. As in several previous studies, three different doses of gp96 were tested, with potentially the lowest dose (2.5 μg/injection) providing the most consistent immune response in patients. Another series of phase II trials in patients with non-Hodgkin's lymphoma also demonstrated safety in all patients and vaccine production feasibility in the majority of patients but was not designed to determine survival benefit or immune response [57, 58]. A small, ten-patient, phase I study in patients with completely resected pancreatic adenocarcinoma treated in the adjuvant setting also demonstrated safety of the approach, with immune responses only in a minority of patients which did not correlate with disease-free survival [59].

To date, over 1,000 patients with multiple tumor types have been safely treated with autologous gp96 but without apparent clinical efficacy. These results in controlled clinical trials are certainly disappointing, but sprinkled throughout these failed trials are individual patients who were observed to have highly unusual "spontaneous" disease remission or subgroups of patients who in post hoc analysis appeared to enjoy a survival benefit. Definitive reasons for these failures are unknown; however, selection of two highly "immunogenic" tumors (melanoma and renal cell carcinoma) for testing in pivotal trials may have played a role [60]. The recent approval studies with anti-CTLA-4 antibodies (ipilimumab) in melanoma support the hypothesis that the most highly immunogenic tumors provide *vaccination* in situ, which predicts the immunoselection of tumor subclones that either display reduced amounts of critical antigens or contribute to local or systemic immunosuppression [12, 48, 49, 60]. The continued growth of tumors that provide *vaccination* in situ indicates that a tumor is progressing in spite of an ongoing immune response and that blocking immune regulatory mechanisms is a more critical first strike than attempting to broaden the scope of the immune response with a vaccine. Combinatorial strategies are in development for these tumor types wherein vaccination may play a secondary role to primary therapy with immune regulatory checkpoint inhibitors such as ipilimumab [61]. The overarching themes from these clinical trials also indicate that autologous gp96 is most effective in patients with earlier stage disease, who generate a positive immune response to the vaccine and for whom sufficient vaccine is produced to extend the treatment period well beyond the first four weekly injections. These predictions are generated from only two large, controlled, phase III clinical trials, and it is unfortunate that controlled studies were never run in phase II clinical trials because some of these concepts may have contributed to improved design of phase III clinical trials and been included in predefined endpoint criteria. An ongoing postsurgical adjuvant therapy trial in patients with >90 % resection of brain and central nervous system tumors (NCT00905060) appears poised to enter a pivotal phase III clinical trial and will hopefully incorporate some of these parameters in future trial design.

3 Allogeneic Cell-Based HSP Vaccines

The initial studies by Srivastava and colleagues clearly indicated that the repertoire of antigens bound to gp96 in purified preparations was sufficiently unique to the parental tumor that immunogenicity did not extend to genetically distinct tumor cell lines [42]. In the years since these initial discoveries, a great deal of progress has been made in understanding the specific nature of tumor antigens and in defining those which may or may not be "shared" by genetically distinct tumors. Two classes of tumor antigens have emerged from this work and are now defined as either "tumor-specific antigens" (TSA) or "abnormal self-antigens" (ASA, also referred to as tumor-associated antigens). TSA are those that arise as a direct result of randomly acquired genetic mutations in somatic genes that contribute as "drivers" or stowaway as "passengers" in the oncogenic process. The Cancer Genome Atlas (TCGA) has in recent years provided definitive evidence that dozens of TSA arise in every tumor type investigated and that at least a handful of those TSA appear to have the appropriate characteristics for binding to and presentation by MHC molecules [62–68]. These studies provide unequivocal evidence that except in very rare cases (such as *kras* in pancreatic adenocarcinoma), somatic mutations do not represent a source of shared antigens between patients with individual tumors. Instead, these studies provide clear evidence that ASA are the much more likely source of shared antigens between patients with related tumors due to common disruptions in core signaling pathways as a result of unique mutations in particular oncogenic "driver" genes [69, 70]. These somatic mutations lead to increases in gene copy number for a range of different proteins that lead to expression patterns not seen in non-transformed cells [71]. It is also clear that acquisition of mutations during oncogenesis leads to re-expression of primitive antigens typically only expressed in germline tissues and which have been broadly named "cancer testis antigens." This group of antigens is widely understood to represent a source of commonly shared antigens between genetically distinct tumors [72–74]. In fact, the world's first FDA-approved cancer vaccine is based upon the principle of antigen sharing between genetically distinct tumors and demonstrates that even a single shared ASA (prostatic acid phosphatase) can provide meaningful clinical efficacy [75]. At the same time, preclinical studies demonstrated that shared antigens between several established multiple myeloma cell lines could provide a basis for HSP gp96-mediated immunoprotection against genetically distinct tumors [76]. The antigenic underpinnings of these observations remain to be mechanistically elucidated; however, it is proposed that the spectrum of antigens from individual cell lines that are potentially shared with the antigens expressed by a patient tumor is increased by combining multiple cell lines into the vaccine preparation. Whether these observations reflect a unique antigenic property of myeloma or whether this phenomenon is generalizable to other tumor types also remains to be experimentally proven.

To date, clinical experience with allogeneic heat-shock protein vaccines is limited to a single approach based on a cell-secreted genetically engineered construct of gp96 [77]. This approach seeks to mimic the natural release of gp96 during necrotic cell death by replacing the KDEL endoplasmic reticulum retention sequence on the C-terminus of gp96 with a secretory molecule, in this case the hinge-CH2-CH3 domain from an IgG1 molecule to create a gp96-Ig fusion protein [78]. When transfected cell lines express and secrete gp96-Ig, it was found to chaperone peptides to the cross-presentation pathway similar to autologous gp96 and lead to CD8+ T cell-, NK cell-, and perforin-dependent antitumor immunity [41, 79–81]. Because this construct of gp96 was transfected into mammalian cells in sterile cell culture, required no purification steps, and provided CD8+ T cell-mediated antigen-specific immunity in vivo, this work finally laid to rest the long-standing criticism that HSP-mediated immune activation was simply a consequence of lipopolysaccharide contamination of autologous preparations. Further, preclinical studies demonstrated that immunization with cell-secreted gp96 led to an approximately tenfold increase in the magnitude of antigen-specific CD8+ T cell activation as compared to immunization with an equivalent quantity of cell-purified gp96 [80]. The reasons for this increase likely relate to increased half-life in vivo of a continuously secreted protein. Similar to autologous gp96, cell-secreted gp96-Ig has been shown to stimulate polyclonal and polyfunctional CD8+ T cell responses against all relevant antigens contained within the transfected cells [61, 82, 83].

A phase I clinical trial in patients with advanced non-small-cell lung cancer has examined the safety and immunogenicity of secreted gp96-Ig. NSCLC was selected as a tumor target for this approach because it represents a comparatively non-immunogenic tumor type as compared to melanoma and renal cell carcinoma and because 5-year survival for patients with NSCLC only increased from 14.2 to 18.0 % from 1975 to 2006, indicating that new treatment modalities are necessary [84]. The phase I study was conducted in a total of 18 patients with stage IIIB/IV NSCLC who had failed at least two prior therapies. The drug consisted of an adeno-carcinoma cell line that secreted gp96-Ig and which was irradiated and frozen prior to administration to patients by intradermal injection. The cell line provided the source of shared NSCLC antigens for delivery by gp96-Ig and was selected on the basis of cancer/testis antigens that are shared between patients with NSCLC [85–87]. All patients had progressive disease at the time of study enrollment and were divided into three different dosing arms which varied on the basis of frequency of injection but not total dose of vaccine administered. This design was based on preclinical studies indicating that increased frequency of vaccination provided increased antitumor immunity and tumor regression [80, 81]. This study demonstrated that administration of cell-secreted gp96-Ig to patients was safe and stimulated a vaccine-specific immune response in 73 % of patients treated. An analysis of correlation between immune response and overall survival demonstrated a significant association between the two, with nonresponders surviving 4.5 months and responders an average of 16.5 months. These findings remain anecdotal but supported progression to phase II clinical trials which are currently ongoing. This phase II study (NCT01504542) includes a randomized placebo control group, which had not been included in any of the previous HSP trials at the phase II stage and may facilitate appropriate prospective endpoint design for a subsequent phase III study.

Additional clinical trials are needed to demonstrate whether allogeneic approaches with gp96 provide clinical benefit. Potential advantages of this approach relate to feasibility of vaccine production for all patients enrolled in the study. Because the product is identical for all patients and easily scalable, concerns over obtaining sufficient material for vaccine production, which limited feasibility in the phase III melanoma trial to just 60 % of enrolled patients, are significantly reduced. Potential disadvantages surround the issue of whether the antigens expressed by the selected cell line are shared between a sufficient proportion of the treated patient population; the success of a single-antigen vaccine somewhat reduces these concerns [75].

In comparison to other allogeneic cell-based vaccines, HSP constructs provide several distinct advantages. First, no other allogeneic cell-based approach in clinical testing facilitates the delivery of antigens specifically to APCs or to the antigen cross-presentation pathway. In all other cases, stimulation of adaptive immunity first requires destruction of the injected cells by an anti-allogeneic immune response.

Killed vaccine cell fragments are then able to be phagocytozed by nearby macrophages, whereupon tumor antigens may be re-presented by those macrophages. In general, this is an antigen presentation pathway that is far more efficient for antigen presentation by MHC II than MHC I and therefore leads to the more potent activation of CD4+ T cells than CD8+ T cells. In addition, because antigens are not delivered to APCs specifically by an HSP, this pathway lacks the efficiency to stimulate CD8+ T cell responses at femto-molar concentrations of antigen as is the case with gp96 and other HSPs. Thus, success of a non-HSP-dependent allogeneic vaccine is predicted to increase the chances that an HSP-dependent approach will also succeed in the clinic.

4 Recombinant and Nucleic Acid-Based HSP Vaccines

The natural immunogenicity of HSP enables the design of recombinant proteins and subsequent loading of those recombinant HSP with antigens of interest. This approach alleviates the feasibility challenges associated with purification of autologous HSP preparations but inherits the efficacy challenges associated with selecting appropriate shared ASA to target. One approach to minimize the ASA-associated shortcoming of this approach is to target cancers with a known viral etiology and where viral antigens may form the foundation of the antitumor immune response. This combination has been examined clinically using a recombinant bacterial Hsp65 (from *M. bovis*) fused to the E7 protein of human papilloma virus 16 [88].

In the phase II clinical trial, a total of 58 women with cervical intraepithelial neoplasia III (CIN III) were treated with a series of three monthly vaccinations of Hsp65–E7 protein and subsequently monitored by colposcopy. A large proportion of patients enrolled in the trial experienced either a complete or a partial pathologic response to treatment (77.5 %); however, this association was not significantly associated with a history of HPV 16 infection. Because the antigenic nature of the vaccine is predicted to stimulate immunity to HPV 16 E7 antigen, it remains unclear how immunity would develop in patients without HPV 16 infection and in the absence of an appropriate control group no definitive determinations could be made. Nonetheless, this approach was extremely well tolerated and warrants additional testing in an appropriately controlled clinical setting to determine efficacy [88].

Yet another approach to utilize HSP to stimulate antitumor immunity involves the in vivo injection of recombinant DNA molecules encoding a particular HSP of interest. This strategy has been tested in a phase I clinical trial for 21 patients with advanced head and neck squamous cell carcinoma (HNSCC) in Brazil. Escalating doses of recombinant DNA hsp65 (*M. bovis*) were injected intratumorally to an accessible lesion every 3 weeks for a total of three injections [89]. This phase I study demonstrated that the approach was generally safe but associated with significant pain and edema in a number of patients. It was not possible to determine efficacy in this small, uncontrolled, study, and there was no association found between patient immune response to the hsp65 protein and overall survival [90].

A related strategy to direct intratumoral injection of HSP DNA sequences is to encode particular HSP within viral vectors and attempt to infect tumor cells in vivo with these HSP-expressing virus particles. This has been examined in a phase I clinical trial where a modified group C type 2 adenovirus was genetically engineered to express HSP70 and repeatedly injected in a dose escalation study to 27 patients with multiple advanced-stage solid tumors [91]. All evaluable patients developed an antibody response to the virus; however, no clear evidence of a cellular immune response was found. As in previous trials, anecdotal evidence of tumor response was observed in a minority of patients treated at the highest dose, but it remains unclear whether these responses were associated with the vaccine administration. The vaccine was safe in most patients, with a large number of patients developing fever and a single patient experiencing grade IV thrombocytopenia following treatment at the highest dose level.

5 Conclusions Based on Clinical Evidence

The initial rise in optimism surrounding the use of heat-shock proteins in cancer vaccines resulted from elegant preclinical studies demonstrating that heat-shock proteins are dual-purpose adjuvants that both chaperone the full antigenic repertoire of tumor cells to the cross-presentation pathway via scavenger receptors and simultaneously provide a maturation signal to the receiving APCs via TLR-2 and -4. The subsequent identification of antigen cross-presentation as a critical process for tumor immunosurveillance provided further support for the scientific validity of this approach [26]. This information, combined with an increased understanding of the molecular participants in "sterile" inflammation, helped to clarify that the name "heat-shock proteins" did not appropriately convey the true role of HSP as DAMPs, which in addition to functioning as protein chaperones provide a critical and potentially non-redundant linkage between sterile inflammation and adaptive immunity. Knowledge that this association is mostly maladaptive and contributes to diseases including atherosclerosis, type 1 diabetes, and Alzheimer's raised the tantalizing possibility that either the linkage between HSP and adaptive immunity was accidental or this association evolved specifically as an immune defense against cellular transformation. Alas, the clinical evidence has clearly demonstrated that the initial wave of optimism was premature.

Incredible effort, expense, and faith on the part of scientists, drug developers, investors, oncologists, and patients have been expended on the development of HSP-based cancer vaccination. Large phase III trial failures in melanoma and renal cell carcinoma may have dampened support for what appeared to be promising early studies in colorectal carcinoma and have no doubt raised the level of skepticism that this approach will eventually lead to an FDA-approved cancer vaccine. Nonetheless, the sporadic and dramatic clinical responses observed in a minority of the patients treated on these trials preserve the belief that HSP-based vaccines will eventually stake their claim as important weapons in a growing immunotherapeutic toolbox available to oncologists in the near future.

These clinical trial results also provide important lessons for how future HSP-based vaccine trials should be designed. In the two largest phase III clinical trials to date, post hoc analysis clearly demonstrated that the dose and duration of vaccination had an important bearing on the clinical response observed in patients and that this clinical response was most apparent in patients with earlier stage disease. Second, the overall absence of placebo-controlled patient groups in phase II clinical trials has likely hampered the clinical success of HSP vaccines. Despite a large number of phase II clinical trials in large number of patients, effectively none of this data provided evidence of an efficacy signal because control groups were not included. This, coupled with the repeated shift in the target patient population between each stage in clinical trials, limited the ability of clinical trial personnel to appropriately select prospective clinical trial endpoints or appropriate patient populations. If controlled phase II studies had been performed in melanoma or renal cell carcinoma they may have enabled phase III designs to determine overall survival in stage M1a/b melanoma patients for whom at least ten doses of vaccine were available or to determine recurrence-free survival in AJCC stage I+II renal cell carcinoma patients. Either of these trials may have led to an FDA-approved HSP-based cancer vaccine and indicate potential strategies for success in future studies.

Ongoing trials may lead to the eventual approval of such a vaccine in the future. The recent approvals of Provenge for treatment of patients with advanced prostate cancer and ipilimumab for patients with advanced melanoma (and potentially with PD-1/PD-L1 blockade in the near future) have renewed enthusiasm in the immunotherapy of cancer [32, 37]. These successes buttress the groundswell of support from the basic scientific community that the immune system plays a dominant role as a cell-extrinsic defense system against cancer [67, 92]. The approval of a single-antigen vaccine also significantly increases the possibility that clinical efficacy of HSP vaccines will not be strictly limited to autologous approaches. If this is indeed the case, then allogeneic, recombinant protein or DNA-based approaches may eventually provide significant advantages in terms of manufacturing cost and scalability given the apparent importance of prolonged treatment for the induction of an effective antitumor immune response. The potential advantages of HSP-based vaccines from a mechanistic perspective provide a compelling rationale for further exploration of the approach. The link between heat-shock proteins and the adaptive immune system may have specifically evolved to provide immunosurveillance against cancer, and through that evolutionary process naturally developed all the core attributes we now understand to be critical for antitumor immunity: poly-antigen specificity, adjuvanticity at physiologic antigen concentrations, and specific stimulation of CD8+ T cell immunity by cross-priming.

References

1. Medzhitov R, Preston-Hurlburt P, Janeway Jr CA. A human homologue of the Drosophila Toll protein signals activation of adaptive immunity. Nature. 1997;388:394–7.
2. Lemaitre B, Nicolas E, Michaut L, Reichhart JM, Hoffmann JA. The dorsoventral regulatory gene cassette spatzle/Toll/cactus controls the potent antifungal response in Drosophila adults. Cell. 1996;86:973–83.
3. Akira S, Uematsu S, Takeuchi O. Pathogen recognition and innate immunity. Cell. 2006;124: 783–801.
4. Beutler B, Jiang Z, Georgel P, Crozat K, Croker B, Rutschmann S, Du X, Hoebe K. Genetic analysis of host resistance: Toll-like receptor signaling and immunity at large. Annu Rev Immunol. 2006;24:353–89.
5. Takeda K, Kaisho T, Akira S. Toll-like receptors. Annu Rev Immunol. 2003;21:335–76.
6. Akira S, Takeda K, Kaisho T. Toll-like receptors: critical proteins linking innate and acquired immunity. Nat Immunol. 2001;2:675–80.
7. Banchereau J, Steinman RM. Dendritic cells and the control of immunity. Nature. 1998;392: 245–52.
8. Reis e Sousa C. Dendritic cells as sensors of infection. Immunity. 2001;14:495–8.
9. Matis LA. The molecular basis of T-cell specificity. Annu Rev Immunol. 1990;8:65–82.
10. McDevitt HO. Discovering the role of the major histocompatibility complex in the immune response. Annu Rev Immunol. 2000;18:1–17.
11. Zinkernagel RM, Pircher HP, Ohashi P, Oehen S, Odermatt B, Mak T, Arnheiter H, Burki K, Hengartner H. T and B cell tolerance and responses to viral antigens in transgenic mice: implications for the pathogenesis of autoimmune versus immunopathological disease. Immunol Rev. 1991;122:133–71.
12. Schreiber RD, Old LJ, Smyth MJ. Cancer immunoediting: integrating immunity's roles in cancer suppression and promotion. Science. 2011;331:1565–70.
13. Smyth MJ, Dunn GP, Schreiber RD. Cancer immunosurveillance and immunoediting: the roles of immunity in suppressing tumor development and shaping tumor immunogenicity. Adv Immunol. 2006;90:1–50.
14. Quintana FJ, Cohen IR. Heat shock proteins as endogenous adjuvants in sterile and septic inflammation. J Immunol. 2005;175:2777–82.
15. Rock KL, Latz E, Ontiveros F, Kono H. The sterile inflammatory response. Annu Rev Immunol. 2010;28:321–42.
16. Chen GY, Nunez G. Sterile inflammation: sensing and reacting to damage. Nat Rev Immunol. 2010;10:826–37.
17. Zitvogel L, Kepp O, Galluzzi L, Kroemer G. Inflammasomes in carcinogenesis and anticancer immune responses. Nat Immunol. 2012;13:343–51.
18. Henao-Mejia J, Elinav E, Strowig T, Flavell RA. Inflammasomes: far beyond inflammation. Nat Immunol. 2012;13:321–4.
19. McDonald B, Pittman K, Menezes GB, Hirota SA, Slaba I, Waterhouse CC, Beck PL, Muruve DA, Kubes P. Intravascular danger signals guide neutrophils to sites of sterile inflammation. Science. 2010;330:362–6.
20. Apetoh L, Ghiringhelli F, Tesniere A, Obeid M, Ortiz C, Criollo A, Mignot G, Maiuri MC, Ullrich E, Saulnier P, Yang H, Amigorena S, Ryffel B, Barrat FJ, Saftig P, Levi F, Lidereau R, Nogues C, Mira JP, Chompret A, Joulin V, Clavel-Chapelon F, Bourhis J, Andre F, Delaloge S, Tursz T, Kroemer G, Zitvogel L. Toll-like receptor 4-dependent contribution of the immune system to anticancer chemotherapy and radiotherapy. Nat Med. 2007;13:1050–9.
21. Belz GT, Vremec D, Febbraio M, Corcoran L, Shortman K, Carbone FR, Heath WR. CD36 is differentially expressed by CD8+ splenic dendritic cells but is not required for cross-presentation in vivo. J Immunol. 2002;168:6066–70.

22. Sancho D, Joffre OP, Keller AM, Rogers NC, Martinez D, Hernanz-Falcon P, Rosewell I, Reis e Sousa C. Identification of a dendritic cell receptor that couples sensing of necrosis to immunity. Nature. 2009;458:899–903.
23. Binder RJ, Srivastava PK. Peptides chaperoned by heat-shock proteins are a necessary and sufficient source of antigen in the cross-priming of CD8+ T cells. Nat Immunol. 2005;6:593–9.
24. Suto R, Srivastava PK. A mechanism for the specific immunogenicity of heat shock protein-chaperoned peptides. Science. 1995;269:1585–8.
25. Binder RJ, Han DK, Srivastava PK. CD91: a receptor for heat shock protein gp96. Nat Immunol. 2000;1:151–5.
26. Hildner K, Edelson BT, Purtha WE, Diamond M, Matsushita H, Kohyama M, Calderon B, Schraml BU, Unanue ER, Diamond MS, Schreiber RD, Murphy TL, Murphy KM. Batf3 deficiency reveals a critical role for CD8alpha+dendritic cells in cytotoxic T cell immunity. Science. 2008;322:1097–100.
27. Sancho D, Mourao-Sa D, Joffre OP, Schulz O, Rogers NC, Pennington DJ, Carlyle JR, Reis e Sousa C. Tumor therapy in mice via antigen targeting to a novel, DC-restricted C-type lectin. J Clin Invest. 2008;118:2098–110.
28. Zhang JG, Czabotar PE, Policheni AN, Caminschi I, San Wan S, Kitsoulis S, Tullett KM, Robin AY, Brammananth R, van Delft MF, Lu J, O'Reilly LA, Josefsson EC, Kile BT, Chin WJ, Mintern JD, Olshina MA, Wong W, Baum J, Wright MD, Huang DC, Mohandas N, Coppel RL, Colman PM, Nicola NA, Shortman K, Lahoud MH. The dendritic cell receptor Clec9A binds damaged cells via exposed actin filaments. Immunity. 2012;36:646–57.
29. Ahrens S, Zelenay S, Sancho D, Hanc P, Kjaer S, Feest C, Fletcher G, Durkin C, Postigo A, Skehel M, Batista F, Thompson B, Way M, Reis ESC, Schulz O. F-actin is an evolutionarily conserved damage-associated molecular pattern recognized by DNGR-1, a receptor for dead cells. Immunity. 2012;36:635–45.
30. Basu S, Binder RJ, Ramalingam T, Srivastava PK. CD91 is a common receptor for heat shock proteins gp96, hsp90, hsp70, and calreticulin. Immunity. 2001;14:303–13.
31. Srivastava P. Interaction of heat shock proteins with peptides and antigen presenting cells: chaperoning of the innate and adaptive immune responses. Annu Rev Immunol. 2002;20: 395–425.
32. Anderson MS, Venanzi ES, Klein L, Chen Z, Berzins SP, Turley SJ, von Boehmer H, Bronson R, Dierich A, Benoist C, Mathis D. Projection of an immunological self shadow within the thymus by the aire protein. Science. 2002;298:1395–401.
33. Beutler B. Neo-ligands for innate immune receptors and the etiology of sterile inflammatory disease. Immunol Rev. 2007;220:113–28.
34. Fuertes MB, Kacha AK, Kline J, Woo SR, Kranz DM, Murphy KM, Gajewski TF. Host type I IFN signals are required for antitumor CD8+ T cell responses through CD8{alpha}+dendritic cells. J Exp Med. 2011;208:2005–16.
35. Lindquist S, Craig EA. The heat-shock proteins. Annu Rev Genet. 1988;22:631–77.
36. Gething MJ, Sambrook J. Protein folding in the cell. Nature. 1992;355:33–45.
37. Parsell DA, Lindquist S. The function of heat-shock proteins in stress tolerance: degradation and reactivation of damaged proteins. Annu Rev Genet. 1993;27:437–96.
38. Ritossa F. Discovery of the heat shock response. Cell Stress Chaperones. 1996;1:97–8.
39. Blachere NE, Li Z, Chandawarkar RY, Suto R, Jaikaria NS, Basu S, Udono H, Srivastava PK. Heat shock protein-peptide complexes, reconstituted in vitro, elicit peptide-specific cytotoxic T lymphocyte response and tumor immunity. J Exp Med. 1997;186:1315–22.
40. Basu S, Srivastava PK. Heat shock proteins: the fountainhead of innate and adaptive immune responses. Cell Stress Chaperones. 2000;5:443–51.
41. Oizumi S, Strbo N, Pahwa S, Deyev V, Podack ER. Molecular and cellular requirements for enhanced antigen cross-presentation to CD8 cytotoxic T lymphocytes. J Immunol. 2007;179: 2310–7.
42. Srivastava PK, DeLeo AB, Old LJ. Tumor rejection antigens of chemically induced sarcomas of inbred mice. Proc Natl Acad Sci U S A. 1986;83:3407–11.

43. Ishii T, Udono H, Yamano T, Ohta H, Uenaka A, Ono T, Hizuta A, Tanaka N, Srivastava PK, Nakayama E. Isolation of MHC class I-restricted tumor antigen peptide and its precursors associated with heat shock proteins hsp70, hsp90, and gp96. J Immunol. 1999;162:1303–9.
44. Tamura Y, Peng P, Liu K, Daou M, Srivastava PK. Immunotherapy of tumors with autologous tumor-derived heat shock protein preparations. Science. 1997;278:117–20.
45. Janetzki S, Palla D, Rosenhauer V, Lochs H, Lewis JJ, Srivastava PK. Immunization of cancer patients with autologous cancer-derived heat shock protein gp96 preparations: a pilot study. Int J Cancer. 2000;88:232–8.
46. Belli F, Testori A, Rivoltini L, Maio M, Andreola G, Sertoli MR, Gallino G, Piris A, Cattelan A, Lazzari I, Carrabba M, Scita G, Santantonio C, Pilla L, Tragni G, Lombardo C, Arienti F, Marchiano A, Queirolo P, Bertolini F, Cova A, Lamaj E, Ascani L, Camerini R, Corsi M, Cascinelli N, Lewis JJ, Srivastava P, Parmiani G. Vaccination of metastatic melanoma patients with autologous tumor-derived heat shock protein gp96-peptide complexes: clinical and immunologic findings. J Clin Oncol. 2002;20:4169–80.
47. Rivoltini L, Castelli C, Carrabba M, Mazzaferro V, Pilla L, Huber V, Coppa J, Gallino G, Scheibenbogen C, Squarcina P, Cova A, Camerini R, Lewis JJ, Srivastava PK, Parmiani G. Human tumor-derived heat shock protein 96 mediates in vitro activation and in vivo expansion of melanoma- and colon carcinoma-specific T cells. J Immunol. 2003;171:3467–74.
48. Hodi FS, Butler M, Oble DA, Seiden MV, Haluska FG, Kruse A, Macrae S, Nelson M, Canning C, Lowy I, Korman A, Lautz D, Russell S, Jaklitsch MT, Ramaiya N, Chen TC, Neuberg D, Allison JP, Mihm MC, Dranoff G. Immunologic and clinical effects of antibody blockade of cytotoxic T lymphocyte-associated antigen 4 in previously vaccinated cancer patients. Proc Natl Acad Sci U S A. 2008;105:3005–10.
49. Hodi FS, O'Day SJ, McDermott DF, Weber RW, Sosman JA, Haanen JB, Gonzalez R, Robert C, Schadendorf D, Hassel JC, Akerley W, van den Eertwegh AJ, Lutzky J, Lorigan P, Vaubel JM, Linette GP, Hogg D, Ottensmeier CH, Lebbe C, Peschel C, Quirt I, Clark JI, Wolchok JD, Weber JS, Tian J, Yellin MJ, Nichol GM, Hoos A, Urba WJ. Improved survival with ipilimumab in patients with metastatic melanoma. New Engl J Med. 2010;363:711–23.
50. Eton O, Ross MI, East MJ, Mansfield PF, Papadopoulos N, Ellerhorst JA, Bedikian AY, Lee JE. Autologous tumor-derived heat-shock protein peptide complex-96 (HSPPC-96) in patients with metastatic melanoma. J Transl Med. 2010;8:9.
51. Pilla L, Patuzzo R, Rivoltini L, Maio M, Pennacchioli E, Lamaj E, Maurichi A, Massarut S, Marchiano A, Santantonio C, Tosi D, Arienti F, Cova A, Sovena G, Piris A, Nonaka D, Bersani I, Di Florio A, Luigi M, Srivastava PK, Hoos A, Santinami M, Parmiani G. A phase II trial of vaccination with autologous, tumor-derived heat-shock protein peptide complexes Gp96, in combination with GM-CSF and interferon-alpha in metastatic melanoma patients. Cancer Immunol Immunother. 2006;55:958–68.
52. Testori A, Richards J, Whitman E, Mann GB, Lutzky J, Camacho L, Parmiani G, Tosti G, Kirkwood JM, Hoos A, Yuh L, Gupta R, Srivastava PK, C. S. Group. Phase III comparison of vitespen, an autologous tumor-derived heat shock protein gp96 peptide complex vaccine, with physician's choice of treatment for stage IV melanoma: the C-100-21 Study Group. J Clin Oncol. 2008;26:955–62.
53. Yedavelli SP, Guo L, Daou ME, Srivastava PK, Mittelman A, Tiwari RK. Preventive and therapeutic effect of tumor derived heat shock protein, gp96, in an experimental prostate cancer model. Int J Mol Med. 1999;4:243–8.
54. Jonasch E, Wood C, Tamboli P, Pagliaro LC, Tu SM, Kim J, Srivastava P, Perez C, Isakov L, Tannir N. Vaccination of metastatic renal cell carcinoma patients with autologous tumour-derived vitespen vaccine: clinical findings. Br J Cancer. 2008;98:1336–41.
55. Wood C, Srivastava P, Bukowski R, Lacombe L, Gorelov AI, Gorelov S, Mulders P, Zielinski H, Hoos A, Teofilovici F, Isakov L, Flanigan R, Figlin R, Gupta R, Escudier B, C. R. S. Group. An adjuvant autologous therapeutic vaccine (HSPPC-96; vitespen) versus observation alone for patients at high risk of recurrence after nephrectomy for renal cell carcinoma: a multicentre, open-label, randomised phase III trial. Lancet. 2008;372:145–54.

56. Mazzaferro V, Coppa J, Carrabba MG, Rivoltini L, Schiavo M, Regalia E, Mariani L, Camerini T, Marchiano A, Andreola S, Camerini R, Corsi M, Lewis JJ, Srivastava PK, Parmiani G. Vaccination with autologous tumor-derived heat-shock protein gp96 after liver resection for metastatic colorectal cancer. Clin Cancer Res. 2003;9:3235–45.
57. Younes A. A phase II study of heat shock protein-peptide complex-96 vaccine therapy in patients with indolent non-Hodgkin's lymphoma. Clin Lymphoma. 2003;4:183–5.
58. Oki Y, McLaughlin P, Fayad LE, Pro B, Mansfield PF, Clayman GL, Medeiros LJ, Kwak LW, Srivastava PK, Younes A. Experience with heat shock protein-peptide complex 96 vaccine therapy in patients with indolent non-Hodgkin lymphoma. Cancer. 2007;109:77–83.
59. Maki RG, Livingston PO, Lewis JJ, Janetzki S, Klimstra D, Desantis D, Srivastava PK, Brennan MF. A phase I pilot study of autologous heat shock protein vaccine HSPPC-96 in patients with resected pancreatic adenocarcinoma. Dig Dis Sci. 2007;52:1964–72.
60. Schreiber TH, Raez L, Rosenblatt JD, Podack ER. Tumor immunogenicity and responsiveness to cancer vaccine therapy: the state of the art. Semin Immunol. 2010;22:105–12.
61. Ascierto PA, Grimaldi AM, Curti B, Faries MB, Ferrone S, Flaherty K, Fox BA, Gajewski TF, Gershenwald JE, Gogas H, Grossmann K, Hauschild A, Hodi FS, Kefford R, Kirkwood JM, Leachmann S, Maio M, Marais R, Palmieri G, Morton DL, Ribas A, Stroncek DF, Stewart R, Wang E, Mozzillo N, Marincola FM. Future perspectives in melanoma research. Meeting report from the"Melanoma research: a bridge from Naples to the World. Napoli, December 5th–6th2011". J Transl Med. 2012;10:83.
62. Parsons DW, Li M, Zhang X, Jones S, Leary RJ, Lin JC, Boca SM, Carter H, Samayoa J, Bettegowda C, Gallia GL, Jallo GI, Binder ZA, Nikolsky Y, Hartigan J, Smith DR, Gerhard DS, Fults DW, VandenBerg S, Berger MS, Marie SK, Shinjo SM, Clara C, Phillips PC, Minturn JE, Biegel JA, Judkins AR, Resnick AC, Storm PB, Curran T, He Y, Rasheed BA, Friedman HS, Keir ST, McLendon R, Northcott PA, Taylor MD, Burger PC, Riggins GJ, Karchin R, Parmigiani G, Bigner DD, Yan H, Papadopoulos N, Vogelstein B, Kinzler KW, Velculescu VE. The genetic landscape of the childhood cancer medulloblastoma. Science. 2011;331:435–9.
63. Jones S, Zhang X, Parsons DW, Lin JC, Leary RJ, Angenendt P, Mankoo P, Carter H, Kamiyama H, Jimeno A, Hong SM, Fu B, Lin MT, Calhoun ES, Kamiyama M, Walter K, Nikolskaya T, Nikolsky Y, Hartigan J, Smith DR, Hidalgo M, Leach SD, Klein AP, Jaffee EM, Goggins M, Maitra A, Iacobuzio-Donahue C, Eshleman JR, Kern SE, Hruban RH, Karchin R, Papadopoulos N, Parmigiani G, Vogelstein B, Velculescu VE, Kinzler KW. Core signaling pathways in human pancreatic cancers revealed by global genomic analyses. Science. 2008;321:1801–6.
64. Parsons DW, Jones S, Zhang X, Lin JC, Leary RJ, Angenendt P, Mankoo P, Carter H, Siu IM, Gallia GL, Olivi A, McLendon R, Rasheed BA, Keir S, Nikolskaya T, Nikolsky Y, Busam DA, Tekleab H, Diaz Jr LA, Hartigan J, Smith DR, Strausberg RL, Marie SK, Shinjo SM, Yan H, Riggins GJ, Bigner DD, Karchin R, Papadopoulos N, Parmigiani G, Vogelstein B, Velculescu VE, Kinzler KW. An integrated genomic analysis of human glioblastoma multiforme. Science. 2008;321:1807–12.
65. Segal NH, Parsons DW, Peggs KS, Velculescu V, Kinzler KW, Vogelstein B, Allison JP. Epitope landscape in breast and colorectal cancer. Cancer Res. 2008;68:889–92.
66. Wood LD, Parsons DW, Jones S, Lin J, Sjoblom T, Leary RJ, Shen D, Boca SM, Barber T, Ptak J, Silliman N, Szabo S, Dezso Z, Ustyanksky V, Nikolskaya T, Nikolsky Y, Karchin R, Wilson PA, Kaminker JS, Zhang Z, Croshaw R, Willis J, Dawson D, Shipitsin M, Willson JK, Sukumar S, Polyak K, Park BH, Pethiyagoda CL, Pant PV, Ballinger DG, Sparks AB, Hartigan J, Smith DR, Suh E, Papadopoulos N, Buckhaults P, Markowitz SD, Parmigiani G, Kinzler KW, Velculescu VE, Vogelstein B. The genomic landscapes of human breast and colorectal cancers. Science. 2007;318:1108–13.
67. Stransky N, Egloff AM, Tward AD, Kostic AD, Cibulskis K, Sivachenko A, Kryukov GV, Lawrence MS, Sougnez C, McKenna A, Shefler E, Ramos AH, Stojanov P, Carter SL, Voet D, Cortes ML, Auclair D, Berger MF, Saksena G, Guiducci C, Onofrio RC, Parkin M, Romkes M, Weissfeld JL, Seethala RR, Wang L, Rangel-Escareno C, Fernandez-Lopez JC, Hidalgo-Miranda A, Melendez-Zajgla J, Winckler W, Ardlie K, Gabriel SB, Meyerson M, Lander ES,

Getz G, Golub TR, Garraway LA, Grandis JR. The mutational landscape of head and neck squamous cell carcinoma. Science. 2011;333:1157–60.

68. Chapman MA, Lawrence MS, Keats JJ, Cibulskis K, Sougnez C, Schinzel AC, Harview CL, Brunet JP, Ahmann GJ, Adli M, Anderson KC, Ardlie KG, Auclair D, Baker A, Bergsagel PL, Bernstein BE, Drier Y, Fonseca R, Gabriel SB, Hofmeister CC, Jagannath S, Jakubowiak AJ, Krishnan A, Levy J, Liefeld T, Lonial S, Mahan S, Mfuko B, Monti S, Perkins LM, Onofrio R, Pugh TJ, Rajkumar SV, Ramos AH, Siegel DS, Sivachenko A, Stewart AK, Trudel S, Vij R, Voet D, Winckler W, Zimmerman T, Carpten J, Trent J, Hahn WC, Garraway LA, Meyerson M, Lander ES, Getz G, Golub TR. Initial genome sequencing and analysis of multiple myeloma. Nature. 2011;471:467–72.
69. Ding L, Getz G, Wheeler DA, Mardis ER, McLellan MD, Cibulskis K, Sougnez C, Greulich H, Muzny DM, Morgan MB, Fulton L, Fulton RS, Zhang Q, Wendl MC, Lawrence MS, Larson DE, Chen K, Dooling DJ, Sabo A, Hawes AC, Shen H, Jhangiani SN, Lewis LR, Hall O, Zhu Y, Mathew T, Ren Y, Yao J, Scherer SE, Clerc K, Metcalf GA, Ng B, Milosavljevic A, Gonzalez-Garay ML, Osborne JR, Meyer R, Shi X, Tang Y, Koboldt DC, Lin L, Abbott R, Miner TL, Pohl C, Fewell G, Haipek C, Schmidt H, Dunford-Shore BH, Kraja A, Crosby SD, Sawyer CS, Vickery T, Sander S, Robinson J, Winckler W, Baldwin J, Chirieac LR, Dutt A, Fennell T, Hanna M, Johnson BE, Onofrio RC, Thomas RK, Tonon G, Weir BA, Zhao X, Ziaugra L, Zody MC, Giordano T, Orringer MB, Roth JA, Spitz MR, Wistuba II B, Ozenberger PJ, Good AC, Chang DG, Beer MA, Watson M, Ladanyi S, Broderick A, Yoshizawa WD, Travis W, Pao MA, Province GM, Weinstock HE, Varmus SB, Gabriel ES, Lander RA, Gibbs MM, Wilson RK. Somatic mutations affect key pathways in lung adenocarcinoma. Nature. 2008;455:1069–75.
70. Cancer Genome Atlas Research N. Comprehensive genomic characterization defines human glioblastoma genes and core pathways. Nature. 2008;455:1061–8.
71. Beroukhim R, Mermel CH, Porter D, Wei G, Raychaudhuri S, Donovan J, Barretina J, Boehm JS, Dobson J, Urashima M, Mc Henry KT, Pinchback RM, Ligon AH, Cho YJ, Haery L, Greulich H, Reich M, Winckler W, Lawrence MS, Weir BA, Tanaka KE, Chiang DY, Bass AJ, Loo A, Hoffman C, Prensner J, Liefeld T, Gao Q, Yecies D, Signoretti S, Maher E, Kaye FJ, Sasaki H, Tepper JE, Fletcher JA, Tabernero J, Baselga J, Tsao MS, Demichelis F, Rubin MA, Janne PA, Daly MJ, Nucera C, Levine RL, Ebert BL, Gabriel S, Rustgi AK, Antonescu CR, Ladanyi M, Letai A, Garraway LA, Loda M, Beer DG, True LD, Okamoto A, Pomeroy SL, Singer S, Golub TR, Lander ES, Getz G, Sellers WR, Meyerson M. The landscape of somatic copy-number alteration across human cancers. Nature. 2010;463:899–905.
72. Van Der Bruggen P, Zhang Y, Chaux P, Stroobant V, Panichelli C, Schultz ES, Chapiro J, Van Den Eynde BJ, Brasseur F, Boon T. Tumor-specific shared antigenic peptides recognized by human T cells. Immunol Rev. 2002;188:51–64.
73. Van den Eynde BJ, van der Bruggen P. T cell defined tumor antigens. Curr Opin Immunol. 1997;9:684–93.
74. Simpson AJ, Caballero OL, Jungbluth A, Chen YT, Old LJ. Cancer/testis antigens, gametogenesis and cancer. Nat Rev Cancer. 2005;5:615–25.
75. Kantoff PW, Higano CS, Shore ND, Berger ER, Small EJ, Penson DF, Redfern CH, Ferrari AC, Dreicer R, Sims RB, Xu Y, Frohlich MW, Schellhammer PF, Investigators IS. Sipuleucel-T immunotherapy for castration-resistant prostate cancer. New Engl J Med. 2010;363:411–22.
76. Qian J, Hong S, Wang S, Zhang L, Sun L, Wang M, Yang J, Kwak LW, Hou J, Yi Q. Myeloma cell line-derived, pooled heat shock proteins as a universal vaccine for immunotherapy of multiple myeloma. Blood. 2009;114:3880–9.
77. Podack ER, Raez LE. Allogeneic tumor-cell-based vaccines secreting endoplasmic reticulum chaperone gp96. Expet Opin Biol Ther. 2007;7:1679–88.
78. Yamazaki K, Nguyen T, Podack ER. Cutting edge: tumor secreted heat shock-fusion protein elicits CD8 cells for rejection. J Immunol. 1999;163:5178–82.
79. Strbo N, Oizumi S, Sotosek-Tokmadzic V, Podack ER. Perforin is required for innate and adaptive immunity induced by heat shock protein gp96. Immunity. 2003;18:381–90.

80. Oizumi S, Deyev V, Yamazaki K, Schreiber T, Strbo N, Rosenblatt J, Podack ER. Surmounting tumor-induced immune suppression by frequent vaccination or immunization in the absence of B cells. J Immunother. 2008;31:394–401.
81. Schreiber TH, Deyev VV, Rosenblatt JD, Podack ER. Tumor-induced suppression of CTL expansion and subjugation by gp96-Ig vaccination. Cancer Res. 2009;69:2026–33.
82. Strbo N, Pahwa S, Kolber MA, Gonzalez L, Fisher E, Podack ER. Cell-secreted Gp96-Ig-peptide complexes induce lamina propria and intraepithelial CD8+ cytotoxic T lymphocytes in the intestinal mucosa. Mucosal Immunol. 2010;3:182–92.
83. Strbo N, Vaccari M, Pahwa S, Kolber MA, Fisher E, Gonzalez L, Doster MN, Hryniewicz A, Felber BK, Pavlakis GN, Franchini G, Podack ER. Gp96 SIV Ig immunization induces potent polyepitope specific, multifunctional memory responses in rectal and vaginal mucosa. Vaccine. 2011;29:2619–25.
84. Raez LE, Rosenblatt JD, Podack ER. Present and future of lung cancer vaccines. Expet Opin Emerg Drug. 2006;11:445–59.
85. Peled N, Oton AB, Hirsch FR, Bunn P. MAGE A3 antigen-specific cancer immunotherapeutic. Immunotherapy. 2009;1:19–25.
86. Lethe B, Lucas S, Michaux L, De Smet C, Godelaine D, Serrano A, De Plaen E, Boon T. LAGE-1, a new gene with tumor specificity. Int J Cancer. 1998;76:903–8.
87. Nakagawa K, Noguchi Y, Uenaka A, Sato S, Okumura H, Tanaka M, Shimono M, Ali Eldib AM, Ono T, Ohara N, Yoshino T, Yamashita K, Tsunoda T, Aoe M, Shimizu N, Nakayama E. XAGE-1 expression in non-small cell lung cancer and antibody response in patients. Clin Cancer Res. 2005;11:5496–503.
88. Einstein MH, Kadish AS, Burk RD, Kim MY, Wadler S, Streicher H, Goldberg GL, Runowicz CD. Heat shock fusion protein-based immunotherapy for treatment of cervical intraepithelial neoplasia III. Gynecol Oncol. 2007;106:453–60.
89. Michaluart P, Abdallah KA, Lima FD, Smith R, Moyses RA, Coelho V, Victora GD, Socorro-Silva A, Volsi EC, Zarate-Blades CR, Ferraz AR, Barreto AK, Chammas MC, Gomes R, Gebrim E, Arakawa-Sugueno L, Fernandes KP, Lotufo PA, Cardoso MR, Kalil J, Silva CL. Phase I trial of DNA-hsp65 immunotherapy for advanced squamous cell carcinoma of the head and neck. Cancer Gene Ther. 2008;15:676–84.
90. Victora GD, Socorro-Silva A, Volsi EC, Abdallah K, Lima FD, Smith RB, Moyses RA, Zarate-Blades CR, Michaluart P, Silva CL, Kalil J, Coelho V. Immune response to vaccination with DNA-Hsp65 in a phase I clinical trial with head and neck cancer patients. Cancer Gene Ther. 2009;16:598–608.
91. Li JL, Liu HL, Zhang XR, Xu JP, Hu WK, Liang M, Chen SY, Hu F, Chu DT. A phase I trial of intratumoral administration of recombinant oncolytic adenovirus overexpressing HSP70 in advanced solid tumor patients. Gene Ther. 2009;16:376–82.
92. Hanahan D, Weinberg RA. Hallmarks of cancer: the next generation. Cell. 2011;144:646–74.

Activation of NK Cell Responses and Immunotherapy of Cancer

George J. Weiner

Abstract Monoclonal antibodies, including rituximab, are a mainstay in the therapy of cancer; however, there is much we do not understand about their mechanisms of action. In vitro analysis, animal models, and clinical trials suggest signaling, complement, and cellular cytotoxicity, each playing a role. Increasing evidence indicates that these mechanisms of action do not operate in isolation and that there are considerable interactions, some synergistic and some antagonistic, between mechanisms that can impact on the efficacy of therapy. An improved understanding of the relative importance of each mechanism, and how these mechanisms interact in various clinical scenarios, is vital if we are to make a highly valuable approach to cancer therapy even better.

Keywords NK cell • Antibody dependent cellular cytotoxicity • Cancer immunotherapy

1 Background and History of NK Cells

Soon after the first blood smear was placed under a microscope, hematologists described a small but clear population of large granular lymphocytes. Decades later, analysis of the function of these cells demonstrated that they were capable of killing some tumor cells [1], hence their designation as natural killer (NK) cells. With the advent of immunophenotyping, it became clear that NK cells represent a distinct lineage of mononuclear cells. Further studies demonstrated that NK cells are heterogeneous and are able to both mediate cytotoxicity and produce a variety of cytokines [2]. NK cells are often thought of as key components of the innate immune

G.J. Weiner (✉)
Holden Comprehensive Cancer Center and Department of Internal Medicine,
University of Iowa, Iowa City, Iowa
e-mail: george-weiner@uiowa.edu

J.D. Rosenblatt et al. (eds.), *Advances in Tumor Immunology and Immunotherapy*,
Current Cancer Research, DOI 10.1007/978-1-4614-8809-5_4,
© Springer Science+Business Media New York 2014

response because of their immediate and nonspecific effects. However, it is increasingly clear that NK cells demonstrate a high degree of specificity and interact extensively with the adaptive immune response. Thus, they represent a vital link between innate and adaptive immunity [3]. In this chapter, we review how activation of NK activation impacts on cancer and cancer immunotherapy.

Our understanding of NK cell biology is evolving rapidly. This biology has been reviewed extensively elsewhere [4, 5] and is not discussed at length here. However, there are aspects of NK cell biology that impact on NK cell activation, NK cell responses to cancer, and NK-based immunotherapy that are worth summarizing.

In humans, NK cells are broadly defined as CD3–, CD56+ lymphocytes. They are divided into CD56 bright and CD56 dim subsets, which differ in function and homing properties. CD56 bright NK cells have effects predominantly mediated by cytokine production, while CD56 dim NK cells express CD16 and have cytotoxic function [2]. NK cells were initially identified in peripheral blood but are now known to be widespread in both lymphoid and non-lymphoid tissues. Most NK cells in the circulation are CD56 dim and express CD16. These cells express perforin, are cytotoxic, and are effective at mediating antibody-dependent cellular cytotoxicity (ADCC). A minority of cells in the circulation, but a larger percentage of NK cells in the tissues, are of the CD56 bright and CD16-negative subset [6]. This population is less effective at mediating cytotoxicity but is very effective at producing cytokines that play a central role in linking innate and adaptive immunity.

2 NK Cell Activation

Both classes of NK cells express a large number of receptors that recognize ligands capable of inducing both activating and inhibitory responses [7]. Activating NK receptors are capable of detecting cells that are stressed. These responses can be mediated by infectious ligands via toll-like receptors (TLRs) [8–10], self-ligands such as CD40 [11], or signaling mediated by antibody-coated target cells via CD16, also known as FcγRIIIa [12]. Maturation and activation of NK cells are influenced by the microenvironment including the type and concentration of a broad range of cytokines including IFNα and cytokines that serve as ligands for receptors with the common gamma chain including IL2, IL7, IL15, and IL21 [13]. The activation of NK cells is enhanced or significantly modified when multiple signals are present [14, 15].

Uncontrolled activation of NK cells is prevented by inhibitory receptors which mediate their function via intracellular inhibitory signaling domains known as immunoreceptor tyrosine-based inhibition motifs (ITIMs) [16]. Killer immunoglobulin-like receptors (KIRs) recognize groups of HLA-A, HLA-B, and HLA-C alleles. Individuals differ in the number and type of inherited KIR genes. The products of these genes are distributed in the NK cell repertoire. Thus, individual NK cells express only some of the potentially many different KIRs. The negative signal mediated by KIRs is abrogated, and the NK cell can be activated, when KIR signaling is reduced as the NK cell encounters target cells that lack class

I MHC [17, 18]. The complex pattern of KIR expression by NK cells allows them to detect cells that lack specific MHC1 molecules [19, 20]. This mechanism helps the immune system respond to infection that might down-regulate class I MHC as a way to avoid a T cell response. A subset of NK cells does not express inhibitory KIRs. These cells generally express CD94-NKG2A. Like the KIRs, CD94 inhibits nonspecific activation of NK cells. Thus, multiple checkpoints impact on the activation or the inhibition of NK cells [21]. These signaling pathways of NK cells are clearly quite complex, and their effect on NK cell activation varies with respect to the baseline phenotype and activation status of the NK cell [22].

When activated, NK cells capable of mediating cytotoxicity exocytose granules containing perforin and granzyme, which results in death of the target cell. Activated NK cells can also express molecules of the TNF superfamily that engage death receptors on target cells [23]. Cytokine-producing NK cells secrete IFNγ, TNF, GMCSF, and other cytokines that can enhance the inflammatory response and support the development of an adaptive immune response. This is mediated in part by secondary activation of a broad variety of other cell populations including monocytes, dendritic cells, granulocytes, and eventually T cells [3, 24, 25].

In summary, whether or not an NK cell is activated is dependent on the phenotype of the NK cell as well as on cellular and soluble factors in the microenvironment. Factors associated with infection and stress can result in NK cell activation, which depending on the type of NK cell can lead to a direct cytotoxic response or cytokine production that can activate other cell populations. These other cells then can impact on induction of inflammation or support development of an adaptive immune response. Thus, NK cells play a crucial role in the relationship between inflammation and both the innate and adaptive immune response.

3 NK Cells and Cancer

As is the case with infection, multiple receptor–ligand interactions impact on how NK cells respond to malignant cells [26]. Among the most extensively studied is the ability of NK cells to mediate the rejection of tumors that lack class I MHC expression. Combinations of MHC class I and KIR variants influence a broad variety of natural and therapeutic responses including the immune response to malignancy. They appear to play a particularly important role after hematopoietic stem cell transplantation with varying degrees of class I MHC mismatch [27]. NK cells also act as regulatory cells and, through cytokine production, influence the anticancer activity of other lymphocyte populations and cell types including dendritic cells and T cells [14, 28]. NK cells can also influence development of an active immune response by having direct cytotoxicity effects on antigen-presenting cells [29]. Killing of tumor cells by NK cells can lead to cross presentation of antigens, and the cytokines produced by NK cells can enhance DC activation and cross presentation—an effect that is enhanced by the ability of activated NK cells to produce cytokines including IFNγ. NK cells can be activated by IFNα that is produced by plasmacytic DCs, thus creating a positive feedback loop. Thus, the effects of NK cells on direct and indirect killing tumor cells are quite complex.

Much of the above work has been done utilizing murine models. Data demonstrating un-manipulated NK cells' impact on the control of human cancer is intriguing but indirect. Higher absolute lymphocyte counts and NK cell numbers correlate with a positive outcome after a variety of treatments for lymphoid malignancies [30–32]. Clinical data with solid tumors is less clear although there is data demonstrating that human NK cells can recognize and kill a variety of tumor cells in vitro [33, 34].

4 Activated NK Cells as a Cancer Immunotherapy

Studies elucidating the biology of NK cell activation have led to exploration of a number of different strategies for activating NK cells as a way to treat cancer. Type I IFN, including IFNα and β, were the first types of cytokine tested as potential cancer therapies [35]. They are known to have a number of biologic effects, including NK cell activation, that could contribute to their modest but clear clinical antitumor activity. Members of the IL2 family of cytokines including IL2, IL12, IL15, IL18, and IL21 can activate NK cells as well as other immune effector cell populations and have been explored in clinical trials [36, 37]. IL2 therapy has demonstrated impressive clinical responses, albeit in a small minority of carefully selected subjects [38]. This and subsequent studies led to the approval by the FDA of high-dose IL2 in melanoma. Non-biologic agents that broadly activate the immune system can activate NK cells including drugs such as lenalidomide [39]. NK cells are activated by nonspecific immunotherapy, such as the use of BCG for treatment of bladder cancer [40, 41]. We have explored the use of immunostimulatory CpG DNA to enhance NK activity in animal models and the clinic [42, 43]. Each of these therapeutic strategies impacts on both NK cells and other cell types including dendritic cells and T cells. Thus, while preclinical studies point to the importance of NK cells, it is difficult to determine to what extent their ability to activate NK cells impacts on their demonstrated or hypothesized clinical therapeutic efficacy.

Rosenberg and colleagues led studies in the 1980s to expand and activate NK cells ex vivo and reinfuse them with the goal of enhancing their antitumor effects [44]. In the absence of additional immunotherapy, the trafficking to tumor and survival of such lymphokine-activated killer (LAK) cells in vivo were limited. This led early on to the addition of in vivo therapy with cytokines, most commonly IL2, following infusion of the ex vivo-activated cells [45]. The infused cells often had a mixed phenotype [46]; thus, it can be questioned whether this approach would be accurately considered a form of NK cell therapy. Follow-up studies suggested that IL2 therapy alone might be as effective as infusion of activated cells followed by IL2 therapy, raising the question of the value of the cellular infusions [47]. Subsequent trials have explored different cell populations generated by selecting the initial cells before expansion (NK cells, NK T cells, unfractionated mononuclear cells) and using different agents to expand and activate the resulting cells. These cells have been given alternative names such as cytokine-induced killer (CIK) cells that are derived from NKT cells [48]. While some clinical responses have been reported, at this point in time, there is little evidence that in vitro expansion of autologous NK cells and their reinfusion is a valuable clinical strategy for the treatment of cancer.

5 NK Cells and Other Immunotherapeutic Approaches

Indirect evidence suggests that ADCC mediated by NK cells is mechanistically involved in clinical response to therapy with monoclonal antibodies (mAb). Correlative studies demonstrate an association between polymorphisms on CD16 (also known as FcγRIIIa) and clinical response to single-agent anti-CD20 (rituximab). CD16 homozygous for valine at 158 (VV) has a higher affinity for IgG1 than does CD16 with phenylalanine at that position (VF or FF) [49]. Patients with lymphoma and the VV genotype have a better clinical response to rituximab than patients that are VF or FF [50–52]. Within 4 h of clinical therapy with rituximab, NK cells in patients with the high-affinity polymorphism are activated and traffic out of the circulation, while NK cells of patients with the low-affinity polymorphism are not activated and remain in the circulation [53]. This evidence that NK cells are central to the mechanisms of action of rituximab has led to the clinical evaluation of novel strategies for enhancing target cell lysis by NK cells including the addition to mAb of immunostimulatory agents designed to activate NK cells [54, 55] and development of anti-CD20 antibodies with stronger affinity for CD16 [56, 57]. Thus far, none of these strategies has been shown to unequivocally superior to standard antibody therapy alone, but evaluation is ongoing.

Different and creative approaches to enhancing NK cell therapy with mAb are under evaluation. One is to block inhibitory KIR with additional antibodies, thereby taking the brakes off and augmenting tumor cell recognition by the NK cell [58]. Another is to combine antitumor mAb with antibody, such as anti-CD137, that can further activate the NK cells [59]. A strategy that has been pursued for a number of years involves the use of bispecific antibodies to target NK cells to tumors in a way that can bypass the usual receptors. Such bispecific antibodies bind with one arm to NK cells such as through CD16 and with tumor cells with the other arm. Such bispecific antibodies are potent in vitro, but their clinical utility remains uncertain [60].

Allogeneic NK cells have also been viewed as a potential effector cell population in mediating the graft vs. leukemia response following stem cell transplantation. When transplantation takes place across HLA class I barriers, it can trigger alloreactive NK cell responses if the recipient lacks HLA class I ligands that contribute to signaling via donor inhibitory KIRs. The most promising results using this approach have been in acute myeloid leukemia patients [61]. Interestingly, stem cell transplant that involved NK cell alloreactivity was associated with higher rates of bone marrow engraftment and reduced rates of GVH [62]. This seems counterintuitive and may be a consequence of limited priming of alloreactive donor T cells because of the ability of the NK cells to eliminate recipient antigen-presenting cells [63]. The clinical data is far from clear, with some studies suggesting the benefit in survival due to KIR ligand mismatch [64, 65] while others failing to show such an effect [66, 67]. These studies differ in the source of the NK cells and conditioning regimens which could impact on the interactions between the NK cells and host cells and explain this apparent discrepancy [68]. Miller and colleagues have been exploring the use of allogeneic haploidentical NK cell infusions in a non-transplant setting. Infused cells generally disappear quickly. Ongoing strategies to address this problem include immunosuppression and ongoing therapy with IL2 [69].

6 Conclusion

NK cells were initially described based on their activity and phenotype and were thought to be a relatively homogeneous population of cells. We now know that NK cells are highly heterogeneous. They were initially considered to be a component of the innate immune system but are now known to play a central role in linking the innate and adaptive immune systems.

NK cells are considered to be important contributors to the efficacy of accepted approaches to cancer immunotherapy such as mAb therapy and treatment with cytokines such as IFNα and IL2. The past 20 years have seen evaluation of a broad variety of additional approaches to treat cancer through manipulation of NK cell activation. Evaluation of the precise role NK cells play in the efficacy of these therapeutic approaches is complicated as our understanding of the heterogeneity of the NK cells themselves, and the variety of different roles played by NK cells, grows. Additional laboratory, translational, and clinical investigation is needed so that we can improve our understanding of the role NK cell activation plays in cancer and use this information to design better approaches to treatment.

References

1. Herberman RB, Nunn ME, Holden HT, Lavrin DH. Natural cytotoxic reactivity of mouse lymphoid cells against syngeneic and allogeneic tumors. II. Characterization of effector cells. Int J Cancer. 1975;16(2):230–9.
2. Cooper MA, Fehniger TA, Turner SC, Chen KS, Ghaheri BA, Ghayur T, et al. Human natural killer cells: a unique innate immunoregulatory role for the CD56(bright) subset. Blood. 2001;97(10):3146–51.
3. Vivier E, Raulet DH, Moretta A, Caligiuri MA, Zitvogel L, Lanier LL, et al. Innate or adaptive immunity? The example of natural killer cells. Science. 2011;331(6013):44–9.
4. Caligiuri MA. Human natural killer cells. Blood. 2008;112(3):461–9.
5. Farag SS, Fehniger TA, Becknell B, Blaser BW, Caligiuri MA. New directions in natural killer cell-based immunotherapy of human cancer. Expert Opin Biol Ther. 2003;3(2):237–50.
6. Ferlazzo G, Munz C. NK cell compartments and their activation by dendritic cells. J Immunol. 2004;172(3):1333–9.

7. Lanier LL. NK cell recognition. Annu Rev Immunol. 2005;23:225–74.
8. Sivori S, Falco M, Della Chiesa M, Carlomagno S, Vitale M, Moretta L, et al. CpG and double-stranded RNA trigger human NK cells by Toll-like receptors: induction of cytokine release and cytotoxicity against tumors and dendritic cells. Proc Natl Acad Sci U S A. 2004;101(27):10116–21.
9. Ballas ZK, Rasmussen WL, Krieg AM. Induction of NK activity in murine and human cells by CpG motifs in oligodeoxynucleotides and bacterial DNA. J Immunol. 1996;157(5):1840–5.
10. Hart OM, Athie-Morales V, O'Connor GM, Gardiner CM. TLR7/8-mediated activation of human NK cells results in accessory cell-dependent IFN-gamma production. J Immunol. 2005;175(3):1636–42.
11. Carbone E, Ruggiero G, Terrazzano G, Palomba C, Manzo C, Fontana S, et al. A new mechanism of NK cell cytotoxicity activation: the CD40-CD40 ligand interaction. J Exp Med. 1997;185(12):2053–60.
12. Bowles JA, Weiner GJ. CD16 polymorphisms and NK activation induced by monoclonal antibody-coated target cells. J Immunol Methods. 2005;304:88–99.
13. Meazza R, Azzarone B, Orengo AM, Ferrini S. Role of common-gamma chain cytokines in NK cell development and function: perspectives for immunotherapy. J Biomed Biotechnol. 2011;2011:861920.
14. Gerosa F, Gobbi A, Zorzi P, Burg S, Briere F, Carra G, et al. The reciprocal interaction of NK cells with plasmacytoid or myeloid dendritic cells profoundly affects innate resistance functions. J Immunol. 2005;174(2):727–34.
15. Gao JX, Liu X, Wen J, Caligiuri MA, Stroynowski I, Zheng P, et al. Two-signal requirement for activation and effector function of natural killer cell response to allogeneic tumor cells. Blood. 2003;102(13):4456–63.
16. Vivier E, Nunes JA, Vely F. Natural killer cell signaling pathways. Science. 2004;306(5701):1517–9.
17. Moretta A, Tambussi G, Bottino C, Tripodi G, Merli A, Ciccone E, et al. A novel surface antigen expressed by a subset of human CD3-CD16+ natural killer cells. J Exp Med. 1990;171:695–714.
18. Moretta A, Locatelli F, Moretta L. Human NK cells: from HLA class I-specific killer Ig-like receptors to the therapy of acute leukemias. Immunol Rev. 2008;224:58–69.
19. Elliott JM, Yokoyama WM. Unifying concepts of MHC-dependent natural killer cell education. Trends Immunol. 2011;32(8):364–72.
20. Yokoyama WM, Kim S. Licensing of natural killer cells by self-major histocompatibility complex class I. Immunol Rev. 2006;214:143–54.
21. Moretta L, Bottino C, Pende D, Vitale M, Mingari MC, Moretta A. Different checkpoints in human NK-cell activation. Trends Immunol. 2004;25(12):670–6.
22. Chiesa S, Mingueneau M, Fuseri N, Malissen B, Raulet DH, Malissen M, et al. Multiplicity and plasticity of natural killer cell signaling pathways. Blood. 2006;107(6):2364–72.
23. Vujanovic NL. Role of TNF superfamily ligands in innate immunity. Immunol Res. 2011;50(2–3):159–74.
24. Raulet DH. Interplay of natural killer cells and their receptors with the adaptive immune response. Nat Immunol. 2004;5(10):996–1002.
25. Raulet DH. Natural killer cells: remembrances of things past. Curr Biol. 2009;19(7):R294–6.
26. Moretta L, Bottino C, Pende D, Castriconi R, Mingari MC, Moretta A. Surface NK receptors and their ligands on tumor cells. Semin Immunol. 2006;18(3):151–8.
27. Parham P. MHC class I molecules and KIRs in human history, health and survival. Nat Rev Immunol. 2005;5(3):201–14.
28. Martin-Fontecha A, Thomsen LL, Brett S, Gerard C, Lipp M, Lanzavecchia A, et al. Induced recruitment of NK cells to lymph nodes provides IFN-gamma for T(H)1 priming. Nat Immunol. 2004;5(12):1260–5.
29. Sivori S, Carlomagno S, Falco M, Romeo E, Moretta L, Moretta A. Natural killer cells expressing the KIR2DS1-activating receptor efficiently kill T-cell blasts and dendritic cells: implications in haploidentical HSCT. Blood. 2011;117(16):4284–92.

30. Palmer S, Hanson CA, Zent CS, Porrata LF, Laplant B, Geyer SM, et al. Prognostic importance of T and NK-cells in a consecutive series of newly diagnosed patients with chronic lymphocytic leukaemia. Br J Haematol. 2008;141(5):607–14.
31. Porrata LF, Ristow K, Habermann TM, Ozsan N, Dogan A, Macon W, et al. Absolute monocyte/lymphocyte count prognostic score is independent of immunohistochemically determined cell of origin in predicting survival in diffuse large B-cell lymphoma. Leuk Lymphoma. 2012;53:2159–65.
32. Porrata LF, Ristow K, Habermann TM, Witzig TE, Colgan JP, Inwards DJ, et al. Peripheral blood lymphocyte/monocyte ratio at diagnosis and survival in nodular lymphocyte-predominant Hodgkin lymphoma. Br J Haematol. 2012;157(3):321–30.
33. Bottino C, Moretta L, Moretta A. NK cell activating receptors and tumor recognition in humans. Curr Top Microbiol Immunol. 2006;298:175–82.
34. Castriconi R, Daga A, Dondero A, Zona G, Poliani PL, Melotti A, et al. NK cells recognize and kill human glioblastoma cells with stem cell-like properties. J Immunol. 2009;182(6):3530–9.
35. Maricic Z, Nola P, Ikic D, Smudj K, Oresic V, Knezevic M, et al. Human leukocyte interferon in therapy of patients with urinary bladder papillomatosis, breast cancer, and melanoma. J Cancer Res Clin Oncol. 1981;101(3):317–23.
36. Colucci F, Caligiuri MA, Di Santo JP. What does it take to make a natural killer? Nat Rev Immunol. 2003;3(5):413–25.
37. Becknell B, Caligiuri MA. Interleukin-2, interleukin-15, and their roles in human natural killer cells. Adv Immunol. 2005;86:209–39.
38. Rosenberg SA. Interleukin-2 and the development of immunotherapy for the treatment of patients with cancer. Cancer J Sci Am. 2000;6 Suppl 1:S2–7.
39. Hayashi T, Hideshima T, Akiyama M, Podar K, Yasui H, Raje N, et al. Molecular mechanisms whereby immunomodulatory drugs activate natural killer cells: clinical application. Br J Haematol. 2005;128(2):192–203.
40. Brandau S, Riemensberger J, Jacobsen M, Kemp D, Zhao W, Zhao X, et al. NK cells are essential for effective BCG immunotherapy. Int J Cancer. 2001;92(5):697–702.
41. Brandau S, Suttmann H. Thirty years of BCG immunotherapy for non-muscle invasive bladder cancer: a success story with room for improvement. Biomed Pharmacother. 2007;61(6):299–305.
42. Ballas ZK, Krieg AM, Warren T, Rasmussen W, Davis HL, Waldschmidt M, et al. Divergent therapeutic and immunologic effects of oligodeoxynucleotides with distinct CpG motifs. J Immunol. 2001;167(9):4878–86.
43. Link BK, Ballas ZK, Weisdorf D, Wooldridge JE, Bossler AD, Shannon M, et al. Oligodeoxynucleotide CpG 7909 delivered as intravenous infusion demonstrates immunologic modulation in patients with previously treated non-hodgkin lymphoma. J Immunother. 2006;29(5):558–68.
44. Lotze MT, Rosenberg SA. Results of clinical trials with the administration of interleukin 2 and adoptive immunotherapy with activated cells in patients with cancer. Immunobiology. 1986;172(3–5):420–37.
45. Rosenberg SA. Immunotherapy of patients with advanced cancer using interleukin-2 alone or in combination with lymphokine activated killer cells. Important Adv Oncol. 1988;58:217–57.
46. LeFor AT, Eisenthal A, Rosenberg SA. Heterogeneity of lymphokine-activated killer cells induced by IL-2. Separate lymphoid subpopulations lyse tumor, allogeneic blasts, and modified syngeneic blasts. J Immunol. 1988;140(11):4062–9.
47. Law TM, Motzer RJ, Mazumdar M, Sell KW, Walther PJ, O'Connell M, et al. Phase III randomized trial of interleukin-2 with or without lymphokine-activated killer cells in the treatment of patients with advanced renal cell carcinoma. Cancer. 1995;76(5):824–32.

48. Nishimura R, Baker J, Beilhack A, Zeiser R, Olson JA, Sega EI, et al. In vivo trafficking and survival of cytokine-induced killer cells resulting in minimal GVHD with retention of antitumor activity. Blood. 2008;112(6):2563–74.
49. Koene HR, Kleijer M, Algra J, Roos D, von dem Borne AE, de Haas M. Fc gammaRIIIa-158V/F polymorphism influences the binding of IgG by natural killer cell Fc gammaRIIIa, independently of the Fc gammaRIIIa-48L/R/H phenotype. Blood. 1997;90(3):1109–14.
50. Cartron G, Dacheux L, Salles G, Solal-Celigny P, Bardos P, Colombat P, et al. Therapeutic activity of humanized anti-CD20 monoclonal antibody and polymorphism in IgG Fc receptor FcgammaRIIIa gene. Blood. 2002;99(3):754–8.
51. Weng WK, Levy R. Two immunoglobulin G fragment C receptor polymorphisms independently predict response to rituximab in patients with follicular lymphoma. J Clin Oncol. 2003;21(21):3940–7.
52. Treon SP, Hansen M, Branagan AR, Verselis S, Emmanouilides C, Kimby E, et al. Polymorphisms in FcgammaRIIIA (CD16) receptor expression are associated with clinical response to rituximab in Waldenstrom's macroglobulinemia. J Clin Oncol. 2005;23(3):474–81.
53. Veeramani S, Wang SY, Dahle C, Blackwell S, Jacobus L, Knutson T, et al. Rituximab infusion induces NK activation in lymphoma patients with the high-affinity CD16 polymorphism. Blood. 2011;118(12):3347–9.
54. Friedberg JW, Neuberg D, Gribben JG, Fisher DC, Canning C, Koval M, et al. Combination immunotherapy with rituximab and interleukin 2 in patients with relapsed or refractory follicular non-Hodgkin's lymphoma. Br J Haematol. 2002;117(4):828–34.
55. Leonard JP, Link BK, Emmanouilides C, Gregory SA, Weisdorf D, Andrey J, et al. Phase I trial of Toll-like receptor 9 agonist PF-3512676 with and following rituximab in patients with recurrent indolent and aggressive non Hodgkin's lymphoma. Clin Cancer Res. 2007;13(20):6168–74.
56. Bowles JA, Wang SY, Link BK, Allen B, Beuerlein G, Campbell MA, et al. Anti-CD20 monoclonal antibody with enhanced affinity for CD16 activates NK cells at lower concentrations and more effectively than rituximab. Blood. 2006;108:2648–54.
57. Robak T. GA-101, a third-generation, humanized and glyco-engineered anti-CD20 mAb for the treatment of B-cell lymphoid malignancies. Curr Opin Investig Drugs. 2009;10(6):588–96.
58. Sheridan C. First-in-class cancer therapeutic to stimulate natural killer cells. Nat Biotechnol. 2006;24(6):597.
59. Kohrt HE, Houot R, Goldstein MJ, Weiskopf K, Alizadeh AA, Brody J, et al. CD137 stimulation enhances the antilymphoma activity of anti-CD20 antibodies. Blood. 2011;117(8):2423–32.
60. Peipp M, Valerius T. Bispecific antibodies targeting cancer cells. Biochem Soc Trans. 2002;30(4):507–11.
61. Curti A, Ruggeri L, D'Addio A, Bontadini A, Dan E, Motta MR, et al. Successful transfer of alloreactive haploidentical KIR ligand-mismatched natural killer cells after infusion in elderly high risk acute myeloid leukemia patients. Blood. 2011;118(12):3273–9.
62. Ruggeri L, Zhang S, Farag SS. Natural killer cell activity and killer immunoglobulin-like receptors in hematopoietic stem cell transplantation. Cancer Treat Res. 2009;144:47–69.
63. Shlomchik WD. Antigen presentation in graft-vs-host disease. Exp Hematol. 2003;31(12):1187–97.
64. Miller JS, Cooley S, Parham P, Farag SS, Verneris MR, McQueen KL, et al. Missing KIR ligands are associated with less relapse and increased graft-versus-host disease (GVHD) following unrelated donor allogeneic HCT. Blood. 2007;109(11):5058–61.
65. Giebel S, Locatelli F, Lamparelli T, Velardi A, Davies S, Frumento G, et al. Survival advantage with KIR ligand incompatibility in hematopoietic stem cell transplantation from unrelated donors. Blood. 2003;102(3):814–9.

66. Davies SM, Ruggieri L, DeFor T, Wagner JE, Weisdorf DJ, Miller JS, et al. Evaluation of KIR ligand incompatibility in mismatched unrelated donor hematopoietic transplants. Killer immunoglobulin-like receptor. Blood. 2002;100(10):3825–7.
67. Farag SS, Bacigalupo A, Eapen M, Hurley C, Dupont B, Caligiuri MA, et al. The effect of KIR ligand incompatibility on the outcome of unrelated donor transplantation: a report from the center for international blood and marrow transplant research, the European blood and marrow transplant registry, and the Dutch registry. Biol Blood Marrow Transplant. 2006;12(8):876–84.
68. Brunstein CG, Wagner JE, Weisdorf DJ, Cooley S, Noreen H, Barker JN, et al. Negative effect of KIR alloreactivity in recipients of umbilical cord blood transplant depends on transplantation conditioning intensity. Blood. 2009;113(22):5628–34.
69. Geller MA, Cooley S, Judson PL, Ghebre R, Carson LF, Argenta PA, et al. A phase II study of allogeneic natural killer cell therapy to treat patients with recurrent ovarian and breast cancer. Cytotherapy. 2011;13(1):98–107.

Induction of Tumor Immunity by Targeted Inhibition of Nonsense-Mediated mRNA Decay

Eli Gilboa

Abstract Whereas tumor progression in cancer patients can elicit a weak immune response which keeps the tumor in check, albeit transiently, the weak antigenicity of the tumor provides the time and opportunity for the tumor to elaborate immune evasion mechanisms. Weak antigenicity is, therefore, the root cause why tumors escape immune control. We have recently described a way to activate the antitumor immune response that is fundamentally different from current strategies collectively referred to as "cancer vaccination," because instead of stimulating immune responses against existing and mostly weak, tumor antigens, novel, and thereby potent, antigens are induced de novo in the disseminated tumor lesions of the patient. The approach is to inhibit a process in the tumor cells known as nonsense-mediated mRNA decay (NMD). The physiological role of NMD is to eliminate defective products generated in the cells, and therefore inhibiting the NMD process will lead to the accumulation of defective products, some of which will encode novel, and thereby potent, antigens to which the immune system has not been tolerized. Inhibition of NMD was accomplished using chemically synthesized siRNAs to downregulate key mediators of the NMD process such as Smg-1 or Upf-2. However, since NMD is a constitutive process that operates in all the somatic cells of the body, global inhibition of NMD could lead to system-wide autoimmune pathology. To obviate the risk of autoimmunity, NMD inhibition was limited to the disseminated tumor lesions by targeted delivery of siRNAs conjugated to oligonucleotide aptamer ligands that bind to receptors expressed preferentially, if not exclusively, on the tumor cells. We have shown that in subcutaneous and metastatic murine tumor models, the tumor-targeted delivery of NMD factor siRNAs led to significant inhibition of tumor growth which was superior to that of a gold standard "conventional" cancer vaccination protocol. Tumor-targeted NMD inhibition forms the basis of a simple,

E. Gilboa (✉)
Department of Microbiology & Immunology, Sylvester Comprehensive Cancer Center, Dodson Interdisciplinary Immunotherapy Institute, Miller School of Medicine, University of Miami, Miami, FL 33136, USA
e-mail: egilboa@med.miami.edu

J.D. Rosenblatt et al. (eds.), *Advances in Tumor Immunology and Immunotherapy*, Current Cancer Research, DOI 10.1007/978-1-4614-8809-5_5,
© Springer Science+Business Media New York 2014

broadly useful, and clinically feasible approach to enhance the antigenicity of disseminated tumors leading to their immune recognition and rejection. The cell-free chemically synthesized oligonucleotide backbone of aptamer–siRNAs reduces the risk of immunogenicity and enhances the feasibility of generating reagents suitable for clinical use.

Keywords Nonsense-mediated mRNA decay • Small interfering RNAs • Oligonucleotide aptamers • Cancer immunotherapy • Tumor antigens

1 Introduction

The recent FDA approval of two immune-potentiating drugs for cancer patients, Sipuleucel-T, a cellular vaccine based on enriched blood APC [1], and Ipilimumab, a CTLA-4-blocking antibody [2], have provided the formal validation for using the immunological modality to treat cancer. Nonetheless, the therapeutic benefit of both drugs was modest, underscoring the need to develop more potent and/or complementary treatments. The main reason why tumors are not eliminated by the immune system is that, unlike pathogens, tumors do not express potent tumor rejection antigens. Whereas tumor progression in cancer patients can elicit a weak immune response which keeps the tumor in check, albeit transiently [3], the weak antigenicity of the tumor provides the time and opportunity for the tumor to elaborate immune evasion mechanisms. Weak antigenicity is, therefore, the root cause why tumors escape immune control.

The general principle and underlying premise of "cancer vaccination," exemplified by the recently approved Sipuleucel-T vaccine for the treatment of advanced prostate cancer, is to administer a tumor antigen(s) to the cancer patient in a manner that it will elicit an immune response of magnitude, duration, and quality that will eliminate the tumor cells expressing the said antigen. The tumor antigen in question needs to be foremost "potent," namely, capable of eliciting a potent immune response, but also it needs to be expressed in the tumors of many patients, because identifying tumor antigens in each patient while feasible is not practical. The problem is that such "potent" antigens are mostly patient specific whereas the shared antigens are by and large "weak." Consequently, current approaches in cancer immunotherapy aim at developing vaccination protocols designed to offset the inherent weakness of the resident endogenous tumor antigens.

An alternative, and arguably superior, approach would be to enhance the antigenicity of tumor cells in situ, namely, to express new, and thereby potent, antigens in the disseminated tumor lesions of the patient. The idea itself is arguably obvious, but the challenge is, and has been, how to do that; how to express new antigens in the disseminated tumor lesions of the patient, lesions that are hard to access, and often we do not know where they are. And of course, how to do that in a cost-effective, broadly applicable, and clinically feasible manner. With this in mind, we have recently described a way to express new antigens in the tumor cells of the patient by inhibiting a process known as nonsense-mediated mRNA decay (NMD) [4].

2 Nonsense-Mediated mRNA Decay: A Primer

Figure 1 depicts how the NMD process prevents the accumulation of mRNAs containing a premature termination codon (PTC) [5–7]. In brief, removal of introns from the pre-mRNA leaves behind an exon-junction complex (EJC) demarcating the splice junctions (Panel A). An NMD complex consisting of several factors including SMG-1, Upf1, Upf2, and Up3 (Panel B) is then assembled on each EJC as shown in Panel C. When the mRNA undergoes the first round of translation, called the "pioneer translation," the EJC/NMD complex is removed, presumably as a result of the translational machinery moving thru the region, thereby rendering the

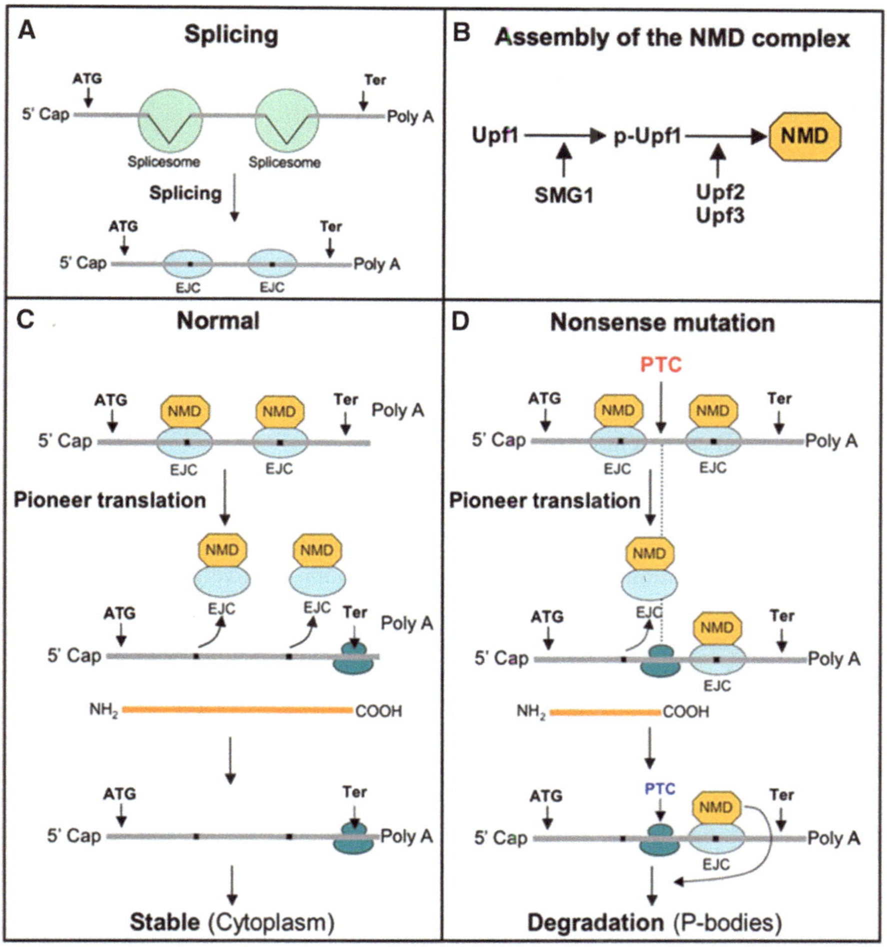

Fig. 1 Nonsense-mediated mRNA decay in eukaryotic cells (see text for details)

mRNA stable and competent for additional rounds of translation (Panel C). However, if a PTC is present in an exon (other than the last exon), for example as a result of aberrant splicing (Panel D), the EJC/NMD complexes downstream to the PTC are not removed from the mRNA. The attached NMD complex then triggers the degradation of the mRNA.

With a few exceptions, the PTC must not reside in the last exon, and often the NMD-triggering PTCs are found at least 50–55 nt upstream of a splice junction (in which case there are many exceptions). There is considerable variability in the efficiency of NMD among various PTC-containing mRNA which cannot be always explained by the these rules. NMD-mediated degradation of mRNA is not limited to instances of mutations or recombinations generating PTCs. Error-free mRNAs containing short 5′ open reading frames (ORFs), mRNAs which are regulated by stop codon read-through, leaky scanning for translation initiation, or regulated frameshifting of mRNA can be also recognized by NMD.

2.1 Physiological Roles of NMD

It was initially thought that the main role of NMD was to maintain the proteome integrity of the cell by eliminating transcripts with nonsense mutations generating PTCs yielding truncated products. Indeed, over 30 % of genetic disorders are caused by PTC [8, 9]. In several instances, e.g., β-thalassemia, the severity of the disease was shown to correlate with the NMD-controlled degradation of the mutant mRNA. Yet, nonsense mutations generating PTCs are rare events, and it is unlikely that the NMD system has evolved to counter their potential deleterious effects. There is in fact accumulating evidence that the main and physiological role of the NMD is to regulate normal gene expression.

An important role of NMD is to maintain splicing integrity. The efficiency and accuracy of splicing are notoriously imperfect. Such transcripts will often contain PTCs and hence become targets for NMD elimination [5, 6]. NMD is also responsible for the elimination of transcripts encoding nonproductively rearranged T cell receptors and immunoglobulin chains [5, 8]. A significant proportion of gene products (>15 %) that are upregulated when NMD is inhibited, such as by targeting Upf1 with siRNA, are involved in amino acid biosynthesis and transcription factors which coordinate cellular responses to starvation [6, 10]. Since starvation also downregulates translation thru phosphorylation and inhibition of eIF2α, which in turn inhibits NMD efficiency, it appears that the response to starvation is in part under NMD control. NMD is also implicated in several instances of products autoregulating alternative splicing (e.g., serine-arginine (SR)-rich proteins and hnRNP splicing factors such as SC35, calpain, CDC-like kinases), biosynthesis of selenoproteins, and telomere synthesis [6, 9].

2.2 *Role of NMD in Cancer*

There is also evidence that cancer cells accumulate elevated level of PTC containing NMD mRNA substrates [11]. About 15 % of cancers exhibit defects in DNA mismatch repair (MMR) often manifested as microsatellite instability (MSI). Such defects affecting many products, including products associated with tumor progression such as TGFβRII, APAF-1, IGFIIR, BAX, PTEN, and RHAMM, give rise to frameshift mutation ending in PTCs. Such PTC-containing transcripts are under NMD control as shown in a study whereby Upf1 siRNA-mediated inhibition of NMD in a human colorectal cancer cell line exhibiting an MSI phenotype stabilized the frameshifted mutant transcripts [12]. Such products could provide a source of tumor-specific antigenic determinants downstream the recombination site [13]. Consistent with this hypothesis, increased immune infiltrates are seen in tumors with MIS phenotype which correlate with the levels of Upf1 in the tumors [12]. Inhibiting NMD could, therefore, theoretically further augment the production of such tumor-specific antigens.

3 Tumor-Targeted NMD Inhibition to Express New Antigens in Disseminated Tumor Lesions

3.1 *The Concept and Rationale*

Several studies have shown that inhibition of NMD in cultured cells using RNAi technology targeted to any of its factors, SMG-1, Upf-1, Upf-2, or Upf3, resulted in the upregulation of multiple products expressed from the PTC-containing mRNA destined for NMD-mediated degradation [10, 14–16] and reviewed in [6]. No adverse impact on cell viability was noted in vitro. The underlying hypothesis of our approach was, therefore, that inhibition of NMD in the tumor cells of the patient will lead to expression of new polypeptides, a proportion of which will encode antigenic determinants that the immune system was not tolerized to, such as products corresponding to the intron regions of alternatively or mis-spliced mRNA but not prematurely terminated polypeptides resulting from in-frame nonsense mutation. NMD inhibition can be readily accomplished using chemically synthesized siRNAs to downregulate any of the known NMD factors, SMG-1, Upf-1, Upf-2, or Upf-3.

Given that the goal is to express new antigens in disseminated tumor lesions the siRNAs have to be administered systemically into the circulation. This raises a problem not uncommon with siRNA therapeutics as well as cancer therapeutics in general. NMD is a constitutive process operating in every somatic cell of the body, tumor cell, as well as normal cells. Inhibiting NMD and consequently expressing new antigens in normal tissues all but certainly will lead to an autoimmune inferno. Limiting NMD inhibition to tumor cells is therefore a paramount requisite to translate this concept into clinical reality. The approach we used was to target the NMD factor siRNA to the tumor cells by conjugation to a targeting ligand that recognizes a product expressed preferentially, not necessarily exclusively, on the surface of the tumor cells. Monoclonal antibodies, a versatile platform for generating ligands with the desired specificity, were the obvious choice for targeting ligands to deliver the NMD factor siRNAs to tumor cells in vivo. Nonetheless, access to monoclonal antibodies, especially for applications, is limited and uncertain at best. The reason is that such protein-based biologicals are cell-based products requiring a complex and costly manufacturing and regulatory approval process. Hence monoclonal antibodies are almost exclusively developed by companies and provided to academic investigators on a selective basis under strict contractual agreement and company oversight [17]. Not less important, chemical conjugation of the targeting antibodies to their therapeutic cargo is complex and costly requiring skill sets that are not readily available, especially in academic settings. Third, monoclonal antibodies, including fully humanized antibodies, run the risk of inducing neutralizing anti-antibody responses that will limit their utility, especially when repeated administration is called for.

With this in mind, we chose to use an alternative platform of targeting ligands in the form of short chemically synthesized, nuclease-resistant, oligonucleotides called aptamers. Aptamers are high-affinity single-stranded nucleic acid ligands, each specific for a given target molecule which can be isolated through a combinatorial chemistry process using iterative in vitro selection techniques, analogous to isolation of high-affinity peptide ligands from phage display libraries. The basic approach named SELEX (systematic evolution of ligands by exponential enrichment) is depicted in Fig. 2 and can be considered an extremely powerful purification method in which very rare binding activities (with frequencies of 1 in 10^{11} to 1 in 10^{13}) are isolated by affinity purification [18, 19]. Aptamers isolated by this method can exhibit remarkable affinity and specificity to their targets comparable to or exceeding those of antibodies. For example, aptamers have been generated that are capable of discriminating between isoforms of protein kinase C that share a high degree of homology [20], and modified-RNA aptamers to coagulation factor VIIa (FVIIa) exhibit a greater than 500-fold specificity for FVIIa relative to coagulation factor Xa and greater than 1,000-fold relative to coagulation factor IXa, although these proteins share a common set of structural domains [21]. Accumulating experience shows that aptamers can be generated against most targets [22, 23] which can inhibit the function of the proteins to which they bind or, as we have recently shown, act in an agonistic fashion to promote the function of their cognate receptors on the cell surface [24, 25]. The first aptamer developed by in vitro selection targeting $VEGF_{165}$ (NX-1838, named Pegaptanib sodium (Macugen)) has been approved for the treatment of macular degeneration, arguably a milestone in the application of aptamer technology [26]. A second aptamer targeted to the coagulation factor IXa is currently tested in phase I/II clinical trials to prevent blood clotting during cardiopulmonary surgery. Phase I clinical trials have demonstrated an excellent safety and functional profile [27].

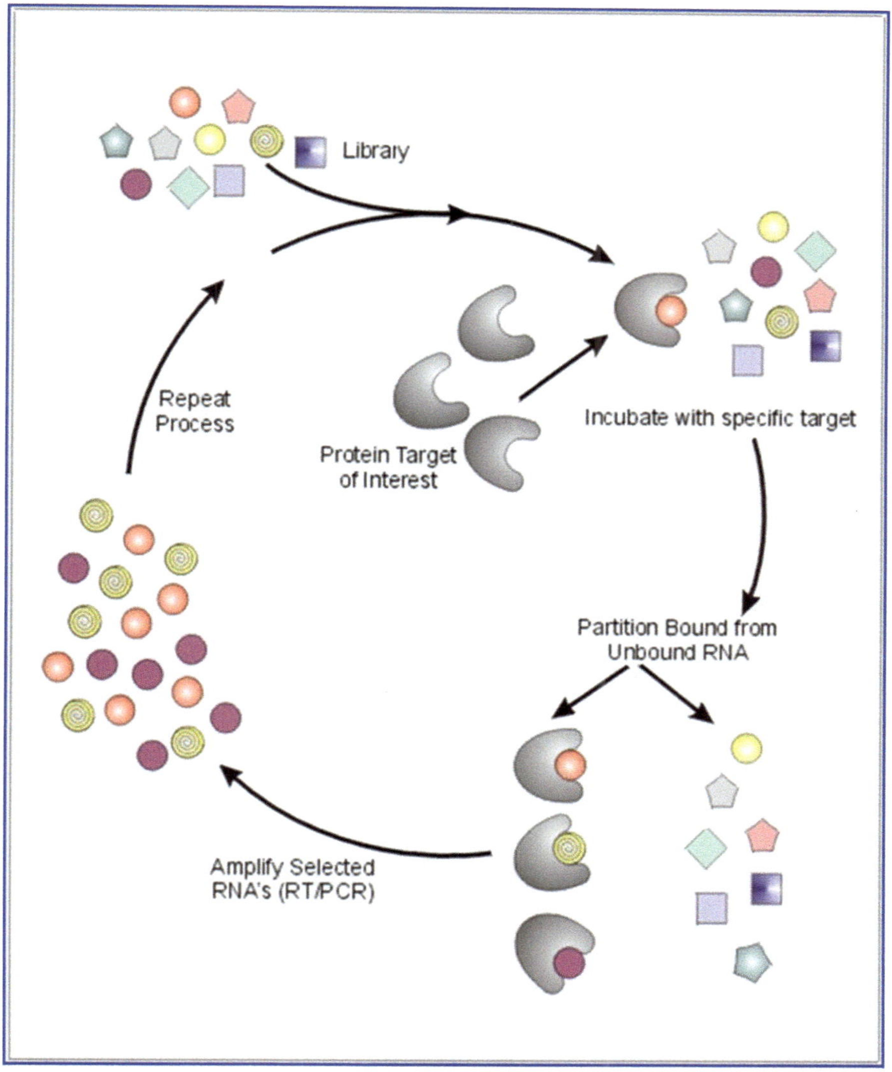

Fig. 2 Systemic evolution of ligands by exponential enrichement (SELEX). A random set of oligonucleotides (ODNs) is incubated with its intended target. Target-bound ODNs are separated from the unbound ODNs, eluted, amplified by PCR, and subjected to a second round of selection. After 8–14 rounds of selection, ODNs which bind its target with high affinity are enriched, cloned, sequenced, and characterized individually. For additional information see refs. [18, 19]

Unlike antibodies, and what is probably a key advantage of aptamers, the 35–55 nt long nuclease-resistant aptamers can be synthesized chemically. Synthesis, purification, and production on large-scale production of short oligonucleotides can be readily carried out under good manufacturing conditions (GMP). Manufacture of clinical grade aptamers, including aptamer–siRNA fusion ODNs, is straightforward

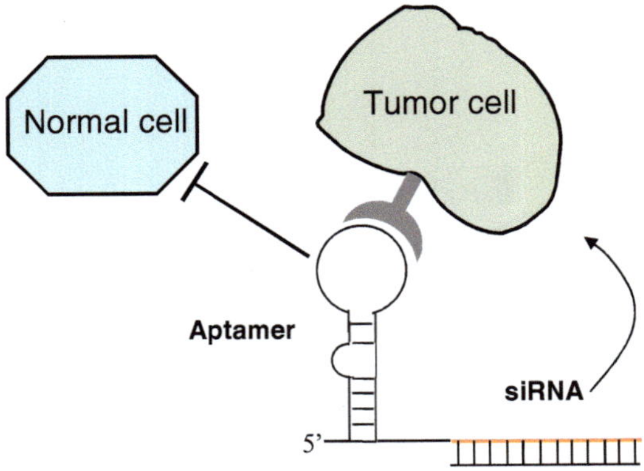

Fig. 3 Aptamer targeting of siRNA to tumor cells. An aptamer, which binds to a specific product expressed on tumor cells but not on normal cells, is conjugated to an siRNA via complementary sequences engineered at the ends of the aptamer and one of the siRNA strands. Binding of the aptamer–siRNA conjugate to the tumor cells triggers its internalization, translocation to the cytoplasm, and siRNA knockdown of its target RNA

and (relatively) cost effective and the regulatory approval process significantly simpler. Conjugation of two oligonucleotides, e.g., aptamer and siRNA, can be accomplished in a simple and straightforward hybridization reaction using short complementary sequences appended to the ends of each oligonucleotide. Lastly, though not experimentally confirmed, short oligonucleotides are not likely to induce significant level of neutralizing immune response.

3.2 *Preclinical Proof-of-Concept Studies in Murine Tumor Models*

This section presents a synopsis of a recently published study showing that aptamer-targeted NMD inhibition is capable of controlling tumor growth in mice. For additional detail see reference 4.

We used aptamers to target the NMD factor siRNAs to tumor cells whereby the NMD factor-specific siRNA was conjugated to an aptamer by hybridization as shown in Fig. 3. Our approach was based on the pioneering studies of Giangrande and her colleagues showing that PSMA-expressing tumor cells can be differentially killed in vitro and in mice by targeting siRNAs corresponding to the broadly expressed survival genes Plk-1 and Bcl-2 fused to a PSMA-specific aptamer [28]. Recent high-profile publications have confirmed the feasibility and therapeutic potential of aptamers as targeting ligands for siRNAs to eradicate tumors [29], sensitize tumor cells to radiation therapy [30], inhibit HIV replication [31, 32], and, as discussed here, potentiate tumor immunity [4].

The first critical test of this approach was to determine whether siRNA-mediated NMD inhibition in tumor cells will lead to the generation of new antigens that will

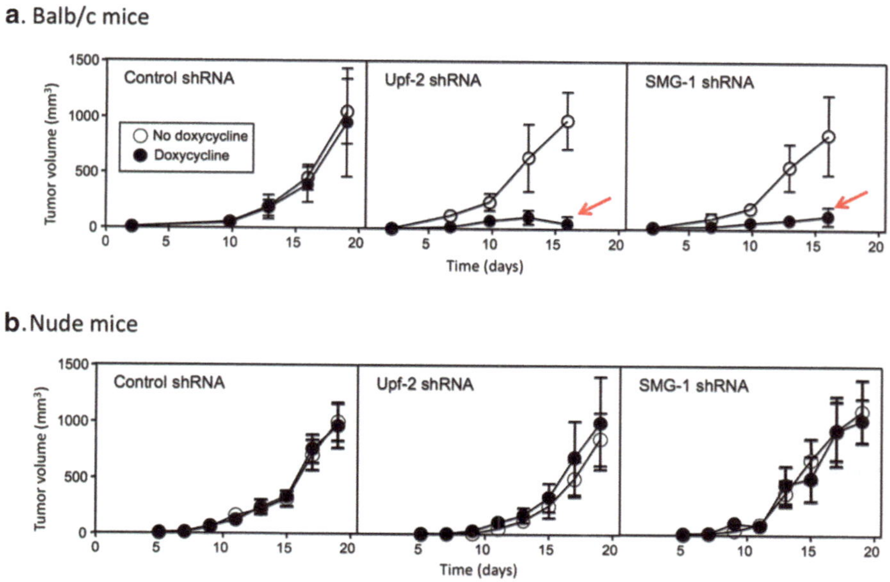

Fig. 4 shRNA inhibition of NMD in tumor cells leads to immune-mediated tumor rejection. (**a**) Balb/c mice were implanted subcutaneously with CT26 tumor cells stably transduced with the doxycycline-inducible lentiviral vectors encoding SMG-1, Upf-2 shRNAs, as well as control shRNA. Each group was divided into two subgroups receiving (*filled circle*) or not receiving (*open circle*) doxycycline in the drinking water. (**b**) Same as panel **a** except that tumor cells were injected into immune-deficient nude mice

elicit an immune response capable of inhibiting tumor growth. To this end, we engineered tumor cells that stably express the NMD siRNAs (used in a configuration called shRNAs). Expression of the siRNA and NMD inhibition was controlled with a drug, doxycycline (DOX). As shown in Fig. 4, tumors harboring the NMD siRNAs Ufp-2 or SMG-1, but not a control siRNA, failed to grow when siRNA expression was turned on (DOX was added to the drinking water of the tumor-bearing mice). But was inhibition mediated by an immune response as we hypothesize or a direct cytotoxic effect of siRNA expression and NMD inhibition? The experiment in Panel B shows that tumor growth was not affected by the siRNAs if the mice were immune compromised. This, and the observation that mice in Panel A that rejected the tumors were resistant to a subsequent challenge with tumor cells, provided fairly compelling evidence that tumor rejection was immune mediated, thereby validating the underlying hypothesis of this approach that siRNA-mediated inhibition of NMD in tumor cells is capable of stimulating a tumor-specific immune response in mice of a magnitude that can negatively impacts on tumor growth.

While providing a proof of concept, the experimental system used in Fig. 4 is not clinically "translatable" because in this experiment NMD was inhibited in all tumor cells from the start. The question, therefore, is whether inhibition of NMD in preexisting tumors will be capable of inducing an immune response of sufficient

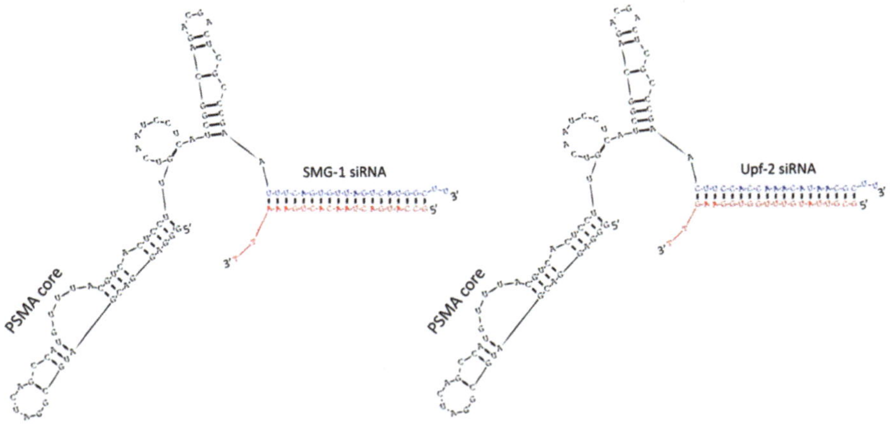

Fig. 5 The sequence and computer-predicted secondary structure of PSMA aptamer–NMD factor siRNAs (see text for details)

magnitude to reverse tumor growth. Moreover, since it is not realistic to expect that we will be able to deliver the aptamer-targeted siRNAs to all, or even the majority, of the tumor cells, the question is whether inhibition of NMD in a proportion of the tumor cells within the tumor lesion will suffice. The second critical test of this approach was, therefore, to determine whether systemic delivery of the aptamer-targeted siRNAs to tumor-bearing mice will be capable of inhibiting tumor growth, and how effectively.

As shown in Fig. 5, two siRNAs corresponding to the NMD factors SMG-1 and Upf-2 were conjugated by hybridization via complementary sequences engineered in the aptamer and siRNA to an aptamer that binds to PSMA, a cell surface product expressed on human prostate tumor cells. The PSMA aptamer, therefore, serves as the targeting ligand to deliver the siRNAs to PSMA-expressing tumor cells. The conjugates were first characterized in vitro in cultured cells to show that they bind only to and inhibit the NMD process in PSMA-expressing cells. Mice were then implanted with tumor cells to establish micro-metastases in the lung and treated with the aptamer–siRNA conjugates that were administered into the circulation by tail vein injection. Since the human PSMA-binding aptamer we used in this study did not bind to murine PSMA the murine tumor cells were engineered to express the human PSMA. As illustrated in Fig. 6, the PSMA aptamer–SMG-1 siRNA inhibited lung metastasis; five out of seven mice showed no evidence of tumor in the lung, assessed both by weighing the lungs or visualizing the metastatic foci.

What this experiment shows is that aptamer-targeted NMD factor siRNA administration to mice bearing disseminated tumor lesion is sufficiently effective to inhibit tumor growth, notwithstanding the fact that mice have already established tumors at the time of treatment and that in all likelihood only a small proportion of the tumor cells in the lesion were successfully targeted with the conjugate to downregulate the NMD process and express new antigens.

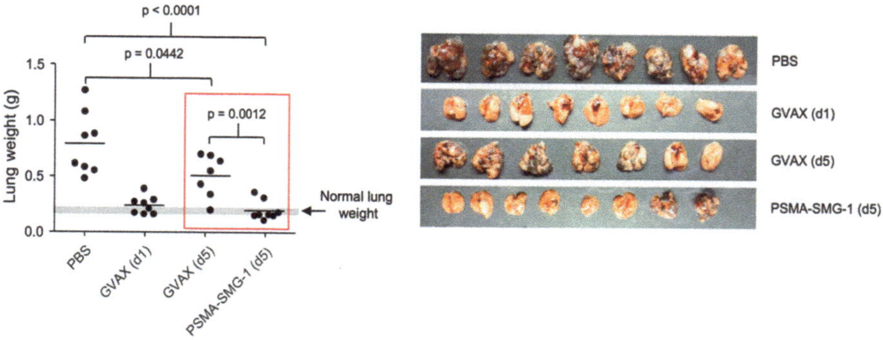

Fig. 6 Comparison of PSMA aptamer–SMG-1 siRNA treatment to vaccination with GM-CSF-expressing irradiated tumor cells. C57BL/6 mice were injected intravenously with B16 melanoma tumor cells and treated with PSMA aptamer–siRNA conjugates starting at day 5 as described or vaccinated with GM-CSF-expressing irradiated B16 tumor cells (GVAX) starting at day 1 or day 5 using the protocol described in reference [39]

But what this and similar experiments do not tell us is how effective is the NMD inhibition approach. The fact that five out of seven mice have cleared the preexisting micro-metastases in the lung, and in parallel experiments remained tumor free, essentially "cured," should not be interpreted to suggest that human patients will experience a similar outcome. A main reason is that conditions of animal experimentation can be readily manipulated that can significantly affect the therapeutic outcome. For example, testing a particular treatment strategy using a more or less susceptible tumor model the proportion of "cured" mice can vary significantly. Tested in isolation, therefore, animal experiments do not teach us how effective is a particular approach compared to a multitude of other approaches. This is, however, critical information because the primary role of animal studies is not, and is not able, to determine which treatment will work in human patients but rather to screen and select for those treatments that are more likely to be effective, prior to engaging in the more challenging clinical trials in human patient. Arguably the most informative way to assess the potential value of a treatment strategy tested in mice is to compare it side by side to a gold standard, in this instance to compare the NMD inhibition approach to a best-in-class "conventional" vaccination protocol. In the experiment shown in Fig. 6 we compared the NMD strategy to vaccination with GVAX, a cell-based vaccine formulation considered to be one of the more effective vaccination protocols in mice [33, 34]. As was also previously noted, in this stringent experimental model of a poorly immunogenic aggressive tumor, GVAX vaccination administered 5 days after tumor implantation had only a modest anti-metastatic impact. Strikingly, under the same condition the NMD inhibition strategy was clearly more effective. Notwithstanding the many limitations of animal models, these experiments clearly establish that the aptamer-targeted NMD inhibition approach is not only capable of inhibition of tumor growth in tumor-bearing mice, but it is also not less effective, if not more so, than "conventional" vaccination strategies. Considering the fact that these were proof-of-concept studies using first-generation aptamer–siRNA conjugates and most likely using a suboptimal treatment protocol, this is not unremarkable.

4 Conclusions and Future Directions

Much of the effort in the field of cancer immunotherapy is devoted to the development of "cancer vaccines," identifying potent and broadly expressed tumor-expressed resident antigens, and methods of vaccination, adjuvants, to stimulate an effective antitumor immune response that also needs to offset the inherent weakness of tumor antigens. Expressing new, and thereby potent, antigens in the disseminated tumor lesions is a new concept that if proven successful could replace the "conventional vaccination" approach. The NMD inhibition approach to express new tumor antigens is a broadly applicable (relatively), cost-effective, and clinically feasible approach that also obviates the need to identify the more potent antigens that are likely to differ from patient to patient. The oligonucleotide-based reagents, aptamer and siRNA, are chemically synthesized which is more cost effective than cell-based products such as antibodies, and the treatment itself consists of simple needle injections. The therapeutic component of the drug, the NMD factor siRNA, is common to all cancer patients. The one limiting factor (today, ideas are being explored to address this as well) is the targeting. The ability to target depends on having identified a product on the surface of the tumor cells. Today we can target PSMA in patient with prostate cancer, Her2 in a proportion of patients with breast cancer, EGFR or preferably its variant EGFRvIII in glioma patient, etc. Thus today a family of 4–7 conjugates will cover about 30 % of the cancer patient population. Suitable targets are likely to be found in all cancers, and clinical success will generate the incentive to discover them.

Which brings up the question, have we cured cancer. Will the sheer expression of new antigens in the disseminated tumor lesions of the cancer patient be able to elicit an immune response of a magnitude that will reverse tumor growth? The answer is unfortunately and of course a definite NO. A main reason, from an immunological standpoint, is that the new antigens will be expressed in tumor lesions that already festered in the patients for many months, during which time they had the opportunity and time to elaborate a plethora of immune-suppressive strategies that will blunt the immune recognition of the NMD inhibition-induced new antigens. Thus in order to elicit a therapeutically effective immune response it will be necessary to develop complementary and synergistic strategies in order to enhance the "immunogenicity" of the tumor lesion, to enhance the potency of the immune response elicited against the new antigens, and to counter the tumor-induced immune-suppressive mechanisms.

To this end we are developing ways to potentiate costimulation at the tumor site, enhance the persistence of (NMD inhibition induced) T cells, protect the tumor-infiltrating T cells from TGFβ, a key mediator of immune suppression, and more (reference 35 and unpublished data). The common denominator of the approaches we are developing is that the therapeutic agent is targeted to the relevant cells in vivo, tumor cells or immune cells, and the use of chemically synthesized oligonucleotides both as therapeutic agents, siRNAs, aptamer, or antagomirs (the latter to control the microRNA world), and as targeting ligands in the form of aptamers as discussed above. In vivo cell targeting will enhance the therapeutic index of the otherwise poorly specific or even nonspecific drugs, arguably a major challenge of cancer therapeutics, and the chemically synthesized ODN-based reagents will enhance the feasibility of their clinical use, a paramount consideration especially if a combination of multiple treatment protocols is called for.

4.1 *Cytotoxic Therapy or Immunotherapy?*

Cytotoxic therapy, chemotherapy or radiation, is the most direct, finite, and broadly used approach to treat cancer. Immunotherapy, to elicit an immune response that will then eliminate the cancer, is indirect and instinctively less appealing. Also active immunotherapy (not counting passive immunotherapy with monoclonal antibodies) has yet to provide compelling evidence of its effectiveness comparable to what has been achieved with cytotoxic therapy (though I believe this is only a matter of time). Indeed, aptamer-targeted therapies to cancer were initially developed to deliver cytotoxic agents, e.g., siRNAs to inhibit survival genes in cancer cells [28]. Notwithstanding, one should bear in mind that the bar for targeting tumors with cytotoxic agents is higher than that of targeting tumor or immune cells for the purpose of stimulating immunity. In the former case it will be necessary to successfully target and eliminate at least 90–95 % of tumor cells within the lesion to exert a therapeutic effect. In the case of immunotherapy a much lower threshold of targeting, perhaps as low as 5–20 %, is likely to suffice, because the activated immune response exerts a dominant effect and acts also on the nontargeted tumor cells. Since increasing the efficiency of targeting is becoming exponentially more difficult (aptamer) targeted immunotherapy may prove to be more effective than cytotoxic therapy.

Recent exciting research, heralding the next generation of successful cancer therapies, suggests that the choice is not between chemotherapy or immunotherapy but rather a judicious combination of both. At the core of this revolution in the making is the recognition that some form of chemotherapies, including the widely used anthracylines and cisplatin family of chemotherapeutic drug, can induce the so-called immunogenic tumor cell death which is not only compatible with but promotes tumor immunity [36, 37].

If so, cytotoxic therapies, irradiation or chemotherapies, will be administered at considerably lower doses well beyond their current dose-limiting toxic range to kill a fraction of tumor cells to provide antigenic debris for the immune therapy-induced immune system. Thus a marriage between aptamer-targeted cytotoxic therapy and immunotherapy is in the cards.

4.2 *What If?*

Are the NMD inhibition-induced antigens unique? Will each tumor or each patient express a unique set of antigens when NMD is inhibited, or are they universal, the same antigens being induced in all cancer patients? The biology of NMD does not offer a clue; the question can, and will, be addressed experimentally, first in mice. If the NMD inhibition antigens are common the therapeutic implications could be far reaching, for example forming the basis of a universal prophylactic cancer vaccine. Cancer immunotherapy is at present developed therapeutically to treat patients that already have cancer. If NMD inhibition-induced antigens are common, they can be isolated and used to vaccinate individuals at risk for cancer, such as women presenting during routine mammography with "high mammographic density" [38]. Vaccination should be well tolerated because the NMD inhibition-induced antigens represent "foreign" antigens not unlike pathogen antigens used in common vaccines. If and when the individuals at risk progress to cancer, at early stages of disease before tumors had the opportunity to establish significant suppression, patients could conceivably be treated with the aptamer–siRNA conjugates to induce the NMD inhibition-specific antigens in their lesions that will be met by an already preexisting, and hence more potent, immune response.

References

1. Kantoff PW, Higano CS, Shore ND, Berger ER, Small EJ, Penson DF, Redfern CH, Ferrari AC, Dreicer R, Sims RB, et al. Sipuleucel-T immunotherapy for castration-resistant prostate cancer. New Engl J Med. 2010;363:411–22.
2. Hodi FS, O'Day SJ, McDermott DF, Weber RW, Sosman JA, Haanen JB, Gonzalez R, Robert C, Schadendorf D, Hassel JC, et al. Improved survival with ipilimumab in patients with metastatic melanoma. New Engl J Med. 2010;363:711–23.
3. Bindea G, Mlecnik B, Fridman WH, Pages F, Galon J. Natural immunity to cancer in humans. Curr Opin Immunol. 2010;22:215–22.
4. Pastor F, Kolonias D, Giangrande PH, Gilboa E. Induction of tumor immunity by targeted inhibition of nonsense mediated mRNA decay. Nature. 2010;465:227–31.
5. Behm-Ansmant I, Kashima I, Rehwinkel J, Sauliere J, Wittkopp N, Izaurralde E. mRNA quality control: an ancient machinery recognizes and degrades mRNAs with nonsense codons. FEBS Lett. 2007;581:2845–53.
6. Isken O, Maquat LE. The multiple lives of NMD factors: balancing roles in gene and genome regulation. Nat Rev Genet. 2008;9:699–712.
7. Muhlemann O, Eberle AB, Stalder L, Zamudio Orozco R. Recognition and elimination of nonsense mRNA. Biochim Biophys Acta. 2008;1779:538–49.
8. Frischmeyer PA, Dietz HC. Nonsense-mediated mRNA decay in health and disease. Hum Mol Genet. 1999;8:1893–900.
9. Holbrook JA, Neu-Yilik G, Hentze MW, Kulozik AE. Nonsense-mediated decay approaches the clinic. Nat Genet. 2004;36:801–8.
10. Mendell JT, Sharifi NA, Meyers JL, Martinez-Murillo F, Dietz HC. Nonsense surveillance regulates expression of diverse classes of mammalian transcripts and mutes genomic noise. Nat Genet. 2004;36:1073–8.

11. Duval A, Hamelin R. Mutations at coding repeat sequences in mismatch repair-deficient human cancers: toward a new concept of target genes for instability. Cancer Res. 2002;62: 2447–54.
12. El-Bchiri J, Guilloux A, Dartigues P, Loire E, Mercier D, Buhard O, Sobhani I, de la Grange P, Auboeuf D, Praz F, et al. Nonsense-mediated mRNA decay impacts MSI-driven carcinogenesis and anti-tumor immunity in colorectal cancers. PLoS ONE. 2008;3:e2583.
13. Saeterdal I, Bjorheim J, Lislerud K, Gjertsen MK, Bukholm IK, Olsen OC, Nesland JM, Eriksen JA, Moller M, Lindblom A, et al. Frameshift-mutation-derived peptides as tumor-specific antigens in inherited and spontaneous colorectal cancer. Proc Natl Acad Sci U S A. 2001;98:13255–60.
14. Mendell JT, ap Rhys CM, Dietz HC. Separable roles for rent1/hUpf1 in altered splicing and decay of nonsense transcripts. Science. 2002;298:419–22.
15. Usuki F, Yamashita A, Kashima I, Higuchi I, Osame M, Ohno S. Specific inhibition of nonsense-mediated mRNA decay components, SMG-1 or Upf1, rescues the phenotype of Ullrich disease fibroblasts. Mol Ther. 2006;14:351–60.
16. Wittmann J, Hol EM, Jack HM. hUPF2 silencing identifies physiologic substrates of mammalian nonsense-mediated mRNA decay. Mol Cell Biol. 2006;26:1272–87.
17. Pardoll D, Allison J. Cancer immunotherapy: breaking the barriers to harvest the crop. Nat Med. 2004;10:887–92.
18. Ellington AD, Szostak JW. In vitro selection of RNA molecules that bind specific ligands. Nature. 1990;346:818–22.
19. Tuerk C, Gold L. Systematic evolution of ligands by exponential enrichment: RNA ligands to bacteriophage T4 DNA polymerase. Science. 1990;249:505–10.
20. Conrad R, Keranen LM, Ellington AD, Newton AC. Isozyme-specific inhibition of protein kinase C by RNA aptamers. J Biol Chem. 1994;269:32051–4.
21. Rusconi CP, Yeh A, Lyerly HK, Lawson JH, Sullenger BA. Blocking the initiation of coagulation by RNA aptamers to factor VIIa. Thromb Haemost. 2000;84:841–8.
22. Keefe AD, Pai S, Ellington A. Aptamers as therapeutics. Nat Rev Drug Discov. 2010;9:537–50.
23. Nimjee SM, Rusconi CP, Sullenger BA. Aptamers: an emerging class of therapeutics. Annu Rev Med. 2005;56:555–83.
24. Dollins CM, Nair S, Boczkowski D, Lee J, Layzer JM, Gilboa E, Sullenger BA. Assembling OX40 aptamers on a molecular scaffold to create a receptor-activating aptamer. Chem Biol. 2008;15:675–82.
25. McNamara JO, Kolonias D, Pastor F, Mittler RS, Chen L, Giangrande PH, Sullenger B, Gilboa E. Multivalent 4-1BB binding aptamers costimulate CD8 T cells and inhibit tumor growth in mice. J Clin Invest. 2008;118:376–86.
26. Ng EW, Shima DT, Calias P, Cunningham Jr ET, Guyer DR, Adamis AP. Pegaptanib, a targeted anti-VEGF aptamer for ocular vascular disease. Nat Rev Drug Discov. 2006;5:123–32.
27. Vavalle JP, Rusconi CP, Zelenkofske S, Wargin WA, Alexander JH, Becker RC. A phase 1 ascending dose study of a subcutaneously administered factor IXa inhibitor and its active control agent. J Thromb Haemost. 2012;10:1303–11.
28. McNamara 2nd JO, Andrechek ER, Wang Y, Viles KD, Rempel RE, Gilboa E, Sullenger BA, Giangrande PH. Cell type-specific delivery of siRNAs with aptamer-siRNA chimeras. Nat Biotechnol. 2006;24:1005–15.
29. Dassie JP, Liu XY, Thomas GS, Whitaker RM, Thiel KW, Stockdale KR, Meyerholz DK, McCaffrey AP, McNamara 2nd JO, Giangrande PH. Systemic administration of optimized aptamer-siRNA chimeras promotes regression of PSMA-expressing tumors. Nat Biotechnol. 2009;27:839–49.
30. Ni X, Zhang Y, Ribas J, Chowdhury WH, Castanares M, Zhang Z, Laiho M, Deweese TL, Lupold SE. Prostate-targeted radiosensitization via aptamer-shRNA chimeras in human tumor xenografts. J Clin Invest. 2011;121:2383–90.
31. Neff CP, Zhou J, Remling L, Kuruvilla J, Zhang J, Li H, Smith DD, Swiderski P, Rossi JJ, Akkina R. An aptamer-siRNA chimera suppresses HIV-1 viral loads and protects from helper CD4(+) T cell decline in humanized mice. Sci Transl Med. 2011;3:66ra66.

32. Wheeler LA, Trifonova R, Vrbanac V, Basar E, McKernan S, Xu Z, Seung E, Deruaz M, Dudek T, Einarsson JI, et al. Inhibition of HIV transmission in human cervicovaginal explants and humanized mice using CD4 aptamer-siRNA chimeras. J Clin Invest. 2011;121:2401–12.
33. Dranoff G, Jaffee E, Lazenby A, Golumbek P, Levitsky H, Brose K, Jackson V, Hamada H, Pardoll D, Mulligan RC. Vaccination with irradiated tumor cells engineered to secrete murine granulocyte-macrophage colony-stimulating factor stimulates potent, specific, and long-lasting anti-tumor immunity. Proc Natl Acad Sci U S A. 1993;90:3539–43.
34. Jinushi M, Hodi FS, Dranoff G. Enhancing the clinical activity of granulocyte-macrophage colony-stimulating factor-secreting tumor cell vaccines. Immunol Rev. 2008;222:287–98.
35. Pastor F, Kolonias D, McNamara 2nd JO, Gilboa E. Targeting 4-1BB costimulation to disseminated tumor lesions with bi-specific oligonucleotide aptamers. Mol Ther. 2011;19:1878–86.
36. Ma Y, Kepp O, Ghiringhelli F, Apetoh L, Aymeric L, Locher C, Tesniere A, Martins I, Ly A, Haynes NM, et al. Chemotherapy and radiotherapy: cryptic anticancer vaccines. Semin Immunol. 2010;22:113–24.
37. Tesniere A, Apetoh L, Ghiringhelli F, Joza N, Panaretakis T, Kepp O, Schlemmer F, Zitvogel L, Kroemer G. Immunogenic cancer cell death: a key-lock paradigm. Curr Opin Immunol. 2008;20:504–11.
38. Kelemen LE, Sellers TA, Vachon CM. Can genes for mammographic density inform cancer aetiology? Nat Rev Cancer. 2008;8:812–23.
39. van Elsas A, Hurwitz AA, Allison JP. Combination immunotherapy of B16 melanoma using anti-cytotoxic T lymphocyte-associated antigen 4 (CTLA-4) and granulocyte/macrophage colony-stimulating factor (GM-CSF)-producing vaccines induces rejection of subcutaneous and metastatic tumors accompanied by autoimmune depigmentation. J Exp Med. 1999;190: 355–66.

Employing T Cell Homeostasis as an Antitumor Strategy

Shawn M. Jensen, Christopher C. Paustain, and Bernard A. Fox

Abstract In the arena of cancer treatments, chemotherapeutic agents and radiotherapy were originally designed to kill rapidly dividing cancer cells and deletion of lymphoid cells was simply considered collateral damage. The last few decades have witnessed a growing appreciation for immunologic control of tumor burdens, and consequently, numerous strategies designed to harness the immune system to combat cancers have been developed. While on the surface the combination of immune-depleting chemo/radiotherapies and immunotherapies may seem counterintuitive, the fact that the immune system has mechanisms in place for compensatory expansion after depletion, an effect called homeostasis-driven T cell expansion, has been exploited in both preclinical models as well as clinical therapies. This chapter examines both.

Keywords Homeostasis • Lymphopenia • T cell • Antitumor immune response • Clinical trial • Antitumor vaccination • Adoptive immunotherapy

---

SM Jensen and CC Paustian contributed equally to this work.

S.M. Jensen • C.C. Paustain
Laboratory of Molecular and Tumor Immunology, Robert W. Franz Cancer Research Center, Earle A. Chiles Research Institute, Providence Cancer Center, Portland, OR 97213, USA

B.A. Fox (✉)
Laboratory of Molecular and Tumor Immunology, Robert W. Franz Cancer Research Center, Earle A. Chiles Research Institute, Providence Cancer Center, Portland, OR 97213, USA

Department of Molecular Microbiology and Immunology, and Knight Cancer Institute, Oregon Health and Science University, Portland, OR 97239, USA
e-mail: foxb@foxlab.org

J.D. Rosenblatt et al. (eds.), *Advances in Tumor Immunology and Immunotherapy*, Current Cancer Research, DOI 10.1007/978-1-4614-8809-5_6,

© Springer Science+Business Media New York 2014

1 Introduction

Biological systems respond to the external environmental cues that either stimulate or inhibit biological processes. However, one of the key aspects of a multicellular organism is its ability to stably regulate its internal environment even when faced with external stimuli. Left unregulated these processes would be detrimental to the organism. In the 1850s Claude Bernard underlined this important concept when he stated, "*The constancy of the internal environment is the condition for a free and independent life.*" Bernard coined the term *milieu intérieur*, which referred to the ability of the living body to be relatively independent of the surrounding environment due to the internal environment of which it is constituted. Walter Cannon further refined this concept of *milieu intérieur* in 1929, developing the theory of homeostasis [1]. He proposed that steady-state conditions require organized mechanisms that resist change anytime there is a tendency to move from constancy. Cannon based this theory on his insights on how the body maintains steady states in glucose concentration and body temperature.

Lymphocytes of the immune system rely on homeostatic regulation to maintain the size and composition of the lymphocyte pool. Any perturbation to the immune system that either expands or decreases the number of lymphocytes is countered by homeostatic mechanisms to keep the number of lymphocytes in the periphery at a relatively constant level. The rapid expansion of T cells after infection with lymphocytic choriomeningitis virus is followed by massive cell death after the insult is cleared in order to reestablish equilibrium conditions [2]. Alternatively, insults that cause depletion of the lymphocyte pool lead to lymphocyte proliferation in order to replenish the lymphocyte compartment. Increased access to homeostatic cytokines and self-peptide/MHC molecules as well as a lack of regulatory T cells are primarily responsible for the lymphopenia-induced proliferation. In this chapter we discuss the mechanisms that maintain homeostasis and review strategies that have employed the lymphopenic environment to augment priming and expansion of tumor-specific lymphocytes in the field of tumor immunology.

2 Homeostasis of T Lymphocytes

Maturation of T cells requires them to pass through positive and negative selection in the thymus. Those T cells that interact with self-peptide/MHC molecules (spMHC) on cortical epithelial cells with sufficient affinity are positively selected and survive. However, T cells with medium to high affinity for spMHC are deleted in the thymus by negative selection ensuring the removal of potentially autoreactive T cells. The surviving T cell population leaves the thymus and becomes part of the peripheral pool of T cells. Immune homeostasis is dependent on two primary pathways: continued generation of new T cells through thymopoiesis and peripheral expansion of T cells by spMHC and homeostatic cytokines. Primary T cell development is dependent on thymopoiesis during the neonatal period; however, due to thymic involution that occurs during puberty, peripheral expansion of T cells becomes more important for maintenance of the peripheral T cell pool over the lifespan of the host [3]. In the periphery, naïve T cells still depend on sub-mitogenic signaling through spMHC and their coreceptors CD4 or CD8 for survival [1, 4, 5]. Using MHC class $II^{-/-}$ mice, Takeda et al. demonstrated that weak interactions between the T cell receptor and MHC class II molecules are required for the long-term survival of $CD4^+$ T cells [2, 6]. Similarly, naïve $CD8^+$ T cells also require MHC class I molecules for their survival [3, 7]. However, homeostasis-driven proliferation is independent of costimulation signals mediated through CD28/B7, CD40L/CD40, or 4-1BB/4-1BBL [8].

Interleukin-7 (IL-7) is a key cytokine that maintains survival of naïve T cells in the periphery [9–11]. IL-7 is a member of the type I cytokine family that includes IL-2, IL-4, Il-9, IL-15, and IL-21 which share the common γ-chain. Although these other cytokines (IL-4, IL-12, and IL-15) can augment homeostasis-driven proliferation, naïve T cells require IL-7 for homeostasis-driven proliferation [11, 12]. IL-7 is produced by stromal cells, keratinocytes, dendritic cells, and epithelial cells and binds to a heterodimer receptor consisting of the common γ-chain and IL-7Rα (CD127) [10, 13–15]. In vivo manipulation of IL-7 cytokine levels has been shown to modulate the overall size of the T cell population [1, 10, 16]. In the absence of IL-7, $IL\text{-}7^{-/-}$ mice or $IL\text{-}7R\alpha^{-/-}$ mice, there is a loss of T cells demonstrating the necessity of this cytokine for normal T cell homeostasis [1, 2, 17].

Various studies have examined where the production of IL-7 is most crucial for naïve T cell homeostasis. There is a reduction in the survival of naïve CD4+ T cells in the absence of secondary lymphoid organs ($NIK^{aly/aly}$ mice) implicating their role in homeostasis [2, 3, 18]. The production of CCL19 and CCL21 by fibroblastic reticular cells in the T cell zones of lymphoid organs is crucial to attract naïve T cells where they can receive survival signaling through IL-7 which is also produced by the fibroblastic reticular cells [1, 3–5, 19]. The production of IL-7 is relatively consistent, and thus T cell responses are regulated by competition for the cytokine as well as expression of the IL-7 receptor (CD127). CD127 is differentially expressed on T cells at all stages of development. Interestingly, naïve T cells were found to downregulate CD127 after IL-7 stimulation and upregulate CD127 in the absence of IL-7 [2, 4–6, 20].

IL-7 promotes cell survival by preventing apoptosis mediated by Bcl-2 family members. IL-7 signaling increases the expression of Bcl-2 which regulates the activity of the apoptotic molecules, Bax and Bad, and contributes to the enhanced survival [3, 6, 7, 21, 22]. Signaling through the IL-7 receptor also activates the Jak/STAT signaling pathways [7, 8, 23]. Activation of these pathways is known to have effects on cell survival, growth, and metabolism [8–11, 24, 25].

In contrast to the quiescent state of naïve T cells, memory T cells undergo slow cell division about once every 2–3 weeks [9–12, 26]. Survival of memory T cells is independent of spMHC but is dependent on common γ chain cytokines, IL-15 and IL-7 [10–15, 27–29]. $CD8^+$ central memory T cells express high levels of CD127

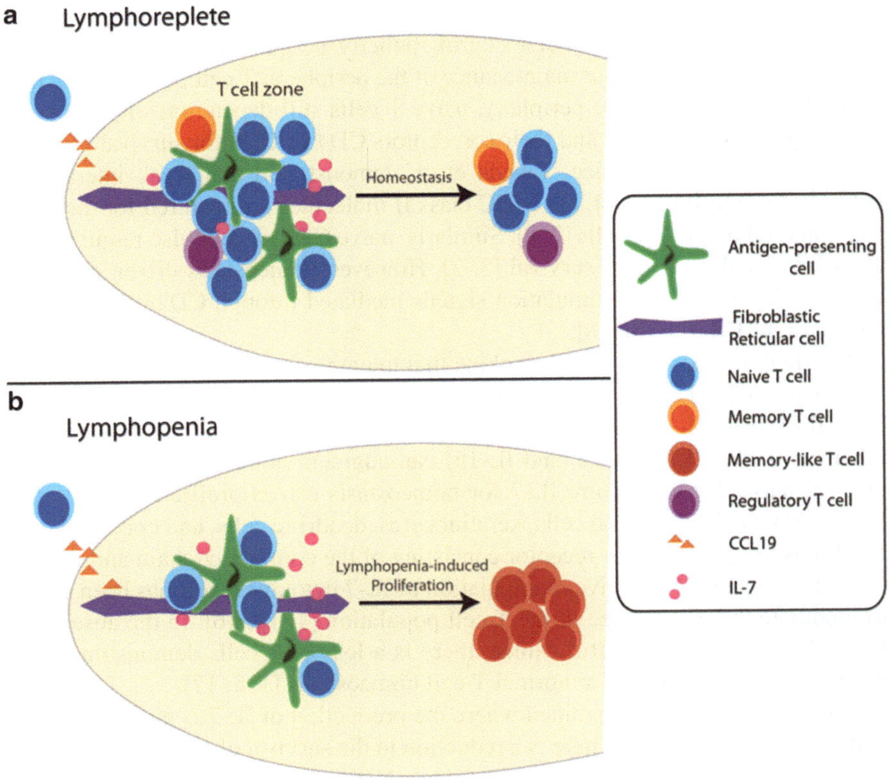

Fig. 1 Lymphopenia leads to the proliferation of T cells. (**a**) Within the T cell zone of lymphoid organs T cells compete for the presence of sp/MHC on antigen-presenting cells as well as for homeostatic cytokine, IL-7, during lymphoreplete conditions. (**b**) In contrast, conditions that cause T cell depletion create a lymphopenic environment in the T cell zone leading to increased access to IL-7 and sp/MHC on antigen-presenting cells. Naïve T cells are also brought from the periphery to the T cell zone of lymphoid organs due to increased access to chemokines, such as CCL19. The resultant lymphopenia-induced proliferation creates memory-like cells that share phenotypically markers and similar function as antigen-induced memory T cells

(IL-7Rα) and CD122 (IL-15Rβ), allowing them to rapidly respond to IL-7 and IL-15 [10, 13–15, 30]. In the absence of IL-15 (IL-15$^{-/-}$ mice) there was a lack of CD8^{+} memory T cells [10, 16, 28, 31]. In contrast, CD4^{+} memory T cells express lower levels of CD122 and are less dependent on IL-15 than CD8^{+} memory T cells [5]. CD4^{+} memory T cells express high amounts of IL-7 receptor and have demonstrated dependence on IL-7 for homeostasis-driven proliferation [32].

Taken together these mechanisms ensure that the T cell compartment within the immune system remains within limits (Fig. 1a). Alterations to these mechanisms can lead to compromised homeostasis, which is detrimental to the host as evidenced by mice deficient in these pathways.

3 Lymphopenia-Induced T Cell Proliferation

The same regulatory mechanisms that maintain a stable number of T cells in the periphery are responsible for reconstituting the T cell pool after a lymphopenic insult [33, 34]. Proliferation of T cells is driven by increased access to IL-7 due to the diminished number of lymphocytes in the lymphopenic environment. This "space" created by the lack of lymphocytes decreases competition between T cells for IL-7, inducing lymphopenic proliferation when they engage spMHC [5] (Fig. 1b). Lymphopenia-induced proliferation of T cells not only increases their numbers but also results in their acquiring a memory-like phenotype ($CD44^{+}Ly6C^{+}$, $CD122^{+}$). These memory-like T cells gain the ability to secrete interferon-γ and become cytotoxic effectors when stimulated with their cognate antigen [35–37].

The role of TCR interactions with spMHC in lymphopenia-induced proliferation might favor T cells with higher affinities for spMHC. Indeed it has been shown that lymphopenia-induced proliferation is driven by the affinity of the TCR for the spMHC and favors T cells with higher affinities for spMHC or T cells that have increased access to relevant spMHC [38, 39]. Various groups have shown skewing of the T cell repertoire due to interclonal competition for homeostatic factors [40–42]. These data suggest that over time low-affinity T cells for spMHC would be lost from the T cell pool; however, this is not entirely true since it was observed that the frequency of low-affinity T cells simply plateaus at later time points [43]. This demonstrates that clonal competition also exists during lymphopenia-induced proliferation limiting the number of T cells expressing the same T cell receptor [44, 45].

Regulatory T cells (T_{reg}) have been shown to have a crucial role in preventing autoimmune disease, limiting damage caused by chronic inflammatory diseases, and are important for the maintenance of peripheral tolerance. The role of T_{reg} cells in controlling homeostasis-driven proliferation has been controversial. Some groups have shown little impact on proliferation if T_{reg} cells are co-transferred with naïve T cells into lymphopenic mice [8, 46], while others have observed that T_{reg} cells can inhibit the proliferation of naïve CD4 T cells but not CD8 T cells transferred into a lymphopenic environment [47]. It also appears that the ratio of T_{reg} cells to naïve T cells impacts the likelihood of the naïve T cells to proliferate [47]. Studies using monoclonal T cells demonstrated that the presence of T_{reg} cells was sufficient to only slightly dampen the lymphopenia-driven proliferation of high-affinity T cells but they were sufficient to prevent the cell division of low-affinity T cells [48]. Together these data suggest that the presence of T_{reg} cells raises the threshold of TCR avidity required for lymphopenic induced proliferation. In addition to preventing lymphopenia-driven proliferation, T_{reg} cells also block the differentiation of T cells to the memory phenotype [48]. Although the exact mechanism by which T_{reg} cells might be regulating homeostasis-driven proliferation is unknown, a number of potential candidates including CTLA4 and TGF-β have been studied [49, 50]. The lymphocyte activation gene-3, LAG-3, has been shown to be important for the negative regulation of homeostasis mediated by T_{reg} cells. Interestingly, T cells deficient for LAG-3 showed enhanced lymphopenia-induced proliferation in lymphopenic hosts [51].

4 Lymphopenia-Induced Pathologies

The recognition of self is important for homeostasis; however, severe lymphodepletion enables spMHC molecules to activate T cells specific for self-peptides to proliferate. Depending on additional factors, this lymphopenia-induced proliferation might result in autoimmunity [52]. A number of studies have implicated lymphopenia-induced proliferation as a contributor to autoimmunity [53–55]. Neonatally thymectomized mice (day 3) of several strains develop autoimmune reactions targeted against multiple organs [56, 57]. This autoimmune reaction has been associated with the loss of thymic derived T_{reg} cells that develop after day 3 [58, 59]. This suggests that the peripheral expansion of neonatal T cells coupled with the absence of T_{reg} cells drives these autoimmune responses. Similarly, the adoptive transfer of T_{reg}-depleted splenocytes into a lymphopenic host induces autoimmune gastritis. The autoimmune pathology is dependent on both the absence of T_{reg} cells as well as induced proliferation as neither on their own was able to recapitulate the disease state [53]. Multiorgan autoimmunity can also be observed in mice that are made lymphopenic by high-dose irradiation. Again this is a result of increasing homeostatic cytokine levels and depleting inhibitory lymphocytes. Adding back $CD4^+$ T cells from the spleen of a non-irradiated mouse was sufficient to prevent the autoimmune disease [60] demonstrating that loss of T_{reg} cells induced proliferation that led to autoimmunity.

Additionally, the method that induces lymphopenia might elicit factors that will enhance the immune response. Total body irradiation results in commensal gut microflora in the mesenteric lymph nodes and elevated LPS levels in the sera. The engagement of toll-like receptor 4 by the LPS resulted in increased dendritic cell activation and $CD8^+$ T cell activation [61]. Total body irradiation also causes the upregulation of VCAM1, ICAM1, and B7-2 that might modulate trafficking and costimulation of T cells [62].

5 Lymphopenia-Induced Antitumor Immune Responses

The potent autoimmune responses that have been observed in lymphopenia-induced proliferation models have been enticing to tumor immunologists, providing evidence that anti-self immune responses can be generated. Most tumor vaccine strategies fail to elicit immune responses that impact tumors likely as a result of the lack of potent stimulation by tumor antigens. Because most tumor antigens are self-proteins, potential high-affinity T cells that would target the tumor are either negatively selected in the thymus or silenced by other peripheral suppressive mechanisms. Since lymphopenia provides a window where homeostatic cytokines can induce the proliferation of T cells specific for low-affinity spMHC molecules while also removing suppressive T_{reg} cells, it is an enticing environment to study for improved antitumor immunotherapy.

Early studies by Mitchison et al. demonstrated that irradiation of the host prior to adoptive transfer of lymphocytes led to improved magnitude and duration of the transferred antiviral protection [63]. This observation has been followed by other groups who have shown that after immune cell depletion, adoptive transfer of T cells displayed increased antitumor efficacy [64–67]. Using cyclophosphamide (150 mg/kg i.v.) to induce immune cell depletion, North and colleagues were able to impact tumor growth by transferring naïve T cells into these lymphopenic mice. Additionally, they showed that tumor regression caused by the adoptive transfer in the lymphopenic environment was abolished if spleen cells from tumor-bearing mice were co-transferred [68]. They reasoned that the augmented immunotherapy was due to the cyclophosphamide-induced elimination of tumor-induced suppressor T cells.

Building off previous work using cyclophosphamide, Machiels et al. examined the dose and timing of cyclophosphamide to determine the best schedule for mediating an enhanced tumor-vaccine immune response. They found that administration of cyclophosphamide 1 day prior to vaccine at doses between 50 and 150 mg/kg provided the best antitumor immune responses [69]. At this dose of cyclophosphamide $CD4^+$ and $CD8^+$ T cells are reduced by 50 %, while T_{reg} cells are even more profoundly impacted [70]. Higher doses of cyclophosphamide (200 mg/kg) did not enhance vaccine efficacy due to the severe decrease in all T cell subsets [69, 70]. It is clear from these experiments that in order to utilize the benefits of lymphopenia that would include lymphopenic induced proliferation, the lymphopenic host needs to be reconstituted with lymphocytes. Reconstitution of lymphopenic mice (600 cGy or $Rag1^{-/-}$) with naïve T cells followed by tumor vaccination led to significantly higher frequencies of tumor-specific T cells in the tumor-vaccine draining lymph nodes compared to normal mice [71, 72]. The increased frequency of tumor-specific T cells was represented in both the CD4 and CD8 T cell compartment and exhibited a type 1 phenotype (interferon-γ secretion). Importantly, vaccination was best when performed concomitant with reconstitution of lymphopenic mice, as delaying vaccination resulted in T cells with less therapeutic activity [71]. Similar findings were also observed in a lymphopenic model using sublethal total body irradiation (500 cGy) [73]. However, if the reconstituting fraction came from a tumor-bearing mouse then vaccination was ineffective in priming an antitumor immune response. Corroborating North's earlier findings, removal of the T_{reg} population from the reconstituting fraction restored the ability to prime an antitumor immune response [74, 75].

An alternative approach to using the benefits of lymphopenia-induced proliferation is to transfer tumor-specific T cells into the lymphopenic recipient. This strategy is useful for transferring tumor-infiltrating lymphocytes (TIL), transgenic T cell receptor-transduced T cells, or chimeric-antigen receptor-transduced T cells. The adoptive transfer of TIL into recipient mice had been treated with cyclophosphamide-mediated elimination of tumor in contrast to transfer of TIL alone [76]. The adoptive transfer of transgenic tumor-specific $CD8^+$ T cells into sublethally irradiated lymphopenic mice also blocked tumor growth better than lymphoreplete mice [77–79]. This enhanced antitumor efficacy was attributed to increased antitumor function [77] and longer persistence of memory T cells [78] augmented by the availability of

IL-7 and IL-15 in the lymphopenic mice. Further work demonstrated that the addition of total $CD4^+$ T cells to the adoptive transfer prevented effective adoptive immunotherapy in lymphopenic recipients. However, removal of T_{reg} cells ($CD4^+CD25^+$) from the $CD4^+$ fraction that was transferred with melanoma-specific transgenic $CD8^+$ T cells restored the ability to regress established melanoma in lymphopenic mice [79]. The lymphopenia-induced proliferation of T_{reg} cells during immune reconstitution [80] and their ability to block potential antitumor immune responses must be considered when determining which fraction of cells to use for reconstitution of lymphopenic hosts.

Recent work has focused on increasing the intensity of the lymphodepletion using myeloablative total body irradiation (900 cGy). Since this dose is myeloablative it is imperative to reconstitute the recipient with a hematopoietic stem cell transplant. This strategy exhibited enhanced antitumor activity compared to mice treated with lower intensities of radiation [81, 82]. The myeloablation significantly reduces the number of surviving host cells, reducing the potential for recovery of host immunoregulatory cells that impede the antitumor immune response at lower radiation intensities.

An alternative strategy to inducing lymphopenia in hosts is to replicate the physiology of lymphopenia in lymphoreplete hosts by providing targeted therapies. The rationale for attempting this strategy is that although T cell depletion in humans over the short term has its benefits for antitumor immune responses, over the long term it can be associated with immune dysfunction [83–85]. The adoptive transfer of antitumor TCR-transgenic $CD8^+$ T cells into lymphoreplete hosts treated with recombinant IL-7 and T_{reg} depletion impacted tumor growth and increased survival. Interestingly, this strategy also supported determinant spreading that was absent in lymphopenic hosts [86, 87]. Other groups have demonstrated that the inhibitory receptors LAG-3 and PD-1 control immune homeostasis and prevent autoimmunity [51, 88]. Mice deficient in both of these inhibitory receptors have autoimmune infiltrates in multiple organs that results in lethality. However, blocking both of these pathways using anti-LAG-3/anti-PD-1 antibodies successfully cured mice of established tumors without the lethal autoimmune disease [89].

The data from preclinical studies support the benefits of the lymphopenic environment in generating and sustaining antitumor immune responses. Clinical translation of these mechanisms requires strategies that mimic the lymphopenic conditions while also being cognizant of the potential for unwanted autoimmune pathologies.

6 Clinical Evidence/The Human Model

The induction of lymphopenia has been used to enhance the efficacy of adoptive T cell and vaccine-based immunotherapies in numerous clinical trials for metastatic melanoma as well as renal, pancreatic, breast, and a growing list of other cancers. Cyclophosphamide is the most commonly used strategy to lymphodeplete patients prior to vaccination, and the combination of cyclophosphamide and fludarabine has provided the greatest therapeutic impact in adoptive T cell immunotherapy studies.

However, several other chemotherapies and total body irradiation have been employed alone or in combination with other agents in some clinical trials [90].

This section covers clinical experience with lymphopenia-induced T cell proliferation in the realms of both vaccines and adoptive immunotherapy for the treatment of patients with cancer. We also examine the evidence taken from phenotyping peripheral blood cells of patients in clinical trials that sheds new light on one of the hypothetical mechanisms of action for homeostasis-driven T cell expansion aiding cancer immunotherapies: that changes in T cell subset proportions might favor antitumor responses after homeostasis is achieved. Additionally, clinical evidence that has accumulated concerning how extensive a deletion regimen is needed to boost antitumor responses is examined. However, it should be noted that just as translating experimental results from mouse models to man may at times mislead researchers, so too can the results from clinical trials be misrepresentative. The lack of definitive control groups and small sample numbers in clinical trials often frustrate our ability to answer basic questions of how to further improve patient care and must be taken into account to avoid overinterpreting data.

7 Adoptive Immunotherapy of Cancer

Adoptive T cell immunotherapy for cancer has employed a number of different approaches, but the majority of studies have employed the passive transfer of autologous tumor-reactive T cells generated from tumor-infiltrating lymphocytes that were expanded to large numbers and infused with IL-2 support [91]. An alternative strategy was to transfer tumor-associated peptide-reactive T cell lines or clones generated from the peripheral blood. With few exceptions, adoptive transfer of TIL, T cell lines, or clones provided limited therapeutic impact, beyond that of IL-2 alone, when T cells were transferred into lymphoreplete hosts.

The first reasonably sized study to combine adoptive immunotherapy and nonmyeloablative conditioning examined the efficacy of adoptively transferring autologous gp100-specific CD8+ T cell clones to HLA-A2+ patients with metastatic melanoma. Following lymphodepletion with cyclophosphamide and fludarabine, patients received CD8 T cell clones alone or in combination with low- or high-dose IL-2 [92]. No patients exhibited an objective response.

Subsequently, this same group evaluated the impact of adoptively transferring autologous TIL lines, including both CD4+ and CD8+ T cells, into 13 HLA-A2^{+} patients with metastatic melanoma patients. These patients received the same nonmyeloablative conditioning regimen specified above [90]. Strikingly, this strategy resulted in the first example of rapid and extensive in vivo expansion and long-term persistence of tumor-specific TIL and was associated with a high rate of clinical efficacy. Six of the thirteen patients (46 %) had an objective clinical response, and four others exhibited mixed responses, with significant shrinkage at one or more metastatic sites. Of those responders, half presented with the melanocyte-associated autoimmune responses vitiligo and anterior uveitis. Two of the responding patients presented with lymphocytosis comprised primarily the transferred TIL cells.

Incredibly, each of these two patients grew out a single tumor-reactive clone representing the majority of their peripheral blood lymphocytes for 4 months to several years after treatment.

A second NCI fludarabine clinical trial enrolled 35 patients with advanced metastatic melanoma that were refractory to conventional treatments [93]. Eighteen of the thirty-five treated patients demonstrated an objective response to treatment, and eight others demonstrated a mixed or a minor response. While 13 of the patients who exhibited an objective response ultimately progressed at one or more sites after treatment, evidence of immune editing of these metastases gave proof to the power of the therapy. Antigen expression by tumor cells was evaluated in pretreatment and recurrent lesions for nine of these patients. Recurrent lesions from four patients did not express HLA-A2 and recurrent lesions from one other patient did not express the MART-1 protein, while lesions from seven evaluated patients who were nonresponders expressed both HLA and MART-1 antigens. Of note, ten patients in this study did not receive G-CSF after lymphodepleting chemotherapy, since that growth factor has been described by some as immunosuppressive [94]. No obvious difference in clinical response was observed; however, G-CSF administration did significantly improve neutrophil recovery.

Studying metastatic melanoma patients treated with lymphodepleting chemotherapy prior to adoptive T cell immunotherapy has shown that the persistence of the transferred cells is related to the length of the telomeres before transfer [95]. Thus, relatively "young" TIL seem to make better therapies than older cells. This observation led to the creation of a new clinical trial utilizing TIL cultured ex vivo for a shorter time span. In order to accommodate the accelerated timing investigators eliminated the individualized tumor-reactivity screening step and thus were able to broaden the number of patients who were actually treated by this therapy. Thirty-three patients were treated with CD8+-enriched young TIL and IL-2 following lymphodepletion. Twenty-three additional patients were treated with CD8+-enriched young TIL and IL-2 after lymphodepleting chemotherapy plus 6 Gy of total body irradiation. Historically, 27 % of patients who were intended for treatment with TIL have actually received adoptive immunotherapy. This failure to treat was due to lack of tumor specificity (release criteria) of the cultured TIL or patient progression during the time it takes to obtain a sufficient number of TIL for adoptive transfer [96]. In contrast 53 % of eligible patients were able to receive the young TIL therapy. Since both treatments resulted in just over 50 % RECIST response rates, this stands as a significant advance in the field. Importantly, 11 of the 30 objective responders in this trial received TIL that would not have been administered in previous trials [96].

8 Vaccine Augmentation

When patients with cancer were vaccinated with KLH, before or after cyclophosphamide-induced lymphopenia, it was found that pretreatment of patients with cyclophosphamide augmented the development of delayed-type hypersensitivity (DTH) responses to KLH [97]. This finding motivated researchers to ask whether pretreatment with cyclophosphamide could help enhance the effects of a cancer vaccine in a clinical trial [98]. Patients with metastatic melanoma were treated with a lethally irradiated autologous melanoma cell vaccine that was admixed with bacille Calmette–Guérin (BCG) as an adjuvant in a buffered salt solution, either given alone or 3 days after a low-dose cyclophosphamide treatment. The chemotherapy was given as a single bolus injection of 300 mg/m^2, which is very nearly equivalent to 8.1 mg/kg in adult humans [99]. The DTH responses of cyclophosphamide-treated patients were significantly greater than those of patients receiving vaccine only. Whereas seven of eight cyclophosphamide-treated patients developed DTH to autologous melanoma cells of at least 5 mm, only two of seven controls did so. Two patients had significant antitumor responses to treatment with cyclophosphamide plus vaccine, with a complete disappearance of skin metastases and a pulmonary nodule in one and the regression of subcutaneous and liver metastases in the other.

A comparison of the combination of busulfan and fludarabine versus 30 or 60 mg/kg cyclophosphamide was examined in a trial with patients with metastatic melanoma. All patients received a melanoma antigen-peptide (MART-1) vaccine following reinfusion with autologous PBMC [100, 101]. Patients receiving cyclophosphamide were also given G-CSF (low dose) or GM-CSF (high dose) to boost neutrophil counts back to normal levels. A high percentage of activated proliferating cells was detectable early after PBMC transfer and remained so over a period of 3 weeks. Cyclophosphamide treatment resulted in enhanced lymphodepletion that in turn led to greater T cell activation and proliferation that plateaued by day 30 when enhanced proliferation was no longer detected. Busulfan plus fludarabine seemed to be less efficient promoters of homeostasis-driven proliferation since patients of that cohort had very low levels of activated and proliferating T cells. Patients receiving cyclophosphamide who presented with EBV-specific CD8 T cells averaged twice as many EBV-specific CD8 T cells after the treatment. However, the percentage of MART-1-specific CD8 T cells that produced interferon-γ prior to treatment was halved after treatment. This could be a complication of the particular antigen chosen, since the MART-1-specific T cell repertoire in healthy HLA-A2 individuals averages 1 in 1,400 blood CD8 T lymphocytes [102]. Phenotypically and functionally these are naive T cells that appear to undergo an unusually high level of positive selection in the thymus with limited expansion in the periphery, thus making their response to the conditions that drive homeostasis-driven T cell expansion possibly aberrant. Researchers strengthened the finding that patient CD8 T cell responses to melanoma-associated cancer-testis antigen were more frequent 30 days after treatment, and thus the only antigen-specific responses measured that were observed to decrease were the MART-1 response to which patients were vaccinated. Of note, the TLR9 agonist, CpG, given as an adjuvant in this vaccine formulation was not included for boosts given post depletion, and this lack of an adjuvant may well have impacted the potential potency of the vaccine.

Another important clinical trial that combined vaccines to lymphodepleting strategies involved 14 patients with pancreatic adenocarcinomas [103]. Eight weeks after pancreatic duodenectomy, patients received between 10 and 500 million irradiated allogeneic GM-CSF-secreting tumor cells as a cancer vaccine. Twelve of fourteen patients then went on to receive a 6-month course of adjuvant radiation and chemotherapy with a variety of agents. One month after completing adjuvant treatment, six patients still in remission received up to three additional monthly vaccinations with the same vaccine dose that they had received originally. Vaccination induced increased DTH responses to autologous tumor cells in three patients who had received at least 100 million vaccine cells. These three patients also seemed to have had an increased disease-free survival time, remaining disease free at least 25 months after diagnosis. A significant change in post-vaccination DTH activity was not noted in patients treated at lower dose levels. While all patients in this study received lymphodepleting chemotherapy, the profound effect of vaccine dose highlighted an important concept in this type of combined therapy that homeostasis-driven T cell expansion may be able to assist vaccination but only if the vaccine reaches above a threshold of potency.

The vaccine schedule can also have profound effects on immune activation when lymphodepletion is involved [104]. Forty-two advanced myeloma patients were divided into four arms of treatment. All patients received ex vivo co-stimulated T cell infusions combined with a pneumococcal conjugate vaccine (PCV) immunizations after chemotherapy-induced lymphopenia. The four arms represented a factorial design for two variables representing two distinct questions the investigators were asking. Does vaccination just prior to apheresis and chemotherapy-induced lymphopenia efficiently prime later post-depletion vaccinations? And should ex vivo-activated T cells be given prior to post-depletion vaccinations or after? Thus two groups were vaccinated prior to lymphodepletion while two were not. Likewise two groups were reinfused with activated autologous T cells between lymphodepletion and post-depletion vaccination (for one group the first vaccine), while two groups were reinfused after the post-depletion vaccination. In this trial pre-depletion priming seemed to be the most important question/variable, since both groups vaccinated prior to apheresis and lymphodepletion showed stronger PVC IgG responses than patients who received no priming vaccine. Should ex vivo-activated T cells be given prior to post-depletion vaccinations or after? Between the two groups that were primed prior to depletion, more patients given activated T cells prior to boost vaccines made higher PVC IgG titers than patients given activated T cells after boosting; however, these two groups had observably dissimilar responses to the prime vaccine—at which time point their treatments were identical. Given the small number of patients studied and the variable pretreatment response, these interesting results will need future confirmation. However, the significant effect priming prior to depletion had on immune response is remarkable considering that previous studies have shown a profound reduction in vaccine responsiveness within the first 2 years of receiving autologous peripheral blood stem cell and bone marrow transplants [105, 106].

A similar finding was announced by a group looking at 214 patients with clinical stage III melanoma that were vaccinated with multiple intradermal injections of autologous tumor cells modified with the hapten, dinitrophenyl (DNP), and mixed with BCG [107]. Four different vaccine dosage schedules were tested, all of which included low-dose cyclophosphamide. While differences were seen between the four schedules, researchers were surprised to find that the timing of a baseline DTH skin test was an efficient predictor for later DTH responses to autologous unmodified melanoma cells. They discovered that patients who had received baseline skin testing 3–8 days prior to chemotherapy generated greater immunity than those who had been skin-tested 1 day prior or on the day of chemotherapy, a variable identified during post hoc analysis. This effect remained significant in a multivariate analysis that included well-known prognostic variables. While the study was not designed to answer such a question, the sheer number of patients involved as well as the fact that this capitulates another finding give cause to study further the effects of priming before lymphodepletion followed by booster vaccinations.

9 Lymphopenia-Induced Changes in T_{reg} Percentages

An increased percentage of T_{regs} in peripheral blood has been associated with several tumor types, including non-small-cell lung cancer, breast cancer, colorectal cancer, esophageal cancer, gastric cancer, hepatocellular carcinoma, lung cancer, and melanoma [108–113]. These T_{reg} represent a major obstacle in the generation of antitumor immune responses [114]. In a seminal study examining the affects of cyclophosphamide-based chemotherapy-induced lymphopenia and IL-2 therapy on 24 patients with pediatric sarcoma, functionally suppressive T_{reg} were shown to preferentially expand under the conditions of homeostasis-driven proliferation [80]. The addition of exogenous IL-2 seemed to enhance this effect. Interestingly, the youngest participant in this trial was the only one to show recovery of the naive CD4 CD45RA compartment, implying thymic contribution to regenerating T cell numbers after chemotherapy does not occur in adults. Additionally, T cell receptor excision circles (TRECs) were more diluted in T_{regs} of IL-2-receiving patients than patients receiving no IL-2, indicating that this conditioning regimen induced T_{reg} proliferation. Ki-67 staining confirmed that T_{reg} expanded preferentially post cyclophosphamide treatment, a finding at odds with mouse models of cyclophosphamide effects [70].

The NCI tested in vivo transfer of autologous CD25-depleted mononuclear populations to lymphopenic patients in combination with high-dose IL-2 to try to work around this conundrum. Five patients with IL-2 refractory metastatic melanoma were given lymphodepleting chemotherapy followed by the autologous transfer of T_{reg} cell-depleted PBMC and high-dose IL-2. High percentages of CD4 cells in peripheral blood expressed FOXP3 within 10 days of depletion [115]. This study highlights an important possibility that homeostasis of the T_{reg} compartment may enable homeostasis-driven T_{reg} expansion in T_{reg}-depleted hosts, an important consideration since several strategies to selectively deplete T_{reg} are current topics of investigation. Another possibility is that the high-dose IL-2, known to activate and expand T_{reg}, is a suboptimal conditioning regimen for such a depletion strategy [80].

10 The Dose Makes the Poison

The maxim "the dose makes the poison" certainly seems to be true with immunomodulatory chemotherapies. One study examined this phenomenon by using a factorial study design to determine the optimum dosing of combined therapy with cyclophosphamide and doxorubicin. The highest dose of doxorubicin tested was 35 mg/m^2 (equivalent to 0.95 mg/kg in adult humans [99]), and this enhanced patients' humoral responses to an human epidermal growth factor receptor-2 (HER-2) vaccine, while the lowest dose of cyclophosphamide best increased HER-2 antibody responses of the patients. Cyclophosphamide doses more than 200 mg/m^2 (equivalent to 5.4 mg/kg in adult humans [99]) abrogated both cellular and humoral responses [116]. These findings were observed in the context of a dual-chemotherapy regimen; therefore, extrapolating to single-agent treatment studies is tenuous. However, these findings hint that, at least in the case of cyclophosphamide, less can be more.

In order to minimize toxicity chemotherapeutics are sometimes given in repetitive but very low doses, a technique called metronomic chemotherapy. This approach has been proposed as a means of minimizing tumor angiogenesis. One recent study looked at T_{reg} and their correlation to clinical outcome in 12 patients with treatment-refractory metastasized breast cancer who received metronomic low-dose cyclophosphamide daily for 3 months. Cyclophosphamide treatment initially caused a significant reduction in circulating T_{reg}. However, T_{reg} numbers completely recovered during the treatment due to increased proliferative activity and maintained their suppressive capacity. T_{reg} depletion significantly correlated with an increase in breast tumor-specific T cells, the numbers of which correlated with disease stabilization and overall survival [117].

A similar strategy was employed by another group seeking to enhance the antitumor properties of an intratumorally injected oncolytic adenovirus [118]. Forty-three patients with a variety of solid tumors refractory to conventional therapies were divided into four cohorts: cyclophosphamide given in oral metronomic dosing (50 mg/day), intravenously (single 1,000 mg dose), with both chemo regimens, or with no chemotherapy. Metronomic cyclophosphamide (both oral and oral + bolus injection) decreased percentages of T_{regs} cells without impairing the generation of antitumor or antiviral T cell responses. The cytokine profile of ex vivo-stimulated peripheral lymphocytes was analyzed before and after treatment. Patients receiving the combination of metronomic cyclophosphamide and the oncolytic adenovirus had an increase of interferon-γ, tumor necrosis factor-α, and interleukin-2 (IL-2) suggesting an ongoing Th1-type immune response. Importantly, all cyclophosphamide regimens resulted in significantly higher rates of disease control than virus only, and the best progression-free and overall survival was seen in the group receiving oral and intravenous cyclophosphamide.

Investigating the possibility that a more extensive depletion strategy may yield better patient responses, recent clinical trials at the NCI investigated adoptive T cell immunotherapy for patients with metastatic melanoma combined with intensive myeloablative chemoradiation preparative regimens [119]. Their historical data of chemotherapy plus adoptive T cell immunotherapy with autologous TIL and IL-2 has yielded about a 50 % objective response rate. When adding 2 or 12 Gy total body irradiation to the preparative regimen of cyclophosphamide and fludarabine they realized slightly higher (though not statistically significant, perhaps due to small group numbers) objective response rates of 52 and 72 %, respectively. Serum levels of IL-7 and IL-15 were statistically higher in the 12-Gy TBI group than chemo only. It is possible that increased availability of these cytokines to TIL cells in patients conditioned with 12-Gy TBI may have increased their proliferative and functional status in these patients.

Myeloablative therapies supported by autologous stem cell transplantation have proven to be effective treatments for certain hematological malignancies. However there is an increased level of risk with such strategies since complete reconstitution of lymphoid and other immune effector cells may take months to years and the side effects of TBI can be substantial [120, 121]. Fortunately, there are increasing numbers of long-term survivors who have undergone myeloablative therapies, and thus knowledge about late effects on the immune system is accumulating.

11 Conclusion

Many studies have given evidence that cancers do alert the host immune system [121]. Unfortunately, many mechanisms exist whereby cancers can subvert this immunologic recognition and induce tolerance. Given such a state, resetting the immune system through depleting regimens of chemo- or radiotherapy has been an active area of study, both in preclinical and clinical settings. This is fortunate, since while these therapies hold promise, many questions remain concerning best clinical practice for combining lymphodepletion-induced homeostasis-driven T cell expansion with either vaccination or adoptive T cell immunotherapy (Fig. 1). One important question not yet addressed in human clinical trials is whether vaccination and adoptive T cell immunotherapy can be combined for potentially synergistic immunological and clinical effects, as mouse models indicate [81]. Likewise, much excitement has been generated with checkpoint-blockade (i.e., Yervoy, PD-1, PD-L1) and co-stimulatory (i.e., OX40) antibodies where preclinical data dominate [122]. Inclusion of these agents with vaccines and/or adoptive T cell immunotherapy in homeostasis-driven T cell expansion strategies may well represent a very important piece in the puzzle of combination immunotherapy (Fig. 2).

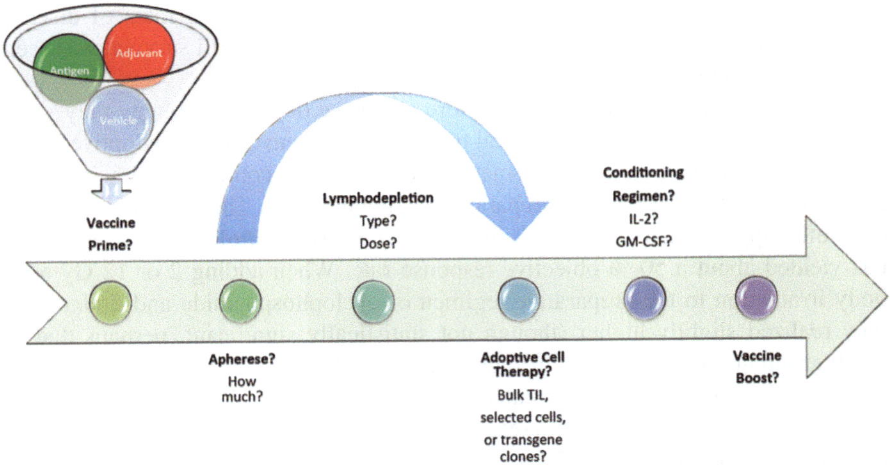

Fig. 2 Variables in immunotherapies employing homeostasis-driven T cell expansion. Many questions are still unanswered concerning how best to utilize homeostasis-driven T cell expansion with cancer immunotherapies. From questions of vaccine choice to whether one uses the patients' pre-depleted blood product to reinfuse patients post depletion. The extent and method of depletion as well as the identity of adoptive cellular therapy product are both major variables for determining success of therapies that have not been sufficiently optimized in clinical trails. Additional "details" that may change patient outcome are the possible use of the proper recombinant hematopoietic growth factors or cytokines as conditioning agents and the timing of booster shots employed in a vaccine modality

References

1. Cannon WB. Organization for physiological homeostasis. Physiol Rev. 1929;9(3):399–431.
2. Badovinac VP, Porter BB, Harty JT. Programmed contraction of CD8(+) T cells after infection. Nat Immunol. 2002;3(7):619–26. doi:10.1038/ni804.
3. Goronzy JJ, Weyand CM. T cell development and receptor diversity during aging. Curr Opin Immunol. 2005;17(5):468–75. doi:10.1016/j.coi.2005.07.020.
4. Martin B. On the role of MHC class II molecules in the survival and lymphopenia-induced proliferation of peripheral CD4+ T cells. Proc Natl Acad Sci U S A. 2003;100(10):6021–6. doi:10.1073/pnas.1037754100.
5. Surh CD, Sprent J. Homeostasis of naive and memory T cells. Immunity. 2008;29(6):848–62. doi:10.1016/j.immuni.2008.11.002.
6. Takeda S, Rodewald HR, Arakawa H, Bluethmann H, Shimizu T. MHC class II molecules are not required for survival of newly generated CD4+ T cells, but affect their long-term life span. Immunity. 1996;5(3):217–28. doi:10.1016/S1074-7613(00)80317-9.
7. Tanchot C, Lemonnier FA, Rarnau BP, Freitas AA, Rocha B. Differential requirements for survival and proliferation of CD8 naÃ¯ve or memory T cells. Science. 1997;276(5321): 2057–62.
8. Prlic M, Blazar BR, Khoruts A, Zell T, Jameson SC. Homeostatic expansion occurs independently of costimulatory signals. J Immunol. 2001;167(10):5664–8.
9. Tan JT, Dudl E, LeRoy E, Murray R, Sprent J, Weinberg KI, Surh CD. IL-7 is critical for homeostatic proliferation and survival of naive T cells. Proc Natl Acad Sci U S A. 2001;98(15):8732–7. doi:10.1073/pnas.161126098.

10. Fry TJ, Mackall CL. The many faces of IL-7: from lymphopoiesis to peripheral T cell maintenance. J Immunol. 2005;174(11):6571–6.
11. Schluns KS, Kieper WC, Jameson SC, Lefrançois L. Interleukin-7 mediates the homeostasis of naïve and memory CD8 T cells in vivo. Nat Immunol. 2000;1(5):426–32. doi:10.1038/80868.
12. Berard M, Brandt K, Bulfone-Paus S, Tough DF. IL-15 promotes the survival of naive and memory phenotype CD8+ T cells. J Immunol. 2003;170(10):5018–26.
13. Heufler C, Topar G, Grasseger A, Stanzl U, Koch F, Romani N, Namen AE, Schuler G. Interleukin 7 is produced by murine and human keratinocytes. J Exp Med. 1993;178(3): 1109–14.
14. Watanabe M, Ueno Y, Yajima T, Iwao Y, Tsuchiya M, Ishikawa H, Aiso S, Hibi T, Ishii H. Interleukin 7 is produced by human intestinal epithelial cells and regulates the proliferation of intestinal mucosal lymphocytes. J Clin Invest. 1995;95(6):2945–53. doi:10.1172/JCI118002.
15. Sorg RV, McLellan AD, Hock BD, Fearnley DB, Hart DN. Human dendritic cells express functional interleukin-7. Immunobiology. 1998;198(5):514–26. doi:10.1016/S0171-2985(98)80075-2.
16. Kieper WCW, Tan JTJ, Bondi-Boyd BB, Gapin LL, Sprent JJ, Ceredig RR, Surh CDC. Overexpression of interleukin (IL)-7 leads to IL-15-independent generation of memory phenotype CD8+ T cells. J Exp Med. 2002;195(12):1533–9.
17. Jacobs SR, Michalek RD, Rathmell JC. IL-7 is essential for homeostatic control of T cell metabolism in vivo. J Immunol. 2010;184(7):3461–9. doi:10.4049/jimmunol.0902593.
18. Dai Z, Lakkis FG. Cutting edge: secondary lymphoid organs are essential for maintaining the CD4, but not CD8, naive T cell pool. J Immunol. 2001;167(12):6711–5.
19. Link A, Vogt TK, Favre S, Britschgi MR, Acha-Orbea H, Hinz B, Cyster JG, Luther SA. Fibroblastic reticular cells in lymph nodes regulate the homeostasis of naive T cells. Nat Immunol. 2007;8(11):1255–65. doi:10.1038/ni1513.
20. Park J-H, Yu Q, Erman B, Appelbaum JS, Montoya-Durango D, Grimes HL, Singer A. Suppression of IL7Ralpha transcription by IL-7 and other prosurvival cytokines: a novel mechanism for maximizing IL-7-dependent T cell survival. Immunity. 2004;21(2):289–302. doi:10.1016/j.immuni.2004.07.016.
21. Kim KK, Lee CKC, Sayers TJT, Muegge KK, Durum SKS. The trophic action of IL-7 on pro-T cells: inhibition of apoptosis of pro-T1, -T2, and -T3 cells correlates with Bcl-2 and Bax levels and is independent of Fas and p53 pathways. J Immunol. 1998;160(12):5735–41.
22. Li WQ, Jiang Q, Khaled AR, Keller JR, Durum SK. Interleukin-7 inactivates the pro-apoptotic protein Bad promoting T cell survival. J Biol Chem. 2004;279(28):29160–6. doi:10.1074/jbc.M401656200.
23. Carrette F, Surh CD. IL-7 signaling and CD127 receptor regulation in the control of T cell homeostasis. Semin Immunol. 2012;24(3):209–17. doi:10.1016/j.smim.2012.04.010.
24. Wofford JA, Wieman HL, Jacobs SR, Zhao Y, Rathmell JC. IL-7 promotes Glut1 trafficking and glucose uptake via STAT5-mediated activation of Akt to support T-cell survival. Blood. 2008;111(4):2101–11. doi:10.1182/blood-2007-06-096297.
25. Rathmell JC, Farkash EA, Gao W, Thompson CB. IL-7 enhances the survival and maintains the size of naive T cells. J Immunol. 2001;167(12):6869–76.
26. Tough DFD, Sprent JJ. Turnover of naive- and memory-phenotype T cells. J Exp Med. 1994;179(4):1127–35.
27. Murali-Krishna K, Lau LL, Sambhara S, Lemonnier F, Altman J, Ahmed R. Persistence of memory CD8 T cells in MHC class I-deficient mice. Science. 1999;286(5443):1377–81.
28. Judge AD, Zhang X, Fujii H, Surh CD, Sprent J. Interleukin 15 controls both proliferation and survival of a subset of memory-phenotype CD8(+) T cells. J Exp Med. 2002; 196(7):935–46.
29. Becker TC, Wherry EJ, Boone D, Murali-Krishna K, Antia R, Ma A, Ahmed R. Interleukin 15 is required for proliferative renewal of virus-specific memory CD8 T cells. J Exp Med. 2002;195(12):1541–8.

30. Boyman O, Purton JF, Surh CD, Sprent J. Cytokines and T-cell homeostasis. Curr Opin Immunol. 2007;19(3):320–6. doi:10.1016/j.coi.2007.04.015.
31. Kennedy MKM, Glaccum MM, Brown SNS, et al. Reversible defects in natural killer and memory CD8 T cell lineages in interleukin 15-deficient mice. J Exp Med. 2000;191(5): 771–80.
32. Lenz DC, Kurz SK, Lemmens E, Schoenberger SP, Sprent J, Oldstone MBA, Homann D. IL-7 regulates basal homeostatic proliferation of antiviral CD4+T cell memory. Proc Natl Acad Sci U S A. 2004;101(25):9357–62. doi:10.1073/pnas.0400640101.
33. Jameson S. Maintaining the norm: T-cell homeostasis. Nat Rev Immunol. 2002;2:547–56. doi:10.1083/nri853.
34. Surh CD, Sprent J. Regulation of naïve and memory T-cell homeostasis. Microbes Infect. 2002;4(1):51–6.
35. Tanchot C, Le Campion A, Martin B, Léaument S, Dautigny N, Lucas B. Conversion of naive T cells to a memory-like phenotype in lymphopenic hosts is not related to a homeostatic mechanism that fills the peripheral naive T cell pool. J Immunol. 2002;168(10):5042–6.
36. Goldrath AW, Bogatzki LY, Bevan MJ. Naive T cells transiently acquire a memory-like phenotype during homeostasis-driven proliferation. J Exp Med. 2000;192(4):557–64.
37. Gudmundsdottir H, Turka LA. A closer look at homeostatic proliferation of CD4+ T cells: costimulatory requirements and role in memory formation. J Immunol. 2001;167(7): 3699–707.
38. Ge Q, Rao VP, Cho BK, Eisen HN, Chen J. Dependence of lymphopenia-induced T cell proliferation on the abundance of peptide/ MHC epitopes and strength of their interaction with T cell receptors. Proc Natl Acad Sci U S A. 2001;98(4):1728–33. doi:10.1073/pnas.98.4.1728.
39. Kieper WC, Burghardt JT, Surh CD. A role for TCR affinity in regulating naive T cell homeostasis. J Immunol. 2004;172(1):40–4.
40. Mackall CL, Bare CV, Granger LA, Sharrow SO, Titus JA, Gress RE. Thymic-independent T cell regeneration occurs via antigen-driven expansion of peripheral T cells resulting in a repertoire that is limited in diversity and prone to skewing. J Immunol. 1996;156(12): 4609–16.
41. Freitas AAA, Agenes FF, Coutinho GCG. Cellular competition modulates survival and selection of CD8+ T cells. Eur J Immunol. 1996;26(11):2640–9. doi:10.1002/eji.1830261115.
42. Gruta N, Driel IR, Gleeson PA. Peripheral T cell expansion in lymphopenic mice results in a restricted T cell repertoire. Eur J Immunol. 2000;30(12):3380–6.
43. Kassiotis G, Zamoyska R, Stockinger B. Involvement of avidity for major histocompatibility complex in homeostasis of naive and memory T cells. J Exp Med. 2003;197(8):1007–16. doi:10.1084/jem.20021812.
44. Troy AE, Shen H. Cutting edge: homeostatic proliferation of peripheral T lymphocytes is regulated by clonal competition. J Immunol. 2003;170(2):672–6.
45. Moses CTC, Thorstenson KMK, Jameson SCS, Khoruts AA. Competition for self ligands restrains homeostatic proliferation of naive CD4 T cells. Proc Natl Acad Sci U S A. 2003;100(3):1185–90. doi:10.2307/3138307.
46. Annacker O, Pimenta-Araujo R, Burlen-Defranoux O, Barbosa TC, Cumano A, Bandeira A. CD25+ CD4+ T cells regulate the expansion of peripheral CD4 T cells through the production of IL-10. J Immunol. 2001;166(5):3008–18.
47. Almeida ARM, Legrand N, Papiernik M, Freitas AA. Homeostasis of peripheral CD4+ T cells: IL-2R alpha and IL-2 shape a population of regulatory cells that controls CD4+ T cell numbers. J Immunol. 2002;169(9):4850–60.
48. Shen S. Control of homeostatic proliferation by regulatory T cells. J Clin Invest. 2005;115(12):3517–26. doi:10.1172/JCI25463DS1.
49. Tivol EAE, Borriello FF, Schweitzer ANA, Lynch WPW, Bluestone JAJ, Sharpe AHA. Loss of CTLA-4 leads to massive lymphoproliferation and fatal multiorgan tissue destruction, revealing a critical negative regulatory role of CTLA-4. Immunity. 1995;3(5):541–7. doi:10.1016/1074-7613(95)90125-6.

50. Lucas PJ, Kim SJ, Melby SJ, Gress RE. Disruption of T cell homeostasis in mice expressing a T cell-specific dominant negative transforming growth factor beta II receptor. J Exp Med. 2000;191(7):1187–96.
51. Workman CJ, Vignali DAA. Negative regulation of T cell homeostasis by lymphocyte activation gene-3 (CD223). J Immunol. 2005;174(2):688–95.
52. Theofilopoulos AN, Dummer W, Kono DH. T cell homeostasis and systemic autoimmunity. J Clin Invest. 2001;108(3):335–40. doi:10.1172/JCI12173.
53. McHugh RS, Shevach EM. Cutting edge: depletion of CD4+CD25+ regulatory T cells is necessary, but not sufficient, for induction of organ-specific autoimmune disease. J Immunol. 2002;168(12):5979–83.
54. Goronzy JJ, Weyand CM. Thymic function and peripheral T-cell homeostasis in rheumatoid arthritis. Trends Immunol. 2001;22(5):251–5.
55. Morrissey PJ, Charrier K, Braddy S, Liggitt D, Watson JD. CD4+ T cells that express high levels of CD45RB induce wasting disease when transferred into congenic severe combined immunodeficient mice. Disease development is prevented by cotransfer of purified CD4+ T cells. J Exp Med. 1993;178(1):237–44.
56. Nishizuka Y, Sakakura T. Thymus and reproduction: sex-linked dysgenesia of the gonad after neonatal thymectomy in mice. Science. 1969;166(3906):753–5. doi:10.1126/science.166.3906.753.
57. Kojima A, Taguchi O, Nishizuka Y. Experimental production of possible autoimmune castritis followed by macrocytic anemia in athymic nude mice. Lab Invest. 1980;42(4):387–95.
58. Sakaguchi S, Sakaguchi N, Asano M, Itoh M, Toda M. Immunologic self-tolerance maintained by activated T cells expressing IL-2 receptor alpha-chains (CD25). Breakdown of a single mechanism of self-tolerance causes various autoimmune diseases. J Immunol. 1995;155(3):1151–64.
59. Asano M, Toda M, Sakaguchi N, Sakaguchi S. Autoimmune disease as a consequence of developmental abnormality of a T cell subpopulation. J Exp Med. 1996;184(2):387–96.
60. Sakaguchi N, Miyai K, Sakaguchi S. Ionizing radiation and autoimmunity. Induction of autoimmune disease in mice by high dose fractionated total lymphoid irradiation and its prevention by inoculating normal T cells. J Immunol. 1994;152(5):2586–95.
61. Paulos CM, Wrzesinski C, Kaiser A, et al. Microbial translocation augments the function of adoptively transferred self/tumor-specific CD8+ T cells via TLR4 signaling. J Clin Invest. 2007;117(8):2197–204. doi:10.1172/JCI32205.
62. Eyrich M, Burger G, Marquardt K, Budach W, Schilbach K, Niethammer D, Schlegel PG. Sequential expression of adhesion and costimulatory molecules in graft-versus-host disease target organs after murine bone marrow transplantation across minor histocompatibility antigen barriers. Biol Blood Marrow Transplant. 2005;11(5):371–82. doi:10.1016/j.bbmt.2005.02.002.
63. Mitchison NAN. Adoptive transfer of immune reactions by cells. J Cell Physiol Suppl. 1957;50 Suppl 1:247–64.
64. North R. Cyclophosphamide-facilitated adoptive immunotherapy of an established tumor depends on elimination of tumor-induced suppressor T cells. J Exp Med. 1982;55:1063–74.
65. Berenson JRJ, Einstein ABA, Fefer AA. Syngeneic adoptive immunotherapy and chemoimmunotherapy of a Friend leukemia: requirement for T cells. J Immunol. 1975;115(1):234–8.
66. Cheever MA, Greenberg PD, Fefer A. Specificity of adoptive chemoimmunotherapy of established syngeneic tumors. J Immunol. 1980;125(2):711–4.
67. Cheever MA, Greenberg PD, Fefer A. Tumor neutralization, immunotherapy, and chemoimmunotherapy of a Friend leukemia with cells secondarily sensitized in vitro: II. Comparison of cells cultured with and without tumor to noncultured immune cells. J Immunol. 1978;121(6):2220–7.
68. Awwad M, North RJ. Cyclophosphamide (Cy)-facilitated adoptive immunotherapy of a Cy-resistant tumour. Evidence that Cy permits the expression of adoptive T-cell mediated immunity by removing suppressor T cells rather than by reducing tumour burden. Immunology. 1988;65(1):87–92.

69. Machiels JP, Reilly RT, Emens LA, Ercolini AM, Lei RY, Weintraub D, Okoye FI, Jaffee EM. Cyclophosphamide, doxorubicin, and paclitaxel enhance the antitumor immune response of granulocyte/macrophage-colony stimulating factor-secreting whole-cell vaccines in HER-2/neu tolerized mice. Cancer Res. 2001;61(9):3689–97.
70. Motoyoshi Y, Kaminoda K, Saitoh O, Hamasaki K, Nakao K, Ishii N, Nagayama Y, Eguchi K. Different mechanisms for anti-tumor effects of low- and high-dose cyclophosphamide. Oncol Rep. 2006;16(1):141–6.
71. Hu H-M, Poehlein CH, Urba WJ, Fox BA. Development of antitumor immune responses in reconstituted lymphopenic hosts. Cancer Res. 2002;62(14):3914–9.
72. Dummer WW, Niethammer AGA, Baccala RR, Lawson BRB, Wagner NN, Reisfeld RAR, Theofilopoulos ANA. T cell homeostatic proliferation elicits effective antitumor autoimmunity. J Clin Invest. 2002;110(2):185–92. doi:10.1172/JCI15175.
73. Ma J, Urba WJ, Si L, Wang Y, Fox BA, Hu H-M. Anti-tumor T cell response and protective immunity in mice that received sublethal irradiation and immune reconstitution. Eur J Immunol. 2003;33(8):2123–32. doi:10.1002/eji.200324034.
74. Poehlein CH, Haley DP, Walker EB, Fox BA. Depletion of tumor-induced Treg prior to reconstitution rescues enhanced priming of tumor-specific, therapeutic effector T cells in lymphopenic hosts. Eur J Immunol. 2009;39(11):3121–33. doi:10.1002/eji.200939453.
75. Turk MJ, Guevara-Patiño JA, Rizzuto GA, Engelhorn ME, Houghton AN. Concomitant tumor immunity to a poorly immunogenic melanoma is prevented by regulatory T cells. J Exp Med. 2004;200(6):771–82. doi:10.1084/jem.20041130.
76. Rosenberg SA, Spiess P, Lafreniere R. A new approach to the adoptive immunotherapy of cancer with tumor-infiltrating lymphocytes. Science. 1986;233(4770):1318–21.
77. Gattinoni L, Finkelstein SE, Klebanoff CA, et al. Removal of homeostatic cytokine sinks by lymphodepletion enhances the efficacy of adoptively transferred tumor-specific CD8+ T cells. J Exp Med. 2005;202(7):907–12. doi:10.1084/jem.20050732.
78. Wang LX. Interleukin-7-dependent expansion and persistence of melanoma-specific T cells in lymphodepleted mice lead to tumor regression and editing. Cancer Res. 2005;65(22): 10569–77. doi:10.1158/0008-5472.CAN-05-2117.
79. Antony PA, Piccirillo CA, Akpinarli A, et al. CD8+ T cell immunity against a tumor/self-antigen is augmented by CD4+ T helper cells and hindered by naturally occurring T regulatory cells. J Immunol. 2005;174(5):2591–601.
80. Zhang H, Chua KS, Guimond M, et al. Lymphopenia and interleukin-2 therapy alter homeostasis of CD4+CD25+ regulatory T cells. Nat Med. 2005;11(11):1238–43. doi:10.1038/nm1312.
81. Wrzesinski C, Paulos CM, Gattinoni L, Palmer DC, Kaiser A, Yu Z, Rosenberg SA, Restifo NP. Hematopoietic stem cells promote the expansion and function of adoptively transferred antitumor CD8 T cells. J Clin Invest. 2007;117(2):492–501. doi:10.1172/JCI30414.
82. Wrzesinski C, Paulos CM, Kaiser A, Muranski P, Palmer DC, Gattinoni L, Yu Z, Rosenberg SA, Restifo NP. Increased intensity lymphodepletion enhances tumor treatment efficacy of adoptively transferred tumor-specific T cells. J Immunother. 2010;33(1):1–7. doi:10.1097/CJI.0b013e3181b88ffc.
83. Lorenzi AR, Clarke AM, Wooldridge T, Waldmann H, Hale G, Symmons D, Hazleman BL, Isaacs JD. Morbidity and mortality in rheumatoid arthritis patients with prolonged therapy-induced lymphopenia: twelve-year outcomes. Arthritis Rheum. 2008;58(2):370–5. doi:10.1002/art.23122.
84. Mackall CL, Fleisher TA, Brown MR, Magrath IT, Shad AT, Horowitz ME, Wexler LH, Adde MA, McClure LL, Gress RE. Lymphocyte depletion during treatment with intensive chemotherapy for cancer. Blood. 1994;84(7):2221–8.
85. Storek J, Gooley T, Witherspoon RP, Sullivan KM, Storb R. Infectious morbidity in long-term survivors of allogeneic marrow transplantation is associated with low CD4 T cell counts. Am J Hematol. 1997;54(2):131–8. doi:10.1002/(SICI)1096-8652(199702)54:2<131::AID-AJH6>3.0.CO;2-Y.

86. Fry TJ, Connick E, Falloon J, et al. A potential role for interleukin-7 in T-cell homeostasis. Blood. 2001;97(10):2983–90. doi:10.1182/blood.V97.10.2983.
87. Cui Y, Zhang H, Meadors J, Poon R, Guimond M, Mackall CL. Harnessing the physiology of lymphopenia to support adoptive immunotherapy in lymphoreplete hosts. Blood. 2009;114(18):3831–40. doi:10.1182/blood-2009-03-212134.
88. Fife BT, Pauken KE, Eagar TN, Obu T, Wu J, Tang Q, Azuma M, Krummel MF, Bluestone JA. Interactions between PD-1 and PD-L1 promote tolerance by blocking the TCR–induced stop signal. Nat Immunol. 2009;10(11):1185–92. doi:10.1038/ni.1790.
89. Woo S-R, Turnis ME, Goldberg MV, et al. Immune inhibitory molecules LAG-3 and PD-1 synergistically regulate T-cell function to promote tumoral immune escape. Cancer Res. 2012. doi:10.1158/0008-5472.CAN-11-1620.
90. Dudley ME, Wunderlich JR, Robbins PF, Yang JC, Hwu P, Schwartzentruber DJ, Topalian SL, Sherry R, Restifo NP, Hubicki AM, Robinson MR, Raffeld M, Duray P, Seipp CA, Rogers-Freezer L, Morton KE, Mavroukakis SA, White DE, Rosenberg SA. Cancer regression and autoimmunity in patients after clonal repopulation with antitumor lymphocytes. Science. 2002;298(5594):850–4. doi:10.1126/science.1076514 1076514 [pii].
91. Rosenberg SA, Restifo NP, Yang JC, Morgan RA, Dudley ME. Adoptive cell transfer: a clinical path to effective cancer immunotherapy. Nat Rev Cancer. 2008;8(4):299–308. doi:nrc2355 [pii] 10.1038/nrc2355.
92. Dudley ME, Wunderlich JR, Yang JC, Hwu P, Schwartzentruber DJ, Topalian SL, Sherry RM, Marincola FM, Leitman SF, Seipp CA, Rogers-Freezer L, Morton KE, Nahvi A, Mavroukakis SA, White DE, Rosenberg SA. A phase I study of nonmyeloablative chemotherapy and adoptive transfer of autologous tumor antigen-specific T lymphocytes in patients with metastatic melanoma. J Immunother. 2002;25(3):243–51.
93. Dudley ME, Wunderlich JR, Yang JC, Sherry RM, Topalian SL, Restifo NP, Royal RE, Kammula U, White DE, Mavroukakis SA, Rogers LJ, Gracia GJ, Jones SA, Mangiameli DP, Pelletier MM, Gea-Banacloche J, Robinson MR, Berman DM, Filie AC, Abati A, Rosenberg SA. Adoptive cell transfer therapy following non-myeloablative but lymphodepleting chemotherapy for the treatment of patients with refractory metastatic melanoma. J Clin Oncol. 2005;23(10):2346–57. doi:23/10/2346 [pii] 10.1200/JCO.2005.00.240.
94. Hoffmann G, Schobersberger W. Anti-inflammatory and nitric oxide-inhibiting properties of granulocyte colony-stimulating factor. Zhongguo Yao Li Xue Bao. 1999;20(8):673–81.
95. Zhou J, Shen X, Huang J, Hodes RJ, Rosenberg SA, Robbins PF. Telomere length of transferred lymphocytes correlates with in vivo persistence and tumor regression in melanoma patients receiving cell transfer therapy. J Immunol. 2005;175(10):7046–52. doi:175/10/7046 [pii].
96. Dudley ME, Gross CA, Langhan MM, Garcia MR, Sherry RM, Yang JC, Phan GQ, Kammula US, Hughes MS, Citrin DE, Restifo NP, Wunderlich JR, Prieto PA, Hong JJ, Langan RC, Zlott DA, Morton KE, White DE, Laurencot CM, Rosenberg SA. CD8+ enriched "young" tumor infiltrating lymphocytes can mediate regression of metastatic melanoma. Clin Cancer Res. 2010;16(24):6122–31. doi:1078–0432.CCR-10-1297 [pii] 10.1158/1078-0432.CCR-10-1297.
97. Berd D, Mastrangelo MJ, Engstrom PF, Paul A, Maguire H. Augmentation of the human immune response by cyclophosphamide. Cancer Res. 1982;42(11):4862–6.
98. Berd D, Maguire Jr HC, Mastrangelo MJ. Induction of cell-mediated immunity to autologous melanoma cells and regression of metastases after treatment with a melanoma cell vaccine preceded by cyclophosphamide. Cancer Res. 1986;46(5):2572–7.
99. Freireich EJ, Gehan EA, Rall DP, Schmidt LH, Skipper HE. Quantitative comparison of toxicity of anticancer agents in mouse, rat, hamster, dog, monkey, and man. Cancer Chemother Rep. 1966;50(4):219–44.
100. Appay V, Voelter V, Rufer N, Reynard S, Jandus C, Gasparini D, Lienard D, Speiser DE, Schneider P, Cerottini JC, Romero P, Leyvraz S. Combination of transient lymphodepletion with busulfan and fludarabine and peptide vaccination in a phase I clinical trial for patients with advanced melanoma. J Immunother. 2007;30(2):240–50. doi:10.1097/01.cji.0000211332.68643.98 00002371-200702000-00011 [pii].

101. Laurent J, Speiser DE, Appay V, Touvrey C, Vicari M, Papaioannou A, Canellini G, Rimoldi D, Rufer N, Romero P, Leyvraz S, Voelter V. Impact of 3 different short-term chemotherapy regimens on lymphocyte-depletion and reconstitution in melanoma patients. J Immunother. 2010;33(7):723–34. doi:10.1097/CJI.0b013e3181ea7e6e.
102. Zippelius A, Pittet MJ, Batard P, Rufer N, de Smedt M, Guillaume P, Ellefsen K, Valmori D, Lienard D, Plum J, MacDonald HR, Speiser DE, Cerottini JC, Romero P. Thymic selection generates a large T cell pool recognizing a self-peptide in humans. J Exp Med. 2002;195(4): 485–94.
103. Jaffee EM, Hruban RH, Biedrzycki B, Laheru D, Schepers K, Sauter PR, Goemann M, Coleman J, Grochow L, Donehower RC, Lillemoe KD, O'Reilly S, Abrams RA, Pardoll DM, Cameron JL, Yeo CJ. Novel allogeneic granulocyte-macrophage colony-stimulating factor-secreting tumor vaccine for pancreatic cancer: a phase I trial of safety and immune activation. J Clin Oncol. 2001;19(1):145–56.
104. Rapoport AP, Stadtmauer EA, Aqui N, Badros A, Cotte J, Chrisley L, Veloso E, Zheng Z, Westphal S, Mair R, Chi N, Ratterree B, Pochran MF, Natt S, Hinkle J, Sickles C, Sohal A, Ruehle K, Lynch C, Zhang L, Porter DL, Luger S, Guo C, Fang HB, Blackwelder W, Hankey K, Mann D, Edelman R, Frasch C, Levine BL, Cross A, June CH. Restoration of immunity in lymphopenic individuals with cancer by vaccination and adoptive T-cell transfer. Nat Med. 2005;11(11):1230–7. doi:nm1310 [pii] 10.1038/nm1310.
105. Gandhi MK, Egner W, Sizer L, Inman I, Zambon M, Craig JI, Marcus RE. Antibody responses to vaccinations given within the first two years after transplant are similar between autologous peripheral blood stem cell and bone marrow transplant recipients. Bone Marrow Transplant. 2001;28(8):775–81. doi:10.1038/sj.bmt.1703239.
106. Guinan EC, Molrine DC, Antin JH, Lee MC, Weinstein HJ, Sallan SE, Parsons SK, Wheeler C, Gross W, McGarigle C, et al. Polysaccharide conjugate vaccine responses in bone marrow transplant patients. Transplantation. 1994;57(5):677–84.
107. Berd D, Sato T, Maguire Jr HC, Kairys J, Mastrangelo MJ. Immunopharmacologic analysis of an autologous, hapten-modified human melanoma vaccine. J Clin Oncol. 2004;22(3):403–15. 10.1200/JCO.2004.06.043 JCO.2004.06.043 [pii].
108. Viguier M, Lemaitre F, Verola O, Cho MS, Gorochov G, Dubertret L, Bachelez H, Kourilsky P, Ferradini L. Foxp3 expressing CD4+CD25(high) regulatory T cells are overrepresented in human metastatic melanoma lymph nodes and inhibit the function of infiltrating T cells. J Immunol. 2004;173(2):1444–53.
109. Wolf AM, Wolf D, Steurer M, Gastl G, Gunsilius E, Grubeck-Loebenstein B. Increase of regulatory T cells in the peripheral blood of cancer patients. Clin Cancer Res. 2003;9(2): 606–12.
110. Audia S, Nicolas A, Cathelin D, Larmonier N, Ferrand C, Foucher P, Fanton A, Bergoin E, Maynadie M, Arnould L, Bateman A, Lorcerie B, Solary E, Chauffert B, Bonnotte B. Increase of CD4+ CD25+ regulatory T cells in the peripheral blood of patients with metastatic carcinoma: a Phase I clinical trial using cyclophosphamide and immunotherapy to eliminate CD4+ CD25+ T lymphocytes. Clin Exp Immunol. 2007;150(3):523–30. doi:CEI3521 [pii] 10.1111/j.1365-2249.2007.03521.x.
111. Ormandy LA, Hillemann T, Wedemeyer H, Manns MP, Greten TF, Korangy F. Increased populations of regulatory T cells in peripheral blood of patients with hepatocellular carcinoma. Cancer Res. 2005;65(6):2457–64. doi:65/6/2457 [pii] 10.1158/0008-5472.CAN-04-3232.
112. Somasundaram R, Jacob L, Swoboda R, Caputo L, Song H, Basak S, Monos D, Peritt D, Marincola F, Cai D, Birebent B, Bloome E, Kim J, Berencsi K, Mastrangelo M, Herlyn D. Inhibition of cytolytic T lymphocyte proliferation by autologous CD4+/CD25+ regulatory T cells in a colorectal carcinoma patient is mediated by transforming growth factor-beta. Cancer Res. 2002;62(18):5267–72.
113. Liyanage UK, Moore TT, Joo HG, Tanaka Y, Herrmann V, Doherty G, Drebin JA, Strasberg SM, Eberlein TJ, Goedegebuure PS, Linehan DC. Prevalence of regulatory T cells is increased in peripheral blood and tumor microenvironment of patients with pancreas or breast adenocarcinoma. J Immunol. 2002;169(5):2756–61.

114. Petrausch U, Poehlein CH, Jensen SM, Twitty C, Thompson JA, Assmann I, Puri S, LaCelle MG, Moudgil T, Maston L, Friedman K, Church S, Cardenas E, Haley DP, Walker EB, Akporiaye E, Weinberg AD, Rosenheim S, Crocenzi TS, Hu HM, Curti BD, Urba WJ, Fox BA. Cancer immunotherapy: the role regulatory T cells play and what can be done to overcome their inhibitory effects. Curr Mol Med. 2009;9(6):673–82.
115. Powell Jr DJ, de Vries CR, Allen T, Ahmadzadeh M, Rosenberg SA. Inability to mediate prolonged reduction of regulatory T Cells after transfer of autologous CD25-depleted PBMC and interleukin-2 after lymphodepleting chemotherapy. J Immunother. 2007;30(4):438–47. doi:10.1097/CJI.0b013e3180600ff9 00002371-200705000-00008 [pii].
116. Emens LA, Asquith JM, Leatherman JM, Kobrin BJ, Petrik S, Laiko M, Levi J, Daphtary MM, Biedrzycki B, Wolff AC, Stearns V, Disis ML, Ye X, Piantadosi S, Fetting JH, Davidson NE, Jaffee EM. Timed sequential treatment with cyclophosphamide, doxorubicin, and an allogeneic granulocyte-macrophage colony-stimulating factor-secreting breast tumor vaccine: a chemotherapy dose-ranging factorial study of safety and immune activation. J Clin Oncol. 2009;27(35):5911–8. JCO.2009.23.3494 [pii] 10.1200/JCO.2009.23.3494.
117. Ge Y, Domschke C, Stoiber N, Schott S, Heil J, Rom J, Blumenstein M, Thum J, Sohn C, Schneeweiss A, Beckhove P, Schuetz F. Metronomic cyclophosphamide treatment in metastasized breast cancer patients: immunological effects and clinical outcome. Cancer Immunol Immunother. 2012;61(3):353–62. doi:10.1007/s00262-011-1106-3.
118. Cerullo V, Diaconu I, Kangasniemi L, Rajecki M, Escutenaire S, Koski A, Romano V, Rouvinen N, Tuuminen T, Laasonen L, Partanen K, Kauppinen S, Joensuu T, Oksanen M, Holm SL, Haavisto E, Karioja-Kallio A, Kanerva A, Pesonen S, Arstila PT, Hemminki A. Immunological effects of low-dose cyclophosphamide in cancer patients treated with oncolytic adenovirus. Mol Ther. 2011;19(9):1737–46. doi:10.1038/mt.2011.113 mt2011113 [pii].
119. Dudley ME, Yang JC, Sherry R, Hughes MS, Royal R, Kammula U, Robbins PF, Huang J, Citrin DE, Leitman SF, Wunderlich J, Restifo NP, Thomasian A, Downey SG, Smith FO, Klapper J, Morton K, Laurencot C, White DE, Rosenberg SA. Adoptive cell therapy for patients with metastatic melanoma: evaluation of intensive myeloablative chemoradiation preparative regimens. J Clin Oncol. 2008;26(32):5233–9. doi:JCO.2008.16.5449 [pii] 10.1200/JCO.2008.16.5449.
120. Ljungman P, Wiklund-Hammarsten M, Duraj V, Hammarstrom L, Lonnqvist B, Paulin T, Ringden O, Pepe MS, Gahrton G. Response to tetanus toxoid immunization after allogeneic bone marrow transplantation. J Infect Dis. 1990;162(2):496–500.
121. Fridman WH, Pages F, Sautes-Fridman C, Galon J. The immune contexture in human tumours: impact on clinical outcome. Nat Rev Cancer. 2012;12(4):298–306. doi:10.1038/nrc3245 nrc3245 [pii].
122. Jensen SM, Maston LD, Gough MJ, Ruby CE, Redmond WL, Crittenden M, Li Y, Puri S, Poehlein CH, Morris N, Kovacsovics-Bankowski M, Moudgil T, Twitty C, Walker EB, Hu HM, Urba WJ, Weinberg AD, Curti B, Fox BA. Signaling through OX40 enhances antitumor immunity. Semin Oncol. 2010;37(5):524–32. doi:S0093-7754(10)00167-3 [pii] 10.1053/j.seminoncol.2010.09.013.

114. Rupprecht [illegible]
MG, Houn[illegible]
Waterman [illegible]
engineered [illegible]

Adoptive Cell Therapy of Systemic Metastases Using erbB-2-Specific T Cells Redirected with a Chimeric Antibody-Based Receptor

Dinorah Friedmann-Morvinski, Tova Waks, Assaf Marcus, and Zelig Eshhar

Abstract Immunotherapy of cancer using adoptive cell transfer combined with the advent of gene-engineering technologies has become an appealing option for a wide spectrum of cancers. In contrast to T cell receptor-based approaches, which are MHC restricted, chimeric antibody-based receptors (CAR), pioneered by our group, allow for a broader application, which are not restricted to individual tissue types. Here, we describe our studies using T cells redirected with CAR specific to the erbB-2 growth factor proto-oncogene as a common tumor target antigen. In a murine model for lung metastasis, we demonstrate that under defined conditions, CAR-expressing T cells (T-bodies) can eliminate systemic lung metastases, which are generally felt to be incurable. The antitumor effect of systemically injected T-bodies was augmented by using increased injected cell doses and repeated administration cycles as well as by pre-vaccination of the tumor-bearing mice. Most importantly, we were able to establish a protocol enabling the use of MHC mismatched T-bodies in a safe and effective manner. We found that a single dose of allogeneic T-bodies under mild immunosuppressive conditions could cure metastases, demonstrating the efficacy of this modality against disseminated disease. These results provide a proof of principle for using allogeneic erbB-2-specific T-bodies as a standard treatment of erbB-2-expressing tumors.

Supported by DoD BCRP and PCRP, ISF and Moross Center for Cancer Research.

D. Friedmann-Morvinski
Laboratory of Genetics, The Salk Institute for Biological Studies, La Jolla, CA, USA

T. Waks • Z. Eshhar (✉)
Department of Immunology, The Weizmann Institute of Science, P.O.Box 26, Rehovot, Israel, 76100
e-mail: Zelig.eshhar@weizmann.ac.il

A. Marcus
Department of Molecular and Cell Biology, University of California Berkeley, Berkeley, CA, USA

J.D. Rosenblatt et al. (eds.), *Advances in Tumor Immunology and Immunotherapy*, Current Cancer Research, DOI 10.1007/978-1-4614-8809-5_7,
© Springer Science+Business Media New York 2014

Keywords Cancer immunotherapy • Adoptive cell therapy • erbB-2 • Chimeric antigen receptor • Allogeneic

1 Introduction

The immune system is a tightly regulated network that is able to maintain a balance of immune homeostasis under normal physiological conditions. Normally, when challenged with foreign antigen, specific and appropriate responses are initiated that are aimed at restoring homeostasis. However under some circumstances, this balance is not maintained and immune responses either under- or overreact. Cancer is an example of a situation in which the immune response can be inefficient or unresponsive, resulting in uncontrolled growth of the cancer cells. This phenomenon is not fully understood, but much evidence suggests that insufficient number of T cells capable of responding to tumor cells, inadequate avidity of these T cells for tumor antigens, and tolerogenic attenuation or suppression induced by the tumor and/or its microenvironment contribute to this immunological failure [30]. At present, the efficacy of conventional therapies, such as chemo- or radiotherapy is limited, and biological therapies that are focused on utilizing the patient's immune response to his/her own disease appear promising. Following the discovery of the first tumor antigens [36], most of the attempts carried out over the past two decades to enhance the immune system by different modes of active vaccination resulted in a very low frequency of durable complete responses against most cancers [15, 37, 38]. Therefore, attempts in immunotherapy of cancer have shifted to passive vaccination, employing cancer-specific antibodies or T cells. While many antibodies specific to tumor-associated antigens (TAA) were generated and several of these have been humanized and applied to the clinic, the antitumor response of the widely used therapeutic antibodies is limited to "soft tumors" such as lymphomas and leukemias (e.g., anti-CD20, rituximab) or antibodies to functional receptors over-expressed on certain solid tumors that are essential for maintaining the transformed phenotype (e.g., anti-erbB-2, herceptin).

The current challenge in the use of antibodies for the immunotherapy of tumor is to increase their antitumor potency especially towards solid tumors. The other effector arm of adaptive immunity that has also been recruited for cancer treatment is that of T cells. T cells recognize tumors through their T cell receptors (TCR) that can bind with relatively low affinity to MHC-bound peptides on the surface of their target cells. The advantage of T cells for tumor therapy is that they target peptides derived from both membrane-bound and intracellular proteins, in contrast to antibodies, which can only target extracellular epitopes. During the last two decades, T cells specific to various cancers were isolated and propagated from resected tumors (collectively termed tumor-infiltrating lymphocytes (TILs)) and, upon reintroduction to the patient, have proven very effective in curing disseminated tumors (such as metastatic melanoma) that are refractory to all other treatments [27]. However, TILs are highly differentiated cells, and it was shown by Rosenberg et al. [14]

that less differentiated T cells are, in practice, more effective. Additionally, the process of isolating TILs is very time consuming and expensive, and in some cases TILs cannot be obtained at all. In recent years, with the advent of gene-transfer technologies, these problems have been circumvented through ectopic expression in patient-derived T cells of gene pairs of TCR chains that encode receptors specific for a given HLA haplotype and peptide complex. In a number of clinical trials targeting melanoma as well as other cancers, such autologous TCR-transduced T cells have been shown to mediate objective clinical responses [28, 29].

The TIL- and the TCR-modified T cell approach are specific to the individual patient and restricted to a given HLA haplotype. In contrast, chimeric antibody-based receptor (CAR)-redirected T cells (the T-body approach [4, 8, 13]) allow for MHC-unrestricted tumor specificity [9, 10, 12]. In its current form, the CAR encompass an extracellular recognition unit made of a single-chain variable region (scFv) of an antitumor antibody linked to a flexible hinge/spacer domain, a transmembrane canonical motif and intracellular co-stimulatory (e.g., CD28 and/or CD137) domains, and stimulatory (e.g., FcRγ or CD3ζ ITAMs) motifs (for recent reviews see [4, 8, 11]). The modular structure of the CAR allows us to introduce various functional moieties and study their effect on the antitumor responses of CAR-modified T cells (e.g., Syk kinase [6]); the transfected cells ("T-bodies") can persist in vivo for an extended period and maintain their function. So far, our group and others [5, 11, 23, 24] have developed the T-body approach as a powerful tool for cancer immunotherapy, in which the CAR-redirected T cells having antibody-type specificity could respond to a variety of tumors and undergo tumor-specific activation to mediate selective rejection and elimination of their tumor targets both in animal and human.

In this chapter, we describe our studies investigating the antitumor reactivity of T cells in vivo. As a TAA of choice we used erbB-2, a member of the erbB-2 growth factor receptor family that is an attractive target for immunotherapy, not only because it is overexpressed on several tumor types (e.g., breast, prostate, ovarian, bladder, pancreatic, colon [1]), but also because it is a growth factor receptor whose expression is required to maintain the transformed phenotype. Overexpression of erbB-2 is associated with increased tumor aggressiveness, increased rates of recurrence, and increased mortality in most of the cancer patients [2, 20, 32].

We generated transgenic mice expressing an erbB-2-specific CAR under the control of CD2 enhancer/promoter, as previously described [7] using an scFv derived from the N29 mAb [33, 34]. All T cells of these mice expressed the CAR on their surface and have a naïve T cell phenotype in addition to the normal repertoire of TCR. Here, we show that naïve T-bodies derived from erbB-2-specific CAR transgenic (Tg) mice can (1) protect the mice from developing s.c. inoculated tumors, (2) protect the mice from developing systemic lung metastasis, and (3) significantly prolong the survival of allogeneic WT mice bearing lung metastasis by the adoptive transfer of T-bodies from these Tg mice.

Finally, we demonstrate the potential of CAR-modified WT cells by showing that fully MHC-mismatched allogeneic T-body cells can, under the appropriate conditions, provide superior therapeutic benefit as compared to syngeneic T-bodies and even cure some mice bearing established lung metastases [18]. These results demonstrate the utility of allogeneic T-bodies as "universal effector cells," which could potentially be used for "off-the-shelf" immunotherapy of cancer.

2 Results and Discussion

2.1 Phenotypic and Functional Profile of the erbB-2-Specific CAR in Transgenic Mice

To study the antitumor reactivity of naïve unprimed lymphocytes, we generated transgenic mice expressing a chimeric receptor composed of an erbB-2-specific scFv derived from N29 mAb [33] fused to the cytoplasmic domains of CD28 and FcRγ chain (Fig. 1a). The transgenic mice were generated as previously described [7] using the CD2 promoter/enhancer vector [39], directing the expression of the

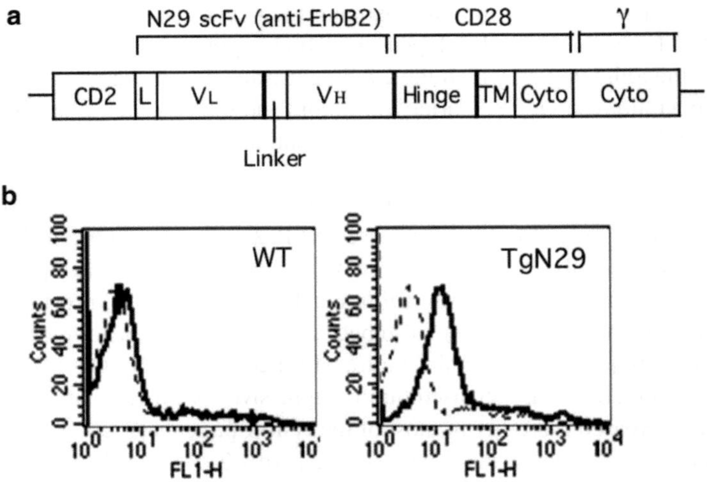

Fig. 1 Expression of erbB-2-specific CAR in transgenic mice. (**a**) *CAR transgene construct*. The construct sequence used to generate the transgenic mice was placed under the control of the human CD2 promoter/enhancer that directs expression only in T and NK cells. Cyto indicates cytoplasmic domain; L, immunoglobulin leader; V_L and V_H, immunoglobulin light- and heavy-chain variable domains, respectively; TM, transmembrane domain. The scFv derived from the anti-erbB-2 mAb, N29, is joined to a portion of the CD28 coding sequence, including its extracellular, transmembrane, and cytoplasmic domains (but lacking the ligand-binding site) fused to the FcRγ chain. (**b**) Surface expression of the CAR in the spleen of transgenic mice. Bulk splenocytes from WT or transgenic mice were double-stained with PE-conjugated rat anti-mouse Thy1.2 and either biotinylated anti-N29 idiotype polyclonal mAb (*bold lines*) or matching biotinylated irrelevant control (*dashed lines*), followed by secondary staining with fluorescein isiothiocyanate (FITC)-conjugated streptavidin. Histograms were generated by gating on Thy1.2$^+$ lymphocytes

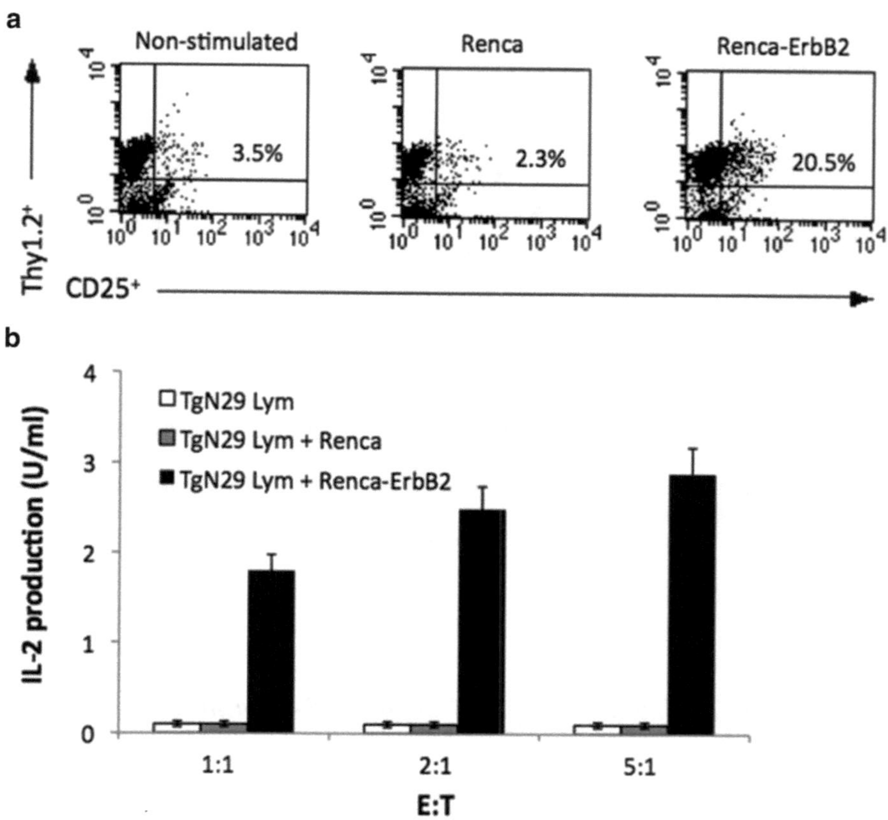

Fig. 2 Stimulation of splenocytes of erbB-2-specific CAR transgenic mice (TgN29). (**a**) Splenocytes from TgN29 mice were co-cultured with the indicated irradiated cell lines. After 48 h, cells were stained with anti-Thy1.2-PE and anti-CD25-biotin followed by streptavidin–FITC and analyzed by flow cytometry. (**b**) IL-2 production in supernatants from the experiment described in (**a**)

CAR in T and NK cells. Splenocytes derived from the transgenic mice express the anti-erbB-2 CAR on practically all T and NK cells as revealed by staining using anti-N29 antibodies (Fig. 1b). A similar pattern was observed in peripheral blood, lymph node, and thymic T cells (not shown). All the T cells of the Tg mice (TgN29) exhibited a naïve phenotype similar to wild-type (WT) mice. The CAR was fully active, as the cells produced IL-2 following incubation with immobilized anti-N29 idiotype antibodies or, when co-cultured with Renca-erbB-2 cells, a spontaneous BALB/c renal carcinoma cell line that was transfected with human erbB-2 [19]. When CAR-expressing splenocytes were co-cultured with Renca-erbB-2 (but not untransfected Renca) cells, a specific and high level of surface CD25 expression was induced, indicating the activation of the transgenic T cells (Fig. 2a). Similarly, elevated levels of IL-2 were secreted into the supernatants (Fig. 2b). All together, these data demonstrate that the CAR expressed in these T cells is indeed functional.

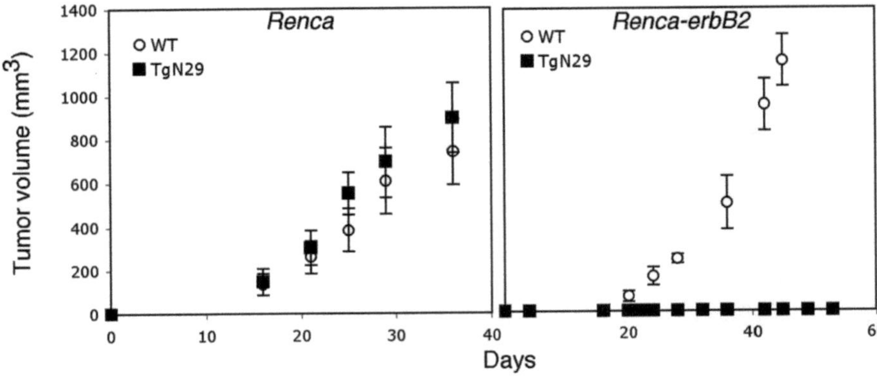

Fig. 3 Prevention of growth of Renca-erbB-2 tumors in TgN29 mice. WT or TgN29 mice ($n=8$) were subcutaneously injected s.c. in the flank with either Renca (*left graph*) or Renca-erbB-2 (*right graph*) tumor cells (5×10^6 cells), and tumor growth was followed. TgN29 injected with Renca-erbB-2 tumor cells did not develop tumors and survived until the end of the experiment (day 120). Results represent the mean size (mm^3) ± SEM of the primary tumor and are representative of two experiments

2.2 Naïve TgN29 Mice Reject Renca-erbB-2 Tumors

To assess the antitumor response of the TgN29 mice, unprimed WT and TgN29 mice were subcutaneously (s.c.) inoculated with either Renca-erbB-2 or Renca cells. As shown in Fig. 3, there was no difference between WT and TgN29 mice, as both developed tumors to a similar extent when inoculated with the parental Renca cells. Similarly, Renca-erbB-2 cells formed tumors in the WT mice. On the other hand, when TgN29 mice were injected with Renca-erbB-2, all the mice completely rejected the erbB-2 tumor cells and remained without evidence of disease for 6 months.

To demonstrate the ability of erbB-2 CAR-specific transgenic (Tg) cells to protect the mice against systemic metastasis formation, we i.v. inoculated Renca-erbB-2 cells to TgN29, WT, and TNP-specific CAR Tg mice (irrelevant specificity control) [7]. In this system, as well, all the TgN29 lungs were free of metastases, while the WT and irrelevant CAR control mice (Tg 8.7) developed pulmonary metastases (Fig. 4a). This observation was confirmed by histopathological examination and weight of the lungs (Fig. 4a, b). As shown above in the subcutaneous model (Fig. 3), parental Renca cells (not expressing erbB-2) injected into WT and TgN29 mice led to a high number of pulmonary metastases (Fig. 4a, b). In contrast, TgN29 mice inoculated i.v. with Renca-erbB-2 survived for at least 6 months (Fig. 4c).

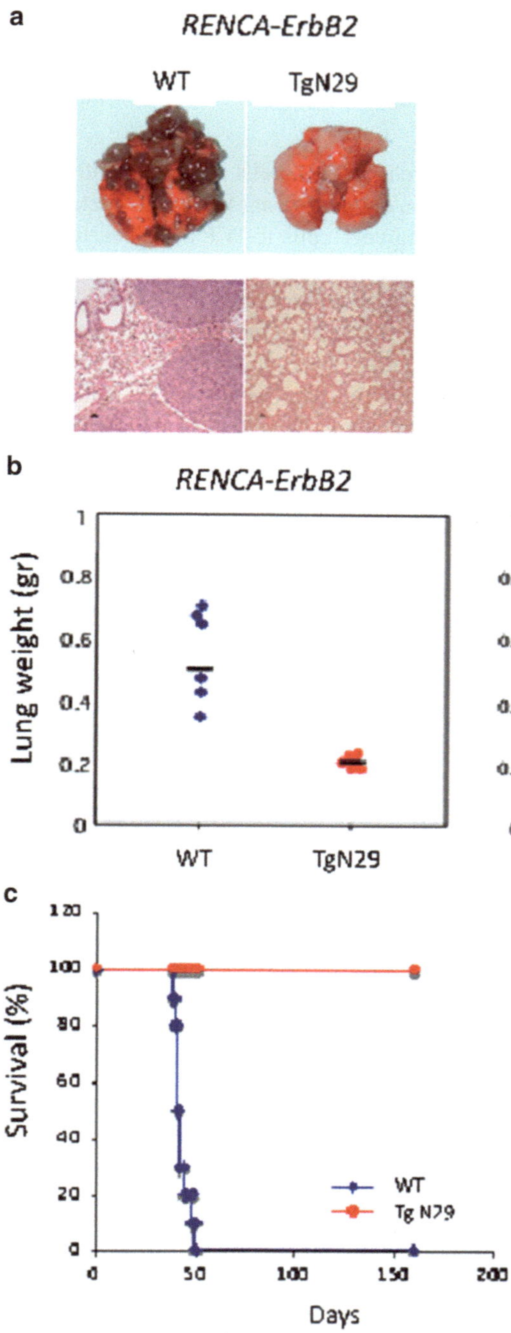

Fig. 4 Rejection of Renca-erbB-2 tumors in TgN29 compared to wild-type mice. (**a**) WT or transgenic mice ($n = 8$) were injected i.v. with 1×10^5 of either Renca or Renca-erbB-2 tumor cells. After approximately 1 month, all the mice were sacrificed and the lungs were isolated. The *lower panel* shows histology of lung sections by hematoxylin and eosin staining. (**b**) Whole lung weight from the WT (*left*) and transgenic (*right*) mice. (**c**) Survival of WT and TgN29 mice injected i.v. with Renca-erbB-2 cells. Results are representative of two experiments

2.3 Adoptive Transfer of Naïve Lymphocytes from TgN29 Mice Extends the Survival of Mice with Systemic Lung Metastases

The most important clinical application of redirected T cells is in the treatment of metastatic disease. To mimic the potential clinical treatment of systemic metastases, we administered different doses of TgN29 naïve T cells to WT mice bearing lung micrometastases. Mice were sublethally irradiated (2 Gy) 1 day before i.v. injection of TgN29 splenocytes (either one or three doses) derived from naïve TgN29 mice. Chest radiographs of two representative mice from each group at day 45 are shown in Fig. 5a. The survival curve derived from this experiment (Fig. 5b) shows that three consecutive administrations of 10×10^6 Tg lymphocytes significantly prolonged survival of the mice. In an attempt to extend the effect of the Tg lymphocytes, this experiment was repeated, and a second course of administration of lymphoyctes was given close to the death of the control group (Fig. 5c). Importantly, the repeated administration of T-bodies extended the median survival time (T_{50}) by twofold.

We next tested whether specific immunization of the recipient mice with killed tumor cells could synergize with the T-body function and thus improve their antitumor activity. As shown in Fig. 6, tumor-free survival was extended for mice that were pre-immunized with irradiated Renca or Renca-erbB-2 cells. Since, in practice, T-bodies for clinical use are prepared by the transduction of the patient's own T cells, a procedure that requires activation of the cells before gene transfer, we tested the effect of pre-activation of the naïve T-bodies before their transfer to the mice. The data presented in Fig. 6 demonstrate that this procedure enhanced the antitumor effect. The process of pre-activation of the T-bodies was required in the case of naïve cells taken from the CAR-transgenic mice in order to compare their activity to CAR-transduced T-bodies that undergo activation with anti-CD3 and CD-28 antibodies to allow their transduction with retro vector.

2.4 Redirected Allogeneic T Cells (Allo-T-Bodies) as Potential Universal Donors

Recent clinical trials have demonstrated that T-bodies can be very effective against various cancers [25, 26]. However, these trials relied on using autologous T cells taken from the patient, transduced with a CAR, and then reinfused to the patient. Relying on autologous T cells is both logistically and economically challenging; we therefore sought a source of T cells that could serve as a universal donor after its modification with CAR. While analyzing different options, we suggested that under conditions of transient lymphodepletion, allogeneic T-bodies could have sufficient time to attack and destroy the tumor before being themselves rejected [18].

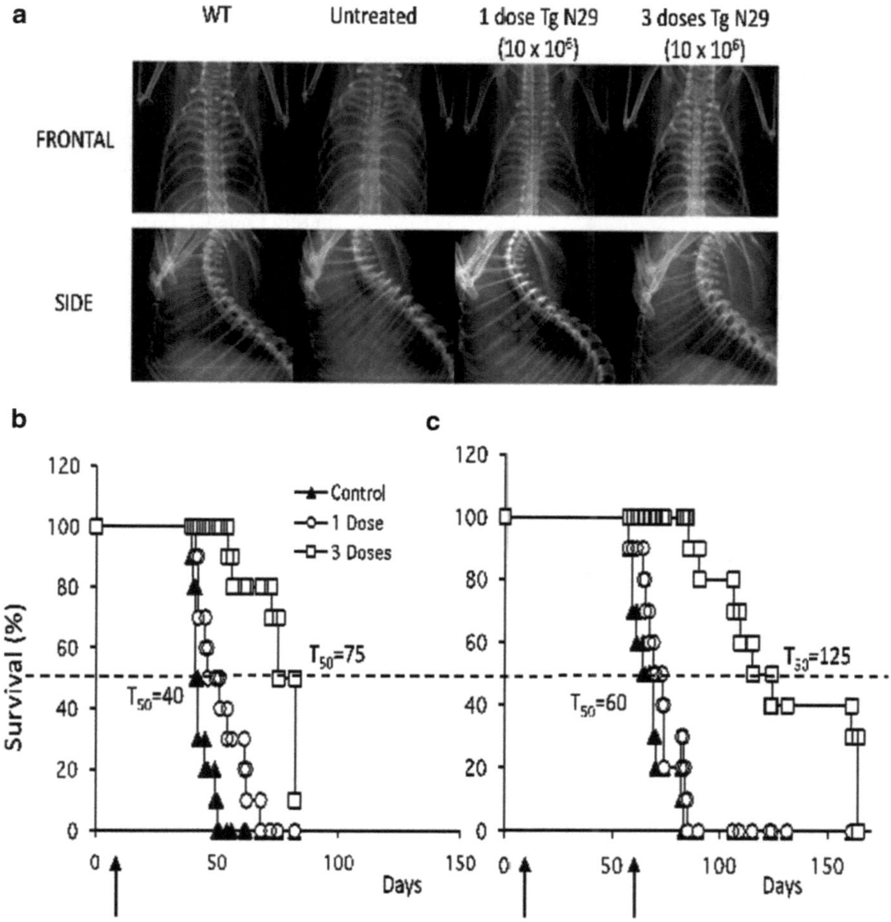

Fig. 5 Growth arrest of lung metastases by adoptive transfer of erbB-2-T-bodies. BALB/c mice ($n=10$ per group) were injected i.v. with 1×10^5 Renca-erbB-2 tumor cells. (**a**) X-ray analysis 40 days after tumor inoculation. The *first column* shows normal lungs in WT mouse. *Second*, "Untreated" mice were injected with Renca-erbB-2 tumor cells only. The *last two columns* were systemically injected with one or three doses of TgN29 cells. (**b**) Survival of mice bearing lung metastases treated i.v. with increasing split doses (three consecutive daily injections) of 1×10^7 TgN29 lymphocytes or medium. All the mice were preconditioned 24 h before the adoptive transfer by a sublethal irradiation (2 Gy). The treated mice received IL-2 (2,000 U, daily) i.p. for 10 days. (**c**) Survival of mice injected i.v. with a second course of three split doses of 1×10^7 TgN29 lymphocytes (*arrows*). In this experiment, all the mice were preconditioned using a combination of sublethal irradiation and cyclophosphamide (200 mg/kg)

The transient persistence of such allogeneic T-bodies would also ensure that no serious graft-versus-host disease (GvHD) would develop. Our initial attempts along this line [18] taught us that a balance between the size of the therapeutic dose of allo-T-bodies and the immunosuppressive regimen can be achieved to create such a therapeutic time window. This assumes that the initial dose of the T-bodies is

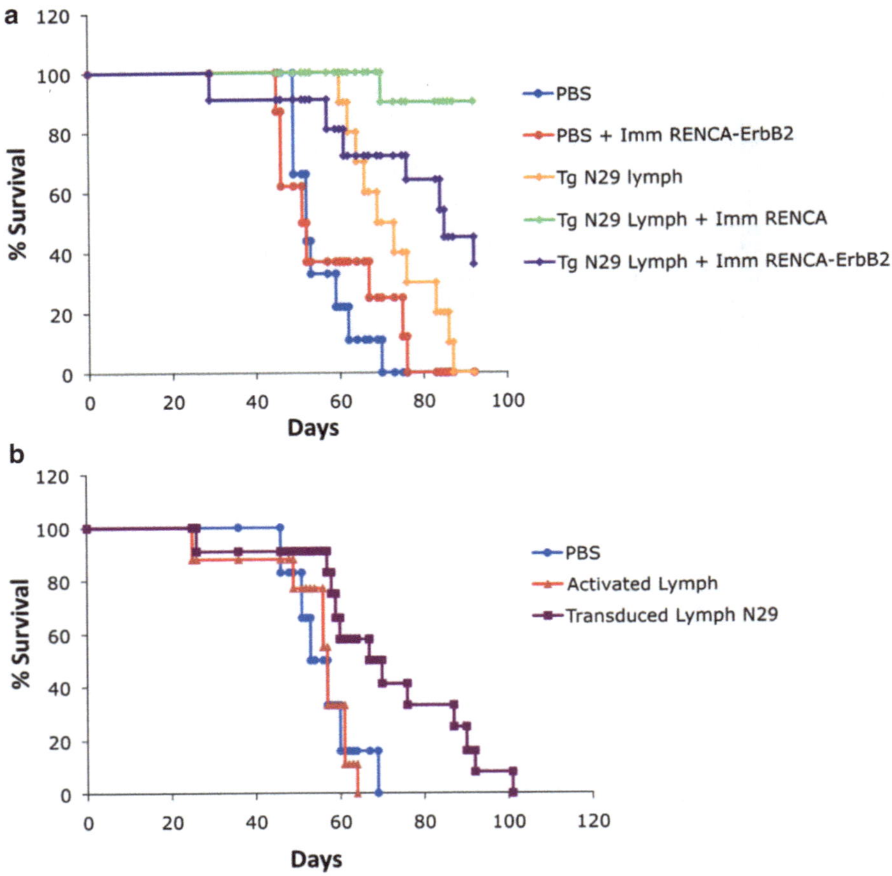

Fig. 6 Pre-immunization of tumor-bearing mice and pre-stimulation of naïve T-bodies enhance the antitumor responses. Balb/c mice bearing Renca-erbB-2 lung metastases were irradiated (2 Gy) and were (**a**) left untreated as a control (PBS) or were either i.v. injected with TgN29 lymphocytes before or after immunization with Renca or Renca-erbB-2 cells (10×10^6 cells/mouse), Tg N29 lymphocytes plus immunization (i.p.) with irradiated Renca (i.p. 1.6×10^4 cells). (**b**) Another group of mice bearing Renca-erbB-2 lung metastases was treated with naïve or in vitro-activated (anti-CD3 + anti-CD28) TgN29 lymphocytes. Mice received IL-2 as described in Fig. 5

sufficient to eradicate most of the tumor. The allo-T-bodies can be administered as adjuvant following conventional antitumor therapy such as chemotherapy, which also creates a niche for the ACT. Figure 7 shows that a single large dose (10^8) of fully mismatched allogeneic non-directed T cells from various mouse strains following mild irradiation (200 rad) can have a beneficial (though modest) antitumor effect without any sign of significant GvHD other than transient weight loss. Doubling the irradiation dose causes severe GvHD that kills the mice [18]. Conditioning the tumor-bearing mice with other lymphodepleting agents such as cyclophosphamide (Fig. 8) also impaired the host-versus-graft (HvG) response

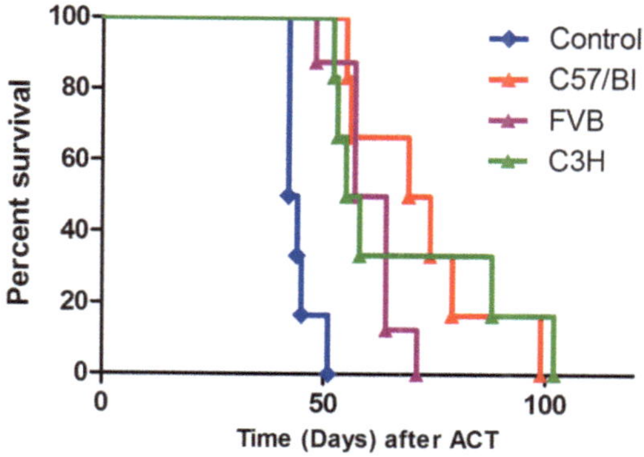

Fig. 7 Non-redirected, allogeneic T cells from multiple strains can extend the survival of tumor-bearing mice. Balb/c mice ($n=6$/group) bearing established Renca-erbB-2 lung metastases were irradiated (2 Gy) and were either left untreated as a control (*blue diamonds*) or injected with 100×10^6 allogeneic T cells (50×10^6 on days 1 and 3). The T cell populations used were allogeneic C57BL6/j T cells ("C57BL," *red triangles*, $P=0.0004$ vs. control), allogeneic FVB T cells ("FVB," *purple triangles* $P=0.0004$ vs. control), or allogeneic C3H T cells ("C3H," *green triangles*, $P=0.0004$ vs. control)

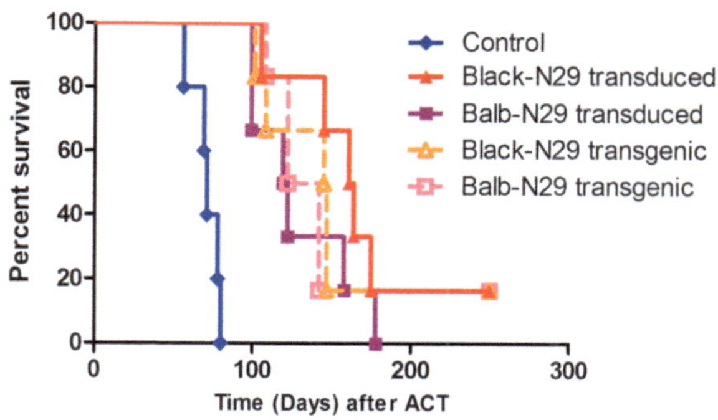

Fig. 8 Comparison of the antitumor activity of preconditioning of syngeneic and allogeneic, naïve and transduced T-bodies. Renca-erbB-2-bearing Balb/c mice ($n=6$/group) were injected with 200 mg/kg cyclophosphamide and 1 day later either left untreated as a control (*blue diamonds*) or injected with 2×10^7 T cells (10^7 on days 1 and 3). The T cell populations used were allogeneic T cells transduced with the N29 CAR ("Black-N29 transduced," *filled red triangles*, $P=0.0007$ vs. control), syngeneic T cells transduced with the N29 CAR ("Balb-N29 transduced," *filled purple squares*, $P=0.0007$ vs. control), allogeneic T cells from N29 transgenic C57BL/6 mice ("C57BL-N29" transgenic, *dashed line*, *open orange triangles*, no significant difference was seen versus transduced cells), or syngeneic T cells from N29 transgenic Balb/c mice ("Balb-N29 transgenic," *dashed line*, *open pink squares*, no significant difference was seen versus transduced cells). Transduction efficiency was about 50 %. In order to simulate the 50 % transduction efficiency, the inoculum of transgenic cells consisted of a mixture of 1:1 transgenic and strain-matched wild-type T cells (so that these mice received 5×10^6 transgenic and 5×10^6 wild-type T cells)

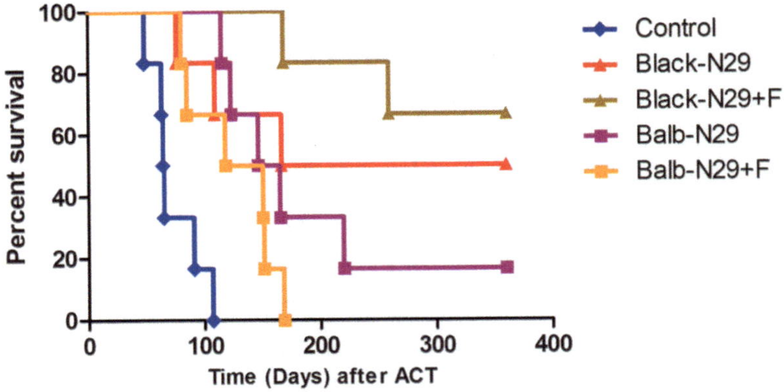

Fig. 9 FTY720 augments allogeneic but not syngeneic adoptive cell therapy. Irradiated (2 Gy), Balb/c mice bearing Renca-erbB-2 lung metastases ($n=6$/group) were a day later either left untreated as a control (*blue diamond*) or injected with 1×10^8 transgenic T-bodies (in a split dose of 5×10^7 cells on days 1 and 3). Indicated groups received FTY720 0.3 mg/kg i.p. for 10 days following transfer. T cells were syngeneic T-bodies (Balb-N29, *purple squares*), syngeneic T-bodies with FTY720 (Balb-N29, *orange squares*), allogeneic T-bodies (C57BL-N29, *red triangles*), or allogeneic T-bodies with FTY720 (C57BL-N29, *brown triangles*)

sufficiently so that the erbB-2-specific C57Bl/6 allo-T-bodies significantly prolonged the survival of the Balb/c tumor-bearing mice, in comparison to mice that received cyclophosphamide alone. In the clinical setting, T-bodies will be generated by transduction of T cells with the CAR, and in this experiment (Fig. 8) and others [18] we directly compared the efficacy of transgenic T-bodies and transduced T-bodies, demonstrating that transduced and transgenic cells can provide comparable therapeutic benefit in both the syngeneic and allogeneic setting. Interestingly the CAR-transduced allogeneic cells were more effective than the syngeneic T-bodies in prolonging the life and causing complete remission of tumor-bearing mice.

To further reduce the HvG response and thereby prolong and substantiate the antitumor response of the allogeneic T-bodies, we treated the mice with FTY720 after the administration of the CAR-modified cells. FTY720 is a sphingosine-1-phosphate (S1P) agonist that causes the internalization of S1P receptor, thus sequestering lymphocytes in the peripheral lymph nodes [3]. In this manner, the allogeneic T-bodies can reach the tumor, but the host cells cannot attack the T-bodies, thereby enhancing the persistence of the allogeneic T cells and their effectiveness. Indeed, as can be seen in Fig. 9, 70 % of the Balb/c mice, bearing Renca-erbB-2 systemic lung metastases that received the allo-T-bodies and FTY720, survived for over a year, in comparison to mice receiving only the allo-T-bodies or syngeneic T-bodies. As expected, FTY720 did not enhance survival of mice receiving syngeneic T-bodies. These results and our previous findings [18] demonstrate that the alloreactivity of the T-bodies can be safely harnessed to potentiate the antitumor response, such that allogeneic T-bodies provide superior therapeutic benefit compared with T-bodies derived from syngeneic (self) T cells.

Table 1 Clinical trials with T-bodies reporting responses

Cancer (group)	CAR specificity	Treated patients	Outcome	Comments
Neuroblastoma (Brenner 2008 [26])	GD2-CD3ζ	19	3 CR, 8 OR	EBV-specific T cells + CAR. Long-term remission >4 years
BCL and CLL (Rosenberg et al. [29])	CD19-CD28-CD3ζ	8	2 CR, 5 OR, 1 TUD	
B cell CLL (June 2011 [25])	CD19-41BB-CD3ζ	3	2 CR, 1 PR	Transduced with lentivectors
B cell CLL + 1ALL	CD19-CD28-CD3ζ	4	0 OR, 1 TUD	No preconditioning
CLL (Sadelain 2011 [40])		4	1 OR	Cyclophosphamide

CR complete remission, *PR* partial remission, *OR* objective remission, *TUD* treatment-unrelated death

3 Conclusions

Our results suggest that T-body ACT is a viable option for the treatment of erbB-2-positive cancer. The first part of our research established the utility of erbB-2-specific T-bodies in the syngeneic setting against both primary and metastatic disease and demonstrated their superiority over conventional T cells. In our subsequent experiments, we extended the use of erbB-2-specific T-bodies to the allogeneic setting and showed that with judicious use of immunomodulation (in this case through FTY720), allogeneic T-bodies could be a superior alternative to syngeneic T-bodies and thus may be preferable not only for their obvious logistical advantages but also due to increased efficacy [17].

So far, clinical application of the T-body approach included transduction of autologous, patient-derived T cells that were reinfused to the patient. Gratifyingly, these pilot trials have shown dramatic success rate in recent clinical trials using GD2-specific T-bodies against neuroblastoma [26] and CD19-specific T-bodies against CLL [16, 25].

Nevertheless, in contrast to the safety seen in these trials, treatment of a patient with a high dose of erbB-2-specific T-body resulted in death that was attributed to the expression of erbB-2 on normal lung and cardiac tissue [21]. The initial successful trials, summarized in Table 1, have demonstrated the great therapeutic potential of T-bodies and highlighted the need for careful evaluation of safety. The growing number of trials listed in the http://clinicaltrials.gov registry together with the ongoing experimental animal models applying T-bodies to additional cancer markers [22, 31, 35] suggests that CAR T-bodies are likely to become an important new therapeutic anticancer approach.

Acknowledgements We are grateful to Dr Shelley Schwarzbaum for scientific editing of the manuscript and to other past and present members of our group who studied and contributed to related aspects described in this chapter.

References

1. Baxevanis CN, Papamichail M. Targeting of tumor cells by lymphocytes engineered to express chimeric receptor genes. Cancer Immunol Immunother. 2004;53:893–903.
2. Choudhury A, Kiessling R. Her-2/neu as a paradigm of a tumor-specific target for therapy. Breast Dis. 2004;20:25–31.
3. Cyster JG, Schwab SR. Sphingosine-1-phosphate and lymphocyte egress from lymphoid organs. Annu Rev Immunol. 2012;30:69–94.
4. Dotti G, Savoldo B, Brenner M. Fifteen years of gene therapy based on chimeric antigen receptors: "are we nearly there yet?". Hum Gene Ther. 2009;20:1229–39.
5. Ertl HC, Zaia J, Rosenberg SA, June CH, Dotti G, Kahn J, Cooper LJ, Corrigan-Curay J, Strome SE. Considerations for the clinical application of chimeric antigen receptor T cells: observations from a recombinant DNA Advisory Committee Symposium held June 15, 2010. Cancer Res. 2011;71:3175–81.
6. Fitzer-Attas CJ, Schindler DG, Waks T, Eshhar Z. Harnessing Syk family tyrosine kinases as signaling domains for chimeric single chain of the variable domain receptors: optimal design for T cell activation. J Immunol. 1998;160:145–54.
7. Friedmann-Morvinski D, Bendavid A, Waks T, Schindler D, Eshhar Z. Redirected primary T cells harboring a chimeric receptor require costimulation for their antigen-specific activation. Blood. 2005;105:3087–93.
8. Gilham DE, Debets R, Pule M, Hawkins RE, Abken H. CAR-T cells and solid tumors: tuning T cells to challenge an inveterate foe. Trends Mol Med. 2012;18(7):377–84.
9. Gross G, Eshhar Z. Endowing T cells with antibody specificity using chimeric T cell receptors. FASEB J. 1992;6:3370–8.
10. Gross G, Waks T, Eshhar Z. Expression of immunoglobulin-T-cell receptor chimeric molecules as functional receptors with antibody-type specificity. Proc Natl Acad Sci U S A. 1989;86:10024–8.
11. Hawkins RE, Gilham DE, Debets R, Eshhar Z, Taylor N, Abken H, Schumacher TN, Consortium A. Development of adoptive cell therapy for cancer: a clinical perspective. Hum Gene Ther. 2010;21:665–72.
12. Hwu P, Shafer GE, Treisman J, Schindler DG, Gross G, Cowherd R, Rosenberg SA, Eshhar Z. Lysis of ovarian cancer cells by human lymphocytes redirected with a chimeric gene composed of an antibody variable region and the Fc receptor gamma chain. J Exp Med. 1993;178:361–6.
13. Jena B, Dotti G, Cooper LJ. Redirecting T-cell specificity by introducing a tumor-specific chimeric antigen receptor. Blood. 2010;116:1035–44.
14. Klebanoff CA, Gattinoni L, Torabi-Parizi P, Kerstann K, Cardones AR, Finkelstein SE, Palmer DC, Antony PA, Hwang ST, Rosenberg SA, et al. Central memory self/tumor-reactive CD8+ T cells confer superior antitumor immunity compared with effector memory T cells. Proc Natl Acad Sci U S A. 2005;102:9571–6.
15. Klebanoff CA, Acquavella N, Yu Z, Restifo NP. Therapeutic cancer vaccines: are we there yet? Immunol Rev. 2011;239:27–44.
16. Kochenderfer JN, Dudley ME, Feldman SA, Wilson WH, Spaner DE, Maric I, Stetler-Stevenson M, Phan GQ, Hughes MS, Sherry RM, et al. B-cell depletion and remissions of malignancy along with cytokine-associated toxicity in a clinical trial of anti-CD19 chimeric-antigen-receptor-transduced T cells. Blood. 2012;119:2709–20.

17. Marcus A, Eshhar Z. Tumor-specific allogeneic cells for cancer therapy. Expert Opin Biol Ther. 2011;11:1551–4.
18. Marcus A, Waks T, Eshhar Z. Redirected tumor-specific allogeneic T cells for universal treatment of cancer. Blood. 2011;118:975–83.
19. Maurer-Gebhard M, Schmidt M, Azemar M, Altenschmidt U, Stocklin E, Wels W, Groner B. Systemic treatment with a recombinant erbB-2 receptor-specific tumor toxin efficiently reduces pulmonary metastases in mice injected with genetically modified carcinoma cells. Cancer Res. 1998;58:2661–6.
20. Moasser MM. The oncogene HER2: its signaling and transforming functions and its role in human cancer pathogenesis. Oncogene. 2007;26:6469–87.
21. Morgan RA, Yang JC, Kitano M, Dudley ME, Laurencot CM, Rosenberg SA. Case report of a serious adverse event following the administration of T cells transduced with a chimeric antigen receptor recognizing ERBB2. Mol Ther. 2010;18:843–51.
22. Morgan RA, Johnson LA, Davis JL, Zheng Z, Woolard KD, Reap EA, Feldman SA, Chinnasamy N, Kuan CT, Song H, et al. Recognition of glioma stem cells by genetically modified T cells targeting EGFRvIII and development of adoptive cell therapy for glioma. Hum Gene Ther. 2012;23:1043–53.
23. Park TS, Rosenberg SA, Morgan RA. Treating cancer with genetically engineered T cells. Trends Biotechnol. 2011;29:550–7.
24. Pegram HJ, Kershaw MH, Darcy PK. Genetic modification of natural killer cells for adoptive cellular immunotherapy. Immunotherapy. 2009;1:623–30.
25. Porter DL, Levine BL, Kalos M, Bagg A, June CH. Chimeric antigen receptor-modified T cells in chronic lymphoid leukemia. N Engl J Med. 2011;365(8):725–33.
26. Pule MA, Savoldo B, Myers GD, Rossig C, Russell HV, Dotti G, Huls MH, Liu E, Gee AP, Mei Z, et al. Virus-specific T cells engineered to coexpress tumor-specific receptors: persistence and antitumor activity in individuals with neuroblastoma. Nat Med. 2008;11:1264–70.
27. Restifo NP, Dudley ME, Rosenberg SA. Adoptive immunotherapy for cancer: harnessing the T cell response. Nat Rev Immunol. 2012;12:269–81.
28. Robbins PF, Morgan RA, Feldman SA, Yang JC, Sherry RM, Dudley ME, Wunderlich JR, Nahvi AV, Helman LJ, Mackall CL, et al. Tumor regression in patients with metastatic synovial cell sarcoma and melanoma using genetically engineered lymphocytes reactive with NY-ESO-1. J Clin Oncol. 2011;29:917–24.
29. Rosenberg SA, Yang JC, Sherry RM, Kammula US, Hughes MS, Phan GQ, Citrin DE, Restifo NP, Robbins PF, Wunderlich JR, et al. Durable complete responses in heavily pretreated patients with metastatic melanoma using T-cell transfer immunotherapy. Clin Cancer Res. 2011;17:4550–7.
30. Schreiber RD, Old LJ, Smyth MJ. Cancer immunoediting: integrating immunity's roles in cancer suppression and promotion. Science. 2011;331:1565–70.
31. Schuberth PC, Jakka G, Jensen SM, Wadle A, Gautschi F, Haley D, Haile S, Mischo A, Held G, Thiel M, et al. Effector memory and central memory NY-ESO-1-specific re-directed T cells for treatment of multiple myeloma. Gene Ther. 2013;20(4):386–95.
32. Sibilia M, Kroismayr R, Lichtenberger BM, Natarajan A, Hecking M, Holcmann M. The epidermal growth factor receptor: from development to tumorigenesis. Differentiation. 2007; 75:770–87.
33. Stancovski I, Hurwitz E, Leitner O, Ullrich A, Yarden Y, Sela M. Mechanistic aspects of the opposing effects of monoclonal antibodies to the ERBB2 receptor on tumor growth. Proc Natl Acad Sci U S A. 1991;88:8691–5.
34. Stancovski I, Schindler DG, Waks T, Yarden Y, Sela M, Eshhar Z. Targeting of T lymphocytes to Neu/HER2-expressing cells using chimeric single chain Fv receptors. J Immunol. 1993;151:6577–82.
35. Tchou J, Wang LC, Selven B, Zhang H, Conejo-Garcia J, Borghaei H, Kalos M, Vondeheide RH, Albelda SM, June CH, et al. Mesothelin, a novel immunotherapy target for triple negative breast cancer. Breast Cancer Res Treat. 2012;133:799–804.

36. van der Bruggen P, Traversari C, Chomez P, Lurquin C, De Plaen E, Van den Eynde B, Knuth A, Boon T. A gene encoding an antigen recognized by cytolytic T lymphocytes on a human melanoma. Science. 1991;254:1643–7.
37. Vesely MD, Kershaw MH, Schreiber RD, Smyth MJ. Natural innate and adaptive immunity to cancer. Annu Rev Immunol. 2011;29:235–71.
38. Westwood JA, Smyth MJ, Teng MW, Moeller M, Trapani JA, Scott AM, Smyth FE, Cartwright GA, Power BE, Honemann D, et al. Adoptive transfer of T cells modified with a humanized chimeric receptor gene inhibits growth of Lewis-Y-expressing tumors in mice. Proc Natl Acad Sci U S A. 2005;102:19051–6.
39. Zhumabekov T, Corbella P, Tolaini M, Kioussis D. Improved version of a human CD2 minigene based vector for T cell-specific expression in transgenic mice. J Immunol Methods. 1995;185:133–40.
40. Brentjens RJ, Rivière I, Park JH, Davila ML, Wang X, Stefanski J, Taylor C, Yeh R, Bartido S, Borquez-Ojeda O, et al. Safety and persistence of adoptively transferred autologous CD19-targeted T cells in patients with relapsed or chemotherapy refractory B-cell leukemias. Blood. 2011;118(18):4817–28.

Part II
Evolving Clinical Immunotherapeutic Strategies

Immunotherapy in Renal Cell Carcinoma

Jennifer Cudris and Jaime R. Merchan

Abstract Renal cell carcinoma (RCC) is a chemotherapy-resistant disease, and current molecularly targeted therapies offer limited clinical benefit but no cures. The observation that RCC is immunogenic led to immune-based strategies for the treatment of this disease. Immunotherapy with high-dose IL-2 can induce long-term, complete responses in a small percentage of patients. IFN has been used as an immune intervention as well but with much less success than IL-2. Currently IFN is used only in combination with the anti-VEGF monoclonal antibody bevacizumab. Further investigation of novel immune interventions in RCC is ongoing with promising results. Dendritic cell vaccines have been tested in single-arm clinical trials suggesting improved survival when added to standard anti-angiogenic therapy. Monoclonal antibodies against PD-1 and PD-L1, novel immune targets, have shown promising response in phase I trials. Peptide vaccines have shown efficacy in phase II trials as well. Phase III trials to test these immune interventions are currently ongoing and have the potential to bring new, effective treatment options for patients with advanced RCC.

Keywords Renal Cell Carcinoma • Immunotherapy • IL-2 • Clinical trials

1 Introduction

An estimated 273,518 new cases of kidney cancer were diagnosed worldwide in 2008, 116,368 of which died of the disease [1]. In the USA, 64,770 new cases will be diagnosed in 2012 and 13,570 deaths are estimated to occur [2]. The incidence has increased every year for both sexes, in part due to increased early detection of small asymptomatic kidney masses. The number of deaths related to RCC has

J. Cudris • J.R. Merchan (✉)
Division of Hematology-Oncology, Department of Medicine, University of Miami Miller School of Medicine, 1475 NW 12 Avenue, Suite 3400, Miami, FL 33136, USA
e-mail: JCudrisMaldonado@med.miami.edu; JMerchan2@med.miami.edu

J.D. Rosenblatt et al. (eds.), *Advances in Tumor Immunology and Immunotherapy*, Current Cancer Research, DOI 10.1007/978-1-4614-8809-5_8,

© Springer Science+Business Media New York 2014

decreased by 0.6 % per year for women and 0.4 % for men [1, 2]. Risk factors associated with kidney cancer include tobacco use, obesity, hypertension, chronic renal failure, exposure to trichloroethylene, and genetic predisposition as in von Hippel–Lindau disease [2]. Because renal tumors can grow without causing symptoms, the disease is diagnosed at a locally advanced or metastatic stage in about 34 % of the cases. Expected survival is highly dependent on the stage at diagnosis, being greater than 90 % at 5 years in stage I tumors that are surgically removed [3] but less than 10 % in patients with distant metastasis [4].

RCC is a chemotherapy-resistant disease. The observation that removal of the primary renal tumor leads in rare sporadic cases to spontaneous remissions of metastatic lesions, as well as very late recurrences after nephrectomy, suggested that this malignancy is immunogenic [5, 6]. Initial clinical trials of immunotherapy were carried in various metastatic malignancies in the 1980s, and it became evident that RCC and melanoma could be responsive to agents such as interferon-α (IFN-α) or interleukin-2 (IL-2) [7, 8]. These therapies, associated with limited—but real—clinical benefit, constituted the standard of care until the beginning of the twenty-first century, when novel targeted agents were developed and became clinically available. The recognition that angiogenic as well as other tumor pathways (e.g., mammalian target of rapamycin—mTOR) [9, 10] are relevant in renal cancer progression led to the development and approval of novel agents for the treatment of this disease. Currently available anti-angiogenic agents mainly target the vascular endothelial growth factor (VEGF) pathway, by binding the VEGF ligand—as the monoclonal antibody bevacizumab [11]—or blocking receptor tyrosine kinases involved with angiogenesis, such as VEGFR-1, VEGFR-2 and /or PDGFR [9]. Examples of currently (USA) approved oral small-molecule receptor tyrosine kinase inhibitors (RTKIs) include sorafenib [12], sunitinib [13], pazopanib [14], and axitinib [15]. Currently approved mTOR inhibitors include the rapamycin analogs temsirolimus [16] and everolimus [17]. The above agents have significantly improved the treatment options for patients with unresectable or metastatic RCC, and current research is focused at individualizing treatment options for these patients.

Even though significant progress has been made in the field by the development of molecularly targeted agents, these treatments are not curative. Furthermore, the majority of patients with advanced RCC eventually progress, leaving them with few therapeutic options. Therefore, development of novel strategies to improve outcomes in patients with RCC is urgently needed.

Published reports of durable, complete responses in subsets of patients with metastatic RCC treated with high-dose IL-2 illustrate the potential utility of immune-based therapies in this disease. Furthermore, the increasing understanding of immune regulation, especially the biology of T cell expansion, memory, and co-stimulation has provided real opportunities for improved immunotherapeutic approaches. This review focuses on past and current immunotherapy strategies for advanced RCC.

2 Standard Immunotherapy Options for Advanced Renal Cell Carcinoma

2.1 Interleukin-2

IL-2 was initially discovered by Gordon and Mc Lean as a mitogenic factor for lymphocytes [18, 19]. It was initially referred to as T cell growth factor (TCGF), and it was the first cytokine fully characterized at a molecular level; it was determined to be a small glycoprotein, and its gene was localized to chromosome 4 [19, 20].

2.1.1 Mechanism of Action

IL-2 enhances both innate and acquired immunity [21, 22]. It has been found to stimulate NK cells upon antigen exposure [21], and it can also support the clonal expansion of activated CD8+ T cells—with cytolytic function [22]—and to a lesser degree that of CD4+ T cells [21, 23] with both effector and regulatory function. In vitro studies have demonstrated IL-2 antitumor effects in different cancer cell lines. Peripheral blood lymphocytes (PBL) from patients with melanoma cultured with IL-2 acquire increased cytotoxic activity against autologous and allogeneic tumor cells [24]. Increased cytotoxic activity of NK cells and PBLs after stimulation with IL-2 against RCC cell lines has also been documented [25]. In vivo administration of IL-2 in syngeneic sarcoma and melanoma models resulted in in vivo generation of lymphokine-activated killer (LAK) cells and potent antitumor effects [26]. Similarly, in vivo studies using a murine renal carcinoma model showed that infusion of IL-2 could enhance tumor control in combination with chemotherapy [27, 28]. These and other studies supported clinical testing of IL-2 in human tumors.

2.1.2 Clinical Activity

Initial phase I trials—reported in 1987—showed feasibility of the use of IL-2 in patients with advanced malignancies, and clinical responses were observed mostly in patients with melanoma and RCC [7]. The activity of IL-2 in RCC was further demonstrated in phase II and III trials [29, 30]. Pooled analysis of seven phase II trials run in the USA showed that after treatment of 255 patients with high-dose IL-2, an overall response rate of 15 %, with a complete remission (CR) of 7 %, was observed [31]. Patients who achieved a CR could have a durable response, over 18 months in initial reports. After longer follow-up, some patients were found to maintain complete remission for more than 10 years [32]. Based on this data, IL-2 was approved by the US Food and Drug Administration (FDA) for the treatment of RCC in 1992. The precise mechanism of action of IL-2 in humans has not been clearly established. Clinical/translational studies in humans with cancer treated with this agent suggest that IL-2 increases the frequency of NK cells in peripheral blood throughout a treatment course with IL-2 [33]. It generates a transient decrease in CD4 and CD8 T cells during the first week of treatment. It also increases the absolute number of circulating iNKT cells, which have been related to antitumor response by inducing IFN-α production. This increase however did not translate into increased production of IFN-α or correlated with clinical response. Therefore, specific immune targets have not been identified.

The high-dose IL-2 regimen used in these trials was 600,000–720,000 IU/kg given as a 15-min IV infusion every 8 h for up to 14 doses over 5 days (days 1–5) as clinically tolerated. Maximal support, including pressors, was frequently required due to significant toxicities; same dose was repeated from days 14 to 19, and this would complete 1 cycle [31]. The treatment could be repeated for up to two more cycles that were given 6–12 weeks apart if tolerance was adequate, and there was evidence of clinical response or stable disease. European trials used a continuous infusion regimen [34]. The dose given was 18 million IU/m2 for 5 days for two induction cycles 1 week apart; if there was no progression, another induction cycle was given and maintenance with three more doses of 5 days was given every 3 weeks. Responses were similar to intermittent bolus schedule with a response rate (RR) of 16 % and CR of 4 %, although no ICU care was necessary in most of the patients. Long-term follow-up confirmed durable responses [35]. Lower doses of IL-2 although better tolerated have been studied with much less success than with high-dose infusions and appear to lead to much lower rates of complete response which are also considerably less durable [36, 37].

High-dose IL-2 was also tested in the postoperative (adjuvant) setting in a randomized trial by the cytokine working group, but the study had to be stopped early after interim analysis evidence that no difference in outcome would be found despite full accrual [38].

2.1.3 IL-2 Combination Therapy

After limited success with single-agent immunotherapy, combination therapies were experimented. Randomized phase II trials have tested combinations of IL-2 and IFN-α with marginal or no added benefit but increase in toxicity [39, 40]. Direct comparisons of high-dose IL-2 versus lower subcutaneous dose plus IFN-α have demonstrated that high-dose IL-2 is a superior regimen with longer survival [29].

Adoptive immunotherapy using combination of high-dose IL-2 and infusion of LAKs or tumor-infiltrating lymphocytes (TILs) has been used with some success in phase II trials. However, randomized studies using combination TIL and low-dose IL-2 failed to increase response rates. Furthermore, obtaining viable TILs was not always technically possible [41]. A randomized comparison of low-dose IL-2 with and without LAK cells did not show difference in response [42]. At this point, there is no evidence of improved clinical activity of combination of TILs and immunotherapy for RCC.

2.1.4 Predictors of Response

Clinical, histological, and molecular predictors have been evaluated.

Clinical Factors

In a retrospective review of clinical trials where IL-2 was used for patients with metastatic RCC, predictive factors associated with response have been variable. An ECOG performance status of 0 has been repeatedly associated with better outcome and tolerance to treatment. Prior nephrectomy and shorter time from diagnosis to treatment have been also suggested as predictors of response [31]. Other variables like number of metastatic sites and location and time of relapse from nephrectomy have been studied with conflicting and inconsistent results [41, 43].

Histopathological Factors

Retrospective data of small studies suggests that tumor histology may be a predictive factor, with sarcomatoid and papillary types being less likely to respond than conventional (clear cell) type [43, 44]. In a study by Upton et al., a review of 265 specimens from patients treated with IL-2 was undertaken [45]. Predictive characteristics besides conventional type were alveolar pattern in more than 50 % of the tumor specimen (28 % response rate compared with 13 % in those with less than 50 % alveolar pattern and 0 % in patients with no alveolar pattern). Granular features on the other hand predicted a poor response. In tumors with granular features in more than 50 %, the response rate was 5 % compared to 19 % response when granular component was less than 50 and 29 % response for tumors with no granular morphology. With these findings, a predictive model that classified patients into three groups was proposed: The group with low probability of response (3 %) included tumors with papillary features of more than 50 %, any granular features, or no alveolar features. In contrast, the group with >50 % alveolar pattern and no granular or papillary features had a 39 % response rate, and patients with no papillary but some granular features (<50 %) had an intermediate 19 % probability of response. According to this model, three distinct survival curves could be obtained showing a 2.8, 1.3, and 0.8 years median survival, respectively.

Molecular Factors

High levels of carbonic anhydrase (CA IX) expression have been found to correlate with response and survival in retrospective studies [46]. It was seen that 78 % of responders had high CA IX expression compared with 51 % of nonresponders. Small studies have suggested that high serum levels of VEGF and fibronectin may be associated with lack of response [47].

A retrospective study by De Martino et al. evaluated single-nucleotide polymorphisms (SNPs) of the CA IX gene in patients treated with IL-2 and found the allele C of rs12553173 (c.249T>C) to be an independent predictor of response and survival, remaining independent upon comparison with high CA IX expression [48]. Patients with the C allele had an improved median survival (27.3 vs. 13.6 months) compared to patients without that variant. Moreover, 57 % of patients with the C variant responded, compared to 22 % of patients without rs12553173. The above results in a limited number of patients warrant further confirmation in prospective randomized trials. The immunological significance of this variant and mechanisms explaining this correlation are not currently understood.

A prospective study to determine the validity of clinical, pathological, and molecular predictors in response to IL-2 has been completed (SELECT trial), and preliminary results presented in an abstract form suggest that no pretreatment clinical factor was able to predict response, but clear cell histology seems to be associated with higher probability of response [49]. Final results from this trial have not been published yet.

2.1.5 Toxicity Profile

The majority of complications from IL-2 therapy are related to capillary leak syndrome (CLS) [50–56]. Treatment-related mortality was found to be 4 % in initial studies. Advances in the understanding of the toxicity and provision of appropriate support during treatment can decrease treatment-related mortality. Fluid retention causes edema and weight gain, which may lead to cardiovascular and/or respiratory complications. Cardiovascular events were seen in 11 % of patients, being life threatening in 1 %. Clinically evident pulmonary edema is observed in 24 % of patients (life threatening in 3 %). Sepsis can also contribute to treatment-related mortality with a 1 % incidence. Other potentially serious effects include hypotension which can be seen in 71 %, fever (21 %), chills (22 %), oliguria (63 %), and anuria (5 %). Life-threatening arrhythmias have also been uncommonly seen (1 %). Nausea (35 %), vomiting (50 %), and diarrhea (67 %) are also common complaints. GI bleed and bowel perforation are rare events. Neurotoxicity is manifested by mental status changes that can be minor like confusion -in 32 % of patients- or can progress to frank coma in 2 %. Elevation of BUN and creatinine are almost universal but almost always reversible upon completion of therapy. Elevation of bilirubin (40 %) and transaminases (23 %) were commonly seen but are generally not dose limiting. Thyroid dysfunction including hypo- or hyperthyroidism can be seen in 40 % of patients; this is resolved after discontinuation of treatment and is associated with antithyroglobulin and antimicrosomal antibodies. The above toxicities, however, are usually reversible upon completion of therapy and many times do not prolong hospital stay. Patients with good performance status (PS) seem to be able to tolerate therapy better than patients with lower PS [31, 34]. Therapy with IL-2 should be discontinued in patients who have experienced angina or myocardial infarction, sustained ventricular tachycardia, intubation for >72 h, uncontrolled supraventricular tachycardia, cardiac tamponade, renal failure requiring dialysis for greater than 72 h, coma or uncontrolled psychosis for >48 h, uncontrolled seizures, bowel ischemia, perforation, or GI bleeding requiring surgery.

Given the potential toxicities associated with this therapy, patients should be carefully selected prior to initiating high-dose IL-2. This therapy is generally reserved to patients with excellent performance status and no evidence of significant cardiac or pulmonary disease, documented by negative stress test and normal pulmonary function tests, and no evidence of brain metastases [57].

2.2 *Interferon Alpha*

Interferon was initially discovered in 1954 by Nagano when he found evidence of a factor that interfered with viral replication (therefore the term interferon). The finding went unnoticed until Isaacs and Lindemmann re-demonstrated it in 1957 [58, 59]. Two families of IFN have been identified: I (alpha and beta) and II (gamma). IFN-α's chemical structure was identified in 1980, and gene was isolated [60, 61] and localized to chromosome 9 one year later [62].

2.2.1 Mechanism of Action

IFN-α is known to be produced by leukocytes upon stimulation by viral antigens and increase cytotoxic activity by activating NK cells and macrophages [63, 64]. The antitumor effect of IFN-α in RCC is poorly understood. However IFN-α is thought to regulate cell proliferation by targeting kinases (JAK1) that activate the signal transducer and transactivator (STAT) proteins and induce expression of different genes that regulate cell proliferation and apoptosis [65]. In addition, IFN may have intrinsic anti-angiogenic effects by blocking fibroblastic growth factor-induced cell proliferation [66] and decreasing endothelial cell proliferation [67]. Several effects of IFN-α in patients with renal cell cancer have been described, including increased T cell proliferation, production of IL-2 and expression of IL-2 receptors, and monocyte production of IL-1 which may correlate with prognosis [68].

2.2.2 Clinical Activity

Phase II trials of IFN-α in RCC showed response rates of less than 10 %, but some complete responses and subcutaneous administration appear to be equally effective and less toxic than intravenous administration [69]. There was a consistent response rate of approximately 15 % and PFS of 4 months; very occasional complete responses were seen, but these were not durable. Addition of IFN-γ to IFN-α showed no improvement in response [70]. The use of IFN-α as a single agent has been largely replaced by targeted agents that carry less toxicity and improve PFS [13, 16]. IFN-α is currently approved by FDA for use in metastatic RCC only *in combination* with bevacizumab (see below), based on results from a randomized trial that demonstrated improved outcomes with the combination [71]. Doses of IFN-α used have ranged from 2 to 10 million IU/m^2. The standard dose used in latest randomized trials is 9 million IU subcutaneously three times a week [11, 69].

Adjuvant treatment with IFN-α after nephrectomy in high-risk patients with T3 and T4 tumors has been proven ineffective in randomized trials [72].

2.2.3 Role of Cytoreductive Nephrectomy

Cytoreductive nephrectomy has shown to improve survival in patients with metastatic disease undergoing systemic therapy with IFN-α in two published studies [73, 74]. Retrospective reviews have also shown that response to IFN-α is better in clear cell RCC [40].

2.2.4 Predictors of Response

Recently, a retrospective study suggested that SNPs of the STAT gene could be predictors of response to IFN. It was found that the CC genotype at rs4796793 had an odds ratio for response of 8.38 compared to GG and GC phenotypes [75]. It has also been suggested that the presence of tumor-infiltrating dendritic cells can predict response to IFN and IL-2 [76].

2.2.5 Prognostic Factors

A retrospective review of trials of IFN-α in advanced RCC at Memorial Sloan Kettering Cancer Center found the following factors to be related to worse outcome [77]:

- LDH >1.5 times the upper limit of normal
- Hb: Less than lower limit of normal
- Karnofsky performance status ≤ 80 %
- Hypercalcemia
- Interval from initial diagnosis to initiation of treatment ≥1 year

Based on these factors, three prognostic groups have been proposed: Low risk: No adverse factors present: 3-year survival of 45 % and median OS 30 months. Intermediate risk: One or two factors: 3-year OS 17 %, and median OS 14 months. Poor risk: Three or more factors: 3-year OS 2 %, and median OS 5 months.

2.2.6 IFN-α Combination Therapies

Two randomized trials have evaluated the efficacy of combination bevacizumab and IFN-α in patients with advanced RCC. The AVOREN trial randomized 649 patients to IFN (9MIU SQ three times a week) and placebo versus IFN plus bevacizumab (10 mg/kg every 2 weeks) [11]. PFS was 5.4 vs. 10 months favoring the combination. OS was similar but likely due to the use of second-line therapies after progression. Common toxicities are fatigue (33 %), asthenia (32 %), neutropenia (7 %), hypertension (26 %), proteinuria (18 %), life-threatening events occurred including rare bowel perforations (1 %), and thromboembolic events (3 %). The CALGB 90206 trial randomized 732 patients to same regimens finding a PFS of 8.5 vs. 5.2 months favoring the addition of bevacizumab, but again no improved survival was seen and toxicities were similar [71].

Randomized studies of interferon have been done in combination with vinblastine, showing improvement in response from 2.5 to 16 % and survival from 9 to 16 months with the combination compared with vinblastine alone [8]. Addition of trans-retinoic acid to IFN therapy has also been attempted in an European trial with small improvement in response and PFS from 3.4 to 5.1 months and OS from 13 to 17 months [78]; however, a similar study at MSKCC failed to reproduce these results and did not confirm any advantage for the combination [79].

2.2.7 Toxicity

IFN therapy is associated with a "flu-like" syndrome in 100 % of the cases, which can be severe in approximately 30 % of the cases. Anorexia, severe somnolence (7 %), severe nausea (15 %), leukopenia (6 %, severe in 2 %), and thrombocytopenia (4 % and severe in 2 %) can also be seen. Severe depression (4 %) and neurological toxicity (2 %) including altered mental status and changes in behavior are less common [72].

3 Investigational Immunotherapy Strategies

3.1 Dendritic Cell-Based Therapy

Dendritic cells (DC) are professional antigen-presenting cells (APCs) that are capable of inducing rejection of tumors by enhancing cytotoxic lymphocyte activity [80]. Dendritic cells are known to take part in the cytotoxic response to malignancy, by activating T cells in a very efficient manner [81]. DCs were found in renal cell tumors but in small numbers and not in activated state, suggesting DC inhibition by local microenvironment [82]. These cells have been successfully activated by incubation with IL-2 [83]. Preclinical studies have proved the concept that manipulating DCs by exposure to known tumor peptides or fusion with tumor cells can induce tumor-specific cytotoxic cells and antitumor activity [84–87].

Phase I and II trials with different schemes of injection of dendritic cells have shown variable immunological responses with evidence of clinical response (Table 1). Most studies have included heavily pretreated patients. Clinical studies have used autologous as well as allogeneic dendritic cells from the peripheral blood or the bone marrow [88]. DCs have been used in an immature state or matured ex vivo with tumor necrosis factor (TNF) [89], prostaglandins, or IL-4 [90] and/or pulsed with tumor lysates [91] or RNA [92]. It has been observed that mature DCs induce better responses than immature cells [93]. Objective responses have been observed in these early studies, indicating that these strategies hold clinical promise. Response rates have ranged from 0 to 50 % and stabilization of disease from 15 to 50 % (Table 1). Addition of IL-2 and/or IFN has been pursued as well, and although responses have been observed, it is not clear if the responses are due to cytokine therapy or addition of dendritic cells [94].

AGS003 is a dendritic cell vaccine prepared from matured monocyte-derived dendritic cells co-electroporated with the subject's own amplified total tumor RNA as well as synthetic CD40 ligand RNA. A phase II study presented at the 2012 American Society of Clinical Oncology (ASCO) meeting used the combination of sunitinib plus AGS003 vs. sunitinib alone in 20 patients with untreated metastatic RCC. Preliminary results showed one patient with a PR and seven with stable disease. Progression-free survival of 11 months for intermediate-risk patients and 6 months for poor-risk patients were reported; overall survival had not been reached in the intermediate-risk group at the time of the report [92]. A randomized trial comparing AGS003 with standard therapy is under way (see Table 2).

3.1.1 Toxicity

The most common side effects seen with these therapies include infusion reactions, erythema at the site of injection, and fever. No life-threatening adverse events have been seen in the use of these vaccines.

3.2 Anti-CTLA4 Therapies

Cytotoxic T lymphocyte antigen 4 (CTLA4) is a membrane receptor that is expressed in T cells and regulates the intensity of the T cell activation by counteracting the activity of CD28. CD28 is the co-stimulatory receptor necessary to initiate T cell activation acting when engaged as signal 2 to complement TCR binding. CTLA4 binds the same CD 28 ligands, CD80 and CD86, but with higher affinity, making CTLA4 an inhibitor of T cell activation by competitive binding of ligands [95–97].

Table 1 Selected published clinical trials on the use of dendritic cell vaccines for renal cell carcinoma

Author	Number of patients	Phase	DC cells	Adjunct	Response rate	Immune response	Survival	AEs
Avigan [89]	24	I/II	Allogeneic mature	None	2PR	Eight had twofold increase in CD4 intracellular IFN-γ	Mean PFS: 18 weeks	Fatigue, cough rigors, skin reaction
					8SD	Six had twofold increase in CD8 IFN-γ	Mean OS: 116 weeks	
Kim [90]	9	I/II	Autologous mature	None	1PR	Increased DTH to DC and KLH, increased lymphocyte proliferation	TTP: 5.2 months	Skin reaction, fever, myalgia, rash
					5SD	Serum IFN-γ, no change	OS: 29 months	
Berntsen [91]	27	I/II	Auto mature	Low-dose IL-2	No PR	Increased IFN-γ to tumor peptide	PFS: 2.7 months	Flu like
					13 SD		OS: 16.6 months	Fatigue, local reaction
Schwaab [94]	18	II	Auto (mature)	IL-2 CIV	3CR	Increased CD8 IFN-γ production	PFS 8 months	IL-2 toxicity
				IFN SQ	6PR 6SD	Increased NK cells	OS not reached	
Wierecky [112]	20	I	Auto	IL-2 low dose	2PR 1CR 5SD	Increased PADRE proliferation	NR	NR
Holtl [113]	20	I/II	Allo (TNF IL1 IL6 prosta E2)	cyclophosphamide	3SD	Increased PBMC proliferation	NR	Flu like
Oosterwijk [114]	12	I	Auto	IL-2 SQ	No PR 1SD	No increased DTH to tumor lysate	NR	IL-2 toxicity Erythema injection site

(continued)

Table 1 (continued)

Author	Number of patients	Phase	DC cells	Adjunct	Response rate	Immune response	Survival	AEs
Marten [115]	15	I	Auto mature	5FU IFN and IL2 in 3	7SD 1PR	Increased proliferation of PBL	NR	None
Marten [116]	12	I/II	Autologous (4) Allo (8)	None	4SD	DTH positive, increased cytotoxicity of PBL	NR	None
Figlin [92]	21	II	Auto	Sunitinib	NR	NR	PFS: 11.9 months OS poor risk: 7.9 months	No grade 3 reported
Su [117]	10	I	Allo immature	None	NR	Increased IFN-γ	19 months	Skin reaction, mild
Gitlitz [118]	14	I	Autologous	None	None	None	NR	Fatigue, mild

Table 2 Ongoing clinical trials with investigational immunotherapeutic agents

Agent name	Identifier number	Class	Phase of study	Investigator/sponsor	Intervention
AGS003	NCT01582672	Autologous ribonucleic acid (RNA) electroporated dendritic cell (DC)-based immunotherapy	Phase 3	Figlin	Standard treatment ± AGS 003 for advanced renal cell carcinoma
IMA901	NCT01265901	Multi-peptide vaccine	Phase 3	Rini	Sunitinib ± IMA 901 vaccine for untreated metastatic RCC
MDX1106	NCT01668784	Anti-PD-1	Phase 3	Bristol Myers Squibb	MDX1106 vs. everolimus after angiogenic therapy in metastatic RCC
DC vaccine + L-2 + IFN + bevacizumab	NCT00913913	Multiple immune interventions	Phase 2	Ernstoff	Combination of four immune interventions in metastatic RCC
CT011 ± DC/RCC fusion vaccine	NCT01441765	Anti-PD-1 (CT011) and DC/RCC fusion vaccine	Phase 2	Avigan	Anti-PD-1 with or without DC vaccine in metastatic RCC
MVA-5T4 + IL-2	NCT00083941	Peptide vaccine	Phase 2	Oxford BioMedica	MVA-5T4 with IL-2 in metastatic RCC
MDPL3280A	NCT01375842	Anti-PD-L1	Phase 1	Genentech	Various malignancies
MDPL3280A + avastin ± chemotherapy	NCT01633970	Anti-PD-L1 Anti-VEGF Cytotoxic chemotherapy	Phase 1	Genentech	Various malignancies
AMP-224	NCT01352884	Anti-PD-1	Phase 1	Glaxo	Various malignancies

Source: www.clinicaltrials.gov

Preclinical studies have demonstrated that blockade of CTLA4 could enhance T cell activation and induce antitumor cytotoxic effects [98]. A phase I trial of ipilimumab, a humanized anti-CTLA4 antibody, showed that this treatment was feasible and clinical responses were observed.

3.2.1 Clinical Activity

Ipilimumab was tested in a phase III trial, where it prolonged survival from 6.4 to 10 months in patients with metastatic melanoma when compared with gp100 vaccine [99]. Ipilimumab has been also tested in RCC in a phase II trial, where 6/40 patients had partial responses [50]. All the responses were seen in patients who had autoimmune manifestations as consequence of the treatment. Tremelimumab, another anti-CTLA4 antibody, failed to show improvement in response in melanoma. It has also been tested in a phase I trial in combination with sunitinib in 28 patients with metastatic RCC [100]. There was one sudden death and dose-limiting toxicities (acute renal failure in three patients), raising concern about the safety of this combination.

3.2.2 Toxicity

Significant autoimmune manifestations are associated with the use of ipilimumab in about 60 % of patients (15 %, grade 3 and 4). Skin toxicity (pruritus and rash) occurs in 40 % of patients (25 % grade 3) and gastrointestinal tract (colitis, diarrhea) in up to 31 % of patients (3.7 % grade 3). In moderate and severe cases, steroids are required to control symptoms and prevent bowel perforation; infliximab, an anti-TNFα monoclonal antibody, may be necessary in severe cases of colitis. Other adverse events included endocrinopathies in 3.9 % including hypophysitis and hypopituitarism and vitiligo in 3.7 %. Phase II trials have shown correlation of autoimmune manifestations with higher clinical response, suggesting that activated autoimmunity increases antitumor activity. In a study by Attia et al., 5 of 14 patients with grade 3 and 4 toxicity had clinical response to ipilimumab, compared to 2 of 42 with no autoimmune toxicity [101]. Ipilimumab has been approved by the FDA for the treatment of metastatic melanoma.

3.3 Anti-Programmed Death-1 Therapies

Programmed cell death 1 (PD-1) is a membrane receptor present in T cells, a subset of B cells, and NK cells. It is known to inhibit the inflammatory activity of lymphocytes in the tissues in response to infection and therefore limits autoimmunity [102, 103]. Its ligand—PD-L1—is a cell membrane-bound protein. Several tumors have been found to express PD-L1, and tumor-associated PD-L1 may be associated with immune evasion mechanisms by inhibiting tumor-specific T cells [104]. In RCC, increased expression of PD-L1 is associated with poor survival, and blockade of PD-L1 augments human tumor-specific T cell responses [105, 106]. These preclinical observations led to the development of strategies aimed at targeting this pathway.

3.3.1 Clinical Activity

The safety and activity of two agents targeting PD-1 or PD-L1 in solid tumors, including RCC, have been reported. A phase I trial of MDX1105-01 (fully humanized anti-PD-L1 monoclonal antibody) in patients with various advanced malignancies, including 17 patients with RCC, was recently reported [107]. Objective response was seen in two patients with RCC (duration of response of 17.4 months) and stable disease in seven RCC patients, with a PFS rate at 6 months of 53 %. Two of 207 patients experienced grade 3 or 4 toxicity with infusion reaction and adrenal insufficiency. The remaining toxicities were mild and most commonly due to infusion reactions (10 %), diarrhea (9 %), and rash (7 %).

At the same time, MDX1106 (fully humanized antibody against the PD-1 receptor) was tested in a large phase I trial where patients with RCC and other malignancies were enrolled [108, 109]. A total of 296 patients, including 33 with metastatic RCC, were accrued. Objective responses were seen in nine patients with RCC and SD in other nine patients. The duration of response was 17 months in the 1 mg/kg cohort and 22 months in the 10 mg/kg group. The PFS at 6 months was 56 %. Toxicity consisted most commonly of diarrhea (10 %), rash (12 %), and pruritus (9 %); grade 3 and 4 events were 1 % or less, and most significant ones were diarrhea, pneumonitis, pruritus, rash, elevated liver enzymes, and thyroid dysfunction. There were three treatment-related deaths due to pneumonitis, two in non-small-cell lung cancer patients and one in colorectal cancer. Pathological studies of a small number of patients including five with RCC suggested that tumor expression of PDL1 may correlate with response. Clinical trials exploring the activity of anti-PD1 in RCC and other malignancies are ongoing (Table 2).

3.4 Peptide Vaccines

Efforts to determine tumor-specific antigens that stimulate a cytotoxic immune response have been facilitated by integrated functional genomics approaches, where candidate tumor-associated peptides (TUMAPs) in RCC tumors were detected by overexpression of RNA and compared with HLA class I ligand epitopes in tumor tissue by mass spectroscopy [110, 111]. A recently published phase I/II trial demonstrated the feasibility of this approach by detecting 10 candidate peptides overexpressed in the tumors of 28 patients with metastatic RCC and naturally presented by

HLA 2 A02+ using a computer-based platform to create a multi-peptide vaccine called IMA 901 [111]. Patients were vaccinated after injection of GM-CSF as immunomodulator and found that specific T cell responses to one or several of the TUMAPs could be detected.

The phase II portion of the study randomized patients to receive vaccination with or without cyclophosphamide pretreatment, under the hypothesis that cyclophosphamide could decrease the number of T regulatory cells that may interfere with the immune response. The rate of disease control (ORR + SD) was 31 % at 6 months, and there was improved survival in patients who received cyclophosphamide, 23.5 versus 14.8 months when the vaccine was given alone. Generation of peptide-specific T cells after vaccination was seen in 64 % of the patients, and it was not affected by the use of cyclophosphamide. Among patients who mounted an immune response to the vaccine, survival was prolonged for those who received cyclophosphamide with an HR of 0.38. In patients who did not mount an immune response, use of cyclophosphamide did not have any effect on survival. Tumor markers APOA1 and CCL17 were found to be predictive for immune response. The treatment was well tolerated with local skin reactions being the most frequent adverse event. A randomized trial comparing sunitinib versus sunitinib plus IMA901 is currently in progress.

In summary, immune-based therapies constitute a viable and promising strategy for advanced RCC. Significant progress has occurred in both the understanding of immune regulatory pathways involved in RCC and novel immune therapies since the initial studies of IL-2 and interferon in the 1980s. An increasing number of clinical trials with novel immune-based therapies, both alone and in combination with standard immune or targeted therapies, are under way and have the potential to significantly improve the outcomes of thousands of patients with advanced RCC.

References

1. Ferlay J, Shin HR, Bray F, Forman D, Mathers C and Parkin DM. GLOBOCAN 2008 v2.0, Cancer Incidence and Mortality Worldwide: IARC CancerBase No. 10 [Internet]. Lyon, France: International Agency for Research on Cancer; 2010. Available from: http://globocan.iarc.fr/factsheets/populations/factsheet.asp (2008) Accessed Aug 2012.
2. American Cancer Society. Cancer facts and figures 2012. Atlanta: American cancer society; 2012.
3. Verhoest G, Avakian R, Bensalah K, Thuret R, Ficarra V, Artibani W, et al. Urinary collecting system invasion is an independent prognostic factor of organ confined renal cell carcinoma. J Urol. 2009;182(3):854–9.
4. Motzer RJ, Mazumdar M, Bacik J, Berg W, Amsterdam A, Ferrara J. Survival and prognostic stratification of 670 patients with advanced renal cell carcinoma. J Clin Oncol. 1999;17(8):2530–40.
5. Elhilali MM, Gleave M, Fradet Y, Davis I, Venner P, Saad F, et al. Placebo-associated remissions in a multicentre, randomized, double-blind trial of interferon gamma-1b for the treatment of metastatic renal cell carcinoma. the Canadian Urologic Oncology Group. BJU Int. 2000;86(6):613–8.

6. Marcus SG, Choyke PL, Reiter R, Jaffe GS, Alexander RB, Linehan WM, et al. Regression of metastatic renal cell carcinoma after cytoreductive nephrectomy. J Urol. 1993;150(2 Pt 1):463–6.
7. Rosenberg SA, Lotze MT, Muul LM, Chang AE, Avis FP, Leitman S, et al. A progress report on the treatment of 157 patients with advanced cancer using lymphokine-activated killer cells and interleukin-2 or high-dose interleukin-2 alone. N Engl J Med. 1987;316(15):889–97.
8. Pyrhonen S, Salminen E, Ruutu M, Lehtonen T, Nurmi M, Tammela T, et al. Prospective randomized trial of interferon alfa-2a plus vinblastine versus vinblastine alone in patients with advanced renal cell cancer. J Clin Oncol. 1999;17(9):2859–67.
9. Escudier B, Albiges L. Vascular endothelial growth factor-targeted therapy for the treatment of renal cell carcinoma. Drugs. 2011;71(9):1179–91.
10. Voss MH, Molina AM, Motzer RJ. mTOR inhibitors in advanced renal cell carcinoma. Hematol Oncol Clin North Am. 2011;25(4):835–52.
11. Escudier B, Bellmunt J, Negrier S, Bajetta E, Melichar B, Bracarda S, et al. Phase III trial of bevacizumab plus interferon alfa-2a in patients with metastatic renal cell carcinoma (AVOREN): final analysis of overall survival. J Clin Oncol. 2010;28(13):2144–50.
12. Escudier B, Eisen T, Stadler WM, Szczylik C, Oudard S, Siebels M, et al. Sorafenib in advanced clear-cell renal-cell carcinoma. N Engl J Med. 2007;356(2):125–34.
13. Motzer RJ, Hutson TE, Tomczak P, Michaelson MD, Bukowski RM, Rixe O, et al. Sunitinib versus interferon alfa in metastatic renal-cell carcinoma. N Engl J Med. 2007;356(2): 115–24.
14. Sternberg CN, Davis ID, Mardiak J, Szczylik C, Lee E, Wagstaff J, et al. Pazopanib in locally advanced or metastatic renal cell carcinoma: results of a randomized phase III trial. J Clin Oncol. 2010;28(6):1061–8.
15. Rini BI, Escudier B, Tomczak P, Kaprin A, Szczylik C, Hutson TE, et al. Comparative effectiveness of axitinib versus sorafenib in advanced renal cell carcinoma (AXIS): a randomised phase 3 trial. Lancet. 2011;378(9807):1931–9.
16. Hudes G, Carducci M, Tomczak P, Dutcher J, Figlin R, Kapoor A, et al. Temsirolimus, interferon alfa, or both for advanced renal-cell carcinoma. N Engl J Med. 2007;356(22): 2271–81.
17. Motzer RJ, Escudier B, Oudard S, Hutson TE, Porta C, Bracarda S, et al. Efficacy of everolimus in advanced renal cell carcinoma: a double-blind, randomised, placebo-controlled phase III trial. Lancet. 2008;372(9637):449–56.
18. Gordon J, MacLean LD. A lymphocyte-stimulating factor produced in vitro. Nature. 1965;208(5012):795–6.
19. Sykora KW, Kolitz J, Szabo P, Grzeschik KH, Moore MA, Mertelsmann R. Human interleukin 2 gene is located on chromosome 4. Cancer Invest. 1984;2(4):261–5.
20. Taniguchi T, Matsui H, Fujita T, Takaoka C, Kashima N, Yoshimoto R, et al. Structure and expression of a cloned cDNA for human interleukin-2. Nature. 1983;302(5906):305–10.
21. Caligiuri MA, Zmuidzinas A, Manley TJ, Levine H, Smith KA, Ritz J. Functional consequences of interleukin 2 receptor expression on resting human lymphocytes. Identification of a novel natural killer cell subset with high affinity receptors. J Exp Med. 1990;171(5): 1509–26.
22. Baker PE, Gillis S, Smith KA. Monoclonal cytolytic T-cell lines. J Exp Med. 1979;149(1): 273–8.
23. Gullberg M, Smith KA. Regulation of T cell autocrine growth. T4+ cells become refractory to interleukin 2. J Exp Med. 1986;163(2):270–84.
24. Hersey P, Bindon C, Edwards A, Murray E, Phillips G, McCarthy WH. Induction of cytotoxic activity in human lymphocytes against autologous and allogeneic melanoma cells in vitro by culture with interleukin 2. Int J Cancer. 1981;28(6):695–703.
25. Kanar MC, Thiele DL, Ostensen M, Lipsky PE. Regulation of human natural killer (NK) cell function: Induction of killing of an NK-resistant renal carcinoma cell line. J Clin Immunol. 1988;8(1):69–79.

26. Rosenberg SA, Mule JJ, Spiess PJ, Reichert CM, Schwarz SL. Regression of established pulmonary metastases and subcutaneous tumor mediated by the systemic administration of high-dose recombinant interleukin 2. J Exp Med. 1985;161(5):1169–88.
27. Salup RR, Back TC, Wiltrout RH. Successful treatment of advanced murine renal cell cancer by bicompartmental adoptive chemoimmunotherapy. J Immunol. 1987;138(2):641–7.
28. Salup RR, Wiltrout RH. Adjuvant immunotherapy of established murine renal cancer by interleukin 2-stimulated cytotoxic lymphocytes. Cancer Res. 1986;46(7):3358–63.
29. McDermott DF, Regan MM, Clark JI, Flaherty LE, Weiss GR, Logan TF, et al. Randomized phase III trial of high-dose interleukin-2 versus subcutaneous interleukin-2 and interferon in patients with metastatic renal cell carcinoma. J Clin Oncol. 2005;23(1):133–41.
30. Figlin R, Gitlitz B, Franklin J, Dorey F, Moldawer N, Rausch J, et al. Interleukin-2-based immunotherapy for the treatment of metastatic renal cell carcinoma: an analysis of 203 consecutively treated patients. Cancer J Sci Am. 1997;3 Suppl 1:S92–7.
31. Fyfe G, Fisher RI, Rosenberg SA, Sznol M, Parkinson DR, Louie AC. Results of treatment of 255 patients with metastatic renal cell carcinoma who received high-dose recombinant interleukin-2 therapy. J Clin Oncol. 1995;13(3):688–96.
32. Fisher RI, Rosenberg SA, Sznol M, Parkinson DR, Fyfe G. High-dose aldesleukin in renal cell carcinoma: long-term survival update. Cancer J Sci Am. 1997;3 Suppl 1:S70–2.
33. van der Vliet HJ, Koon HB, Yue SC, Uzunparmak B, Seery V, Gavin MA, et al. Effects of the administration of high-dose interleukin-2 on immunoregulatory cell subsets in patients with advanced melanoma and renal cell cancer. Clin Cancer Res. 2007;13(7):2100–8.
34. von der Maase H, Geertsen P, Thatcher N, Jasmin C, Mercatello A, Fossa SD, et al. Recombinant interleukin-2 in metastatic renal cell carcinoma–a European multicentre phase II study. Eur J Cancer. 1991;27(12):1583–9.
35. Negrier S, Maral J, Drevon M, Vinke J, Escudier B, Philip T. Long-term follow-up of patients with metastatic renal cell carcinoma treated with intravenous recombinant interleukin-2 in Europe. Cancer J Sci Am. 2000;6 Suppl 1:S93–8.
36. Vlasveld LT, Horenblas S, Hekman A, Hilton AM, Dubbelman AC, Melief CJ, et al. Phase II study of intermittent continuous infusion of low-dose recombinant interleukin-2 in advanced melanoma and renal cell cancer. Ann Oncol. 1994;5(2):179–81.
37. Yang JC, Topalian SL, Parkinson D, Schwartzentruber DJ, Weber JS, Ettinghausen SE, et al. Randomized comparison of high-dose and low-dose intravenous interleukin-2 for the therapy of metastatic renal cell carcinoma: an interim report. J Clin Oncol. 1994;12(8):1572–6.
38. Clark JI, Atkins MB, Urba WJ, Creech S, Figlin RA, Dutcher JP, et al. Adjuvant high-dose bolus interleukin-2 for patients with high-risk renal cell carcinoma: A cytokine working group randomized trial. J Clin Oncol. 2003;21(16):3133–40.
39. Gore ME, Griffin CL, Hancock B, Patel PM, Pyle L, Aitchison M, et al. Interferon alfa-2a versus combination therapy with interferon alfa-2a, interleukin-2, and fluorouracil in patients with untreated metastatic renal cell carcinoma (MRC RE04/EORTC GU 30012): an open-label randomised trial. Lancet. 2010;375(9715):641–8.
40. Dutcher JP, de Souza P, McDermott D, Figlin RA, Berkenblit A, Thiele A, et al. Effect of temsirolimus versus interferon-alpha on outcome of patients with advanced renal cell carcinoma of different tumor histologies. Med Oncol. 2009;26(2):202–9.
41. Figlin RA, Thompson JA, Bukowski RM, Vogelzang NJ, Novick AC, Lange P, et al. Multicenter, randomized, phase III trial of CD8(+) tumor-infiltrating lymphocytes in combination with recombinant interleukin-2 in metastatic renal cell carcinoma. J Clin Oncol. 1999;17(8):2521–9.
42. Law TM, Motzer RJ, Mazumdar M, Sell KW, Walther PJ, O'Connell M, et al. Phase III randomized trial of interleukin-2 with or without lymphokine-activated killer cells in the treatment of patients with advanced renal cell carcinoma. Cancer. 1995;76(5):824–32.
43. Mani S, Todd MB, Katz K, Poo WJ. Prognostic factors for survival in patients with metastatic renal cancer treated with biological response modifiers. J Urol. 1995;154(1):35–40.

44. Herrmann E, Brinkmann OA, Bode ME, Bierer S, Kopke T, Bogemann M, et al. Histologic subtype of metastatic renal cell carcinoma predicts response to combined immunochemotherapy with interleukin 2, interferon alpha and 5-fluorouracil. Eur Urol. 2007;51(6):1625,31. discussion 1631-2.
45. Upton MP, Parker RA, Youmans A, McDermott DF, Atkins MB. Histologic predictors of renal cell carcinoma response to interleukin-2-based therapy. J Immunother. 2005;28(5): 488–95.
46. Atkins M, Regan M, McDermott D, Mier J, Stanbridge E, Youmans A, et al. Carbonic anhydrase IX expression predicts outcome of interleukin 2 therapy for renal cancer. Clin Cancer Res. 2005;11(10):3714–21.
47. Sabatino M, Kim-Schulze S, Panelli MC, Stroncek D, Wang E, Taback B, et al. Serum vascular endothelial growth factor and fibronectin predict clinical response to high-dose interleukin-2 therapy. J Clin Oncol. 2009;27(16):2645–52.
48. de Martino M, Klatte T, Seligson DB, LaRochelle J, Shuch B, Caliliw R, et al. CA9 gene: single nucleotide polymorphism predicts metastatic renal cell carcinoma prognosis. J Urol. 2009;182(2):728–34.
49. McDermott DF. The high-dose aldesleukin (HD IL-2) “SELECT” trial in patients with metastatic renal cell carcinoma. J Clin Oncol. 2010;28 Suppl 15:4514.
50. Yang JC, Hughes M, Kammula U, Royal R, Sherry RM, Topalian SL, et al. Ipilimumab (anti-CTLA4 antibody) causes regression of metastatic renal cell cancer associated with enteritis and hypophysitis. J Immunother. 2007;30(8):825–30.
51. Yang JC, Sherry_RM, Steinberg SM, Topalian SL, Schwartzentruber DJ, Hwu P, et al. Randomized study of high-dose and low-dose interleukin-2 in patients with metastatic renal cancer. J Clin Oncol. 2003;21(16):3127–32.
52. Yang JC, Rosenberg SA. An ongoing prospective randomized comparison of interleukin-2 regimens for the treatment of metastatic renal cell cancer. Cancer J Sci Am. 1997;3 Suppl 1:S79–84.
53. Weiss GR, Margolin KA, Aronson FR, Sznol M, Atkins MB, Dutcher JP, et al. A randomized phase II trial of continuous infusion interleukin-2 or bolus injection interleukin-2 plus lymphokine-activated killer cells for advanced renal cell carcinoma. J Clin Oncol. 1992;10(2):275–81.
54. Rosenberg SA, Lotze MT, Muul LM, Leitman S, Chang AE, Ettinghausen SE, et al. Observations on the systemic administration of autologous lymphokine-activated killer cells and recombinant interleukin-2 to patients with metastatic cancer. N Engl J Med. 1985;313(23):1485–92.
55. Negrier S, Perol D, Ravaud A, Bay JO, Oudard S, Chabaud S, et al. Randomized study of intravenous versus subcutaneous interleukin-2, and IFNalpha in patients with good prognosis metastatic renal cancer. Clin Cancer Res. 2008;14(18):5907–12.
56. Negrier S, Philip T, Stoter G, Fossa SD, Janssen S, Iacone A, et al. Interleukin-2 with or without LAK cells in metastatic renal cell carcinoma: a report of a european multicentre study. Eur J Cancer Clin Oncol. 1989;25 Suppl 3:S21–8.
57. Aldesleukin prescribing information. United States: U.S Department of Health & Human Services [updated 03/08/2010]. http://www.fda.gov/Drugs/DevelopmentApprovalProcess/HowDrugsareDevelopedandApproved/ApprovalApplications/TherapeuticBiologicApplications/ucm080733.htm (2010). Accessed 23 Aug 2012.
58. NAGANO Y, KOJIMA Y. Inhibition of vaccinia infection by a liquid factor in tissues infected by homologous virus. C R Seances Soc Biol Fil. 1958;152(11):1627–9.
59. Isaacs A, Lindenmann J. Virus interference I. The interferon. Proc R Soc Lond B Biol Sci. 1957;147(927):258–67.
60. Knight Jr E, Hunkapiller MW, Korant BD, Hardy RW, Hood LE. Human fibroblast interferon: amino acid analysis and amino terminal amino acid sequence. Science. 1980;207(4430):525–6.

61. Derynck R, Content J, DeClercq E, Volckaert G, Tavernier J, Devos R, et al. Isolation and structure of a human fibroblast interferon gene. Nature. 1980;285(5766):542–7.
62. Owerbach D, Rutter WJ, Shows TB, Gray P, Goeddel DV, Lawn RM. Leukocyte and fibroblast interferon genes are located on human chromosome 9. Proc Natl Acad Sci U S A. 1981;78(5):3123–7.
63. Herberman RB, Ortaldo JR, Mantovani A, Hobbs DS, Kung HF, Pestka S. Effect of human recombinant interferon on cytotoxic activity of natural killer (NK) cells and monocytes. Cell Immunol. 1982;67(1):160–7.
64. Herberman RR, Ortaldo JR, Bonnard GD. Augmentation by interferon of human natural and antibody-dependent cell-mediated cytotoxicity. Nature. 1979;277(5693):221–3.
65. Caraglia M, Marra M, Pelaia G, Maselli R, Caputi M, Marsico SA, et al. Alpha-interferon and its effects on signal transduction pathways. J Cell Physiol. 2005;202(2):323–35.
66. Fidler IJ. Regulation of neoplastic angiogenesis. J Natl Cancer Inst Monogr. 2001;28:10–4.
67. Avnet S, Cenni E, Perut F, Granchi D, Brandi ML, Giunti A, et al. Interferon-alpha inhibits in vitro osteoclast differentiation and renal cell carcinoma-induced angiogenesis. Int J Oncol. 2007;30(2):469–76.
68. Kosmidis PA, Baxevanis CN, Tsavaris N, Papanastasiou M, Anastasopoulos E, Bacoyiannis C, et al. The prognostic significance of immune changes in patients with renal cell carcinoma treated with interferon alfa-2b. J Clin Oncol. 1992;10(7):1153–7.
69. Muss HB, Costanzi JJ, Leavitt R, Williams RD, Kempf RA, Pollard R, et al. Recombinant alfa interferon in renal cell carcinoma: a randomized trial of two routes of administration. J Clin Oncol. 1987;5(2):286–91.
70. De Mulder PH, Oosterhof G, Bouffioux C, van Oosterom AT, Vermeylen K, Sylvester R. EORTC (30885) randomised phase III study with recombinant interferon alpha and recombinant interferon alpha and gamma in patients with advanced renal cell carcinoma. The EORTC Genitourinary Group. Br J Cancer. 1995;71(2):371–5.
71. Rini BI, Halabi S, Rosenberg JE, Stadler WM, Vaena DA, Archer L, et al. Phase III trial of bevacizumab plus interferon alfa versus interferon alfa monotherapy in patients with metastatic renal cell carcinoma: final results of CALGB 90206. J Clin Oncol. 2010;28(13): 2137,2143.
72. Messing EM, Manola J, Wilding G, Propert K, Fleischmann J, Crawford ED, et al. Phase III study of interferon alfa-NL as adjuvant treatment for resectable renal cell carcinoma: an Eastern Cooperative Oncology Group/Intergroup trial. J Clin Oncol. 2003;21(7):1214–22.
73. Flanigan RC, Salmon SE, Blumenstein BA, Bearman SI, Roy V, McGrath PC, et al. Nephrectomy followed by interferon alfa-2b compared with interferon alfa-2b alone for metastatic renal-cell cancer. N Engl J Med. 2001;345(23):1655–9.
74. Mickisch GH, Garin A, van Poppel H, de Prijck L, Sylvester R. Radical nephrectomy plus interferon-alfa-based immunotherapy compared with interferon alfa alone in metastatic renal-cell carcinoma: a randomised trial. Lancet. 2001;358(9286):966–70.
75. Ito N, Eto M, Nakamura E, Takahashi A, Tsukamoto T, Toma H, et al. STAT3 polymorphism predicts interferon-alfa response in patients with metastatic renal cell carcinoma. J Clin Oncol. 2007;25(19):2785–91.
76. Kobayashi M, Suzuki K, Yashi M, Yuzawa M, Takayashiki N, Morita T. Tumor infiltrating dendritic cells predict treatment response to immmunotherapy in patients with metastatic renal cell carcinoma. Anticancer Res. 2007;27(2):1137–41.
77. Motzer RJ, Bacik J, Murphy BA, Russo P, Mazumdar M. Interferon-alfa as a comparative treatment for clinical trials of new therapies against advanced renal cell carcinoma. J Clin Oncol. 2002;20(1):289–96.
78. Aass N, De Mulder PH, Mickisch GH, Mulders P, van Oosterom AT, van Poppel H, et al. Randomized phase II/III trial of interferon alfa-2a with and without 13-cis-retinoic acid in patients with progressive metastatic renal cell carcinoma: the European Organisation for Research and Treatment of Cancer Genito-Urinary Tract Cancer Group (EORTC 30951). J Clin Oncol. 2005;23(18):4172–8.

79. Motzer RJ, Murphy BA, Bacik J, Schwartz LH, Nanus DM, Mariani T, et al. Phase III trial of interferon alfa-2a with or without 13-cis-retinoic acid for patients with advanced renal cell carcinoma. J Clin Oncol. 2000;18(16):2972–80.
80. Dudley ME, Wunderlich JR, Robbins PF, Yang JC, Hwu P, Schwartzentruber DJ, et al. Cancer regression and autoimmunity in patients after clonal repopulation with antitumor lymphocytes. Science. 2002;298(5594):850–4.
81. Mayordomo JI, Zorina T, Storkus WJ, Zitvogel L, Celluzzi C, Falo LD, et al. Bone marrow-derived dendritic cells pulsed with synthetic tumour peptides elicit protective and therapeutic antitumour immunity. Nat Med. 1995;1(12):1297–302.
82. Troy AJ, Summers KL, Davidson PJ, Atkinson CH, Hart DN. Minimal recruitment and activation of dendritic cells within renal cell carcinoma. Clin Cancer Res. 1998;4(3):585–93.
83. Thurnher M, Radmayr C, Ramoner R, Ebner S, Bock G, Klocker H, et al. Human renal-cell carcinoma tissue contains dendritic cells. Int J Cancer. 1996;68(1):1–7.
84. Gong J, Chen D, Kashiwaba M, Kufe D. Induction of antitumor activity by immunization with fusions of dendritic and carcinoma cells. Nat Med. 1997;3(5):558–61.
85. Celluzzi CM, Mayordomo JI, Storkus WJ, Lotze MT, Falo Jr LD. Peptide-pulsed dendritic cells induce antigen-specific CTL-mediated protective tumor immunity. J Exp Med. 1996;183(1):283–7.
86. Hayashi T, Tanaka H, Tanaka J, Wang R, Averbook BJ, Cohen PA, et al. Immunogenicity and therapeutic efficacy of dendritic-tumor hybrid cells generated by electrofusion. Clin Immunol. 2002;104(1):14–20.
87. Lambert LA, Gibson GR, Maloney M, Durell B, Noelle RJ, Barth Jr RJ. Intranodal immunization with tumor lysate-pulsed dendritic cells enhances protective antitumor immunity. Cancer Res. 2001;61(2):641–6.
88. Lemoine FM, Cherai M, Giverne C, Dimitri D, Rosenzwajg M, Trebeden-Negre H, et al. Massive expansion of regulatory T-cells following interleukin 2 treatment during a phase I-II dendritic cell-based immunotherapy of metastatic renal cancer. Int J Oncol. 2009;35(3):569–81.
89. Avigan DE, Vasir B, George DJ, Oh WK, Atkins MB, McDermott DF, et al. Phase I/II study of vaccination with electrofused allogeneic dendritic cells/autologous tumor-derived cells in patients with stage IV renal cell carcinoma. J Immunother. 2007;30(7):749–61.
90. Kim JH, Lee Y, Bae YS, Kim WS, Kim K, Im HY, et al. Phase I/II study of immunotherapy using autologous tumor lysate-pulsed dendritic cells in patients with metastatic renal cell carcinoma. Clin Immunol. 2007;125(3):257–67.
91. Berntsen A, Trepiakas R, Wenandy L, Geertsen PF. thor Straten P, Andersen MH, et al. Therapeutic dendritic cell vaccination of patients with metastatic renal cell carcinoma: a clinical phase 1/2 trial. J Immunother. 2008;31(8):771–80.
92. Figlin RA. Phase II, study combining personalized dendritic cell -based therapy AGS 003, with sunitinib in metastatic renal cell carcinoma. J Clin Oncol. 2012;30 Suppl 4:348.
93. Ridolfi R, Riccobon A. Comparison between immature and mature dendritic cells in a vaccination trial. J Clin Oncol. 2004;22(14S):2562.
94. Schwaab T, Schwarzer A, Wolf B, Crocenzi TS, Seigne JD, Crosby NA, et al. Clinical and immunologic effects of intranodal autologous tumor lysate-dendritic cell vaccine with aldesleukin (interleukin 2) and IFN-{alpha}2a therapy in metastatic renal cell carcinoma patients. Clin Cancer Res. 2009;15(15):4986–92.
95. Linsley PS, Greene JL, Tan P, Bradshaw J, Ledbetter JA, Anasetti C, et al. Coexpression and functional cooperation of CTLA-4 and CD28 on activated T lymphocytes. J Exp Med. 1992;176(6):1595–604.
96. Linsley PS, Wallace PM, Johnson J, Gibson MG, Greene JL, Ledbetter JA, et al. Immunosuppression in vivo by a soluble form of the CTLA-4 T cell activation molecule. Science. 1992;257(5071):792–5.
97. Schwartz RH. Costimulation of T lymphocytes: The role of CD28, CTLA-4, and B7/BB1 in interleukin-2 production and immunotherapy. Cell. 1992;71(7):1065–8.

98. Leach DR, Krummel MF, Allison JP. Enhancement of antitumor immunity by CTLA-4 blockade. Science. 1996;271(5256):1734–6.
99. Hodi FS, O'Day SJ, McDermott DF, Weber RW, Sosman JA, Haanen JB, et al. Improved survival with ipilimumab in patients with metastatic melanoma. N Engl J Med. 2010;363(8): 711–23.
100. Rini BI, Stein M, Shannon P, Eddy S, Tyler A, Stephenson Jr JJ, et al. Phase 1 dose-escalation trial of tremelimumab plus sunitinib in patients with metastatic renal cell carcinoma. Cancer. 2011;117(4):758–67.
101. Attia P, Phan GQ, Maker AV, Robinson MR, Quezado MM, Yang JC, et al. Autoimmunity correlates with tumor regression in patients with metastatic melanoma treated with anti-cytotoxic T-lymphocyte antigen-4. J Clin Oncol. 2005;23(25):6043–53.
102. Ishida Y, Agata Y, Shibahara K, Honjo T. Induced expression of PD-1, a novel member of the immunoglobulin gene superfamily, upon programmed cell death. EMBO J. 1992;11(11): 3887–95.
103. Freeman GJ, Long AJ, Iwai Y, Bourque K, Chernova T, Nishimura H, et al. Engagement of the PD-1 immunoinhibitory receptor by a novel B7 family member leads to negative regulation of lymphocyte activation. J Exp Med. 2000;192(7):1027–34.
104. Dong H, Strome SE, Salomao DR, Tamura H, Hirano F, Flies DB, et al. Tumor-associated B7-H1 promotes T-cell apoptosis: a potential mechanism of immune evasion. Nat Med. 2002;8(8):793–800.
105. Blank C, Kuball J, Voelkl S, Wiendl H, Becker B, Walter B, et al. Blockade of PD-L1 (B7-H1) augments human tumor-specific T cell responses in vitro. Int J Cancer. 2006;119(2): 317–27.
106. Thompson RH, Dong H, Kwon ED. Implications of B7-H1 expression in clear cell carcinoma of the kidney for prognostication and therapy. Clin Cancer Res. 2007;13(2 Pt 2):709s–15.
107. Brahmer JR, Tykodi SS, Chow LQ, Hwu WJ, Topalian SL, Hwu P, et al. Safety and activity of anti-PD-L1 antibody in patients with advanced cancer. N Engl J Med. 2012; 366(26):2455–65.
108. Topalian SL, Hodi FS, Brahmer JR, Gettinger SN, Smith DC, McDermott DF, et al. Safety, activity, and immune correlates of anti-PD-1 antibody in cancer. N Engl J Med. 2012;366(26): 2443–54.
109. Brahmer JR, Drake CG, Wollner I, Powderly JD, Picus J, Sharfman WH, et al. Phase I study of single-agent anti-programmed death-1 (MDX-1106) in refractory solid tumors: safety, clinical activity, pharmacodynamics, and immunologic correlates. J Clin Oncol. 2010; 28(19):3167–75.
110. Weinschenk T, Gouttefangeas C, Schirle M, Obermayr F, Walter S, Schoor O, et al. Integrated functional genomics approach for the design of patient-individual antitumor vaccines. Cancer Res. 2002;62(20):5818–27.
111. Walter S, Weinschenk T, Stenzl A, Zdrojowy R, Pluzanska A, Szczylik C, et al. Multipeptide immune response to cancer vaccine IMA901 after single-dose cyclophosphamide associates with longer patient survival. Nat Med. 2012;18(8).
112. Wierecky J, Muller MR, Wirths S, Halder-Oehler E, Dorfel D, Schmidt SM, et al. Immunologic and clinical responses after vaccinations with peptide-pulsed dendritic cells in metastatic renal cancer patients. Cancer Res. 2006;66(11):5910–8.
113. Holtl L, Ramoner R, Zelle-Rieser C, Gander H, Putz T, Papesh C, et al. Allogeneic dendritic cell vaccination against metastatic renal cell carcinoma with or without cyclophosphamide. Cancer Immunol Immunother. 2005;54(7):663–70.
114. Oosterwijk-Wakka JC, Tiemessen DM, Bleumer I, de Vries IJ, Jongmans W, Adema GJ, et al. Vaccination of patients with metastatic renal cell carcinoma with autologous dendritic cells pulsed with autologous tumor antigens in combination with interleukin-2: a phase 1 study. J Immunother. 2002;25(6):500–8.
115. Marten A, Flieger D, Renoth S, Weineck S, Albers P, Compes M, et al. Therapeutic vaccination against metastatic renal cell carcinoma by autologous dendritic cells: preclinical results

and outcome of a first clinical phase I/II trial. Cancer Immunol Immunother. 2002; 51(11–12):637–44.
116. Marten A, Renoth S, Heinicke T, Albers P, Pauli A, Mey U, et al. Allogeneic dendritic cells fused with tumor cells: preclinical results and outcome of a clinical phase I/II trial in patients with metastatic renal cell carcinoma. Hum Gene Ther. 2003;14(5):483–94.
117. Su Z, Dannull J, Heiser A, Yancey D, Pruitt S, Madden J, et al. Immunological and clinical responses in metastatic renal cancer patients vaccinated with tumor RNA-transfected dendritic cells. Cancer Res. 2003;63(9):2127–33.
118. Gitlitz BJ, Belldegrun AS, Zisman A, Chao DH, Pantuck AJ, Hinkel A, et al. A pilot trial of tumor lysate-loaded dendritic cells for the treatment of metastatic renal cell carcinoma. J Immunother. 2003;26(5):412–9.

Adoptive T-Cell Transfer as a Clinical Antitumor Strategy for Hematologic Malignancies

Aaron P. Rapoport and Nadia Ijaz

Abstract Allogeneic stem cell transplantation remains the only widely accepted and effective form of T-cell immunotherapy for blood cancers including lymphoma, myeloma, and leukemia. However this therapy carries substantial risks and is available to only a minority of patients who have suitable donors. The goal of harnessing autologous (patient derived) T-cells to treat blood cancers has been elusive. Nonetheless, new insights into T-cell biology and advances in vaccine and T-cell culture technology have provided a foundation for the development and clinical application of autologous T-cell immunotherapy. Two major but intersecting strategies have been used to stimulate antitumor immunity in patients: therapeutic or "active" immunization using putative cancer-based vaccines and "passive" immunization chiefly referring to the transfer of autologous (or allogeneic) T-cells into tumor-bearing hosts. This chapter briefly reviews the early studies that formed the basis for adoptive T-cell immunotherapy and then focuses on the growing clinical experience of using adoptive T-cell transfer therapy for immune reconstitution and treatment of hematological malignancies. Historically, most of this experience involves the transfer of cultured, poly-specific T-cells obtained from tumor-bearing tissues or peripheral blood. However, advances in the efficiency and safety of gene-transfer technology are driving efforts to generate T-cells with predetermined specificity for known tumor antigens and enhanced functional properties as well. Recent clinical success using adoptive transfer of genetically altered T-cells in the setting of chronic lymphocytic leukemia and pediatric acute lymphoblastic leukemia, although limited to a small number of patients, has generated increasing interest and has validated the therapeutic potential inherent in T-cell transfer strategies.

Keywords Adoptive T-cell Transfers • Autologous T-cell immunotherapy • Cellular Immunotherapy • Gene-modified T-cells • Chimeric Antigen Receptors • CART cells

A.P. Rapoport, M.D. (✉) • N. Ijaz, M.D.
Department of Medicine, University of Maryland School of Medicine,
Marlene and Stewart Greenebaum Cancer Center, Baltimore, MD 21201, USA
e-mail: Arapoport@umm.edu

J.D. Rosenblatt et al. (eds.), *Advances in Tumor Immunology and Immunotherapy*, Current Cancer Research, DOI 10.1007/978-1-4614-8809-5_9,

© Springer Science+Business Media New York 2014

1 Background

Despite impressive advances in the treatment of nearly all types of hematological malignancies, cures remain uncommon for the majority of patients with myeloma and relapsed or refractory lymphoma and leukemia. Dose-intensive chemotherapy/radiotherapy followed by autologous (patient derived) stem cell transplantation leads to complete remissions and extended (~5 years) disease-free survival in about 20–40 % of myeloma patients, but the 10-year disease-free survival is <20 % and the likelihood of cure is < 10 % [1–4]. Autologous stem cell transplants induce cures in about 40 % of patients with relapsed lymphoma [5]. Allogeneic (donor derived) stem cell transplants induce cures in about 20–60 % of patients with acute leukemia depending on remission status and may increase the likelihood of cure for patients with myeloma and high-risk aggressive lymphoma largely through a T-cell-mediated graft-vs.-tumor effect [6–11]. However, the benefit of the graft-vs.-tumor effect is offset to a significant extent by increased treatment-related morbidity and mortality from graft-vs.-host disease (GVHD) wherein donor-derived T-cells attack certain healthy cells and tissues in the patient (e.g., skin, intestinal tract, and liver in the acute phase). Furthermore, immune depletion after all forms of high-dose chemotherapy may be long-lasting and increases the risk for serious bacterial and viral infections [12–14].

Enhanced immune cell number and/or function may be associated with better outcomes after the treatment of a variety of hematologic malignancies. For example, higher lymphocyte counts at diagnosis and after transplantation predicted better disease-free and overall survival for patients with myeloma [15, 16]. Higher lymphocyte counts at diagnosis and relapse have also been associated with improved progression-free and/or overall survivals for patients with lymphoma and myelodysplastic syndromes [17–21], while a few studies have not demonstrated an association between lymphocyte recovery and outcome [22]. In the case of myeloma, tumor-reactive T-cells have been detected at low frequencies in the marrow or the blood of untreated patients [23, 24]. Furthermore, CD4+ and CD8+ T-cells directed against epitopes from the mutated region of NPM1 can be detected in about 30–40 % of patients with NPM1-mutated AML, and in vitro studies reveal that these cells can elicit specific lysis of leukemic blasts [25]. These lines of indirect evidence suggest that tumor-reactive T-cells may be found in a significant proportion of patients with a variety of hematologic malignancies and also provide a justification for the notion that forced increases in the number and function of these tumor-reactive T-cells may contribute to better tumor control. Adoptive transfer of functionally enhanced T-cells which are either poly specific or preferably tumor specific may help repair the immunodepletion that inevitably follows the treatment of hematologic malignancies with standard-dose or high-dose chemotherapy and may exert antitumor effects. While infusion of allogeneic T-cells is a widely accepted and effective if potentially toxic form of adoptive cellular therapy, recent clinical experience suggests that autologous T-cell transfers may also exhibit clinical benefits. These benefits include accelerated immune recovery, protection from infections, enhanced responses to microbial and putative cancer vaccines, and possibly antitumor effects as well. There is growing hope that further developments will allow autologous adoptive T-cell immunotherapy to become a new and highly effective therapeutic branch of transfusion medicine.

2 Allogeneic (Donor) Lymphocyte Infusions

Weiden et al. were among the first to recognize the therapeutic impact of passenger lymphocytes in marrow/stem cell products when they discovered a significantly lower rate of leukemia relapse among recipients of allogeneic marrow grafts vs. recipients of marrow grafts from syngeneic (identical twin) donors [26]. A logical extension of this donor lymphocyte-mediated "graft-vs.-leukemia" effect has been the development of therapeutic donor lymphocyte infusions (DLI). DLI involves the transfer of lymphocytes from the original stem cell donor in an effort to treat relapse of the hematologic malignancy after prior allogeneic stem cell transplantation. DLI can be given alone or following chemotherapy, monoclonal antibody therapy, or other form of cytoreductive treatment to achieve a lower burden of disease prior to DLI. DLI induces durable complete remissions in the majority of patients with chronic myelogenous leukemia (CML) in early-stage relapse. However DLI induces remission in less than 30 % of patients with relapsed acute leukemia, myelodysplastic syndrome, and multiple myeloma, and the majority of these patients eventually relapse again.

Preemptive DLI has also been used for patients with hematologic malignancies who have not formally relapsed with the intention of generating full donor chimerism (complete donor stem cell engraftment in the recipient's blood and bone marrow) and potentiating the graft-vs.-tumor effect.

However the success of DLI comes at the price of GVHD and sometimes marrow suppression with frequencies of 50–60 and 20–40 %, respectively. Several groups have studied different strategies to overcome these complications including combining DLI with chemotherapy, using lymphocyte subset selection, or genetically modifying T-cells to express suicide genes which can be activated in the event of serious GHVD.

2.1 Efficacy of DLI in Various Hematologic Malignancies

2.1.1 Chronic Myeloid Leukemia

The most favorable outcomes after DLI occur in patients with relapsed chronic-phase CML. A large multicenter study showed complete cytogenetic remission in 60 % of relapsed CML patients without pre-DLI cytoreduction [27]. The best response to DLI was evident in chronic-phase CML patients with molecular and/or cytogenetic relapse only. Nearly all of these patients had a complete cytogenetic response, defined as complete absence of the Philadelphia chromosome on standard cytogenetic testing. Patients with cytogenetic relapses or chronic-phase CML at the time of relapse had a complete cytogenetic response rate of 75.7 vs. 33.3 and 16.7 % in patients with accelerated or blast-phase relapses, respectively. Complete responses when achieved were durable with a projected probability of 89 % for remaining in complete remission at 2 years of follow-up. By multivariate analysis, predictors of complete response to DLI included chronic GVHD after the original transplant, chronic-phase disease at relapse, and a time interval of 2 years or less between transplant and DLI. Furthermore, the development of acute and chronic GVHD post DLI also correlated significantly with disease response ($P<0.00001$).

2.1.2 Acute Myeloid Leukemia

Table 1 summarizes the response rates to DLI for a variety of hematological malignancies including CML, AML, acute lymphoblastic leukemia (ALL), lymphoma, and myeloma. From this table it is evident that patients with other hematologic malignancies respond less frequently and durably to DLI. For example, the complete remission rate is about 21 % for patients with relapsed AML, and the long-term survival for AML patients treated with DLI is less than 20 %.

DLI in AML from unrelated donors is associated with a higher response rate when compared to related donors, with one series reporting that 42 % of patients achieved a complete remission after unrelated DLI [29]. A retrospective analysis of DLI in AML performed by the European Group for Blood and Marrow Transplantation showed an estimated survival of 21 % among 171 patients who received DLI vs. a 9 % 2-year overall survival for 228 patients who did not receive DLI for post-transplant relapse [33] After adjustment for all the pertinent clinical variables in the two groups, DLI administration appeared to be associated with improved outcome in younger patients and in those patients who relapsed more than 5 months after transplantation. Bone marrow blast count at the time of relapse, female gender, favorable cytogenetics, and disease remission at the time of DLI were predictive of survival by multivariate analysis. For patients who received DLI in remission and had favorable cytogenetics, the 2-year overall survival was estimated at 56 vs. 9–20 % for those who received DLI with active leukemia. The reasons for reduced DLI efficacy in acute myeloid leukemia as compared to CML may be due to rapid growth kinetics of the acute leukemia cells. Other potential mechanisms for decreased efficacy of DLI in AML include lack of surface expression of costimulatory molecules, defective tumor antigen presentation, involvement of immunologically privileged sites, or down regulation of HLA molecules and especially patient-specific major or minor histocompatibility antigens. In this regard, a study of 43 patients who received haploidentical bone marrow transplants and donor T-cell infusions for acute myeloid leukemia or high-risk myelodysplastic syndrome reported that 5 of the 17 patients (29 %) who relapsed had developed resistance to donor lymphocytes due to genomic loss of the mismatched patient-specific HLA haplotype in the leukemic cells [43].

Table 1 Studies of DLI for relapses after SCT

Disease	Ref.	Patients	Other treatments	DLI dose (per kg)	Responses	Survival
CML	[28]	84	None	3×10^8	Cyto relapse: 82 % Hematological:78 % Accel/blast: 12.5 %	67 % at 2 years
	[27]	56	None	$1–8.2 \times 10^8$	Cyto relapse: 100 % Hematologic: 73.5 % Accel/blast: 33 %	60 % at 2 years
	[29]	25	None	0.85×10^8	CR 46 %	53 % for early phase, 12 % for late phase
	[30]	66	None	1.5×10^8	CR 68 %	91 % at 2 years in responders
	[31]	23	Five patients received IFN alpha	3×10^8	91 % in chronic phase	82 % in chronic phase 16 % in active chase
AML	[28]	23	Eight patients received chemotherapy	$2.4\ (0.25–12.3) \times 10^8$	CR 29 %	15 % at 2 years
	[27]	44	Seven patients received chemotherapy	$1–8.2 \times 10^8$	15.4 % CR in patients without chemotherapy	17 % at 2 years
	[29]	23	Four patients were in remission prior to receiving DLI	1.34×10^8	42 %	21 % at 1.4 years
	[31]	21	None	2.3×10^8	CR in 38 %	7 % at 2 years
	[32]	16	All patients received pre DLI chemotherapy	4.5×10^8	CR in 63 %	31 % at 2 years
	[33]	171	124 patients received pre-DLI chemotherapy	2.8×10^8	CR in 35 %	20 % at 3 year

(continued)

Table 1 (continued)

Disease	Ref.	Patients	Other treatments	DLI dose (per kg)	Responses	Survival
ALL	[28]	22	17 patients received chemotherapy	$2.9\ (0.3–11) \times 10^8$	CR in 9 patients after chemotherapy, 0 % CR after DLI alone	12 % AT 1 year
	[27]	15	Four patients received chemotherapy	$1–8.2 \times 10^8$	CR in 18.2 %	18 % at 1.5 years
	[29]	7	Three patients in CR prior to DLI	0.9×10^8	Two out of four not in CR after chemotherapy went into CR	25 % at 3 years
	[34]	44	28 patients received chemotherapy	$0.01–8.8 \times 10^8$	5 of 16 patients not receiving chemotherapy had CR	12.5 % at 2 years for patients receiving DLI
	[31]	23	None	2.1×10^8	CR in 25 %	5 % at 2 years
	[35]	10	All patients received chemotherapy	$2.9–7 \times 10^8$	CR in 70 %	
Lymphoma	[36]	22/26 relapses	16/26 relapses treated with chemotherapy	$0.01–1.0 \times 10^8$	CR in 77 %	Not provided
	[37]	14	Eight patients received chemotherapy	$0.01–1 \times 10^8$	CR in 57 %	35 % at 2 years
	[38]	17	Seven patients received chemotherapy	$0.01–1 \times 10^8$	CR in 76 %	88 %
Multiple myeloma	[27]	5	None	$1–8.2 \times 10^8$	CR in 50 %	40 % at 2 years
	[39]	13	None	$0.01–3.3 \times 10^8$	CR in 31 %	5–38 months
	[40]	27	13 patients received chemotherapy	$0.01–5 \times 10^8$	CR in 30 %	40 % in 5 year
	[41]	25	Four patients received chemotherapy	$0.02–5.55 \times 10^8$	CR in 28 %	48 % at 1 year
	[42]	63	None	$0.01–3 \times 10^8$	Response seen in 38 %	50 % at 2 years

2.1.3 Other Hematologic Malignancies Including ALL, NHL, Myeloma, CLL, and HD

Pre-B cell or B cell ALL appear to respond even less favorably to DLI than myeloid leukemias perhaps due to the rapid proliferation of the leukemia cells and a variety of immunologic escape mechanisms. Multiple studies showed very low response rates to DLI for relapses after either related or unrelated SCT even when chemotherapy was given before DLI with survival rates of less than 20 % at 1–2 years of follow-up [27–29, 31, 34, 35].

For lymphoma patients with relapsed or progressive disease after allogeneic SCT, DLI with or without chemotherapy resulted in about 50–70 % response rates, but published studies are limited to relatively small number of patients [36–38]. Serial PET scanning after allogeneic SCT may allow more selective and earlier application of DLI leading to higher response rates [36]. In aggregate, these studies indicate that indolent lymphomas may have a better response rate to DLI compared to aggressive lymphomas. Myeloma also appears to be amenable to DLI with response rates of about 30–50 % and survival rates of about 40 % at 1–5 years of follow-up [27, 39–42]. For patients who achieve a PR after DLI, the median progression-free survival (PFS) is only about 7 months while for patients who achieve a CR, the median PFS is about 2 years [42]. Even so, the majority of patients who receive DLI for post-allogeneic SCT relapses of myeloma eventually develop disease progression.

There is very limited published experience for the use of DLI in patients with relapsed chronic lymphocytic leukemia (CLL) or Hodgkin's disease (HD). In one study of DLI for residual or relapsed lymphoid neoplasms after allogeneic SCT, three of four patients with CLL had a CR after DLI [44]. A CLL patient was among the 8 patients (of 18) who achieved a CR after receiving anti-CD3/anti-CD28 costimulated or "activated" DLI for relapsed disease, and this patient remained in CR for 53+ months [45]. Also, new and expanded $CD8^+$ T-cell clonotypes were demonstrated in serial peripheral blood samples taken from a CLL patient who received DLI for recurrent CLL, and the emergence of these clonotypes coincided with disease remission [46]. An anecdotal experience may also be illustrative: A patient with fludarabine-resistant CLL relapsed with nodal disease about 1 year after an unrelated allogeneic SCT. After no response to treatment with rituximab and lenalidomide, the patient received 1×10^7 $CD3^+$ T-cells/kg body weight from the unrelated donor and had a partial response. About 4 months later, a second DLI of 2.8×10^7 $CD3^+$ T-cells/kg body weight was administered. About 1 month later, acute skin GVHD developed which required a course of glucocorticoids. Coincident with the clinical GVHD, the lymphadenopathy regressed and a complete response ensued which has been sustained for more than 2 years. Despite limited data, it is fair to conclude that DLI has the potential to reinduce long-lasting clinical remissions for select patients with recurrent CLL after allogeneic stem transplantation. Data regarding the efficacy of DLI for recurrent HD after allogeneic SCT is also very limited. One study reported on 9 HD patients who received a median of

7.75×10^7 $CD3^+$ T-cells (range 0.5–28.5) [47]. The response rate was 44 % (4/9) with a median duration of 7 months (range 4–9). Three of the four responders developed GVHD and also received pre-DLI chemotherapy. The role of DLI for relapsed HD remains unclear.

2.1.4 Preemptive DLI in Hematologic Disease

The role of preemptive DLI in patients with hematologic malignancies was explored in a prospective study of 82 patients with a variety of hematological malignancies (AML, ALL, CML, and MDS) who were considered to be at high risk of relapse after partially T-depleted allogeneic SCT [48]. DLI was given prophylactically to 31 patients at a median of 22 weeks after transplantation. The first six patients received 0.7×10^8 CD3+ cells/kg body weight with five patients developing acute GVHD. The next 25 patients received a dose of 0.1×10^8 CD3+ cells/kg with eight patients developing acute GVHD and three patients developing limited chronic GVHD. The projected 3-year probability of disease-free survival was 77 % for the 35 patients who were eligible for DLI and 45 % for the 47 patients in the comparison group who were considered to be at high risk for relapse but did not receive DLI due to previous grade 2 or higher acute GVHD and/or chronic GVHD ($P=0.024$). The relapse rate at 36 months after transplantation was 18 % in the patients who were eligible for treatment with DLI and 44 % in the comparison group ($P=0.026$). Thus preemptive, low-dose DLI may be a worthy option for patients who are considered to be at high risk for relapse.

2.2 *Strategies for Optimizing Clinical Benefit of DLI and Minimizing the Risks*

2.2.1 Dosing of DLI

It has been postulated that a dose level or a range of T-cells exists which can induce disease remission without triggering GVHD. This dosing window is likely influenced by the type of hematological malignancy (indolent vs. aggressive) as well as the donor source (matched sibling vs. unrelated donor). One study included 22 patients with relapsed CML after SCT who were treated with escalating doses of DLI ranging from 1×10^5 to 5×10^8 $CD3^+$ T-cells/kg (8 dose levels) at a median of every 6 weeks (4–33 weeks) between infusions [49]. Remissions were seen at T-cell doses at or above 1×10^7 $CD3^+$ T-cells/kg. Nineteen of the 22 patients achieved disease remission (most became PCR negative) with 8 patients receiving just 1 dose of 1×10^7 CD3/kg, and only 1 patient out of these 8 developed chronic GVHD. However, 8 out of the 11 patients who responded and received a T-cell dose of $\geq 5 \times 10^7$/kg developed GVHD. Neither GVL nor GVHD effects were evident at T-cell doses below 1×10^7 $CD3^+$ T-cells/kg. This study demonstrated that the incidence of GVHD correlated to the T-cell dose and for CML, the graft-vs.-leukemia effect can be partially separated from clinically significant GVHD. A large multicenter retrospective study evaluated three dosing regimens of less than 0.2, 0.2–2, and greater than 2×10^8 mononuclear cells/kg in 298 patients with CML and found no difference in response rates at these dose levels, but the incidence of GVHD was lower in patients who received the lower initial dose [50]. Another non-randomized study examined the effect of a bulk dose DLI regimen (BDR) vs. an escalating dose DLI regimen (EDR) in 48 patients with cytogenetic or hematologic relapse of CML after SCT. Twenty-eight patients received the BDR at a median of 1×10^8 cells/kg, whereas 20 received the EDR using a median total cell dose of 1.9×10^8 cells/kg starting at 1×10^7 cells/kg for HLA-related donors and 1×10^6 cells/kg for HLA-unrelated donors. The median interval between the sequential DLIs was 20 weeks. There was no statistical difference in the response rates of the two cohorts (67 % in the BDR and 91 % in the EDR); however, grade II–IV GVHD was seen in 45 % of the BDR compared to 10 % in the EDR. This study implies that a low dose of DLI followed by graduated dose escalation may be the preferred strategy for patients with CML and possibly other hematological malignancies if tumor growth kinetics allow.

2.2.2 Combination of DLI with Chemotherapy or Other Antineoplastic Agents

In addition to lowering the disease burden that must be targeted by the T-cells, pre-DLI cytoreductive chemotherapy may also deplete residual host T-cells and help create "immunological space" for the donor cells to expand. This is potentially a more effective approach for patients who are relatively resistant to DLI alone such as those with acute leukemia or advanced CML. In a prospective trial of 65 myeloid leukemia patients with hematologic relapse after HLA-matched BMT 65 patients were prospectively treated with cytarabine at a dose of 100 mg/m^2/day for 7 days and daunorubicin at 30 mg/m^2/day for 3 days followed by G-CSF-primed DLI at 10–14 days after the initiation of chemotherapy [51]. A complete response was seen in 27 patients albeit with treatment-associated mortality of 23 %. The overall survival was 19 % at 2 years. This study did not appear to show any increased incidence of GVHD with cytoreductive chemotherapy and DLI. In contrast, a small study in which 15 patients with relapsed non-CML malignancies who received cyclophosphamide at a dose of 50 mg/kg on day −6 and fludarabine 25 mg/m^2 for 5 consecutive days from −6 to −2 followed by DLI (1×10^8/kg) 48 h after the last dose of fludarabine were compared to 63 control patients who received DLI without chemotherapy suggested that cytoreductive therapy might contribute to worsening of GVHD [52]. All the patients who received chemotherapy developed lymphodepletion to promote donor lymphocyte expansion and a more effective graft-vs.-tumor effect but also developed significant acute GVHD. Mortality in the DLI-only group was due to either persistent disease or disease recurrence with only 5 % of deaths due to GVHD. On the other hand, 5 of 11 deaths (45 %) in the chemotherapy + DLI group were attributed to GVHD, leading to premature termination of the study.

Another phase I–II study investigated the effect of low-dose thalidomide (100 mg/day) followed by DLI in 18 myeloma patients after allogeneic SCT with progressive or residual disease and previous failure of DLI alone. Complete remission was seen in 22 % of the patients with an overall response rate of 67 %. Two patients developed grade I acute GVHD of the skin, and two patients had chronic GVHD. This study indicated that low-dose thalidomide and DLI may have a clinically significant synergistic effect with a low incidence of GVHD [53].

2.2.3 DLI with CD8 Depletion

Earlier studies suggested that cytotoxic $CD8^+$ T-cells are the principal effectors of GVHD, therefore leading to studies of $CD8^+$-depleted stem cell grafts and eventually $CD8^+$-depleted DLI for disease relapse after SCT. A notable study included 40 patients with relapsed hematologic malignancies after SCT, who were treated with $CD8^+$-depleted DLI at 0.3, 1.0, and 1.5×10^8 $CD4^+$ cells/kg dose levels [54]. Fifteen of 19 patients (79 %) with early-phase relapsed CML responded to treatment, whereas 5 of 6 patients (83 %) with relapsed multiple myeloma and 1 patient with myelodysplasia also developed a response. Complete cytogenetic remission was seen in 87 % of CML patients, and a complete molecular response was seen in 78 % at 1 year after receiving DLI. Two CML patients who did not show a response at dose level 1 later achieved complete cytogenetic remission after a second infusion of CD8-depleted cells at dose level 2. All the patients who developed GVHD demonstrated tumor regression, but 48 % of patients who responded to treatment never developed GVHD. Acute GVHD was evident in 24 % of the patients, while chronic GVHD was seen in 16 %, with only one death due to either GVHD or infection. Also noted in this study was a delay in time to development of GVHD and disease response (median of 11 weeks) when compared to conventional DLI. Due to the relatively low risk of toxicity associated with the infusion of defined number of CD4(+) donor cells, further studies may be warranted to prevent relapse after allogeneic BMT in the setting of persistent minimal residual disease.

Another small randomized trial involving the administration of conventional DLI versus CD8+-depleted cells was conducted in patients with disease remission in an effort to prevent relapse [55]. Acute GVHD developed in six of the nine patients (67 %) undergoing conventional DLI as opposed to no cases of acute GVHD among nine patients receiving CD8-depleted DLI. In the CD8-depleted cohort, there were no toxic deaths and only one relapse. T-cell recovery patterns evaluated by T-cell receptor spectratyping were similar in both groups. This study showed that CD8-depleted DLI led to immune-mediated tumor responses without significant GVHD. Although CD8 depletion appears to reliably reduce GVHD, whether CD8+-depleted DLI will ultimately prove equally effective as a means of inducing GVL is not yet known.

2.2.4 DLI Using Lymphocytes Engineered to Express "Suicide Genes"

Investigators have sought to genetically engineer donor lymphocytes to express thymidine kinase (TK) "suicide" genes which can mediate lymphocyte inactivation upon exposure to ganciclovir. The thymidine kinase encoded by the herpes simplex virus type 1 phosphorylates ganciclovir to an active metabolite which inhibits DNA synthesis and causes cell death. Incorporation of the HSV TK gene into T-cells can lead to the killing of actively dividing cells particularly when these cells are mediating serious GHVD. In one study, 23 patients received TK gene-transduced donor T-cells for relapse of malignancy after SCT and 11/17 evaluable patients had significant clinical benefit including 6 complete responders [56]. Seven patients received ganciclovir which eliminated the TK+cells and appeared to selectively treat the GVHD.

3 Of Mice, Men, and Melanoma: Lessons from Mouse and Human Models of Autologous Immunotherapy

Autologous immunotherapy of cancer can be categorized into three major strategies: (1) general immune cell activation (e.g., IL-2 administration) based on the notion that tumor-directed T-cells exist in the patient but in an inactive state which can be overcome through pharmacologic manipulation; (2) active immunization of the patient with tumor-associated antigen vaccines designed to specifically elicit T-cell and or B-cell responses against the tumor; and (3) adoptive T-cell therapy (ACT) in which autologous T-cells are first removed from the tumor-bearing patient, then otherwise activated, expanded and/or genetically modified to enhance functionality, and then transferred back to the patient to attack the remaining cancer cells. As "stand-alone" therapies, the first two strategies have thus far yielded limited clinical benefits with an objective response rate of 3.3 % among more than 1,300 patients who received a variety of cancer vaccines both at the NIH Surgery Branch and in the published literature [57, 58]. In contrast, ACT has been shown to induce regression of cancer in 50–70 % of patients with advanced and refractory malignancy [59, 60] and offers the potential for sustained responses and application to a wide variety of human cancers.

Much of the early work and success in the field of autologous T-cell immunotherapy were focused on patients with advanced melanoma and EBV-driven tumors including lymphoma and nasopharyngeal carcinoma. Several important principles which would likely apply to the treatment of hematological malignancies with cellular immunotherapy have emerged from this body of work and are summarized below.

3.1 The Importance of Lymphodepletion Before Adoptive Transfers

In order to kill tumor cells in the patient, T-cells must (1) be present in sufficient number, (2) possess adequate affinity for the tumor antigen target, (3) traffic to the tumor bed, and (4) exert a cytotoxic effect on the cancer cells. In addition to the depletion of immune cells which usually accompanies repeated courses of chemoradiotherapy for cancer, a major impediment to effective cellular immunotherapy of cancer is the profound suppression of antitumor reactivity that occurs when T-cells encounter the tumor microenvironment. Indeed, a transgenic murine model in which >95 % of the CD8 cells were specific for a melanoma target antigen (gp100) failed to suppress growth of gp100+ melanoma tumors [61]. Early efforts to isolate, expand, and reinfuse tumor-infiltrating lymphocytes (TILs) to treat metastatic melanoma used either no preparative regimen or low-dose cyclophosphamide (25 mg/kg) yielding objective responses in about 30 % of patients, most of which were short-lived [62, 63]. Based on animal models that suggested that the results of ACT might be improved following more effective lymphodepletion, a series of consecutive trials were conducted that utilized increasingly intensive chemoradiotherapy. Using higher dose cyclophosphamide plus fludarabine (FluCy), FluCy plus low-dose (2 Gy) total body irradiation (TBI), and FluCy plus high-dose TBI (12 Gy), the rate of objective clinical responses after adoptive transfer of about 10^{10}–10^{11} tumor-reactive cultured TILs increased progressively to 49, 52, and 72 %, respectively, by RECIST criteria [64]. Furthermore, responses occurred in a variety of tissues and organs, and the majority of complete responses were durable. The mechanisms whereby intensive lymphodepletion leads to improved survival and clinical impact of adoptively transferred T-cells include (1) liberation of γ_c cytokines including IL-7, IL-15, and IL-21 from "sinks" associated with T/NK cell populations, (2) depletion of CD4+CD25+ regulatory T-cells (Tregs), and (3) enhanced tumor antigen presentation through tumor cell apoptosis and antigen-presenting cell (APC) activation [65, 66]. Whether lymphodepletion and the so-called homeostatic expansion should be routinely incorporated to augment adoptive T-cell transfer strategies requires additional study.

3.2 The Importance of Memory for Optimal ACT

While CD8+ cytotoxic T-cells appear to be the principal actors in the response to ACT, CD4+ T-cells likely provide critical help for CD8+ cells through elaboration of growth factors such as interleukin-2 (IL-2) and IL-21 and expression of CD40-ligand [67–71]. In a cellular vaccine model, CD4+ T-cells also played a broader role in orchestrating an effective antitumor response through recruitment of eosinophils and macrophages. Indeed anecdotally at least one patient with metastatic melanoma achieved a long-term complete remission after infusion of autologous CD4+ T-cell clones that recognized the cancer–testis antigen (CTAg) NY-ESO-1 [72]. The major subsets from which CD8+ T-cells for ACT can be drawn include naïve T-cells (T_N) and memory T-cells (T_M) which can be separated into central memory (T_{CM}) and effector memory (T_{EM}) populations that exhibit distinctive phenotypes, homing properties, and function [73]. CD8+ T_{CM} cells express CD62L and CCR7 which cause homing to lymph nodes, and they activate and expand rapidly upon secondary exposure to cognate antigen. CD8+ T_{EM} cells are negative for CD62L, circulate to infected or inflamed tissues, and more rapidly exert effector functions upon antigen reexposure. Both types of CD8+ T-cells can generate potent effector T-cells (T_E) which kill tumor targets through lytic mechanisms that involve granzyme and perforin release. While highly cytolytic effector cells may exert more potent antitumor activity, memory CD8+ T-cells appear to be the preferred choice for ACT due to higher proliferation potential and survival in vivo [74]. Furthermore, in a primate model, adoptive transfer of effector CD8+ T-cells derived only from CD8+ T_{CM} persisted for a long term, reestablished a memory pool, and responded to rechallenge with a viral (CMV) antigen [75]. However, naïve CD8+ T (T_N)-cells possess characteristics such as higher CD27 expression and longer telomeres that may make them more suitable for ACT when using genetically modified T-cells which have been engineered to recognize and react to tumor targets [76]. The optimal T-cell subpopulations for adoptive transfer have not yet been definitively characterized, and protocols for in vitro expansion and differentiation have not been optimized for clinical use. Improved understanding of T-cell maturation and memory should help further improve ACT protocols.

It should also be noted that while most of the clinical experience of ACT for melanoma has involved TILs, antigen-specific CD8+ T-cell clones derived from the peripheral blood have also yielded durable objective clinical responses [77]. The ability to use tumor antigen-specific peripheral blood lymphocytes for ACT may expand the clinical reach of this form of immunotherapy to the significant proportion of patients whose tumors do not yield adequate TILs for culture and cloning. Recent studies using short-term cultures of enriched but unscreened (for tumor reactivity) CD8+ TILs may also simplify and accelerate the procedure for preparing TILs for successful ACT without sacrificing the high rate of objective responses observed in melanoma patients (50–60 %) [78, 79].

3.3 ACT Can Mediate Regression of Large Tumors: Strategies for Augmenting Responses

An important but perhaps unexpected lesson from studies in melanoma is that ACT can induce regression of very large tumor masses that are well vascularized and metastatic to multiple organs including the lung, liver, adrenal glands, muscle lymph nodes, and skin [64, 80]. Indeed, analysis of large ACT experiences has revealed little or no correlation between tumor bulk and clinical response [81]. Anecdotally, our group has also observed dramatic—albeit transient—regression of advanced, refractory myeloma with nearly 100 % replacement of marrow cellularity by malignant plasma cells and plasmablasts in a patient who received about 5×10^{10} ex vivo costimulated autologous T-cells (unpublished observations). Serial marrow examinations over a period of about 5 weeks showed a progressive decline in marrow plasmacytosis from 100 to 15 % accompanied by a progressive increase in marrow-infiltrating CD8+ T-cells from <5 % to more than 70 %. Taken together, these observations appear to challenge the prevalent notion that cancer immunotherapy is primarily effective for patients with minimal residual disease or only applicable to the adjuvant setting. Factors that correlate to better clinical responses after ACT include long-term persistence of the transferred cells, longer telomere length, and re-expression of CD27 [80]. CD27 expression is a molecular feature which is associated with increased proliferation, IL-2 production, and more resistance to apoptosis of CD8+ T-cells in HIV-infected patients [82]. In a murine model of ACT for large tumors, higher T-cell dose, a T_{CM} phenotype, and post-transfer administration of IL-2, IL-7, IL-15, or IL-21 also predicted better tumor responses [83]. In another murine model, administration of antiangiogenic agents such as vascular endothelial growth factor (VEGF) antibody or VEGFR2 (VEGF-receptor) antibodies increased responses to ACT due in part to increased access of the transferred T-cells to the tumor bed [84].

3.4 *ACT Can Be Used to Treat Viral Infections in Immunocompromised Hosts (e.g., EBV) and EBV-Driven Neoplasms*

Another important application of adoptive T-cell transfer is in the treatment or the prevention of viral infections which arise as a result of loss of immune surveillance in patients who become severely immunocompromised in the course of intensive chemotherapy and/or allogeneic stem cell transplantation. For example, infusions of EBV-specific cytotoxic T lymphocytes (CTLs) generated through gene transfer led to durable (18 + months) immunity against viral challenges [85]. CMV-specific T-cells which were generated by repetitive ex vivo stimulation with CMV antigen led to clearance of CMV viremia in 5/7 evaluable patients who had not responded to antiviral chemotherapy [86]. Newer culture techniques have extended this form of therapy to post-transplant adenoviral infections as well [87]. Given that EBV can cause life-threatening lymphoproliferative disorders after allogeneic stem cell transplantation including up to 25 % of pediatric recipients of T-cell-depleted unrelated or HLA-mismatched donor transplants, EBV-specific CTLs have also been tested in this setting. An early study of 39 patients who were at high risk for EBV-induced lymphoproliferative disorders received 2–4 infusions of polyclonal donor-derived T-cells that were selected and cultured for anti-EBV activity [88]. Six patients with high levels of EBV-DNA had 2–4 log reductions in viral DNA, and none developed lymphoma while two patients who did not receive EBV CTLs and subsequently developed lymphoma exhibited complete responses after T-cell therapy. EBV-specific CTLs were successfully derived from 11 of 15 patients with relapsed EBV+Hodgkin disease and generated temporary clinical responses in 2 of 3 treated patients [89]. Immunoassays from this early study indicated that LMP2 was a frequent target of these CTLs and could elicit homing to tumors. Using gene-marked CTLs raised against EBV-transformed autologous lymphoblastoid cell lines as APCs and a novel strategy for accelerated expansion, 14 patients with relapsed HD were treated with ACT leading to complete responses in five patients, two of whom had measurable disease prior to cell transfer and remained in remission for >9 months and >27 months [90]. Five additional patients exhibited stable disease, and studies of the gene-marked cells clearly showed trafficking of the CTLs to tumor sites. The frequency of LMP2-directed CTLs could be increased about 100-fold by using LMP2 gene-modified APCs as stimulator cells, and these LMP2-specific and expanded CTLs were used to treat 16 patients with EBV+HD or NHL [91]. Nine of ten patients who were treated while in remission remained free of disease, while five of six patients with active disease just prior to ACT had an objective tumor response by RECIST criteria, four of which were complete and sustained for >9 months. One notable patient with marrow involvement with chemotherapy-resistant HD remained in remission for >34 months. ACT with donor-derived viral antigen-specific CTLs has also been used in the allogeneic transplant setting to treat reactivations of EBV, CMV, or adenovirus as well as EBV-driven lymphoproliferative disorders in 153 recipients while incurring acute GVHD in 6.5 % of patients, all of whom had earlier episodes [92]. Notably, there were no differences in the frequency of GVHD between patients who received CTLs from HLA-matched vs. HLA-mismatched donors. At least one patient with protracted and drug-resistant CMV encephalitis had viral suppression and clinical improvement after receiving graduated doses of unmanipulated donor lymphocytes while developing only grade II skin GVHD after the fifth infusion which was steroid responsive [93].

3.5 *Safety and Tolerance of T-Cell Infusions*

Adverse events early after infusions of autologous T-cells for ACT are generally mild and infrequent. The Baylor group recently conducted a review of 381 T-cell products given to 180 patients who were enrolled in 18 clinical trials over a 10-year period [94]. These patients received ex vivo-expanded T-cells that were selected and cultured for tumor or viral antigen specificity and/or were gene-modified. No grade 3–4 infusion reactions were identified during 24 h of observation after infusion. About 12.5 % of patients had grade 1–2 reactions within 24 h of infusion, including nausea/vomiting, hypotension, pain, dyspnea or hypoxia, fever, and chills. It should be noted that the cell doses in these studies were generally low (from 10^4/kg body weight up to $2\times10^8/m^2$). Early and later adverse effects of activated and expanded autologous T-cell transfers appear to be more frequent and more clinically significant in patients who receive higher T-cell doses, undergo more intensive lymphodepletion (e.g., high-dose chemotherapy for autologous stem cell transplants), and/or receive T-cell products which are genetically modified to introduce new target specificities and functional properties. For example, a patient with bulky CLL died from multiorgan failure after receiving gene-modified T-cells engineered to express a chimeric antigen receptor (CAR) which recognized CD19, a common normal B-cell and B-cell lymphoma antigen [95]. A second patient with colon cancer metastatic to the lungs developed fulminant respiratory failure within 15 min of receiving T-cells which had been genetically modified to express a CAR that recognized ERBB2—the tumor-associated antigen which is targeted by the widely used monoclonal antibody Trastuzumab (Herceptin®) and died 5 days later [96]. The intracellular portion of this CAR contained signaling domains derived from CD28, CD3ζ, and 4-1BB which likely provided a strong activation and proliferation signal after antigen encounter. Additional toxicities associated with ACT in hematological neoplasms are discussed in later sections. Caution and vigilant clinical monitoring are clearly warranted for any T-cell products or T-cell stimulants that are being newly tested in humans. Even preclinical models including nonhuman primates failed to predict the nearly fatal widespread T-cell activation and cytokine storm that occurred after giving a superagonistic anti-CD28 monoclonal antibody (TGN1412) to normal human volunteers [97]. Historically, ACT has been avoided in patients with known brain metastases due to safety concerns and uncertainty about whether tumor-directed T-cells could successfully cross the blood–brain barrier. However, a recent analysis of 264 patients with metastatic melanoma who received ACT at the NCI Surgery Branch retrospectively identified 26 patients who had both untreated brain metastases and extracranial disease prior to ACT [98]. Seven of seventeen patients (41 %) who received TILs had a complete response in the brain accompanied by partial extracranial responses in six, while two of nine patients (22 %) who received gene-modified T-cells had a complete response, one of whom also had a partial extracranial response. One patient developed a subarachnoid hemorrhage in a brain tumor while thrombocytopenic but was successfully treated by resection. These data suggest that brain metastases are not beyond the reach of ACT and should not necessarily be a basis for routine exclusion from treatment. A recent trial involving transfer of CAR-modified T-cells into pediatric patients with relapsed childhood ALL shows that modified cells may cross the blood–brain barrier and further raises the possibility of ACT efficacy against CNS disease as well as the potential for CNS toxicity.

3.6 ACT with Gene-Modified T-Cells Is Effective and Potentially Widely Applicable

Despite the great promise of ACT and its demonstrated ability to induce regression of tumors in patients with advanced melanoma, there are at least two important limitations of this approach: (1) patients must have relatively large tumors from which TILs can be isolated and expanded; this procedure occurs successfully in about

50 % of eligible patients, and (2) in many other forms of cancer, tumor-reactive T-cells are much more difficult to identify, isolate, and expand. Work by Eshhar and others has shown that T-cells can be genetically engineered to express novel antigen recognition receptors composed of the variable binding domains of an immunoglobulin molecule fused to the constant, signaling domains of the T-cell receptor (TCR) [99]. These "chimeric TCR"- or "CAR"-expressing T-cells then become functionally redirected to the specific antigen which is recognized by the immunoglobulin portion of the molecule and can proliferate and mediate non-MHC-restricted cytotoxicity against cells expressing the antigenic target. An alternative approach is to isolate and clone native TCRs or generate "affinity-enhanced" TCRs for a specific tumor antigen epitope and then genetically modify T-cells to express these native or affinity-enhanced TCRs in order to redirect them to tumor cells that are known to express the tumor antigen target. This latter approach will be limited to patients who carry the HLA antigens (usually A-0201, A01, or other relatively common class I antigens) which are recognized by the TCRs. Advances in vector technology, specifically the advent of lentiviral vectors which can efficiently target both dividing and nondividing lymphocytes, have facilitated the recent clinical testing and development of these technologies.

Using a retroviral vector which was optimized to express the alpha and beta chains of an anti-MART-1 TCR, HLA-A0201^{+} patients with refractory, metastatic melanoma received ACT with gene-modified autologous T-cells [100]. Among 15 patients who received short-term cultured cells (6–9 days of ex vivo stimulation with anti-CD3 antibody), all showed strong persistence of gene-modified cells with engraftment levels above 10 % of peripheral blood lymphocytes for 2 months or more after infusion. Two patients who had rapid progression of disease prior to ACT had partial responses by RECIST criteria which were sustained at 21 and 20 months of follow-up. Both of these patients had high levels of gene-marked cells at 1 year post treatment as well as evidence of proliferation in the peripheral blood. An emerging principle from both tumor and viral immunology is that higher avidity interactions between T-cells and target antigens may lead to more effective immune responses [101, 102]. In an effort to increase the affinity of native tumor antigen-specific TCRs for their target antigens, one or two amino acid substitutions have been introduced into the complementarity determining regions (CDRs) of TCRs for MART-1 (amino acids 27–35) and the CTAg NY-ESO-1 (amino acids 157–165), leading to enhanced TCR function without apparently sacrificing binding specificity [103]. A clinical trial of ACT using gene-modified autologous T-cells which were engineered to express an affinity-enhanced TCR for the NY-ESO-1 CTAg enrolled 17 patients with metastatic synovial cell sarcoma and melanoma [104]. Objective clinical responses by RECIST criteria were observed in 4/6 sarcoma patients and 5/11 melanoma patients, including 2 complete responses in the latter group which persisted for more than 1 year. Based on murine models, a safety concern that has been raised about the use of TCR gene-modified T-cells is the occurrence of serious autoimmune complications which may arise from the generation of new (self-directed) TCR specificities that result from mixed pairing of exogenous (transferred) and endogenous TCR chains [105]. However, no cases of GVHD nor autoimmune pathology have been observed in more than 100 patients who received gene-modified T-cells that were engineered to express a variety of tumor antigen TCRs derived from both human and mouse origin [106]. This disparity again highlights the potential limitations of using animal models to predict the toxicities (and efficacy) of immunotherapeutic interventions in humans.

4 Clinical Studies of ACT for Hematologic Malignancies

4.1 Background and General Principles

Extensive rationale has led to the ongoing testing of ACT in the setting of hematologic malignancies. Immune cell depletion after chemotherapy, especially high-dose chemotherapy or radiotherapy, can be prolonged and leads to an increased risk for infections [12–14]. In addition, higher lymphocyte levels may be associated with lower rates of relapse and higher rates of survival after allogeneic or autologous stem cell transplantation for hematologic malignancies [107, 108]. Indeed one study of AML patients who received allogeneic transplants showed a 3-year likelihood of relapse of 16 % if the absolute lymphocyte count (ALC) was >200 cells/μl at day +29 vs. a relapse rate of 42 % for patients who exhibited an ALC of ≤200 cells/μl [107]. In a second study of allogeneic bone marrow transplantation for a variety of hematologic malignancies, the overall survival was 79 % at 1 year for patients who had an ALC at day 17 of ≥500/μl vs. 19 % for patients with an ALC <500 cells/μl ($p=0.002$) [108]. Porrata and colleagues examined 230 autograft recipients with myeloma or NHL and showed that day-15 ALC correlated to overall survival [15]. For 126 myeloma patients, an ALC ≥500 on day 15 was associated with median overall (OS) and progression-free survivals of 33 and 16 months, respectively, while an ALC <500 was associated with an OS of 12 months ($P<0.0001$) and a PFS of 8 months ($P<0.0003$) [15]. Among 104 NHL patients the median OS and PFS durations were also significantly longer for patients with an ALC of 500 cells/μl vs. patients with an ALC <500: For OS, not reached vs. 6 months, $P<0.0001$; for PFS, not reached vs. 4 months, $P<0.0001$. Additionally in this study, multivariate analysis revealed that the day-15 ALC level was an independent predictor of OS and PFS.

ACT may result in more predictable and robust patterns of immune cell recovery. However, initial or induction chemotherapy for hematological malignancies often results in profound immune cell depletion which may impair the ability to collect sufficient number of lymphocytes for transfer. Early studies explored whether ex vivo stimulation and expansion of patient-derived lymphocytes followed by adoptive transfer might influence in vivo immune recovery. An early phase I study of CD4+-enriched peripheral blood mononuclear cells (PBMCs) which were expanded ex vivo using anti-CD3 antibody for 4 days and then transferred into 31 patients who then received IL-2 for 7 days demonstrated a statistically significant increase in

CD4+ T-cells, CD4+ subsets, and CD4+/CD8+ ratio [109]. This study included 4 lymphoma patients and 14 melanoma patients, some with subcutaneous tumors to which 111-indium-labeled CD4+ T-cells showed trafficking. Another phase I trial included eight patients with various solid tumors who received multiple infusions of T-cells which were costimulated using anti-CD3/anti-CD28-coated bead cells in the presence of IL-2 [110]. PBMCs from recipients of the bead-costimulated T-cells showed enhanced production of interferon-γ and GM-CSF indicating possible functionality. However tumor responses in both of these studies were infrequent and partial perhaps due to inadequate lymphodepletion prior to T-cell transfers resulting in persistence of T regulatory cells and myeloid suppressor populations. In addition, T-cell responses against specific target antigens could not be evaluated.

In order to be useful in the treatment of hematological malignancies, ACT must likely enhance both T-cell numbers and function. Recent developments in the technology of ex vivo T-cell expansion have allowed about 100-fold expansion of lymphocytes obtained by leukapheresis, enabling even heavily pretreated patients to receive this form of therapy. While isolation and repetitive stimulation of tumor antigen-specific T-cells from peripheral blood or tumor samples may increase the likelihood of tumor recognition and targeting, the procedure is costly, labor intensive, and not infrequently unsuccessful. A second approach based on polyclonal stimulation of T-cells with immunomagnetic beads to which anti-CD3 and anti-CD28 monoclonal antibodies have been conjugated has consistently yielded high number of functional T-cells in support of numerous clinical trials. Key properties of this system are (1) the absence of "feeder" cell layers which facilitates conformity with FDA requirements, (2) ease of clinical scale-up to rapidly produce large number of mature T-cells, and (3) induction of telomerase to minimize the risk of replicative senescence [111, 112]. The rationale for this "polyclonal" approach is predicated in part on the notion that patient immune systems may already be "primed" to their tumors and that augmentation of this endogenous immune response will be clinically beneficial. Evidence for tumor priming seems to be particularly compelling in the area of hematological malignancies [23–25].

4.2 *ACT Using Polyclonal T-Cell Populations*

Early clinical applications of anti-CD3/anti-CD28-costimulated autologous T-cells to the treatment of hematological malignancies involved adoptive transfers after high-dose chemotherapy and autologous stem cell transplantation for patients with relapsed or refractory non-Hodgkin's B-cell lymphoma (NHL) and patients with CML who lacked a suitable donor for allogeneic transplantation. Sixteen patients with relapsed or refractory NHL received 2.5, 5.0, or 10×10^9 costimulated T-cells on day +14 after high-dose BCNU/cytarabine/etoposide/cyclophosphamide (BEAC) and CD34-selected autologous stem cell transplantation [113]. Five patients exhibited a delayed lymphocytosis between days 30 and 120 post transplant, and the procedure partially improved T-cell function as measured by IFN-γ production after

PMA or ionomycin stimulation. Four patients with chronic-phase CML participated in a small pilot study of anti-CD3/anti-CD28-costimulated T-cell transfers following autologous stem cell transplantation [114]. Three of the four patients are long-term survivors including one patient who remains in a complete molecular remission 13 years following autotransplantation, without having received any tyrosine kinase inhibitor therapy for her CML.

To test the feasibility of combining adoptive T-cell transfers with active immunizations and whether such a combined approach could induce vaccine-specific T-cell responses, a randomized trial was conducted in the setting of autologous stem cell transplantation for 54 patients with relapsed or refractory myeloma [115]. The selected vaccine was a heptavalent pneumococcal conjugate vaccine (®Prevnar, PCV) composed of saccharide antigens for the seven most common pneumococcal subtypes linked to a protein carrier (CRM-197) that is derived from diphtheria toxin. The choice of this vaccine allowed both antibody and T-cell responses to be evaluated, while the randomized design allowed different schedules of vaccination (pre- and post-transplant vs. post-transplant only) and T-cell infusion (day +12 vs. day +100 post transplant) to be compared. The optimal schedule (group 1) which yielded the most robust and only sustained antibody responses to the pneumococcal saccharide antigens and the most robust and sustained T-cell responses to the carrier protein was the following: pre-transplant immunization about 10 days before steady-state T-cell collection → early infusion of vaccine-primed and anti-CD3/CD28 antibody-costimulated autologous T-cells at day +12 post transplant → post-transplant booster immunizations at days 30 and 90 post transplantation. The T-cell/vaccine schedules for the other treatment groups including patients who did not receive costimulated T-cells until day +100 (groups 2 and 4) or received no priming (pre-transplant) vaccination (group 3) yielded significantly lower levels of vaccine-directed immune responses which were short-lived. Figure 1 illustrates the flow of this combined vaccine and T-cell strategy. The patients who were randomly assigned to receive up to 1×10^{10} costimulated T-cells at day +12 post transplant had significantly higher CD4 and CD8 T-cell counts at day +42 post transplant than the patients who received T-cells at day +100. In addition, only the patients who were randomized to receive pre- and post-transplant PCV immunizations along with the "early" day +12 infusion of costimulated T-cells generated and maintained protective levels of pneumococcal specific antibodies along with vaccine (CRM-197)-specific CD4+ T-cell responses as early as day +42 post transplant. This randomized pilot study provided convincing evidence that the severe quantitative and qualitative immune deficiencies which prevail after high-dose chemotherapy could be substantially rectified leading to clinically relevant immune function. A similar combination strategy using pre- and post-transplant immunizations using an influenza vaccine plus vaccine-primed and costimulated T-cells also proved effective for generating protective levels of anti-influenza antibodies early after autologous stem cell transplantation for myeloma [116].

To test whether this combination strategy of pre- and post-transplant immunizations plus early transfer of vaccine-primed and ex vivo-costimulated autologous T-cells could induce early immune responses to a cancer-related antigen, a

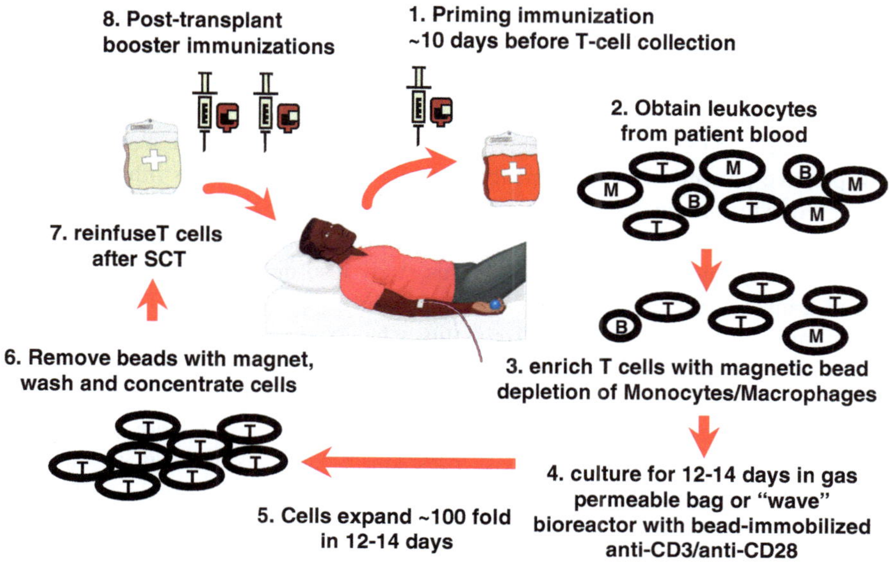

Fig. 1 Combination T-cell and vaccine immunotherapy for hematologic malignancies. Patients with hematologic malignancies who are candidates for autologous stem cell transplantation (ASCT) receive priming tumor and/or microbial antigen immunizations about 10 days before steady-state mononuclear cell collection from the peripheral blood (*1*,*2*). The mononuclear cells are enriched in T-cells by depletion of monocytes and macrophages which can inhibit ex vivo T-cell expansion (*3*). The T-cells are cultured for 12–14 days in gas-permeable bags or in a "wave" bioreactor system with anti-CD3/anti-CD28 monoclonal antibodies conjugated to immunomagnetic beads +/− low-dose IL-2 (*4*). The cells expand about 100-fold after which the magnetic beads are removed, the cells are concentrated, and then prepared for reinfusion after meeting release criteria for sterility and viability (*5*,*6*). Around day +2 after high-dose chemotherapy and autologous stem cell transplantation, patients receive the vaccine-primed and costimulated T-cell product. The product can be shipped fresh and infused on the same day or it can be viably frozen, shipped, and thawed/infused at a later time (*7*). Patients receive two or more post-transplant booster immunizations using the same tumor and/or microbial antigen vaccine that was administered earlier (*8*)

follow-up phase II two-arm trial was conducted using a tumor antigen vaccine composed of peptides derived from the human telomerase reverse transcriptase (hTERT) and the antiapoptotic protein survivin, two potential "universal" tumor antigens [117]. A total of 54 patients with myeloma were enrolled in this phase I/II study including 28 patients who were HLA-A2 positive and therefore eligible to receive the HLA-A2-restricted hTERT/survivin multipeptide tumor antigen vaccine. In an effort to further improve functional immune recovery this new study contained a variety of modifications: First, as a result of technical improvements in the T-cell expansion procedures, patients received up to 5×10^{10} costimulated T-cells which was ~5-fold higher than in the previous study. Second, costimulated T-cells were adoptively transferred on day +2 post transplant rather than day +12 to take better advantage of the stimulatory cytokine milieu induced by severe lymphopenia. Third, the multipeptide vaccine was emulsified in the adjuvant Montanide ISA 51 and coinjected with GM-CSF. Fourth, patients received a total of four vaccinations including one prior to T-cell collection and three vaccinations post transplant at days +14, +42, and +90. In this trial, 36 % of the A2-positive patients exhibited positive immune responses to the hTERT/survivin tumor antigen vaccine as assayed by tetramer analysis. Interestingly, the event-free survival for the group of A2-positive patients who received the tumor antigen vaccine was inferior to that observed in the A2-negative group although this difference appeared to be primarily due to a higher frequency of post-transplant maintenance therapy using thalidomide in the A2-negative (no vaccine) arm. This study also demonstrated that adoptive T-cell transfers resulted in significantly lower levels of regulatory T-cells (Tregs) and significantly higher Teffector/Treg ratios when compared to autograft recipients who did not receive T-cell transfers. Increased Teff/Treg ratios are associated with enhanced tumor necrosis in clinical trials involving immune modulation [118]. Non-myeloma polyclonal immunoglobulins appeared to recover more quickly and robustly in patients who received post-transplant T-cell transfers. Day +2 transfers of up to 5×10^{10} costimulated T-cells led to dramatically higher median CD4 and CD8 counts of about 1,500 cells/μl and nearly 3,000 cells/μl, respectively, at day +14 post transplant. Notably, ~16 % of patients also developed clinically significant autologous GVHD involving the gut and skin which required treatment with systemic glucocorticoids resulting in rapid and complete responses of the GVHD [119]. The patient who had the most severe case of autologous GVHD (grade II skin and grade III gut) remained in complete remission (CR) at 4 years post transplant despite enrolling in the study with advanced and treatment-refractory disease.

Strategies for increasing the frequency and potential clinical impact of post-transplant immune responses to a tumor antigen vaccine may include the use of more effective vaccine adjuvants to enhance priming and boosting of the T-cell responses as well as the incorporation of immunostimulatory drugs (e.g., lenalidomide, anti-CTLA4 antibodies, anti-PD1 antibodies). Along these lines, a recent study was conducted which included 27 patients who were autografted for myeloma. Using a similar pre- and post-transplant immunization scheme plus day +2 infusion of vaccine-primed and ex vivo-costimulated autologous T-cells, this study examined whether the addition of a toll-like receptor-3 (TLR-3) agonist called Poly-ICLC (®Hiltonol) to the vaccine formulation (in addition to GM-CSF and Montanide) would help elicit more robust immune responses [120]. The cancer antigen vaccine employed in this study was a multipeptide vaccine based on the CTAg called MAGE-A3. The vaccine (Orphan Drug Designation GL-0817) is composed of two HLA-A2-restricted class I epitopes and one relatively HLA-unrestricted class II epitope. Early clinical response rates have been encouraging, and importantly, 71 % of patients have exhibited functional vaccine-specific T-cell responses by IFN-γ production on CD4+ T-cells, CD8+ T-cells, or both. In this study, low-dose lenalidomide (10 mg per day) starting at day +100 post transplant was used as a maintenance drug and also as an immunomodulator based on extensive literature suggesting that it has immunostimulatory properties [121–123]. A recent randomized study also demonstrated that lenalidomide enhanced both B- and T-cell immune responses to the 7-valent pneumococcal conjugate vaccine (®Prevnar) in patients with myeloma and appeared to increase myeloma-specific INF-γ-producing T-cells while decreasing Th-17 cells [124].

Potential drawbacks to using tumor antigen vaccines in order to generate tumor specificity are that the success of this approach depends on the existence of naturally occurring tumor-specific T-cell populations that are present in low frequency and even if expanded the T-cell receptors on these tumor antigen-specific T-cells are likely to exhibit low binding affinity as a result of normal T-cell ontogeny. Furthermore, the surface expression level of many tumor antigen epitopes is thought to be extremely low. In particular, the widely studied HLA-A2-restricted epitope $NY\text{-}ESO_{157-165}$ (SLLMWITQC), which is naturally expressed on primary myeloma cells, is estimated to have an expression density of only ~10–50 copies per cell, which is too low to activate conventional cytotoxic lymphocytes [125]. Some investigators have attempted to get around this problem by isolating and activating marrow-infiltrating lymphocytes ("MILs") from patients with myeloma which are akin to "TILs" in that these lymphocyte populations may be self-selected for enhanced tumor antigen specificity and affinity, although tolerized to the myeloma tumor by the immunologically suppressive microenvironment. Recent literature also suggests that the bone marrow is a specific homing site for effector memory T-cells, CD8+ memory cells being the preferred cell type for adoptive immunotherapy as discussed earlier [126]. Indeed, when T-cells were isolated from the marrow of myeloma patients and costimulated with anti-CD3/anti-CD28 to reverse tolerized function, these cells showed significantly higher myeloma-directed cytotoxicity as compared to activated peripheral blood lymphocytes taken from the same patients and also appeared to target clonogenic precursors [24]. A randomized clinical trial of activated MILs alone or in combination with an allogeneic GM-CSF-based myeloma cellular vaccine in the setting of autologous stem cell transplantation for myeloma is in progress.

4.3 Clinical Trials Using Gene-Modified Autologous T-Cells

As described earlier, another strategy to address the challenge of relying on tumor antigen vaccines and activation strategies to enhance endogenous cellular immune responses which are typically low in frequency and antigen affinity is to redirect T-cells to known tumor antigen targets through gene modification. The two major approaches that have been utilized for patients with hematological malignancies is to engineer T-cells to express affinity-enhanced TCRs or CARs, the latter of which are composed of binding domains from the variable regions of antibodies fused to the constant, signaling domains of the TCR (Fig. 2). In one ongoing study based on the first approach, patients receive gene-modified autologous T-cells at day +2 after autologous stem cell transplantation for myeloma [127]. Eligibility for the study requires that patients be HLA-0201 positive and that their myeloma cells express NY-ESO-1 or LAGE-1 by PCR. The T-cells were transduced with a lentiviral vector which encodes an affinity-enhanced TCR for the HLA-A201-restricted epitope

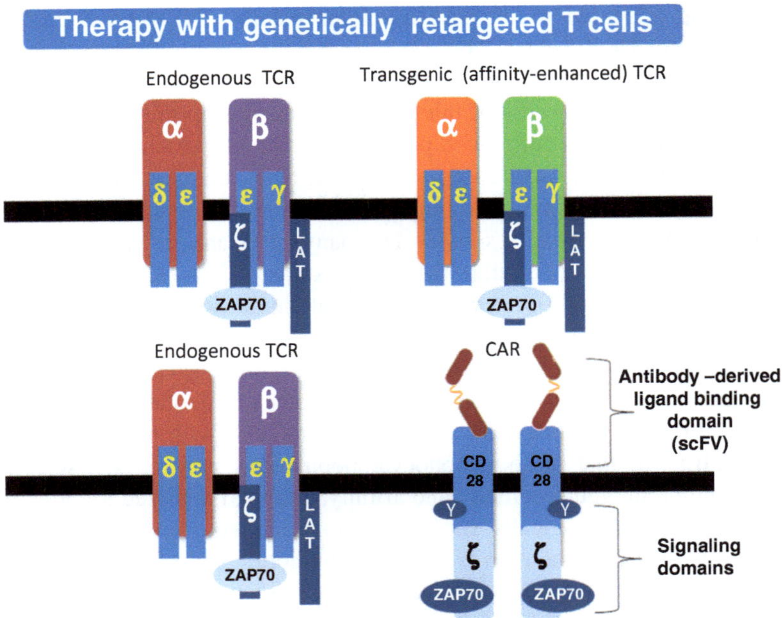

Fig. 2 Therapy with genetically retargeted T-cells. The *top panel* shows a genetically modified T-cell engineered to express an affinity-enhanced T-cell receptor (TCR). This transgenic TCR is coexpressed with the endogenous TCR. The *bottom panel* shows a genetically modified T-cell engineered to express a chimeric antigen receptor (CAR) along with the endogenous TCR. The CAR consists of a ligand or tumor antigen-binding domain derived from the variable regions of the heavy and light chains of an antibody molecule fused to signaling domains that may be derived from the CD3 ζ chain, CD28, 4-1BB, or a combination thereof. A simplified representation of the TCR complex is shown with the α and β subunits, components of CD3 (δ,ε,γ), and downstream signaling effectors (ZAP70 and the transmembrane adapter protein linker for the activation of T-cell—LAT)

NY-ESO$_{157-165}$ (SLLMWITQC) which is also shared by the LAGE-1 CTAg and then activated and expanded using anti-CD3/anti-CD28 immunomagnetic beads. To date, 16 patients have received the gene-modified T-cells, and 13 have reached the day 100 restaging timepoint. Infusions of the gene-modified T-cells have been well tolerated, and ten patients (77 %) have achieved a very good partial response (VGPR) or better, while 11/16 patients continue to show evidence of response with no myeloma progression. Complete and durable clinical responses have also been observed in patients with advanced, refractory, and extramedullary disease [127]. Importantly, the gene-modified T-cells persist for as long as 1 year post infusion and demonstrate marrow trafficking and antigen-specific targeting as NY-ESO-1/Lage-1 expression is extremely low or undetectable in patients with blood and/or marrow persistence of gene-modified T-cells [128].

In contrast to the approach of using affinity-enhanced TCRs, gene modification of T-cells using CARs offers the possibility of redirecting T-cells toward specific tumor antigens without major histocompatibility antigen (MHA) restriction.

Based on groundbreaking work by Eshhar, June, and others, clinical trials of CARs for hematological malignancies are in progress at multiple academic medical centers [99, 129]. The most advanced clinic trials have focused on CD19 which is restricted in its expression to normal and malignant B-cells. Major impediments to the clinical development of CAR technology have been the limited in vivo persistence and expansion of CAR-modified T-cells [130]. Preclinical work has established that addition of the CD137 (4-1BB) cytoplasmic signaling domain to the CD3-ζ chain results in significantly higher persistence, proliferation, and antitumor activity compared to CARs that carry the CD3-ζ chain alone [131]. Translational application of this work led to a pilot clinical trial using autologous T-cells genetically engineered to express an anti-CD19 CAR (CART-19 cells) for patients with relapsed, refractory CLL [132, 133]. Among the first three patients treated on this trial, two achieved a durable complete response and one had a durable partial response. The engineered T-cells expanded more than 1,000-fold in vivo, homed to the bone marrow, killed CD19-expressing target cells, and persisted for at least 6 months. In addition, while the CART19 CD8+ T-cells exhibited an effector memory phenotype ($CCR7^-$, $CD27^-$, $CD28^-$) during and soon after the tumor killing phase, by 6 months post infusion a portion of the CART19 $CD8^+$ T-cells showed a central memory phenotype with coexpression of CCR7 and increased levels of CD27 and CD28. One of the three patients who was described in greater detail had bulky adenopathy and extensive marrow involvement with CLL that carried a 17p deletion with loss of the TP53 locus, a cytogenetic feature which confers a very poor prognosis and is associated with resistance to chemotherapy. This patient received 3×10^8 T-cells over 3 days in escalating doses, of which 5 % were transduced for a total of 1.42×10^7 CART-19+ T-cells. At day 22 post infusion the patient developed dramatic clinical and laboratory signs of tumor lysis syndrome including transient kidney injury requiring hospitalization. This clinical syndrome coincided with peak (3-log) expansion of the CART-19+ T-cells at which time the CART19 cells comprised more than 20 % of the circulating lymphocytes. A complete regression of pathologic lymphadenopathy and marrow and blood involvement ensued which is now reported to be ongoing for 2 years.

This clinical trial experience was recently expanded to include ten patients including nine adults with refractory CLL (3/9 with P53 deletions) and one 7-year-old child with ALL in refractory relapse [134, 135]. All of the CLL patients received lymphodepleting chemotherapy prior to T-cell transfer while the ALL patients did not. The median T-cell dose was 7.5×10^8 (1.7–50) including 1.45×10^8 $CART19^+$ cells (0.14–5.9). With a median follow-up of nearly 6 months, four of nine evaluable patients had a CR (none of whom has relapsed) including three CLL patients and one ALL patient, while two CLL patients had partial responses lasting 3 and 5 months and three patients did not respond. In the four CR patients, the CART19+ cells expanded an average of 27-fold [21–40] in the blood with the peak expansion occurring between days 10 and 31 post infusion. An important and somewhat unexpected finding was that the CART19 cells trafficked to the cerebrospinal fluid in the child with ALL presumably due to the presence of unrecognized CNS involvement with leukemia. Of note, all responding patients developed a "cytokine release syndrome" (CRS) characterized by high fevers and grade III/IV hypotension and hypoxia [136]. The child with ALL exhibited the most severe degree of CRS which culminated in grade IV hypotension and respiratory failure necessitating mechanical ventilatory and pressor support. After glucocorticoid administration led to no improvement, cytokine analysis revealed that IFN-γ, IL-6, IL-2, and TNFα levels were 6,040, 988, 163, and 17 times higher than baseline measured levels. The TNF and IL-6 receptor antagonists etanercept and tocilizumab were given to the patient followed by rapid and complete clinical improvement. Additional laboratory and clinical findings include dramatic elevations of the ferritin levels (44,000–605,000), hepatosplenomegaly unrelated to primary disease, and a moderate degree of disseminated intravascular coagulation (DIC). This constellation of findings suggested that the CRS syndrome had features of macrophage activation syndrome (MAS) and hemophagocytic lymphohistiocytosis (HLH). The 7-year-old ALL patient subsequently entered a complete blood/marrow and CNS remission which is ongoing at 8 months post treatment. This syndrome was subsequently recognized in three CLL patients and treated successfully with the IL-6 receptor antibody tocilizumab alone. Studies to define the optimal time to block the CRS so as not to interfere with the antitumor cellular immune response are under way. A long-term but expected consequence of successful treatment with the CART-19 cells is profound B-cell depletion and hypogammaglobulinemia.

Other groups have reported successful treatment of progressive CD19+ B-cell malignancies including follicular lymphoma using CD19-CAR T-cells in which the signaling domain was derived from CD3-ζ only [137, 138]. Using this construct six of eight patients obtained remissions and four had major elevations of inflammatory cytokines including IFNγ and TNF most likely derived from the gene-modified T-cells. Treatment-related toxicities correlated with the levels of these inflammatory cytokines.

5 Summary

Cellular immunotherapy is the latest to join the three principal systemic therapeutic modalities for hematologic malignancies of chemotherapy, targeted therapy, and antibody therapy. However, the potent cytotoxic potential of T-cells combined with their remarkable capacities for proliferation, trafficking, and sustainability ensures that their role in the treatment of advanced and aggressive blood cancers will likely expand. Although cellular immunotherapy has long been part of the curative mechanism of allogeneic stem cell transplantation, this form of T-cell therapy has been difficult to modulate and separate from serious complications such as GVHD and is limited to a minority of patients in need. The advent of effective and reliable expansion technologies for autologous T-cells and the ability to "redirect" these cells to specific tumor antigen targets through potent vaccine formulations and genetic engineering offer a highly effective and potentially safer approach for a wider spectrum of patients. Future work will likely follow these directions: (1) identification of additional tumor antigens to serve as targets of new high-affinity TCRs or CARs; (2) application of immunomodulatory pharmacologic agents (e.g., IL-15, IL-7, anti-CTLA4, anti-PD1 antibodies, lenalidomide) to further enhance and sustain T-cell growth and function in vivo; and (3) refinement of strategies to ameliorate some of the toxicities associated with activated T-cell therapy including CAR-modified T-cells.

References

1. Barlogie B, Jagannath S, Vesole DH, et al. Superiority of tandem autologous transplantation over standard therapy for previously untreated multiple myeloma. Blood. 1997;89:789–93.
2. Attal M, Harousseau JL, Stoppa AM, et al. A prospective, randomized trial of autologous bone marrow transplantation and chemotherapy in multiple myeloma. Intergroupe Francais du Myelome. N Engl J Med. 1996;335:91–7.
3. Child JA, Morgan GJ, Davies FE, et al. High-dose chemotherapy with hematopoietic stem-cell rescue for multiple myeloma. N Engl J Med. 2003;348:1875–83.
4. Barlogie B, Tricot GJ, van Rhee F, et al. Long-term outcome results of the first tandem auto-transplant trial for multiple myeloma. Br J Haematol. 2006;135:158–64.
5. Rapoport AP, Rowe JM, Kouides PA, Duerst RA, Abboud CN, Liesveld JL, et al. One hundred autotransplants for relapsed or refractory Hodgkin's disease and lymphoma: value of pretransplant disease status for predicting outcome. J Clin Oncol. 1993;11:2351–61.
6. Tricot G, Vesole DH, Jagannath S, Hilton J, Munshi N, Barlogie B. Graft-versus-myeloma effect: proof of principle. Blood. 1996;87:1196–8.
7. Alyea E, Weller E, Schlossman R, et al. T-cell-depleted allogeneic bone marrow transplantation followed by donor lymphocyte infusion in patients with multiple myeloma: induction of graft-versus-myeloma effect. Blood. 2001;98:934–9.
8. Lokhorst HM, Wu K, Verdonck LF, et al. The occurrence of graft-versus-host disease is the major predictive factor for response to donor lymphocyte infusions in multiple myeloma. Blood. 2004;103:4362–4.
9. Garban F, Attal M, Michallet M, et al. on behalf of the IFM group. Prospective comparison of autologous stem cell transplantation followed by a dose-related allograft (IFM99-03 trial) with tandem autologous stem cell transplantation (IFM99-04) trial in high-risk de novo multiple myeloma. Blood. 2006;107:3474–80.
10. Gupta V, Tallman MS, Weisdorf DJ. Allogeneic hematopoietic cell transplantation for adults with acute myeloid leukemia: myths, controversies and unknowns. Blood. 2011;117(8):2307–18.
11. Bacher U, Klyuchnikov E, Le-Rademacher J, Carreras J, Armand P, Bishop MR, et al. Conditioning regimens for allotransplants for diffuse large B-cell lymphoma: myeloablative or reduced intensity? Blood. 2012;120(20):4256–62.
12. Rapoport AP. Immunity for tumors and microbes after autotransplantation: if you build it, they will (not) come. Bone Marrow Transplant. 2006;37:239–47.
13. Youssef S, Rodriguez G, Rolston KV, Champlin RE, Raad II, Safdar A. Streptococcus pneumoniae infections in 47 hematopoietic stem cell transplantation recipients: clinical characteristics of infections and vaccine-breakthrough infections, 1989–2005. Medicine. 2007;86:69–77.
14. Frère P, Pereira M, Fillet G, Beguin Y. Infections after CD34-selected or unmanipulated autologous hematopoietic stem cell transplantation. Eur J Haematol. 2006;76:102–8.
15. Porrata LF, Gertz MA, Inwards DJ, et al. Early lymphocyte recovery predicts superior survival after autologous hematopoietic stem cell transplantation in multiple myeloma or non-Hodgkin lymphoma. Blood. 2001;98:579–85.

16. Ege H, Gertz MA, Markovic SN, et al. Prediction of survival using absolute lymphocyte count for newly diagnosed patients with multiple myeloma: a retrospective study. Br J Haematol. 2008;141(6):792–8.
17. Joao C, Porrata LF, Inwards DJ, et al. Early lymphocyte recovery after autologous stem cell transplantation predicts superior survival in mantle-cell lymphoma. Bone Marrow Transplant. 2006;37(9):865–71.
18. Porrata LF, Inwards DJ, Ansell SM, et al. Early lymphocyte recovery predicts superior survival after autologous stem cell transplantation in non-Hodgkin lymphoma: a prospective study. Biol Blood Marrow Transplant. 2008;14(7):807–16.
19. Porrata LF, Inwards DJ, Ansell SM, et al. New-onset lymphopenia assessed during routine follow-up is a risk factor for relapse postautologous peripheral blood hematopoietic stem cell transplantation in patients with diffuse large B-cell lymphoma. Biol Blood Marrow Transplant. 2010;16(3):376–83.
20. Jacobs NL, Holtan SG, Porrata LF, Markovic SN, Tefferi A, Steensma DP. Host immunity affects survival in myelodysplastic syndromes: Independent prognostic value of the absolute lymphocyte count. Am J Hematol. 2010;85(3):160–3.
21. Porrata LF, Ristow K, Habermann TM, Witzig TE, Inwards DJ, Markovic SN. Absolute lymphocyte count at the time of the first relapse predicts survival in patients with diffuse large B-cell lymphoma. Am J Hematol. 2009;84(2):93–7.
22. Tiwari D, Gao F, Hidalgo J, et al. Prognostic significance of early lymphocyte recovery after post-autografting administration of GM-CSF in non-Hodgkin's lymphoma. Bone Marrow Transplant. 2007;40:671–5.
23. Dhodapkar MV, Krasovsky J, Olson K. T cells from the tumor microenvironment of patients with progressive myeloma can generate strong, tumor-specific cytolytic responses to autologous, tumor-loaded dendritic cells. Proc Natl Acad Sci U S A. 2002;99:13009–13.
24. Noonan K et al. Activated marrow-infiltrating lymphocytes effectively target plasma cells and their clonogenic precursors. Cancer Res. 2005;65:2026–34.
25. Greiner J, Ono Y, Hofmann S, et al. Mutated regions of nucleophosmin 1 elicit both CD4+ and CD8+ responses in patients with acute myeloid leukemia. Blood. 2012;120:1282–9.
26. Weiden PL, Flournoy N, Thomas ED, et al. Antileukemic effect of graft-versus-host disease in human recipients of allogeneic-marrow grafts. N Engl J Med. 1979;300:1068–73.
27. Collins Jr RH, Shpilberg O, Drobyski WR, Porter DL, Giralt S, Champlin R, et al. Donor leukocyte infusions in 140 patients with relapsed malignancy after allogeneic bone marrow transplantation. J Clin Oncol. 1997;15(2):433–44.
28. Kolb HJ, Schattenberg A, Goldman JM, Hertenstein B, Jacobsen N, Arcese W, et al. European group for blood and marrow transplantation working party chronic leukemia graft-versus-leukemia effect of donor lymphocyte transfusions in marrow grafted patients. Blood. 1995;86(5):2041–50.
29. Porter DL, Collins Jr RH, Hardy C, Kernan NA, Drobyski WR, Giralt S, et al. Treatment of relapsed leukemia after unrelated donor marrow transplantation with unrelated donor leukocyte infusions. Blood. 2000;95(4):1214–21.
30. Dazzi F, Szydlo RM, Craddock C, Cross NC, Kaeda J, Chase A, et al. Comparison of single-dose and escalating-dose regimens of donor lymphocyte infusion for relapse after allografting for chronic myeloid leukemia. Blood. 2000;95(1):67–71.
31. Shiobara S, Nakao S, Ueda M, Yamazaki H, Takahashi S, Asano S, et al. Donor leukocyte infusion for Japanese patients with relapsed leukemia after allogeneic bone marrow transplantation: lower incidence of acute graft-versus-host disease and improved outcome. Bone Marrow Transplant. 2000;26(7):769–74.
32. Choi SJ, Lee JH, Kim S, Seol M, Lee YS, Lee JS, et al. Treatment of relapsed acute myeloid leukemia after allogeneic bone marrow transplantation with chemotherapy followed by G-CSF-primed donor leukocyte infusion: a high incidence of isolated extramedullary relapse. Leukemia. 2004;18(11):1789–97.
33. Schmid C, Labopin M, Nagler A, Bornhäuser M, Finke J, Fassas A, et al. Donor lymphocyte infusion in the treatment of first hematological relapse after allogeneic stem-cell transplantation

in adults with acute myeloid leukemia: a retrospective risk factors analysis and comparison with other strategies by the EBMT Acute Leukemia Working Party. J Clin Oncol. 2007;25(31):4938–45.
34. Collins Jr RH, Goldstein S, Giralt S, Levine J, Porter D, Drobyski W, et al. Donor leukocyte infusions in acute lymphocytic leukemia. Bone Marrow Transplant. 2000;26(5):511–6.
35. Choi SJ, Lee JH, Kim S, Lee YS, Seol M, Ryu SG, et al. Treatment of relapsed acute lymphoblastic leukemia after allogeneic bone marrow transplantation with chemotherapy followed by G-CSF-primed donor leukocyte infusion: a prospective study. Bone Marrow Transplant. 2005;36(2):163–9.
36. Lambert JR, Bomanji JB, Peggs KS, Thomson KJ, Chakraverty RK, Fielding AK, et al. Prognostic role of PET scanning before and after reduced-intensity allogeneic stem cell transplantation for lymphoma. Blood. 2010;115(14):2763–8.
37. Peggs KS, Sureda A, Qian W, Caballero D, Hunter A, Urbano-Ispizua A, et al. Reduced-intensity conditioning for allogeneic haematopoietic stem cell transplantation in relapsed and refractory Hodgkin lymphoma: impact of alemtuzumab and donor lymphocyte infusions on long-term outcomes. Br J Haematol. 2007;139(1):70–80.
38. Bloor AJ, Thomson K, Chowdhry N, Verfuerth S, Ings SJ, Chakraverty R, et al. High response rate to donor lymphocyte infusion after allogeneic stem cell transplantation for indolent non-Hodgkin lymphoma. Biol Blood Marrow Transplant. 2008;14(1):50–8.
39. Lokhorst HM, Schattenberg A, Cornelissen JJ, Thomas LL, Verdonck LF. Donor leukocyte infusions are effective in relapsed multiple myeloma after allogeneic bone marrow transplantation. Blood. 1997;90(10):4206–11.
40. Lokhorst HM, Schattenberg A, Cornelissen JJ, van Oers MH, Fibbe W, Russell I, et al. Donor lymphocyte infusions for relapsed multiple myeloma after allogeneic stem-cell transplantation: predictive factors for response and long-term outcome. J Clin Oncol. 2000;16:3031–7.
41. Salama M, Nevill T, Marcellus D, Parker P, Johnson M, Kirk A, et al. Donor leukocyte infusions for multiple myeloma. Bone Marrow Transplant. 2000;26(11):1179–84.
42. Van de Donk NW, Kroger N, Hegenbart U, Corradini P, San Miguel JF, Goldschmidt H, et al. Prognostic factors for donor lymphocyte infusions following non-myeloablative allogeneic stem cell transplantation in multiple myeloma. Bone Marrow Transplant. 2006;37(12): 1135–41.
43. Vago L, Perna SK, Zanussi M, Mazzi B, Barlassina C, Stanghellini MTL, et al. Loss of mismatched HLA in leukemia after stem-cell transplantation. N Engl J Med. 2009;361:478–88.
44. Russell NH, Byrne JL, Faulkner RD, Gilyead M, Das-Gupta EP, Haynes AP. Donor lymphocyte infusions can result in sustained remissions in patients with residual or relapsed lymphoid malignancy following allogeneic haemopoietic stem cell transplantation. Bone Marrow Transplant. 2005;36(5):437–41.
45. Porter DL, Levine GL, Bunin N, Stadtmauer EA, Luger SM, Goldstein S, et al. A phase I trial of donor lymphocyte infusions expanded and activated ex vivo via CD3/CD38 costimulation. Blood. 2006;107(4):1325–31.
46. Kollgaard T, Petersen SL, Hadrup SR, Masmas TN, Seremet T, Andersen MH, et al. Evidence for involvement of clonally expanded CD8+ T cells in anticancer immune responses in CLL patients following nonmyeloablative conditioning and hematopoietic cell transplantation. Leukemia. 2005;19(12):2273–80.
47. Anderlini P, Acholonu SA, Okoroji GJ, Andersson BS, Couriel DR, De Lima MJ, et al. Donor leukocyte infusions in relapsed Hodgkin's lymphoma following allogeneic stem cell transplantation : CD3+ cell dose, GVHD and disease response. Bone Marrow Transplant. 2004;34(6):511–4.
48. Schaap N, Schattenberg A, Bär B, Preijers F, Wiel V, Kemenade E, et al. Induction of graft-versus-leukemia to prevent relapse after partially lymphocyte-depleted allogeneic bone marrow transplantation by pre-emptive donor leukocyte infusions. Leukemia. 2001;15(9): 1339–46.
49. Mackinnon S, Papadopoulos EB, Carabasi MH, Reich L, Collins NH, Boulad F, et al. Adoptive immunotherapy evaluating escalating doses of donor leukocytes for relapse of chronic

myeloid leukemia after bone marrow transplantation: separation of graft-versus-leukemia responses from graft-versus-host disease. Blood. 1995;86(4):1261–8.
50. Guglielmi C, Arcese W, Dazzi F, Brand R, Bunjes D, Verdonck LF, et al. Donor lymphocyte infusion for relapsed chronic myelogenous leukemia: prognostic relevance of the initial cell dose. Blood. 2002;100(2):397–405.
51. Levine JE, Braun T, Penza SL, Beatty P, Cornetta K, Martino R, et al. Prospective trial of chemotherapy and donor leukocyte infusions for relapse of advanced myeloid malignancies after allogeneic stem-cell transplantation. J Clin Oncol. 2002;20(2):405–12.
52. Miller JS, Weisdorf DJ, Burns LJ, Slungaard A, Wagner JE, Verneris MR, et al. Lymphodepletion followed by donor lymphocyte infusion (DLI) causes significantly more acute graft-versus-host disease than DLI alone. Blood. 2007;110(7):2761–3.
53. Kröger N, Shimoni A, Zagrivnaja M, Ayuk F, Lioznov M, Schieder H, et al. Low-dose thalidomide and donor lymphocyte infusion as adoptive immunotherapy after allogeneic stem cell transplantation in patients with multiple myeloma. Blood. 2004;104(10):3361–3.
54. Alyea EP, Soiffer RJ, Canning C, Neuberg D, Schlossman R, Pickett C, et al. Toxicity and efficacy of defined doses of CD4(+) donor lymphocytes for treatment of relapse after allogeneic bone marrow transplant. Blood. 1998;91(10):3671–80.
55. Soiffer RJ, Alyea EP, Hochberg E, Wu C, Canning C, Parikh B, et al. Randomized trial of CD8+ T-cell depletion in the prevention of graft-versus-host disease associated with donor lymphocyte infusion. Biol Blood Marrow Transplant. 2002;8(11):625–32.
56. Ciceri F, Bonini C, Marktel S, Zappone E, Servida P, Bernardi M, et al. Antitumor effects of HSV-TK-engineered donor lymphocytes after allogeneic stem-cell transplantation. Blood. 2007;109(11):4698–707.
57. Rosenberg SA et al. Treatment of 283 consecutive patients with metastatic melanoma or renal cell cancer using high-dose bolus interleukin-2. J Am Med Assoc. 1994;271:907–13.
58. Rosenberg SA, Yang JC, Restifo NP. Cancer immunotherapy: moving beyond current vaccines. Nat Med. 2004;10:909–15.
59. Dudley ME et al. Cancer regression and autoimmunity in patients following clonal repopulation with anti-tumor lymphocytes. Science. 2002;298:850–4.
60. Dudley ME et al. Adoptive cell transfer therapy following non-myeloablative but lymphodepleting chemotherapy for the treatment of patients with refractory metastatic melanoma. J Clin Oncol. 2005;23:2346–57.
61. Overwijk WW, Theoret MR, Finkelstein SE, Surman DR, de Jong LA, Vuth-Dreese FA. Tumor regression and autoimmunity after reversal of a functionally tolerant state of self-reactive CD8+ T cells. J Exp Med. 2003;198:569–80.
62. Rosenberg SA et al. Use of tumor infiltrating lymphocytes and interleukin-2 in the immunotherapy of patients with metastatic melanoma. Preliminary report. NEJM. 1998;319: 1676–80.
63. Rosenberg SA et al. Treatment of patients with metastatic melanoma using autologous tumor-infiltrating lymphocytes and interleukin-2. J Natl Cancer Inst. 1994;86:1159–66.
64. Rosenberg SA, Dudley ME. Adoptive cell therapy for the treatment of patients with metastatic melanoma. Curr Opin Immunol. 2009;21:233–40.
65. Gattinoni L, Finkelstein SE, Klebanoff CA, Antony PA, Palmer DC, Spiess PJ, et al. Removal of homeostatic cytokine sinks by lymphodepletion enhances the efficacy of adoptively transferred tumor-specific CD8+ T cells. J Exp Med. 2005;202:907–12.
66. Klebanoff CA, Khong HT, Antony PA, Palmer DC, Restifo NP. Sinks, suppressors and antigen presenters: how lymphodepletion enhances T cell-mediated tumor immunotherapy. Trends Immunol. 2005;26:111–7.
67. Greenberg PD. Adoptive T, cell therapy of tumors: mechanisms operative in the recognition and elimination of tumor cells. Adv Immunol. 1991;49:281–355.
68. Romerdahl CA, Kripke ML. Role of helper T-lymphocytes in rejection of UV-induced murine skin cancers. Cancer Res. 1988;48:2325–8.
69. Hung K, Hayashi R, Lafond-Walker A, Lowenstein C, Pardoll D, Levitsky H. The central role of CD4(+) T cells in the antitumor immune response. J Exp Med. 1998;188:2357–68.

70. Li Y, Bleakley M, Yee C. IL-21 influences the frequency, phenotype, and affinity of the antigen-specific CD8 T cell response. J Immunol. 2005;175:2261–9.
71. Schoenberger SP, Toes RE, van der Voort EI, Offringa R, Melief CJ. T-cell help for cytotoxic T lymphocytes is mediated by CD40-CD40L interactions. Nature. 1998;393:480–3.
72. Hunder NN, Wallen H, Cao J, Hendricks DW, Reilly JZ, Rodmyre R, et al. Treatment of metastatic melanoma with autologous CD4+ T cells against NY-ESO-1. N Engl J Med. 2008;358:2698–703.
73. Sallusto F, Geginat J, Lanzavecchia A. Central memory and effectory memory T cell subsets: function, generation and maintenance. Annu Rev Immunol. 2004;22:745–63.
74. Perret R, Ronchese F. Memory T cells in cancer immunotherapy: which CD8 T-cell population provides the best protection against tumours? Tissue Antigens. 2008;72:187–94.
75. Berger C, Jensen MC, Landsdorp PM, Gough M, Elliott C, Riddell SR. Adoptive transfer of effector CD8+ T cells derived from central memory cells establishes persistent T cell memory in primates. J Clin Invest. 2008;118:294–305.
76. Hinrichs CS, Borman ZA, Gattinoni L, Yu Z, Burns WR, Huang J. Human effector CD8+ T cells derived from naïve rather than memory subsets possess superior traits for adoptive immunotherapy. Blood. 2011;117:808–14.
77. Yee C, Thompson JA, Byrd D, Riddell SR, Roche P, Celis E, et al. Adoptive T cell therapy using antigen-specific CD8+ T cell clones for the treatment of patients with metastatic melanoma: In vivo persistence, migration and antitumor effect of transferred T cells. PNAS. 2002;99:16168–73.
78. Besser MJ, Shapira-Frommer R, Treves AJ, Zippel D, Itzhaki O, Hershkovitz L, et al. Clinical responses in a phase II study using adoptive transfer of short-term cultured tumor infiltration lymphocytes in metastatic melanoma patients. Clin Cancer Res. 2010;16:2646–55.
79. Dudley ME, Gross CA, Langhan MM, Garcia MR, Sherry RM, Yang JC, et al. CD8+ enriched "young" tumor infiltrating lymphocytes can mediate regression of metastatic melanoma. Clin Cancer Res. 2010;16:6122–31.
80. Rosenberg SA, Yang JC, Sherry RM, Kammula US, Hughes MS, Phan GQ, et al. Durable complete responses in heavily pretreated patients with metastatic melanoma using T cell transfer immunotherapy. Clin Cancer Res. 2011;17:4550–7.
81. Rosenberg SA, Dudley ME, Restifo NP. Letter to the Editor. N Engl J Med. 2008;359:1072.
82. Ochsenbein AF, Riddell SR, Brown M, Corey L, Baerlocher GM, Landsdorp PM, et al. CD27 expression promotes long-term survival of functional effector-memory CD8+ cytotoxic T lymphocytes in HIV-infected patients. J Exp Med. 2004;200:1407–17.
83. Klebanoff CA, Gattinoni L, Palmer DC, Muranski P, Ji Y, Hinrichs CS, et al. Determinants of successful CD8+ T cell adoptive immunotherapy for large established tumors in mice. Clin Cancer Res. 2011;17:5343–52.
84. Shrimali RK, Yu Z, Theoret MR, Chinnasamy D, Restifo NP, Rosenberg SA. Antiangiogenic agents can increase lymphocyte infiltration into tumor and enhance the effectiveness of adoptive immunotherapy of cancer. Cancer Res. 2010;70:6171–80.
85. Heslop HE, Ng CY, Li C, Smith CA, Loftin SK, Krance RA, et al. Long-term restoration of immunity against Epstein-Barr virus infection by adoptive transfer of gene-modified virus-specific T lymphocytes. Nat Med. 1996;2:551–5.
86. Einsele H, Roosnek E, Rufer N, Sinzger C, Riegler S, Löffler J, et al. Infusion of cytomegalovirus (CMV)-specific T cells for the treatment of CMV infection not responding to antiviral chemotherapy. Blood. 2002;99:3916–22.
87. Leen AM, Myers GD, Sili U, Huls MH, Weiss H, Leung KS, et al. Monoculture-derived T lymphocytes specific for multiple viruses expand and produce clinically relevant effects in immunocompromised individuals. Nat Med. 2006;12:1160–6.
88. Rooney CM, Smith CA, Ng CY, Loftin SK, Sixbey JW, Gan Y, et al. Infusion of cytotoxic T cells for the prevention and treatment of Epstein-Barr virus-induced lymphoma in allogeneic transplant recipients. Blood. 1998;92:1549–55.
89. Rooney CM, Roskrow MA, Suzuki N, Ng CY, Brenner MK, Heslop H. Treatment of relapsed Hodgkin's disease using EBV-specific cytotoxic T cells. Ann Oncol. 1998;9 Suppl 5:S129–32.

90. Bollard CM, Aguilar L, Staathof KC, Gahn B, Huls MH, Rousseau A, et al. Cytotoxic T lymphocyte therapy for Epstein-Barr Virus+Hodgkin disease. J Exp Med. 2004;200: 1623–33.
91. Bollard CM, Gottschalk S, Leen AM, Weiss H, Straathof KC, Carrum G, et al. Complete responses of relapsed lymphoma following genetic modification of tumor-antigen presenting cells and T-lymphocyte transfer. Blood. 2007;110:2838–45.
92. Melenhorst JJ, Leen AM, Bollard CM, Quigley MF, Price DA, Rooney CM, et al. Allogeneic virus-specific T cells with HLA alloreactivity do not produce GVHD in human subjects. Blood. 2010;116:4700–2.
93. Akpek G, Mikulski M, Kleinberg M, Badros A, Yanovich S, Rapoport AP. Cellular therapy with sequential unmanipulated donor lymphocyte infusions in drug-resistant cytomegalovirus (CMV) encephalitis. Blood. 2011;117:5772–4.
94. Cruz CR, Hanley PJ, Liu H, Torrano V, Lin Y-F, Arce JA, et al. Adverse events following infusión of T cells for adoptive immunotherapy: a 10 year experience. Cytotherapy. 2010;12:743–9.
95. Brenjens RJ, Riviere I, Hollyman D, Taylor C, Nikhamin Y, Stefanski J, et al. Unexpected toxicity of cyclophosphamide followed by adoptively transferred CD19-targeted T cells in a patient with bulky CLL. Mol Ther. 2009;17 Suppl 1:S157.
96. Morgan RA, Yang JC, Kitano M, Dudley ME, Laurencot CM, Rosenberg SA. Case report of a serious adverse event following the administration of T cells transduced with a chimeric antigen receptor recognizing ERBB2. Mol Ther. 2010;18:843–51.
97. Suntharalingam G, Perry MR, Ward S, Brett SJ, Castello-Cortes A, Brunner MD, et al. Cytokine storm in a phase I trial of the anti-CD28 monoclonal antibody TGN1412. N Engl J Med. 2006;355:1018–28.
98. Hong JJ, Rosenberg SA, Dudley ME, Yang JC, White DE, Butman JA, et al. Successful treatment of melanoma brain metastases with adoptive cell therapy. Clin Cancer Res. 2010;16:4892–8.
99. Gross G, Waks T, Eshhar Z. Expression of immunoglobulin-T-cell receptor chimeric molecules as functional receptors with antibody-type specificity. Proc Natl Acad Sci U S A. 1989;86:10024–8.
100. Morgan RA, Dudley ME, Wunderlich JR, Hughes MS, Yang JC, Sherry RM, et al. Cancer regression in patients after transfer of genetically engineered lymphocytes. Science. 2006; 314:126–9.
101. Zeh 3rd HJ, Perry-Lalley D, Dudley ME, Rosenberg SA, Yang JC. High avidity CTLs for two self-antigens demonstrate superior in vitro and in vivo antitumor efficacy. J Immunol. 1999; 162:989–94.
102. Trautmann L, Rimbert M, Echasserieau K, Saulquin X, Neveu B, Dechanet J, et al. Selection of T cell clones expressing high-affinity public TCRs within human cytomegalovirus-specific CD8 T cell responses. J Immunol. 2005;175:6123–32.
103. Robbins PF, Li YF, El-Gamil M, Zhao Y, Wargo JA, Zheng Z, et al. Single and dual amino acid substitutions in TCR CDRs can enhance antigen-specific T cell functions. J Immunol. 2008;180:6116–31.
104. Robbins PF, Morgan RA, Feldman SA, Yang JC, Sherry RM, Dudley ME, et al. Tumor regression in patients with metastatic synovial cell sarcoma and melanoma using genetically engineered lymphocytes reactive with NY-ESO-1. J Clin Oncol. 2011;29:917–24.
105. Bendle GM, Linneman C, Hooijkaas AI, Bies L, de Witte MA, Jorritsma A, et al. Lethal graft-versus-host disease in mouse models of T cell receptor gene therapy. Nat Med. 2010;16:565–70.
106. Rosenberg SA. Of mice, not men: no evidence for graft-versus-host disease in humans receiving T-cell receptor-transduced autologous T cells. Mol Ther. 2010;18:1744–5.
107. Powles R, Singhal S, Treleaven J, et al. Identification of patients who may benefit from prophylactic immunotherapy after bone marrow transplantation for acute myeloid leukemia on the basis of lymphocyte recovery early after transplantation. Blood. 1998;91:3481–6.

108. Pavletic ZS, Joshi SS, Perruccello SJ, et al. Lymphocyte reconstitution after allogeneic blood stem cell transplantation for hematologic malignancies. Bone Marrow Transplant. 1998;21: 33–41.
109. Curti BD, Ochoa AC, Powers GC, Kopp WC, Alvord WG, Janik JE, et al. Phase I trial of anti-CD3-stimulated CD4+ T cells, infusional interleukin-2, and cyclophosphamide in patients with advanced cancer. J Clin Oncol. 1998;16:2752–60.
110. Lum LG, LeFever AV, Treisman JS, Garlie NK, Hanson JP. Immune modulation in cancer patients after adoptive transfer of anti-CD3/anti-CD28-costimulated T cells-phase I clinical trial. J Immunother. 2001;24:408–19.
111. Levine BL, Bernstein WB, Connors M, Craighead N, Lindsten T, Thompson CB, et al. Effects of CD28 costimulation on long-term proliferation of CD4+ T cells in the absence of exogenous feeder cells. J Immunol. 1997;159:5921–30.
112. Weng N, Levine BL, June CH, Hodes RJ. Regulation of telomerase RNA template expression in human T lymphocyte development and activation. J Immunol. 1997;158:3215–20.
113. Laport GG, Levine BL, Stadtmauer EA, Schuster SJ, Luger SM, Grupp S, et al. Adoptive transfer of costimulated T cells induces lymphocytosis in patients with relapsed/refractory non-Hodgkin lymphoma following CD34+-selected hematopoietic cell transplantation. Blood. 2003;102:2004–13.
114. Rapoport AP, Levine BL, Badros A, Meisenberg B, Ruehle K, Nandi A, et al. Molecular remission of C ML after autotransplantation followed by adoptive transfer of costimulated autologous T cells. Bone Marrow Transplant. 2004;33:53–60.
115. Rapoport AP, Stadtmauer EA, Aqui N, Badros A, Cotte J, Chrisley L, et al. Restoration of immunity in lymphopenic individuals with cancer by vaccination and adoptive T-cell transfer. Nat Med. 2005;11:1230–7.
116. Stadtmauer EA, Vogl DT, Prak EL, Boyer J, Aqui NA, Rapoport AP, et al. Reinfusion of influenza vaccine-primed co-stimulated autologous T-cells after stem cell transplantation for multiple myeloma leads to reconstitution of influenza immunity: results of a randomized clinical trial. Blood. 2011;117:63–71.
117. Rapoport AP, Aqui N, Stadtmauer EA, Vogl DT, Fang HB, Cai L, et al. Combination immunotherapy using adoptive T-cell transfer and tumor antigen vaccination on the basis of hTERT and survivin following ASCT for myeloma. Blood. 2011;117:788–97.
118. Dougan M, Dranoff G. Immune therapy of cancer. Ann Rev Immunol. 2009;27:83–117.
119. Rapoport AP, Stadtmauer E, Aqui N, Vogl D, Chew A, Fang HB, et al. Rapid immune recovery and GVHD-like engraftment syndrome following adoptive transfer of costimulated autologous T Cells. Clin Cancer Res. 2009;15(13):4499–507.
120. Rapoport AP, Aqui N, Stadtmauer E, Badros AZ, Vogl DT, Xu Y, et al. Combination immunotherapy after ASCT for multiple myeloma (MM) using MAGE-A3/poly-ICLC immunizations followed by vaccine-primed and activated autologous T-cells. Blood (ASH Annual Meeting Abstracts). 2012;120:352.
121. Shafer PH, Gandhi AK, Loveland MA, Chen RS, Man H-W, et al. Enhancement of cytokine production and AP-1 transcriptional activity in T cells by thalidomide-related immunomodulatory drugs. J Pharmacol Exp Ther. 2003;305:1222–32.
122. Galustian C, Meyer B, Labarthe MC, Dredge K, Klaschka D, Henry J, et al. The anti-cancer agents lenalidomide and pomalidomide inhibit the proliferation and function of T regulatory cells. Cancer Immunol Immunother. 2009;58(7):1033–45.
123. Ramsay AG, Clear AJ, Kelly G, Fatah R, Matthews J, Macdougall F, et al. Follicular lymphoma cells induce T-cell immunologic synapse dysfunction that can be repaired with lenalidomide: implications for the tumor microenvironment and immunotherapy. Blood. 2009;114(21):4713–20.
124. Noonan K, Rudraraju L, Ferguson A, Emerling A, Pasetti MF, Huff CA, et al. Lenalidomide-induced immunomodulation in multiple myeloma: impact on vaccines and antitumor responses. Clin Cancer Res. 2012;18(5):1426–34.
125. Purbhoo MA, Sutton DH, Brewer JE, Mullings RE, Hill ME, Mahon TM, et al. Quantifying and imaging NY-ESO-1/LAGE-1-derived epitopes on tumor cells using high-affinity T-cell receptors. J Immunol. 2006;176:7308–16.

126. Letsch A, Keilholz U, Assfalg G, Mailander V, Thiel E, Scheinbenbogen C. Bone marrow contains melanoma-reactive CD8+ effector T cells and, compared with peripheral blood, enriched numbers of melanoma-reactive CD8+ memory T cells. Cancer Res. 2003;63(17):5582–6.
127. Rapoport AP, Stadtmauer EA, Vogl DT, Weiss BM, Binder-Scholl GK, Brewer JE, et al. Adoptive transfer of gene-modified T-Cells engineered to express high-affinity TCRs for cancer-testis antigens (CTAs) NY-ESO-1 or Lage-1, in MM patients post Auto-SCT. Blood (ASH Annual Meeting Abstracts). 2012;120:472.
128. Kalos M, Rapoport AP, Stadtmauer EA, Vogl DT, Weiss BM, Binder-Scholl GK, et al. Prolonged T cell persistence, homing to marrow and selective targeting of antigen positive tumor in multiple myeloma patients following adoptive transfer of T Cells genetically engineered to express an affinity-enhanced T Cell receptor against the cancer testis antigens NY-ESO-1 and Lage-1. Blood (ASH Annual Meeting Abstracts). 2012;120:755.
129. Kohn DB, Dotti G, Brentjens R, Savoldo B, Jensen M, Cooper LJ, et al. CARS on track in the clinic. Mol Ther. 2011;19:432–8.
130. Sadelain M, Brentjens R, Rivière I. The promise and pitfalls of chimeric antigen receptors. Curr Opin Immunol. 2009;21:215–23.
131. Milone MC, Fish JD, Carpenito C, Carroll RG, Binder GK, Teachey D, et al. Chimeric receptors containing CD137 signal transduction domains mediate enhanced survival of T cells and increased antileukemic efficacy in vivo. Mol Ther. 2009;17:4353–64.
132. Porter DL, Levine BL, Kalos M, Bagg A, June CH. Chimeric antigen receptor-modified T cells in chronic lymphoid leukemia. N Engl J Med. 2011;365:725–33.
133. Kalos M, Levine BL, Porter DL, Katz S, Grupp SA, Bagg A, et al. T cells with chimeric antigen receptors have potent antitumor effects and can establish memory in patients with advanced leukemia. Sci Transl Med. 2011;3:95ra73.
134. Porter DL, Grupp SA, Kalos M, Loren AW, Lledo L, Gilmore J, et al. Chimeric antigen receptor T cells directed against CD19 induce durable responses and transient cytokine release syndrome in relapsed, refractory CLL and ALL. Blood (ASH Annual Meeting Abstracts). 2012;120:717.
135. Kalos M, Levine BL, Macatee TL, Kulikovskaya I, Suppa E, Jena B, et al. Sustained functional T Cell persistence and B Cell aplasia following CD19-targeting adoptive T Cell immunotherapy for relapsed, refractory CD19+ malignancy. Blood (ASH Annual Meeting Abstracts). 2012;120:756.
136. Grupp SA, Porter DL, Teachey DT, Barrett DM, Chew A, Suppa E, et al. CD19-Redirected chimeric antigen receptor T (CART19) cells induce a cytokine release syndrome (CRS) and induction of treatable macrophage activation syndrome (MAS) that Can Be managed by the IL-6 antagonist tocilizumab (toc). Blood (ASH Annual Meeting Abstracts). 2012;120:2604.
137. Kochenderfer JN, Wilson WH, Janik JE, Dudley E, Stetler-Stevenson M, Feldman SA, et al. Eradication of B-lineage cells and regression of lymphoma in a patient treated with autologous T cells genetically engineered to recognize CD19. Blood. 2010;116(20):4099–102.
138. Kochenderfer JN, Dudley ME, Feldman SA, Wilson WH, Spaner DE, Maric I, et al. B-cell depletion and remissions of malignancy along with cytokine-associated toxicity in a clinical trial of anti-CD19 chimeric-antigen-receptor-transduced T cells. Blood. 2012;119(12):2709–20.

Bifunctional Antibodies: Preclinical and Clinical Applications

Casey W. Shuptrine and Louis M. Weiner

Abstract Treating malignancies with antibody-based immunotherapy has revolutionized the concept of targeted therapy. Rituximab and Trastuzumab, two monoclonal antibodies approved in the 1990s by the FDA, elucidated the potential of harnessing the immune system to eliminate transformed cells. As with any cancer therapy, a significant proportion of patients relapse, driving the development of non-traditional antibody-based therapies. Therefore, in an effort to enhance the ability of antibodies to retarget immune cells toward cancer cells, bispecific antibodies were born. Created through a variety of techniques they conform to an assortment of structures, recapitulating the basic structure of an antibody or deconvoluting the antigen-binding domains into unique designs. The European Union's approval in 2009 of Catumaxomab, a bispecific antibody that links cells of the innate and adaptive immune system to EpCAM + cells for the treatment of malignant ascites, marks the first clinically approved dual-targeting antibody. Blinatumomab, a bispecific T-cell engager (BiTE), links T-cells directly to malignant cells, activating target-cell apoptosis through perforin-granzyme release. Early clinical results of Blinatumomab show a remarkable 80 % response rate in a heavily pretreated ALL patient subgroup. These enticing clinical results represent the forefront of the bispecific antibody field but evidence exists that point to the clinical success of numerous bispecific antibody formats. Although it is unknown which format will exhibit the highest clinical efficacy, it is clear that dual-targeting antibodies represent the future of immunotherapy for the treatment of cancer.

C.W. Shuptrine (✉)
Tumor Biology Training Program, Lombardi Comprehensive Cancer Center, Georgetown University Medical Center, 3800 Reservoir Rd NW, Washington, DC 20007, USA
e-mail: shuptrine128@gmail.com

L.M. Weiner
Department of Oncology, Lombardi Comprehensive Cancer Center, Georgetown University Medical Center, 3800 Reservoir Rd NW, Washington, DC 20007, USA

J.D. Rosenblatt et al. (eds.), *Advances in Tumor Immunology and Immunotherapy*, Current Cancer Research, DOI 10.1007/978-1-4614-8809-5_10,
© Springer Science+Business Media New York 2014

Keywords Bispecific antibody • Triomab • Diabody • Tandab • Tetrabody • Triplebody • Bispecific T-cell engager • Quadroma • Dock-and-lock technique • CovX Body

1 Introduction

The clinical and commercial success of monoclonal antibodies has proven the hypothesis established by Paul Erhlich in the 1900s that the immune system could provide a magic bullet for the treatment of cancer. While these single target antibodies have vastly improved survival for patients with HER2+ breast cancer, CD20+ lymphoma, and CD33 lymphoma, inevitably a significant proportion of patients relapse. With the proof of principle for immunotherapies, a revolution in the tumor immunology world began, with the goal of designing and developing techniques to overcome the current limitations of cancer targeting monoclonal antibodies (mAbs). This has led to the enhancement of effector functions through Fc region modifications, as well as the direct delivery of toxins to transformed cells through toxin–mAb conjugation (trastuzumab-DM1) [68]. A viable alternative method to enhance the efficacy of tumor immunotherapy is the design of antibodies or recombinant proteins that target multiple antigens and/or induce cancer cell destruction through the redirection of lytic immune cells. These dual-targeting antibodies are created through chemical conjugation, fusion of two mAb-producing hybridomas, and genetic recombination. The resulting bispecific antibody (bsAb) field has expanded immensely, with dozens currently undergoing various phases of clinical trials for the treatment of cancer and many more in preclinical studies. Of particular interest are trifunctional antibodies (Triomabs) developed by Trion Pharma and bispecific T-cell engagers (BiTEs) developed by Micromet. Other less clinically developed bsAbs include single-chain Fv (scFv) fusion proteins, diabodies, tribodies, bispecific CovX bodies, and random site mutation bsAbs. Although the structure and function of these bsAbs differ, they share antigen targets. On the tumor cell, they recognize members of the EGFR family, CD19, CD20, CD33, MCSPs, and EpCAM. For those that redirect effector cells, the antigen targets include CD3 on T-cells, CD16 on NK cells, monocytes, macrophages, and neutrophils, and CD64 on macrophages and monocytes. In this chapter, we describe the development of bispecific antibodies for the treatment of cancer in a historical perspective, highlighting the bsAbs that have entered clinical trials.

2 First Generation bsAbs

Before the development of advanced genetic recombination, bsAbs were created by the direct chemical crosslinking of antibody domains or through the fusion of two mAb producing hybridomas, called quadromas (Fig. 1) [56, 82]. Both methods

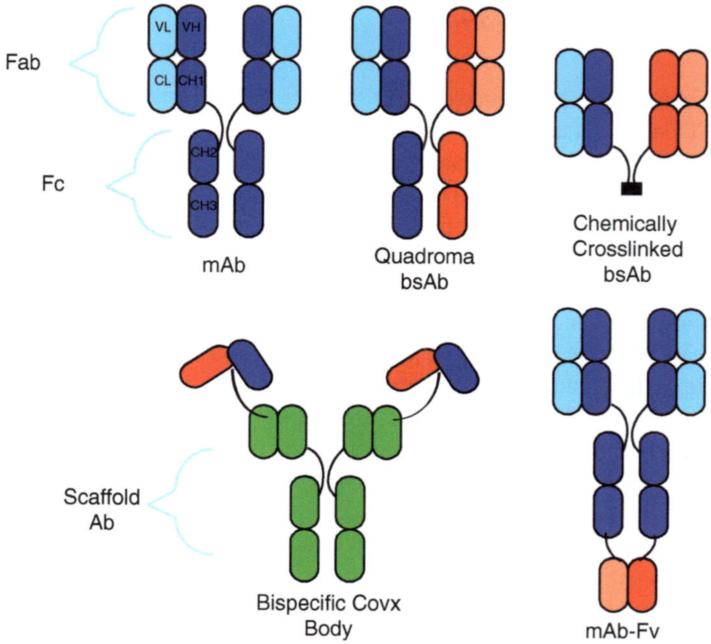

Fig. 1 First generation bispecific antibodies. *Dark regions* correspond to heavy chains, while *light regions* correspond to light chains. A monoclonal antibody is depicted in, with the Fab domain binding to an antigen and the Fc domain binding to FcγRs. *Red* domains represent regions with a different antigen specificity. The *green* antibody domain symbolizes the scaffold antibody for a bs-CovX body. *Black lines* represent linker domains. Bispecific antibodies of the quadroma, chemical crosslinking, bs-CovX body, and mAb-Fv formats are shown

produce a full-length antibody that can effectively bind to multiple antigens, either manipulating the downstream signals of the target or conjugating immune effector cells directly to the target cell. In the 1990s and early 2000s, several of these first generation bsAbs entered phase I clinical trials with limited success [26, 27, 92, 94, 116, 119]. For chemical crosslinking, the production of large quantities of purified bsAbs was cost prohibitive, as each reaction created numerous inert and unusable proteins. For the quadroma bsAbs, which were of murine or rat origin, the development of human anti-mouse antibodies (HAMA) or human anti-rat antibodies (HARA) precluded multiple dosing regimes in patients, severely limiting their clinical applicability. Also, quadromas created from the same species secrete ten possible combinations of light-chain and heavy-chain antibodies, with only one having the correct dual-targeting functionality [69]. A novel discovery was made in 1995 by Horst Lindhofer, that the fusion of a rat hybridoma with a murine hybridoma resulted in the preferential creation of the correct bsAb formation, increasing the yield from quadromas by 3.5-fold [69].

2.1 Chemical Conjugation

The first chemically cross-linked bsAb to enter clinical trials targeted HER2 and FcγRI (CD64), in an attempt to utilize macrophages and monocytes to lyse cancer cells. HER2 is one of the most targeted antigens by immunotherapy, as ~30 % of all breast cancers overexpress this potent tyrosine kinase receptor and is the target for the FDA approved mAb trastuzumab [11]. The murine bsAb, called MDX-210, was formed through the reduction of the two murine parental mAbs into Fab' fragments, chemically cross-linked using *o*-phenylenedimaleimide, acetylated with the alkylating agent iodoacetamide, and then purified through chromatography. Therefore, this molecule mimics the structure of a HER2 mAb, with two antigen-binding arms recognizing HER2 and one region recognizing an FcγR. The major difference compared to standard mAbs is the unique antigen-binding target of CD64, instead of FcγRIII (CD16), which IgG1 molecules recognize through their Fc region. MDX-210 was delivered intravenously to ten patients with HER2+ advanced breast or ovarian cancer, at a dose ranging from 0.35 to 10.0 mg/m^2. The bsAb was well tolerated in the ten evaluable patients, never reaching the maximum tolerated dose (MTD). Most patients only experienced grade 1 and 2 adverse events but two experienced the grade 3 adverse event hypotension. Although the goal was only to test the toxicity of the molecule, MDX-210 treatment resulted in one partial and one mixed tumor response. As expected, HAMA was detectable in six of the ten patients [116]. This observed limiting factor prompted the development of a humanized version of the bsAb, MDX-H210, which was tested in patients with metastatic HER2+ breast cancer in two phase I trials. To enhance the proportion of immune cells with lytic capabilities, these investigators then coadministered MDX-H210 with granulocyte-colony-stimulating factor (G-CSF), which has been shown to induce the expression of CD64 on neutrophils. In the first clinical trial, of the 23 patients enrolled, the majority of patients experienced fevers or diarrhea, while no MTD was reached. No objective clinical responses were observed and all patients had circulating antibodies that recognized the bsAb [92]. The second phase I trial of MDX-H210 was delivered to 30 stage IV HER2+ breast cancer patients in 2003. Similar to the previous trials, no MTD was reached, the molecule was well tolerated, no objective responses were seen, and a majority of patients developed anti-bsAb antibodies [94]. Another chemically conjugated bsAb, MDX-447, which targets EGFR and CD64, was evaluated with and without G-CSF in 64 patients with advanced solid tumors. Although the addition of G-CSF caused dose-limiting toxicities, MDX-447 was relatively tolerated and resulted in no objective clinical responses, halting its further development [34].

The lack of clinical activity in the patients treated with these conjugated molecules might be explained by the strong pre-stimulation of polymorph nuclear neutrophils (PMN) cells with IFN-γ and G-CSF, and the high effector to target ratio of PMNs to tumors cells (50–200:1) that is required for in vitro lysis by MDX-210 and MDX-H210 [57]. Moreover, the development of neutralizing antibodies or the lower lytic capability of CD64 expressing immune cells might have attributed to the lack of clinical efficacy.

2.2 *Quadromas*

The first generation of quadroma bsAbs recognized CD16 or CD3 to link lytic immune cells directly to tumor cells. The resulting bsAbs use one Fab arm to recognize the tumor antigen, another Fab to bind to CD16 or CD3, and use an intact Fc domain to bind to CD16 and FcRn. Therefore, CD16 × tumor antigen bsAbs have two unique binding domains for CD16 on innate immune cells, theoretically enhancing their ability to mediate antibody-dependent cellular cytotoxicity (ADCC). This design was utilized for two murine bsAbs that entered phase I clinical trials in the 1990s, 2B1 and HRS-3/A9. 2B1, which targets HER2/neu and CD16, was utilized in two clinical trials for patients with HER2+ tumors. Preclinical data suggested that the 2B1 bsAb derived from the 520C9 and 3G8 fusion quadroma was effective in eliminating HER2+ target cells in vitro and potentiating their growth in vivo [117, 118]. Similar to MDX-210, the effector cells required significant stimulation and high E:T ratios (25–50:1). Minimal clinical activity was observed following 2B1 therapy, with a total of 33 out of 34 patients developing HAMA [15, 119]. Of particular interest was the induction of an adaptive immune response to HER2/neu, suggesting that 2B1 enhanced antigen presentation for HER2. However, this adaptive immunity did not translate to clinical responses. HRS-3/A9 was created through the fusion of the murine hybridomas HRS-3, which produces a mAb for CD30, and A9, which produces a mAb against CD16 [52]. CD30, a marker for Hodgkin lymphomas, represents a valid target for selective targeting of lymphoma cells [111]. Preclinical studies with HRS-3/A9 were promising, as it was shown to cure mice with CD30+ Hodgkin's lymphomas after only one injection [52]. In 1997, HRS-3/A9 was given to 15 patients with refractory Hodgkin's disease, was well tolerated, and resulted in the first clinical responses seen with a bispecific antibody, with one complete response (CR), one partial response (PR), and three minor responses [43]. Similar results were seen in a second phase I trial, with one CR, three PRs, and four patients with stable disease (SD) [44]. While these results elucidated the potential of bsAbs for the treatment of cancer, 15 of 31 patients developed HAMAs, prohibiting subsequent clinical use [43, 44].

In an effort to enhance the effector functions of antibody therapy, many groups sought to link the most powerful arm of the adaptive immune system to cancer cells. By conjugating CTLs through CD3, directly to a tumor cell through a tumor-associated or -specific antigen, effective lysis can occur. After being primed in the lymph nodes through ligation of CD3 and a second activating signal, CTLs disseminate throughout the body. Through the T-cell receptor (TCR), educated CTLs recognize their "primed antigen" presented on the surface of a cell through major histocompatibility complex (MHC) class I. Upon conjugation, CTLs release perforin and granzymes, activating the apoptotic pathway inside the target cell [81]. Therefore, the creation of a second antigen-binding domain of an antibody to recognize the activating T-cell receptor CD3 could effectively utilize the cytotoxic arm of the adaptive immune system to eliminate cancer cells. Unfortunately, when given to patients, T-cell retargeting bsAbs resulted in a systemic cytokine release induced by

T-cell activation. This, on top of the development of HAMA, significantly limited the bsAb dose, reducing their clinical efficacy.

The first T-cell retargeting quadroma was SHR-1, a rat/murine hybrid that recognized CD3 and the B-cell lymphoma marker, CD19. Preclinical studies found that SHR-1 could lyse CD19+ B-cell lines and B-cells taken directly from lymphoma patients with activated T-cells [39, 40]. SHR-1 was capable of mediating significant lysis of transformed B-cells with T-cells isolated from patients with lymphoma, proving that CD3 could serve as a potent activator of previously tolerant T-cells. Further in vitro studies demonstrated complete cell growth inhibition at a relatively low E:T ratio of 9:1 when SHR-1 was combined with Il-2 stimulated peripheral blood mononuclear cells (PMBCs) [41]. These promising results led to a phase I clinical trial in 1995, where three non-Hodgkin's lymphoma (NHL) patients were exposed to increasing doses of SHR-1. Although the bsAb was well tolerated with little observed toxicity, clinical activity was minimal [26, 27]. HEA125×OKT3, another first generation quadroma bsAb of murine origin, retargeted T-cells to EpCAM (CD326) positive tumors. EpCAM expression is commonly associated with poor prognosis, is expressed on a broad range of carcinomas, and is often used as a marker for stem cell-like properties [83, 86, 109]. EpCAM is also expressed on normal cells but is generally confined to intracellular spaces, making it an attractive target for anticancer therapy. In 2002 HEA125×OKT3 was evaluated in ten EpCAM+ovarian carcinoma patients with malignant ascites. At the time, patients with malignant ascites, which are tumor cells that metastasize to the peritoneal cavity causing pain and swelling, had limited options for palliative treatment. Diuretics or direct fluid drainage through paracentesis were the only viable options to improve quality of life. Since the malignant epithelial cells in ascites caused by ovarian carcinoma are often EpCAM +, treatment with HEA125×OKT3 was considered to potentially fill a significant unmet need in cancer palliative care. When injected intraperitoneally, HEA125×OKT3 resulted in the complete inhibition of ascites formation in eight patients and reduced ascites formation in two patients. However, 80 % of the patients developed HAMAs, seemingly slowing its further clinical development [77].

2.3 Triomabs

2.3.1 Early Generation Triomabs

Triomabs, the most successful bsAb created using the quadroma technique, are the only type of bispecific antibody used to treat cancer. Since first generation quadromas produced ten antibody formations randomly, it was difficult to purify the correct dual-targeting antibody. Utilizing the discovery of preferential pairing of bsAbs in mouse IgG2a/rat IgG2b quadromas and a single step pH elution on protein A, the desired bsAb could be isolated with previously unimagined ease [69]. Surprisingly, the Fc region of these triomabs bound only to activating FcγRs (Fcγ RI and Fcγ RIII) on effector cells and not to inhibitory receptors (Fcγ RIIB) [123]. This prompted the development of numerous commercially viable bsAbs, targeting EpCAM, HER2,

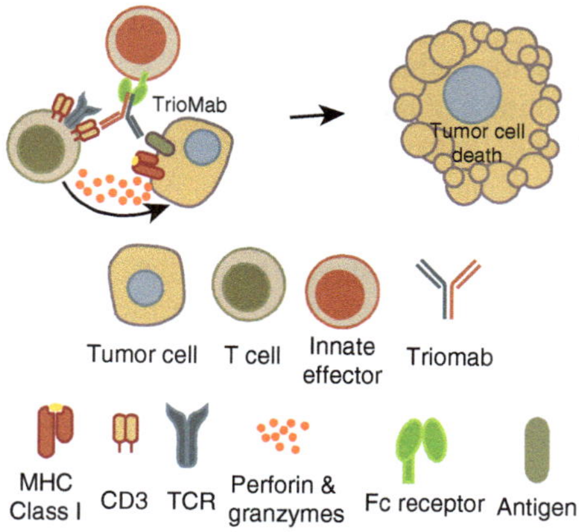

Fig. 2 Triomab's mechanism of action. Trifunctional antibodies, such as catumaxomab, ertumaxomab, and Bi20, lyse tumor cells by retargeting T-cells to antigen expressing tumor cells. The Fc region of the triomab binds to cells of the innate immune system, such as NK cells, which can induce ADCC of the tumor cell as well as supplying stimulatory signals to the retargeted T-cells. Once conjugated, T-cells or NK cells release perforin and granzymes to induce apoptosis of the tumor cell

CD20, melanoma-associated proteoglycans, and the melanoma-associated gangliosides GD2 and GD3, all of which utilize CD3 as their secondary binding target [70]. The first proof of principle triomab targeted against EpCAM, called BiUII, could mediate lysis of PCL-1 and FaDu, squamous carcinoma cells of the head and neck, with unstimulated PBMCs [122]. This was evident at relatively low concentrations of BiUII (5 ng/ml) and could mediate higher lysis of target cells than a combination of both parental CD3 and EpCAM antibodies. Therefore, the direct linkage of T-cells, NK cells, and tumor cells appears to impart a cytotoxic advantage, possibly due to the secondary activation of T-cells by NK cells or macrophages (Fig. 2). Although a high E:T ratio of 20:1 was required to reach specific lysis near 90 %, BiUII was capable of mediating 60 % and 25 % lysis at the conservative E:T ratios of 5:1 and 1:1, respectively [122]. Other preclinical EpCAM triomabs were shown to mediate significant lysis of EpCAM positive prostate cancer cell lines as well as protect 100 % of the mice from secondary challenge with B16 melanoma cells 144 days after initial inoculation [96, 98]. The induction of an adaptive immune response was likely due to the triomab's ability to activate dendritic cells, T-cells, and macrophages [123]. These trifunctional antibodies overcame the limitations of large-scale purification and were able to link the innate and adaptive together in a common anticancer goal, prompting their clinical development.

2.3.2 Catumaxomab (Removab)

Learning from the design of previous EpCAM triomabs, catumaxomab (Removab®) was developed specifically for the clinic and similar to HEA125×OKT3, was utilized for the treatment of malignant ascites. Initial phase I results demonstrated limited toxicity of catumaxomab therapy when delivered intraperitoneally to seven patients in 2005, prompting a phase I/II trial with 23 women presenting with malignant ascites [46]. Patients received 4–5 regimens of catumaxomab at increasing doses starting from 10 μg and ending at 200 μg. Although a significant proportion of patients experienced grade 3 adverse events, the majority of events were reversible. Remarkably after the 37 day trial, only one of the twenty-three patients required paracentesis, a significant improvement from the median time to paracentesis of 7–11 days commonly seen in this patient subgroup [21]. After the final treatment, those treated with catumaxomab saw a 99.9 % reduction in the mean EpCAM + tumor cell numbers in the peritoneal fluid, clearly demonstrating the antitumor ability of catumaxomab [21]. Using the dose established in this trial, a second phase II trial was conducted for 13 patients with malignant ascites to determine the pharmacokinetics and efficacy of catumaxomab. At days 0, 3, 6 or 7, and 10, patients received doses of 10, 20, 50, and 150 μg of the triomab intraperitoneally. The half-life was determined to be 2.13 days and although peritoneal concentrations were consistently high ranging from 552 to 6,121 ρg/ml, the systemic levels in the serum remained extremely low, with a maximum concentration of 403 ρg/ml [100]. While the low systemic concentration could limit the efficacy of Catumaxomab, it likely reduced the toxicity of this therapy. After a single 10 μg dose of Catumaxomab, the median EpCAM + tumor cell count reduced from 9,362 tumor cells per million ascites cells to only 49 [100].

A landmark phase II/III trial (NCT 00836654) with 258 patients with recurrent symptomatic malignant ascites caused by ovarian or non-ovarian cancer proved that intraperitoneal treatment of catumaxomab leads to a significant enhancement in puncture-free survival, median time to next paracentesis, and higher overall survival in gastric cancer patients. Utilizing the same increasing dose regimen as the previous phase II trial, patients were separated into two groups: paracentesis and catumaxomab (treatment) or paracentesis alone (control). Catumaxomab's addition resulted in an increase in puncture-free survival from 11 days in the control group to 46 days and enhanced the median time to paracentesis from 13 days to 77 days [47]. Catumaxomab also completely eliminated the EpCAM + tumor cell count in the ascites fluid in 95 of the 115 evaluable samples. The adverse events associated with catumaxomab were widespread, affecting 98 % of the patients. Toxicities from cytokine release were well controlled and reversible. Eight days after the last infusion, 76 % of all patients (85/112) presented with HAMA even though only 5 % (6/124) of patients had detectable HAMAs before the last infusion of 150 μg [47]. In a post hoc analysis, the induction of HAMA did not adversely influence clinical benefits, but instead suggested that the development of HAMA could effectively be used as a biomarker for responders to catumaxomab treatment [89]. A second post hoc analysis demonstrated that peritoneal samples from catumaxomab-treated patients had significantly lower tumor cell counts, no stem cell-like tumor cells (CD133+/EpCAM+), lower VEGF levels, and double the number of activated CD4+ and CD8+ T-cells compared to the control group [54]. Early results of this Phase II/III trial prompted the European Union to approve the use of catumaxomab for the treatment of malignant ascites in 2009, as no effective therapeutic existed for this patient group. Catumaxomab is the first and only bispecific antibody to receive approval for clinical use as a cancer therapeutic.

However, as EpCAM is expressed on such a broad range of carcinomas, it could be utilized for the treatment of numerous different cancers. As the most similar indication to malignant ascites, catumaxomab has been used in a phase II trial to treat patients with malignant pleural effusions caused by breast cancer or NSCLC. Three escalating intra-pleural doses of 5–200 μg in the 24 patients led to significant adverse events, with two dose limiting toxicities (DLTs). Although the trial was stopped early due to the high number of serious adverse events (23) and dropouts, one CR and four PRs associated with pleural effusion, occurred in the breast cancer group. Not surprisingly, most patients developed HAMA [107]. Since catumaxomab has the potential to eliminate solid tumors, one phase I and one phase II trial have been performed for NSCLC and epithelial ovarian cancer, respectively. The phase I trial represents the only instance where catumaxomab was delivered intravenously to patients. Utilizing an increasing dosing regimen of 2–7.5 μg, the maximal tolerable dose was determined to be 5 μg when administered with 40 mg of dexamethasone, a potent anti-inflammatory agent [106]. Surprisingly, no patients developed HAMA or HARA when exposed to catumaxomab, although one patient, who had preexisting HARA before treatment, had elevated levels by the end of the trial. In an effort to directly treat patients with epithelial ovarian cancer, catumaxomab was delivered intraperitoneally to 45 patients in 2011. Stratified into two groups, the low dose group of four infusions of 10 μg resulted in two patients with stable disease. The high dose group received infusions of 10, 20, 50, and 100 μg of catumaxomab, leading to one partial response and five patients with stable disease. Every patient exhibited a treatment-related adverse event, 17 of 45 patients developed HAMA or HARA, and no difference in progression-free survival was seen between the two groups [12]. Additional trials are being performed to determine the efficacy of catumaxomab as an anticancer therapeutic for indications different from malignant ascites. As of 2012, catumaxomab is being utilized in close to a dozen clinical trials with the most notable being a phase III trial for malignant ascites with or without the anti-inflammatory drug prednisolone (NCT 00822809).

2.3.3 Ertumaxomab (Rexomum)

The second triomab, ertumaxomab, was developed with the same CD3 binding arm of catumaxomab, to retarget T-cells and innate killer cells to HER2+ tumor cells. When compared to trastuzumab at a high E:T ratio of 20:1, ertumaxomab-mediated maximum lysis of high HER2 expressing cells, classified as HER2 3+, at a fivefold lower concentration (1 ng/ml vs. 5 ng/ml). Reducing the E:T ratio to 5:1 to closer reflect in vivo conditions, trastuzumab only mediated 40 % lysis of tumor cells at maximum concentrations of 1–5 μg, while ertumaxomab was able to mediate total tumor lysis at 25 ng/ml [53]. One major limitation of trastuzumab therapy is its inability to lyse tumor cells that express low levels of HER2. In the same preclinical study, trastuzumab only lysed 10 % of 1+ HER2 cells at a concentration of 5 μg/ml, while ertumaxomab mediated 100 % tumor cell killing at 5 ng/ml, at an E:T ratio of 20:1. This potency was maintained when the effector cells were significantly reduced [53]. Therefore, ertumaxomab mediates significantly improved lysis of HER2+ cancer cells at low E:T ratios and can promote the lysis of cells that are typically resistant to trastuzumab-promoted ADCC. As of 2012, ertumaxomab has been studied in two phase I clinical trials, in order to determine its toxicity profile. The first phase I trial, with four malignant ascites patients, demonstrated that ertumaxomab was well tolerated, resulting mainly in flu-like symptoms, including fever, chills, and fatigue [46]. This prompted a second phase I trial for 15 patients with HER2 expressing metastatic breast cancer. Utilizing a similar dosing regimen as catumaxomab, ertumaxomab was administered i.v. on days 1.7 ± 1 and 13 ± 1 with an initial dose of 10 μg and a final dose of 200 μg. Again, most adverse events were associated with flu-like symptoms. A few adverse events were considered serious, based on grade 3 and 4 lymphocytopenia and an increase in liver enzymes. All adverse events were reversible and the MTD was determined to be 100 μg. Of the 15 evaluable patients, one patient experienced a CR, two had PR, and two had SD [59]. Measurement of cytokine levels revealed that ertumaxomab elicited a strong Th1 cytokine response, as IL-6, IL-2, TNF-α, and IFN-γ were all elevated. Also, surprisingly, only five of the fifteen patients developed HAMA or HARA. Currently, ertumaxomab is being studied in one phase I/II clinical trial for the treatment of HER2+ solid tumors (NCT 01569412).

2.3.4 Bi20 (FBTA20)

A third Triomab, Bi20 or FBTA20, targets CD20 on lymphoma cells, linking T-cells and innate immune cells through the same CD3 domain and the intact Fc domain, respectively, as the other two triomabs. Preclinical data demonstrated the potent ability of Bi20 to mediate cytotoxicity of CD20+ B-cell lines at E:T ratios of 5:1. At a concentration of 50 ng/ml, Bi20 killed 95–100 % of B-cells, while rituximab, the FDA approved mAb to treat CD20 cancers, only mediated 65 % of B-cell lysis at 50 μg/ml [110]. In contrast to rituximab, Bi20 mediated enhanced T-cell and monocyte/macrophage activation and proliferation, a strong Th1 cytokine response, and lysed low expressing CD20 B-cells. These findings were replicated using B-cells isolated from patients with chronic lymphocytic leukemia, where Bi20 mediated efficient lysis even when CD20 expression was extremely low [14]. A phase I trial of i.v. delivered Bi20 for CLL and NHL patients in combination with donor lymphocytes, demonstrated mild adverse events of fever, chills, and bone pain. None of the six patients developed HAMA with Bi20 treatment and survival ranged from 38 to 486 days [20]. Bi20 is currently not being tested in any clinical trials but could prove to be efficacious in B-cell malignancies.

Also of interest are two triomabs created in 2004 that target melanoma-associated proteoglycans (TRBs02) and the melanoma-associated gangliosides GD2 and GD3 (TRBs07). The parental hybridomas B5 and Me361 were each fused with the CD3 hybridoma 26II6 to create TRBs02 and TRBs07, respectively. Both Triomabs were capable of inducing a Th1 cytokine response when exposed to tumor cells and PBMCs, associated with TNF-α, IL-2, IL-6, and IFN-γ, as well as the immunosuppressive cytokines IL-10. TRBs02 and TRBs07 induced the proliferation of CD8+ and CD4+ T-cells but reduced the number of NK cells and monocytes [99]. Lysis of antigen presenting cells was modest compared to other triomabs but combining both bsAbs was especially potent against cells expressing both tumor antigen targets.

2.4 Alternative Full-Length BsAbs

With the first clinical approval of a bsAb as well as extremely promising preclinical and clinical results of other bsAbs, there has been a renewed interest in developing methods to produce non-immunogenic, production-scalable bsAbs. These include two novel redox reactions, a knobs-into-holes method, a CDR mutational method, bispecific CovX bodies, and a mAb with an extra Fv domain. Both redox reactions take existing mAbs and expose them to either reducing agent, 2-mercaptoethanesulfonic acid sodium salt (MESNA) or glutathione (GSH), respectively [22, 112]. These methods result in the relatively quick formation of a bsAb with one binding domain for each antigen. Strop and colleagues mutated the hinge region with oppositely charged amino acids and the CH3 domain of each separately expressed mAb. This method facilitates the stabilization of the bispecific antibody format. As a proof of principle, using this method, they created a HER2×EGFR and a CD20×CD3 bsAb, which have hybrid IgG1/IgG2 Fc domains [112]. The CD20/CD3 bsAb mediated 80 % lysis of the CD20 positive cell line, A20, at 1 μg/ml with a low E:T ratio of 5:1 and could mediate a depletion of CD19+ A20 cells in vivo. The proof of principle bsAbs created from Heath's group demonstrated that the redox method could create bsAbs in 6–10 days of same species or cross species fusions [22].

Another unique method utilizes the knobs-into-holes technology originally hypothesized by Watson and Crick and developed in the 1990s. By replacing a small amino acid (AA) side-chain with a large AA side-chain, or "knob," in the CH3 domain of one antibody and replacing a large AA side-chain with a small AA side-chain, or "hole," in the CH3 domain of another antibody, the yield of bsAbs can be significantly increased [95]. This discovery enhances the heterodimerization of dual-targeting antibodies and reduces the different types of possible isomers to four. As one example, they created a bsAb targeted against VEGF-A and Ang-2, showing that the bsAb bound to both antigens with the same affinity as the parental mAbs. This bsAb also inhibited in vivo growth of Colo205 cells by 92 %, while the combination of both mAbs were somewhat less efficient, inhibiting growth by 78 % [101, 102]. Therefore, targeting two growth factors with one antibody may impart an enhanced antitumor effect.

One group, in an effort to approach the bi-specificity from a different angle, developed an intriguing method that results in two different antigen-binding domains on each Fab arm. Starting with a full-length mAb, this group creates a library of variants with mutated light-chain (LC) complementarity determining regions (CDRs). All variants are then analyzed for binding to the two antigens of interest, with the goal of isolating a variant with strong affinity for two targets. The first of these "two-in-one" bsAbs was created from trastuzumab and mutated to also bind to VEGF. The best dual-targeting variant bH1 underwent a second round of mutations to enhance the affinity for each antigen. The resulting high affinity variant, hB1-44, was able to inhibit the growth of Colo205 cells in vivo better than either parental antibody alone [16]. Another two-in-one antibody, MEHD7945A, was created using a phage display library of mutated Fab domains to target HER3 and EGFR. As before, this bsAb has identical Fab arms and is capable of binding either antigen with high affinity. MEHD7945A was capable of inactivating the EGFR and ERK pathway at an IC50 = 0.03 and 0.16 μg/ml, respectively, inhibiting growth of EGFR + lines in vitro, and stunting the growth of EGFR+/HER3+ cells in vivo. This was compared to the combination of the two parental mAbs [101, 102]. Also, this bsAb could mediate ADCC and when tested in cynomolgous monkeys, elicited significantly less dermatological toxicity than the FDA approved EGFR parental antibody, cetuximab. The clinical dose was determined to be 8–12 mg/kg of MEHD7945A and is currently being evaluated in a phase I trial for patients with epithelial tumors (NCT01577173) [55].

Other promising chemical conjugation techniques are bispecific CovX bodies and mAb-Fv fusions. The bispecific CovX body is a unique method that utilizes the same Fc backbone, a so-called scaffold antibody CVX-2000, with interchangeable antigen-binding domains, allowing for rapid creation of mAbs or bsAbs. The antigen binding domains are chemically linked using an azetidione linker to the scaffold antibody after the antigen peptides are fused together using maleimidethiol ligation. The first of these bs-CovX bodies, CVX-241 targeted Ang-2 and VEGF-A, with bivalent binding on each Fab arm, as each arm of the antibody can bind to either antigen [30]. CVX-241 was capable of inhibiting the growth of Colo205 cells in a xenograft model, compared to the combination of Ang-2 and VEGF-A monoclonal CovX bodies. Of particular interest, the bispecific antibody synergized with the common chemotherapeutic agent irinotecan to significantly inhibit in vivo growth. The first phase I trial with CVX-241 was terminated due to poor pharmacological properties at the highest dose of 25 mg/kg (NCT 01004822). Instead of trying to manipulate the basic binding structure of mAbs to allow for a second binding site, another method fuses an Fv region to the Fc domain of a mAb. If the Fv domain targets CD3, then the resulting bispecific antibody, called a mAb-Fv, can mediate antigen binding, ADCC, and retargeting of T-cells, similar to triomabs. The first set of these antibodies targeted HER2 × CD3 × CD16 and HM 1.24 × CD3 × CD16. Surprisingly the HER2 mAb-Fv variant bound to CD16 with higher affinity and mediated greater than sevenfold higher lysis via ADCC than the parental mAb trastuzumab [85]. Moreover, the mAb-Fvs still bound to FcRn with similar affinity as the parental antibodies, suggesting that serum half-life of the fusion antibodies will not be compromised.

3 Recombinant Bispecific Antibodies

3.1 Tandem scFv

As an alternative approach to creating full-length bsAbs, many groups have chosen to manipulate the inherent structure of the antibody itself, creating a plethora of unique molecules. The basic design of these recombinant proteins involves deconvoluting the structure of an antibody down to the elements that are vital for antigen recognition and binding. With two binding sites for antigens and no Fc domain, these proteins retarget immune cells to tumor cells through CD3 or CD16. Utilizing T-cells or innate killer cells, they can mediate significant lysis of antigen expressing cells (Fig. 3). Expressed in bacterial or mammalian cells, the recombinant proteins are purified using a variety of techniques. The first developed technique fused two single-chain variable regions (scFvs) together using a peptide linker usually between 15 and 20 AA in length, creating a tandem scFv (TaFv). The AA linker length imparted flexibility for the scFvs, allowing for the correct domains to form together. Early designs demonstrated the lytic capability of these immune cell retargeting antibodies, as they were more cytotoxic than their parental mAbs [28, 37]. One TaFv, developed in an effort to circumvent the lack of success seen by the quadroma 2B1, targeted HER2 and CD16. The protein-mediated significant lysis of HER2 overexpressing cells and demonstrated good tumor retention in vivo [79]. rM28, a unique TaFv, targeted the melanoma-associated proteoglycan (NG2) and redirected T-cells through CD28 activation. Therefore, rM28 links tumor cells to T-cells while

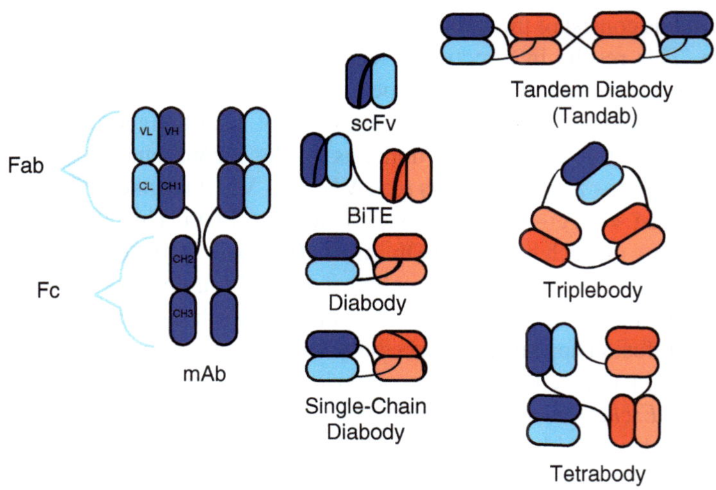

Fig. 3 Recombinant bsAbs. The antigen binding components of a mAb are isolated to create smaller antibodies, reducing their stability and immunogenicity. *Black lines* represent linker domains. Bispecific antibodies of the diabody, single-chain diabody, BiTE, tandab, triplebody, and tetrabody formats are shown

simultaneously providing them with a potent activating signal, resulting in "targeted supra-agonistic CD28 stimulation" directly at the tumor site [36]. Exciting preclinical results moved this bsAb to a phase I/II clinical trial in 2005 (NCT 00204594). Unfortunately, this trial was terminated due to the significant adverse events seen in a phase I trial of the CD28 mAb TGN1412, which caused life-threatening cytokine storm in treated volunteers [113]. A successor TaFv that targets CD20 and CD28 was then created using the same CD28 scFv. r2820 eliminated CD20+ lymphoma cells at modest antibody concentrations (0.5 μg/ml) [90]. E3Bi, another TaFv created using a 14 AA linker sequence, targeted EpCAM and CD3. This molecule was capable of eliminating EpCAM+cells both in vitro at extremely low E:T ratios of 1–2.5:1, and in vivo, where it significantly inhibited tumor growth [93]. An alternative approach to the retargeting of immune cells is the inhibition of growth factor receptor signaling. One example of this method is the scFv fusion protein, MM-111, which recognizes HER2 and HER3, inhibiting the intracellular signaling of both tyrosine kinase receptors [80]. This fusion protein differs in the basic structure from other TaFvs, as it is also bound to modified human serum albumin, in an effort to enhance MM-111 serum stability. Further studies need to be done to determine if this type of scFv fusion has antitumor capabilities, as it lacks any effector cell-mediated lytic potential. It is currently involved in three phase I clinical trials for HER2-amplified cancers.

3.2 *Diabody*

Diabodies (Db) are another recombinant bsAb that have been intensively studied. These proteins consist of the same scFv domains as TaFvs but utilize a shorter linker sequence. This results in a reduced yield of homodimers, essentially driving the formation of the bispecific format. Specifically, the heavy-chain variable domain (VH) and the light-chain variable domain (VL) of each antigen binding chain are forced to connect with respective domains on the second antigen chain. In other words, for antigens A and B, TaFvs read VH(A)—VL(A) (linker) VH(B)—VL(B), while Dbs read VH(A)—VL(B) (linker) VH(B)—VL(A). This allows for bivalent antigen binding on each half of the Db. As of 2012, over 40 different types of bispecific Dbs have been developed in preclinical studies, but none have entered human trials. This is mainly due to the short half-life seen with these small molecules, as continuous infusion appears to be necessary for adequate serum concentrations. The first Db design targeted the hapten phenyloxazone and hen egg lysozyme, was expressed in *Escherichia coli* (*E. coli*), and purified using affinity chromatography, yielding 0.3–1 mg/L [49]. The first Db to be tested in vivo targeted HER2, was almost cleared from the blood within 4 h but was retained in the tumor for close to a day [1]. Holliger and colleagues also developed the first Db that retargeted T-cells to tumor cells, using CD3 to link T-cells to BCL-1+lymphoma cells. At a molecular weight of 50 kDa, this Db was capable of mediating 80 % lysis of lymphoma cells at the extremely low concentration of 63 ng/ml [50]. It also induced significantly higher lysis than a CD3 × BCL-1 quadroma bsAb, showing for the first time that the Db format could mediate higher tumor lysis than a similar quadroma bsAb.

Of the CD3 T-cell retargeting Dbs CD19, CEA, EGFR, Endoglin, and PSMA Dbs are of particular interest. All five of these Dbs were expressed in *E. coli*, with a yield ranging from 0.1 to 3 mg/L [33, 45, 51, 60, 65]. The CD19 × CD3 Db-mediated lysis of CD19+ lymphoma cells at a tenfold lower concentration than a CD19 × CD3 quadroma bsAb, although the E:T ratios and maximum lysis were modest [60]. Targeting CEA expressing colon carcinoma cells with IL-2 stimulated PBMCs and 100 ng/ml of the respective Db, resulted in 50 % lysis at the moderate E:T ratio of 10:1 [51]. The EGFR Db, Ex3, only mediated 60 % lysis at 1 μg/ml with 100 times more lymphokine-activated killer cells than EGFR expressing bile duct carcinoma cells [45]. Therefore, the group attempted to enhance the lytic capacity by humanizing the diabody, creating hEx3. This Db was able to mediate 100 % tumor inhibition at 0.5 ρmol/ml at an E:T of 5:1 and enhanced in vivo survival from 10 weeks (control) to 23 weeks [6]. The endoglin targeting Db-mediated 50–60 % maximum lysis of endothelial cells at high LAK levels [65]. Lastly, the PSMA single-chain Db (scDb), which conforms to a slightly different shape with the binding domain for PSMA and CD3 existing on opposite sides of the molecule, was able to significantly inhibit tumor formation of prostate carcinoma cells in mice [33]. The remaining immune retargeting Dbs bind to CD16 and CD19, CD30, or EGFR. Not surprisingly, these Dbs required significantly high E:T ratios to mediate effective lysis of target cells [5, 8, 62].

3.3 Multi-Targeting Antibodies

In an effort to enhance the serum stability of these recombinant proteins, increase the avidity for an antigen, or increase the number of targets, groups added additional antigen binding domains. Similar to the CD3 x CD19 Db, Kipriyanov et al. created a Tandab, or tandem diabody, that targeted the same antigens. This format results in a protein that's double the size of Dbs (~114 kDa), increasing half-life, with four Vh–Vl domains instead of two [61]. This Tandab was able to stimulate T-cells, elicit higher lysis, and significantly inhibit the growth of in vivo lymphoma cells compared to the CD19 × CD3 Db [24, 61]. Another group developed a similar molecule, called a tetrabody, from the humanized Ex3 Db. Although this molecule has four binding domains, similar to Tandabs, it is arranged in a circular format instead of a linear one. This hEx3 tetrabody was 113 kDa and could mediate the same lysis as the Db but at a 100-fold lower concentration, resulting in an extremely low EC50 of 0.5 fmol/ml at an E:T of 5:1 with LAK cells [7]. The triplebody, another bsAb format which binds to three antigens, is created by linking three scFvs together. Four promising candidates, CD19 × CD16 × CD19, CD33 × CD123 × CD16, CD123 × CD16 × CD123, CD33 × CD19 × CD16, exhibited enhanced stability, were expressed in mammalian cells, and induced half-maximum lysis in the low picomolar range [58, 67, 105]. As these molecules have the potential to form aggregates when in suspension, it remains to be seen if their potent lytic capabilities will translate safely into humans.

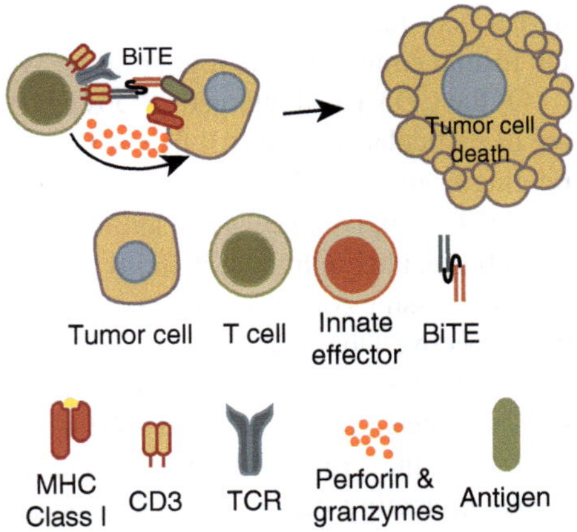

Fig. 4 BiTE's mechanism of action. Bispecific T-cell engager's function by linking T-cells directly to tumor cells through CD3 on T-cells. Conjugation of T-cells to tumor cells results in the release of perforin and granzyme, inducing apoptosis in the target cells. BiTEs exist that target CD19, EpCAM, EGFR, CD33, MCSPs, CEA, and EphA2

3.4 Bispecific T-*Cell Engagers*

3.4.1 Early Generation BiTEs

Even though BiTEs, or bispecific T-cell engagers, have not been evaluated in phase III clinical trials, they may represent the future of the bsAb field. The concentrations required to induce significant lysis in vitro and in vivo are some of the lowest seen for any anticancer therapy. By redirecting T-cells to antigen positive tumor cells, this approach is not unique. What is unique, is the ability to eliminate cancer cells at E:T ratios that are orders of magnitude lower than other bsAbs (1:1 or 1:10) with PBMCs that do not require pre-stimulation with IL-2 or CD28 activation [66, 121]. As two scFvs bound together with a short gly$_4$-ser$_1$ linker, the bispecific molecules are only approximately 55 kDa and are capable of binding only one antigen on each arm (Fig. 4). Currently, Micromet is in various stages of preclinical and clinical tests involving ten BiTEs that target eight different antigens. They are CD19, EpCAM, HER2/neu, EGFR, CEA, CD33, EphA2, and MCSPs [9]. One of the most surprising features of these bispecific molecules is their ability to mediate potent lysis without the need for MHC Class I [87]. Therefore, these molecules can utilize T-cells to target any type of cell, regardless of the T-cell's ability to inherently recognize the target cell. Importantly, BiTEs address previous toxicity limitations seen with earlier CD3-based bsAbs by utilizing a lower binding affinity to CD3, allowing for T-cell activation only at tumor sites. Therefore, BiTEs lead to specific antitumor effects without potentially life-threatening host toxicity caused by excessive cytokine release.

MT103 and MT110, which target CD19 and EpCAM, respectively, are the only two BiTEs in clinical trials but many more will follow soon, as all published results for these molecules are promising. The EpCAM-targeted BiTE is only undergoing a phase I clinical trial, when it was the first developed. In 1995, Mack et al.

developed the scFv fusion protein targeting CD3 and EpCAM. This molecule was capable of only being expressed in CHO cells, as *E. coli* expression resulted in inert protein [75]. Fortunately, the harvest of the EpCAM scFv fusion was significantly higher than other recombinant bsAbs, yielding 12–15 mg of protein per liter of media. This early generation BiTE was capable of inducing significant lysis at only 8 ng/ml and was stable in PBS for 6 months and serum for 56 h [66, 75]. Not surprisingly, CD8+ and CD4+ T-cells were required for the antitumor lysis [66]. The early generation EpCAM BiTEs could induce substantial lysis at concentrations near or below 1 ng/ml, all utilizing unstimulated PBMCs from healthy and cancer patients [76, 103, 120]. One in vivo study found that 1 μg of the EpCAM BiTE could protect all six mice from challenge with SW480 colon carcinoma cells and even eliminate growth in some mice with established tumors. This same study discovered that the bsAb could utilize tumor infiltrating T-cells to eliminate tumors engrafted in mice when isolated directly from patients at only 5 μg/mouse [103]. This experiment, where three of six mice treated with the BiTE survived challenge, proved that this molecule could utilize a patients' own T-cells to modulate an antitumor effect.

Early generation CD19 BiTEs showed similar promising results. First created in 2000, Loffler et al. demonstrated that the CD19 BiTE could retarget T-cells to lymphoma cells, eliciting significant lysis at low E:T ratios (2:1 or 4:1) at concentrations between 10 and 100 ρg/ml, a 10–100-fold lower concentration than even the EpCAM BiTE and 1–10,000-fold lower than a quadroma CD19×CD3 bsAb [71]. Interestingly, short-term addition of IL-2 to PBMCs did not drastically enhance the lysis of B-cells by the CD19 BiTEs, although long-term exposure of IL-2 resulting in LAK effector cells enhanced the EC_{50} by tenfold [31, 72]. Even at E:T ratios of 1:4, the CD19 BiTE could eliminate all CD19+ B-cells at a low concentration of 5 ng/ml [72]. An in vivo study found that, similar to the EpCAM BiTE, the CD19 BiTE could protect mice from tumor challenge and even eliminate large establish tumors [32]. The BiTEs appear to require T-cells to release perforin to mediate lysis, as cells treated with the perforin inhibitor Oncanamycin A (OMA), had significantly reduced lysis [38].

3.4.2 MT103 (Blinatumomab)

Learning from previous designs, Micromet designed and created MT103, the CD19×CD3 BiTE currently in clinical trials. MT103 exhibited significant preclinical potency to CD19+ autologous B-cells, with an EC_{50} of 130 ρg/ml with human PBMCs and 150 ρg/ml with chimpanzee PBMCs [104]. When the BiTE was given to chimpanzees, the molecule was well tolerated, with an increase in Th1 cytokines and T-cell activation. After a dose of 0.1 μg/kg in chimpanzees, MT103 peaked around 1 ng/ml and reduced to 50 ρg/ml within 10–24 h after treatment [104]. As MT103 can induce the release of the Th1 cytokines IFN-γ, TNF-α, and IL-2, it would most likely require coadministration with an anti-inflammatory agent. Therefore, Micromet analyzed the functionality of MT103 with the clinically used anit-inflammatory agent dexamethasone [17, 19]. Fortunately, the anit-inflammatory agent did not reduce lysis or T-cell activation but did attenuate cytokine release [17]. When compared to a CD19×CD3 tandab, MT103 was 1,000 times more potent, when unstimulated T-cells were used, highlighting for the first time, that the BiTE format was more potent than similarly designed recombinant bsAbs [84]. Another comparison study found that MT103 mediated 150–450 times more efficient lysis than rituximab to CD19+ CD20+ cells but found that even in optimal conditions for rituximab, MT103's addition could still enhance tumor cell apoptosis [25]. Even with extremely low E:T ratios, MT103 was capable of inducing significant cell death, implying that T-cells can mediate serial killing of target cells [25].

These encouraging results led to a phase I trial for MT103 for patients with non-Hodgkin's B-cell lymphoma. Of the 38 patients treated, 11 exhibited objective responses, with four CRs and seven PRs. All six patients treated at the highest dose of 0.06 mg/m^2 showed a response to treatment. Overall, the adverse events were mild, including chills, pyrexia, lymphopenia, and leukopenia and occurred in the first week of treatment. No antidrug antibodies were seen in any of the 38 patients [10]. A phase II trial, published in 2011, demonstrated an 80 % response rate in 21 patients with adult B-cell lineage ALL, treated with a dose of 0.015 mg/m^2. After a single cycle of MT103, 16 of 20 evaluable patients were switched from minimum residual disease (MRD) positive status to negative. As MRD is a common indicator of relapse and these patients were heavily pretreated, these results are promising. Overall, the estimate of relapse-free survival was 78 % [114]. As in the phase I trial, MT103 was well tolerated, with similar adverse events. A secondary analysis of the immunological responses to MT103 revealed that most patients responded with similar trends after treatment. Within a single day, the number of circulating B-cells dropped to one B-cell/μL of blood, and did not increase throughout the treatment cycles. The percentage of activated CD8+ and CD4+ T-cells increased from 19.47 to 48.78 % and 12.32 to 35.63 %, respectively, elucidating MT103's potent effects on T-cells. Fortunately, no patient developed HAMA [64]. With these results, MT103 is currently being evaluated in six phase I or phase II clinical trials, and phase III trials results are awaited with interest.

3.4.3 MT110

Similar to MT103, Micromet used previous EpCAM BiTE designs to enhance the potency of the bispecific molecule being tested in clinical trials. The resulting BiTE, MT110, is ~55 kDa, can redirect PBMCs to tumor cells with an EC_{50} of 230 ρg/ml, can eliminate tumor initiating cells and is not affected by circulating levels of EpCAMs ectodomain, EpEx [18, 19, 48, 91]. MT110 was also capable of killing primary pancreatic cells at concentrations of 1–100 ng/ml [23]. In vivo treatment of 1 μg MT110 resulted in the complete prevention of tumor growth in both challenge and established tumors [18]. Interestingly, MT110 was able to induce tumor elimination in mice utilizing only the T-cells that infiltrated the tumor before removal from patients, again elucidating the potency of retargeting T-cells to fight cancer.

In an attempt to determine if an EpCAM BiTE would be toxic to normal EpCAM expressing cells, Brischwein and colleagues performed a series of preclinical studies using a murine EpCAM BiTE analog in immune-competent mice. MuS110 could recognize murine CD3 and murine EpCAM and has an EC_{50} similar to MT110, albeit slightly worse [2, 19]. At doses of 15 μg/kg, MuS110 was well tolerated in mice and was capable of inhibiting syngeneic tumor growth. Increasing the dose to 50 μg/kg or 500 μg/kg resulted in cytokine release syndrome or death in mice, respectively [2, 3]. In the 15 μg/kg treated mice, MuS110 caused a fivefold drop in B-cell numbers and an eightfold drop in T-cell numbers [3]. Unlike humans, mice have EpCAM+lymphocytes, which might be contributing to side effects such as lymphopenia. Therefore, it is possible that initially eliminating this subpopulation of cells could enhance the tolerability of MuS110. Initial low doses of 0.4–10 μg/kg tolerized mice to doses of MuS110 up to 500 μg/kg [3, 4]. MuS110 did not damage EpCAM+tissues or organs and long-term dosing did not result in T-cell anergy, strengthening the clinical utility of an EpCAM BiTE. All of these results led to an ongoing phase I clinical trial in patients with EpCAM+solid tumors.

3.4.4 Other BiTEs

The remaining BiTEs in clinical trials target CEA, EphA2, EGFR, CD33, and MCSPs. The CEA BiTE was found from a panel of CEA BiTEs created from three CEA mAbs and thirteen scFvs directed against CEA, all with the same CD3 binding domain. The most potent protein, MT111, had an EC_{50} of 200–500 pg/ml with unstimulated PBMCs and an EC_{50} of 2.3 pg/ml using stimulated human T-cells. It inhibited tumor xenograft growth and had similar lysis across 12 different CEA expressing tumor lines [73]. As many patients with CEA+tumors have circulating soluble CEA (sCEA), it was important to discover that sCEA did not inhibit tumor cell lysis by MT111 [73, 88]. On top of this, a murine analog of MT111 was capable of inhibiting metastatic lung lesions in a syngeneic mouse model [73]. Both of these findings underscore the clinical potential of this BiTE.

EphA2 is a tyrosine kinase receptor that is often overexpressed in aggressive epithelial cancers. The EphA2 BiTE developed by Micromet is unique from others in its class, as it only recognizes EphA2 on malignant cells, sparing any T-cell elimination of normal cells. The BiTE was capable of eliminating tumor cells at EC_{50} concentrations of about 6 ng/ml and could mediate maximal lysis at an E:T ratio of 1:5 with 7 ng/ml of the bsAb. Confirmatory results were seen in vivo [42]. The remaining BiTEs targeting EGFR, CD33, and MCSPs offer promising further preclinical and clinical results. C-BiTE and P-BiTE, developed from the binding domains of cetuximab and panitumumab, two FDA approved EGFR mAbs, were able to lyse KRAS- and BRAF-mutated colorectal cells [74]. The MCSP BiTE recognizes the D3 domain of the heavily glycosylated human melanoma chondroitin sulfate proteoglycan (MCSP) [13]. The bsAb-mediated significant lysis of 33

MCSP+melanoma cell lines with PBMCs isolated from healthy and melanoma patients, albeit reduced with the latter cell sources [115]. The CD33 BiTE, MT114, exhibits similar potent lysis, with EC_{50} values as low as 5 pg/ml and mediates lysis across numerous CD33+AML cell lines [29, 63].

4 Imaging

There is an evolving area of the tumor immunology field that is utilizing bsAbs for cancer imaging. Since the second target can be engineered to bind to a radiolabeled agent, these bsAbs are simpler to create than radiolabeled mAbs. One of the most common methods for creating radiolabeled bsAbs is the dock-and-lock (DNL) technique. Originally developed in 2006, the DNL method can be used to efficiently create bsAbs for any target but as of 2012 was entirely devoted to the creation of radiolabeled bsAbs [97]. TF2, which targets CEA and the hapten histamine-succinyl-glycine (HSG), is currently undergoing three phase I trials and one phase I/II trial for imaging colorectal or lung cancers [78]. After injection and clearance of the bsAb, ^{99m}Tc-labeled hapten is infused into the patient, resulting in radioactive labeling of only bsAb bound cells. TF4 and TF10 are two other DNL bsAbs directed against CD20×HSG hapten and MUC1×HSG hapten, respectively [35, 108].

5 Conclusions

The clinical efficacy of catumaxomab and blinatumomab highlight the potential of bispecific antibody therapy modalities. The progress seen 25 years following the production of the first such molecules augurs well for the future of the field (Table 1). Learning from previous designs and trials, researchers have developed molecules that overcome problems like the development of HAMA, by creating bsAbs that work at increasingly low concentrations, precluding the need for excessive doses or humanization. First generation bsAbs required such high ratios of effector to tumor cells that could never translate into clinical efficacy. The efficiency of newer compounds permits them to be used at low concentrations that require potentially physiological effector: target ratios. Moreover, by targeting hematologic malignancies, the potential barriers of access of effector cells to tumor targets may be minimized. Challenges remain; the need for prolonged continuous infusion makes BiTEs inconvenient and expensive for patients. Additional modifications to promote prolonged half-lives may be required for these reagents to achieve their full potential. Moreover, the ability of BiTEs to effectively treat solid human tumors in the clinical setting remains unproven. However, the presence of these challenges should not obscure the fact that bispecific antibodies can work to effectively treat cancer. The challenge to the field is to build upon the exciting findings for the benefit of patients with diverse forms of cancer.

Table 1 A list of bsAbs that have entered clinical trials

Name	Design	Target	Species	Indication	Phase	References
MDX-210	$(Fab')_2$	HER2 × CD64	Murine	Breast	I	[116]
MDX-H210	$(Fab')_2$	HER2 × CD64	Humanized	Breast	I	[94]
MDX-447	$(Fab')_2$	EGFR × CD64	Humanized	EGFR tumors	I	[34]
2B1	Quadroma	HER2 × CD16	Murine	HER2 tumors	I	[15]
HRS-3/A9	Quadroma	CD30 × CD16	Murine	Lymphoma	I/II	[44]
SHR-1	Quadroma	CD19 × CD3	Rat/murine	Lymphoma	I	[26, 27]
HEA125 × OKT3	Quadroma	EpCAM × CD3	Murine	Malignant ascites	I	[77]
Catumaxomab	Triomab	EpCAM × CD3	Rat/murine	Malignant ascites	EU approval/III	[47]
Ertumaxomab	Triomab	HER2 × CD3	Rat/murine	HER2 tumors	I/II	[59]
Bi20	Triomab	CD20 × CD3	Rat/murine	Lymphoma	I	[20]
MEHD794A	Two-in-one	HER3 × EGFR	Human	Solid tumors	I/II	NCT01577173
CVX-241	CovX body	VEGF-A × Ang-2	Human	Solid tumors	I	NCT01004822
rM28	TaFv	NG2 × CD28	Murine	Melanoma	I/II	NCT00204594
MM-111	TaFv-albumin	HER2 × HER3	Human	HER2 tumors	I	NCT00911898
MT103	BiTE	CD19 × CD3	Murine	Lymphoma	II	[114]
MT110	BiTE	EpCAM × CD3	Murine	EpCAM tumors	I	NCT00635596

Citations represent the most recently published trial. If a reference isn't cited, the clinical trial is currently in progress

References

1. Adams GP, Schier R, McCall AM, Crawford RS, Wolf EJ, Weiner LM, Marks JD. Prolonged in vivo tumour retention of a human diabody targeting the extracellular domain of human HER2/Neu. Br J Cancer. 1998;77(9):1405–12.
2. Amann M, Brischwein K, Lutterbuese P, Parr L, Petersen L, Lorenczewski G, Krinner E, et al. Therapeutic window of MuS110, a single-chain antibody construct bispecific for murine EpCAM and murine CD3. Cancer Res. 2008;68(1):1–10. doi:10.1158/0008-5472.CAN-07-2182.
3. Amann M, Friedrich M, Lutterbuese P, Vieser E, Lorenczewski G, Petersen L, Brischwein K, Kufer P, et al. Therapeutic window of an EpCAM/CD3-specific BiTE antibody in mice is determined by a subpopulation of EpCAM-expressing lymphocytes that is absent in humans. Cancer Immunol Immunother. 2009;58(1):1–15. doi:10.1007/s00262-008-0529-y.
4. Amann M, D'Argouges S, Lorenczewski G, Brischwein K, Kischel R, Lutterbuese R, Mangold S, Rau D, et al. Antitumor activity of an EpCAM/CD3-bispecific BiTE antibody during long-term treatment of mice in the absence of T-cell anergy and sustained cytokine release. J Immunother. 2009;32(5). 10.1097/CJI.0b013e3181a1c097.
5. Arndt MA, Krauss J, Kipriyanov SM, Pfreundschuh M, Little M. A bispecific diabody that mediates natural killer cell cytotoxicity against xenotransplantated human Hodgkin's tumors. Blood. 1999;94(8):2562–8.
6. Ryutaro A, Sone Y, Makabe K, Tsumoto K, Hayashi H, Katayose Y, Unno M, Kudo T, Kumagai I. Humanization of the bispecific epidermal growth factor receptor X CD3 diabody and its efficacy as a potential clinical reagent. Clin Cancer Res. 2006;12(13):1–8. doi:10.1158/1078-0432.CCR-06-0059.
7. Ryutaro A, Ikoma K, Sone Y, Kawaguchi H, Taki S, Hayashi H, Nakanishi T, et al. Highly enhanced cytotoxicity of a dimeric bispecific diabody, the hEx3 tetrabody. J Biol Chem. 2010;285(27):1–6. doi:10.1074/jbc.M110.120444.
8. Ryutaro A, Nakayama M, Kawaguchi H, Kubota T, Nakanishi T, Umetsu M, Hayashi H, et al. Construction and humanization of a functional bispecific EGFR×CD16 diabody using a refolding system. FEBS J. 2012;279(2):223–33. doi:10.1111/j.1742-4658.2011.08417.x.
9. Baeuerle PA, Kufer P, Bargou R. BiTE: teaching antibodies to engage T-cells for cancer therapy. Curr Opin Mol Ther. 2009;11(1):22–30.
10. Bargou R, Leo E, Zugmaier G, Klinger M, Goebeler M, Knop S, Noppeney R, et al. Tumor regression in cancer patients by very low doses of a T cell-engaging antibody. Science. 2008;321(5891):1–5. doi:10.1126/science.1158545.
11. Baselga J, Swain SM. Novel anticancer targets: revisiting ERBB2 and discovering ERBB3. Nat Rev Cancer. 2009;9(7):463–75. doi:10.1038/nrc2656.
12. Baumann K, Pfisterer J, Wimberger P, Burchardi N, Kurzeder C, du Bois A, Loibl S, et al. intraperitoneal treatment with the trifunctional bispecific antibody catumaxomab in patients with platinum-resistant epithelial ovarian cancer: a phase IIa study of the AGO Study Group. Gynecol Oncol. 2011;123(1):1–6. doi:10.1016/j.ygyno.2011.06.004.
13. Bluemel C, Hausmann S, Fluhr P, Sriskandarajah M, Stallcup WB, Baeuerle PA, Kufer P. Epitope distance to the target cell membrane and antigen size determine the potency of T cell-mediated lysis by BiTE antibodies specific for a large melanoma surface antigen. Cancer Immunol Immunother. 2010;59(8):1–13. doi:10.1007/s00262-010-0844-y.
14. Boehrer S, Schroeder P, Mueller T, Atz J, Chow KU. Cytotoxic effects of the trifunctional bispecific antibody FBTA05 in ex-vivo cells of chronic lymphocytic leukaemia depend on immune-mediated mechanism. Anticancer Drugs. 2011;22(6):519–30. doi:10.1097/CAD.0b013e328344887f.
15. Borghaei H, Alpaugh RK, Bernardo P, Palazzo IE, Dutcher JP, Venkatraj U, Wood WC, Goldstein L, Weiner LM. Induction of adaptive anti-HER2/Neu immune responses in a phase 1B/2 trial of 2B1 bispecific murine monoclonal antibody in metastatic breast cancer (E3194):

a trial coordinated by the Eastern Cooperative Oncology Group. J Immunother. 2007;30(4):455–67. doi:10.1097/CJI.0b013e31803bb421.

16. Bostrom J, Yu S-F, Kan D, Appleton BA, Lee CV, Billeci K, Man W, et al. Variants of the antibody herceptin that interact with HER2 and VEGF at the antigen binding site. Science. 2009;323(5921):1610–4. doi:10.1126/science.1165480.
17. Brandl C, Haas C, d'Argouges S, Fisch T, Kufer P, Brischwein K, Prang N, et al. The effect of dexamethasone on polyclonal T cell activation and redirected target cell lysis as induced by a CD19/CD3-bispecific single-chain antibody construct. Cancer Immunol Immunother. 2007;56(10):1551–63. doi:10.1007/s00262-007-0298-z.
18. Brischwein K, Schlereth B, Guller B, Steiger C, Wolf A, Lutterbuese R, Offner S, et al. MT110: a novel bispecific single-chain antibody construct with high efficacy in eradicating established tumors. Mol Immunol. 2006;43(8):1–15. doi:10.1016/j.molimm.2005.07.034.
19. Brischwein K, Parr L, Pflanz S, Volkland J, Lumsden J, Klinger M, Locher M, et al. Strictly target cell-dependent activation of T Cells by bispecific single-chain antibody constructs of the BiTE class. J Immunother. 2007;30(8). 10.1097/CJI.0b013e318156750c.
20. Buhmann R, Simoes B, Stanglmaier M, Yang T, Faltin M, Bund D, Lindhofer H, Kolb H-J. Immunotherapy of recurrent B-cell malignancies after allo-SCT with Bi20 (FBTA05), a trifunctional anti-CD3 X anti-CD20 antibody and donor lymphocyte infusion. Bone Marrow Transplant. 2009;43(5):1–15. doi:10.1038/bmt.2008.323.
21. Burges A, Wimberger P, Kümper C, Gorbounova V, Sommer H, Schmalfeldt B, Pfisterer J, et al. Effective relief of malignant ascites in patients with advanced ovarian cancer by a trifunctional anti-EpCAM X anti-CD3 antibody: a phase I/II study. Clin Cancer Res. 2007;13:1–8. doi:10.1158/1078-0432.CCR-06-2769.
22. Carlring J, de Leenheer E, Heath AW. A novel redox method for rapid production of functional bi-specific antibodies for use in early pilot studies. PLoS One. 2011;6(7):1–6. doi:10.1371/journal.pone.0022533.
23. Cioffi M, Dorado J, Baeuerle PA, Heeschen C. EpCAM/CD3-bispecific T-cell engaging antibody MT110 eliminates primary human pancreatic cancer stem cells. Clin Cancer Res. 2012;18(2):1–11. doi:10.1158/1078-0432.CCR-11-1270.
24. Cochlovius B, Kipriyanov SM, Stassar MJ, Schuhmacher J, Benner A, Moldenhauer G, Little M. Cure of Burkitt's lymphoma in severe combined immunodeficiency mice by T cells, tetravalent CD3 X CD19 tandem diabody, and CD28 costimulation. Cancer Res. 2000; 60(16):4336–41.
25. D'Argouges S, Wissing S, Brandl C, Prang N, Lutterbuese R, Kozhich A, Suzich J, et al. Combination of rituximab with blinatumomab (MT103/MEDI-538), a T cell-engaging CD19-/CD3-bispecific antibody, for highly efficient lysis of human B lymphoma cells. Leuk Res. 2009;33(3):1–9. doi:10.1016/j.leukres.2008.08.025.
26. De Gast GC, Van Houten AA, Haagen IA, Klein S, De Weger RA, Van Dijk A, Phillips J, Clark M, Bast BJ. Clinical experience with CD3 X CD19 bispecific antibodies in patients with B cell malignancies. J Hematother. 1995;4(5):433–7.
27. de Gast GC, Haagen IA, van Houten AA, Klein SC, Duits AJ, de Weger RA, Vroom TM, Clark MR, Phillips J, van Dijk AJ. CD8 T cell activation after intravenous administration of CD3 X CD19 bispecific antibody in patients with non-hodgkin lymphoma. Cancer Immunol Immunother. 1995;40(6):390–6.
28. de Jonge J, Heirman C, de Veerman M, van Meirvenne S, Moser M, Leo O, Thielemans K. In vivo retargeting of T cell effector function by recombinant bispecific single chain Fv (anti-CD3 X anti-idiotype) induces long-term survival in the murine BCL1 lymphoma model. J Immunol. 1998;161(3):1454–61.
29. Dhimolea E. World bispecific antibody summit, 27–28 Sept 2011, Boston, MA. mAbs. 2012;
30. Doppalapudi VR, Huang J, Liu D, Jin P, Liu B, Li L, Desharnais J, et al. Chemical generation of bispecific antibodies. Proc Natl Acad Sci U S A. 2010;107(52):22611–6. doi:10.1073/pnas.1016478108.
31. Dreier T, Lorenczewski G, Brandl C, Hoffmann P, Syring U, Hanakam F, Kufer P, Riethmuller G, Bargou R, Baeuerle PA. Extremely potent, rapid and costimulation-independent cytotoxic

T-cell response against lymphoma cells catalyzed by a single-chain bispecific antibody. Int J Cancer. 2002;100(6):690–7. doi:10.1002/ijc.10557.
32. Dreier T, Baeuerle PA, Fichtner I, Grün M, Schlereth B, Lorenczewski G, Kufer P, et al. T cell costimulus-independent and very efficacious inhibition of tumor growth in mice bearing subcutaneous or leukemic human B cell lymphoma xenografts by a CD19-/CD3- bispecific single-chain antibody construct. J Immunol. 2003;170(8):1–7.
33. Fortmüller K, Alt K, Gierschner D, Wolf P, Baum V, Freudenberg N, Wetterauer U, Elsässer-Beile U, Bühler P. Effective targeting of prostate cancer by lymphocytes redirected by a PSMA × CD3 bispecific single-chain diabody. Prostate. 2011;71(6):588–96. doi:10.1002/pros.21274.
34. Fury MG, Lipton A, Smith KM, Winston CB, Pfister DG. A phase-I trial of the epidermal growth factor receptor directed bispecific antibody MDX-447 without and with recombinant human granulocyte-colony stimulating factor in patients with advanced solid tumors. Cancer Immunol Immunother. 2008;57(2):1–9. doi:10.1007/s00262-007-0357-5.
35. Gold DV, Goldenberg DM, Karacay H, Rossi EA, Chang C-H, Cardillo TM, McBride WJ, Sharkey RM. A novel bispecific, trivalent antibody construct for targeting pancreatic carcinoma. Cancer Res. 2008;68(12):1–9. doi:10.1158/0008-5472.CAN-08-0232.
36. Grosse-Hovest L, Hartlapp I, Marwan W, Brem G, Rammensee H-G, Jung G. A recombinant bispecific single-chain antibody induces targeted, supra-agonistic CD28-stimulation and tumor cell killing. Eur J Immunol. 2003;33(5):1–7. doi:10.1002/eji.200323322.
37. Gruber M, Schodin BA, Wilson ER, Kranz DM. Efficient tumor cell lysis mediated by a bispecific single chain antibody expressed in *Escherichia coli*. J Immunol. 1994;152(11): 5368–74.
38. Gruen M, Bommert K, Bargou RC. T-cell-mediated lysis of B cells induced by a CD19xCD3 bispecific single-chain antibody is perforin dependent and death receptor independent. Cancer Immunol Immunother. 2004;53(7):625–32. doi:10.1007/s00262-003-0496-2.
39. Haagen IA, van de Griend R, Clark M, Geerars A, Bast B, de Gast B. Killing of human leukaemia/lymphoma B cells by activated cytotoxic T lymphocytes in the presence of a bispecific monoclonal antibody (Alpha CD3/Alpha CD19). Clin Exp Immunol. 1992;90(3): 368–75.
40. Haagen IA, Geerars AJ, de Lau WB, Clark MR, van de Griend RJ, Bast BJ, de Gast BC. Killing of autologous B-lineage malignancy using CD3 X CD19 bispecific monoclonal antibody in end stage leukemia and lymphoma. Blood. 1994;84(2):556–63.
41. Haagen IA, Geerars AJ, de Lau WB, Bast BJ, de Gast BC. The efficacy of CD3 X CD19 bispecific monoclonal antibody (BsAb) in a clonogenic assay: the effect of repeated addition of BsAb and Interleukin-2. Blood. 1995;85(11):3208–12.
42. Hammond SA, Lutterbuese R, Roff S, Lutterbuese P, Schlereth B, Bruckheimer E, Kinch MS, et al. Selective targeting and potent control of tumor growth using an EphA2/CD3-bispecific single-chain antibody construct. Cancer Res. 2007;67(8):1–10. doi:10.1158/0008-5472.CAN-06-2760.
43. Hartmann F, Renner C, Jung W, Deisting C, Juwana M, Eichentopf B, Kloft M, Pfreundschuh M. Treatment of refractory Hodgkin's disease with an anti-CD16/CD30 bispecific antibody. Blood. 1997;89(6):1–8.
44. Hartmann F, Renner C, Jung W, da Costa L, Tembrink S, Held G, Sek A, et al. Anti-CD16/CD30 bispecific antibody treatment for Hodgkin's disease: role of infusion schedule and costimulation with cytokines. Clin Cancer Res. 2001;7(7):1873–81.
45. Hayashi H, Asano R, Tsumoto K, Katayose Y, Suzuki M, Unno M, Kodama H, et al. A highly effective and stable bispecific diabody for cancer immunotherapy: cure of xenografted tumors by bispecific diabody and T-LAK cells. Cancer Immunol Immunother. 2004;53(6):497–509. doi:10.1007/s00262-003-0465-9.
46. Heiss MM, Ströhlein MA, Jäger M, Kimmig R, Burges A, Schoberth A, Jauch K-W, Schildberg F-W, Lindhofer H. Immunotherapy of malignant ascites with trifunctional antibodies. Int J Cancer. 2005;117(3):1–9. doi:10.1002/ijc.21165.

47. Heiss MM, Murawa P, Koralewski P, Kutarska E, Kolesnik OO, Ivanchenko VV, Dudnichenko AS, et al. The trifunctional antibody catumaxomab for the treatment of malignant ascites due to epithelial cancer: results of a prospective randomized phase II/III trial. Int J Cancer. 2010;127(9):2209–21. doi:10.1002/ijc.25423.
48. Herrmann I, Baeuerle PA, Friedrich M, Murr A, Filusch S, Rüttinger D, Majdoub MW, et al. Highly efficient elimination of colorectal tumor-initiating cells by an EpCAM/CD3-bispecific antibody engaging human T cells. PLoS One. 2010;5(10):1–10. doi:10.1371/journal.pone.0013474.
49. Holliger P, Prospero T, Winter G. Diabodies: small bivalent and bispecific antibody fragments. Proc Natl Acad Sci U S A. 1993;90(14):6444–8.
50. Holliger P, Brissinck J, Williams RL, Thielemans K, Winter G. Specific killing of lymphoma cells by cytotoxic T-cells mediated by a bispecific diabody. Protein Eng. 1996;9(3): 299–305.
51. Holliger P, Manzke O, Span M, Hawkins R, Fleischmann B, Qinghua L, Wolf J, et al. Carcinoembryonic antigen (CEA)-specific T-cell activation in colon carcinoma induced by anti-CD3 X anti-CEA bispecific diabodies and B7 X anti-CEA bispecific fusion proteins. Cancer Res. 1999;59(12):2909–16.
52. Hombach A, Jung W, Pohl C, Renner C, Sahin U, Schmits R, Wolf J, Kapp U, Diehl V, Pfreundschuh M. A CD16/CD30 bispecific monoclonal antibody induces lysis of Hodgkin's cells by unstimulated natural killer cells in vitro and in vivo. Int J Cancer. 1993;55(5): 830–6.
53. Jäger M, Schoberth A, Ruf P, Hess J, Lindhofer H. The trifunctional antibody ertumaxomab destroys tumor cells that express low levels of human epidermal growth factor receptor 2. Cancer Res. 2009;69(10):1–8. doi:10.1158/0008-5472.CAN-08-2861.
54. Jäger M, Schoberth A, Ruf P, Hess J, Hennig M, Schmalfeldt B, Wimberger P, et al. Immunomonitoring results of a phase II/III study of malignant ascites patients treated with the trifunctional antibody catumaxomab (anti-EpCAM X anti-CD3). Cancer Res. 2012;72(1):1–10. doi:10.1158/0008-5472.CAN-11-2235.
55. Kamath AV, Lu D, Gupta P, Jin D, Xiang H, Wong A, Leddy C, et al. Preclinical pharmacokinetics of MEHD7945A, a novel EGFR/HER3 dual-action antibody, and prediction of its human pharmacokinetics and efficacious clinical dose. Cancer Chemother Pharmacol. 2012;69(4):1063–9. doi:10.1007/s00280-011-1806-6.
56. Karpovsky B, Titus JA, Stephany DA, Segal DM. Production of target-specific effector cells using hetero-cross-linked aggregates containing anti-target cell and anti-Fc gamma receptor antibodies. J Exp Med. 1984;160(6):1–16.
57. Keler T, Graziano RF, Mandal A, Wallace PK. Bispecific antibody-dependent cellular cytotoxicity of HER2/Neu-overexpressing tumor cells by Fcγ receptor type I-expressing effector cells. Cancer Res. 1997.
58. Kellner C, Bruenke J, Stieglmaier J, Schwemmlein M, Schwenkert M, Singer H, Mentz K, et al. A novel CD19-directed recombinant bispecific antibody derivative with enhanced immune effector functions for human leukemic cells. J Immunother. 2008;31(9):871–84. 10.1097/CJI.0b013e318186c8b4.
59. Kiewe P, Hasmüller S, Kahlert S, Heinrigs M, Rack B, Marmé A, Korfel A, et al. Phase I trial of the trifunctional anti-HER2 X anti-CD3 antibody ertumaxomab in metastatic breast cancer. Clin Cancer Res. 2006;12(10):3085–91. doi:10.1158/1078-0432.CCR-05-2436.
60. Kipriyanov M, Moldenhauer G, Strauss G, Little M. Bispecific CD3 X CD19 diabody for T cell-mediated lysis of malignant human B cells. Int J Cancer. 1998;77(5):763–72.
61. Kipriyanov SM, Moldenhauer G, Schuhmacher J, Cochlovius B, von der Lieth CW, Matys ER, Little M. Bispecific tandem diabody for tumor therapy with improved antigen binding and pharmacokinetics. J Mol Biol. 1999;293(1):41–56. doi:10.1006/jmbi.1999.3156.
62. Kipriyanov SM, Cochlovius B, Schäfer HJ, Moldenhauer G, Bähre A, Le Gall F, Knackmuss S, Little M. Synergistic antitumor effect of bispecific CD19 X CD3 and CD19 X CD16 diabodies in a preclinical model of non-Hodgkin's lymphoma. J Immunol. 2002;169(1).

63. Kischel R, Raum T, Hausmann S, Rau D. Characterization in primates of MCSP-and CD33-specific human BiTE antibodies for treatment of melanoma and AML. Proc Am Assoc Cancer Res. 2008.
64. Klinger M, Brandl C, Zugmaier G, Hijazi Y, Bargou RC, Topp MS, Gökbuget N, et al. Immunopharmacological response of patients with B-lineage acute lymphoblastic leukemia to continuous infusion of T cell-engaging CD19/CD3-bispecific BiTE antibody blinatumomab. Blood. 2012. doi:10.1182/blood-2012-01-400515.
65. Korn T, Müller R, Kontermann RE. Bispecific single-chain diabody-mediated killing of endoglin-positive endothelial cells by cytotoxic T lymphocytes. J Immunother. 2004;27(2): 99–106.
66. Kufer P, Mack M, Gruber R, Lutterbüse R, Zettl F, Riethmüller G. Construction and biological activity of a recombinant bispecific single-chain antibody designed for therapy of minimal residual colorectal cancer. Cancer Immunol Immunother. 1997;45(3–4).
67. Kügler M, Stein C, Kellner C, Mentz K, Saul D, Schwenkert M, Schubert I, et al. A recombinant trispecific single-chain Fv derivative directed against CD123 and CD33 mediates effective elimination of acute myeloid leukaemia cells by dual targeting. Br J Haematol. 2010;150(5):574–86. doi:10.1111/j.1365-2141.2010.08300.x.
68. Lazar GA, Dang W, Karki S, Vafa O, Peng JS, Hyun L, Chan C, et al. Engineered antibody Fc variants with enhanced effector function. Proc Natl Acad Sci U S A. 2006;103(11):4005–10. doi:10.1073/pnas.0508123103.
69. Lindhofer H, Mocikat R, Steipe B, Thierfelder S. Preferential species-restricted heavy/light chain pairing in rat/mouse quadromas. Implications for a single-step purification of bispecific antibodies. J Immunol. 1995;155(1):1–7.
70. Linke R, Klein A, Seimetz D. Catumaxomab: clinical development and future directions. mAbs. 2010;2(2):1–8.
71. Löffler A, Kufer P, Lutterbüse R, Zettl F, Daniel PT, Schwenkenbecher JM, Riethmüller G, Dörken B, Bargou RC. A recombinant bispecific single-chain antibody, CD19 X CD3, induces rapid and high lymphoma-directed cytotoxicity by unstimulated T lymphocytes. Blood. 2000;95(6):1–7.
72. Löffler A, Gruen M, Wuchter C, Schriever F, Kufer P, Dreier T, Hanakam F, et al. Efficient elimination of chronic lymphocytic leukaemia B cells by autologous T cells with a bispecific anti-CD19/anti-CD3 single-chain antibody construct. Leukemia. 2003;17(5):900–9. doi:10.1038/sj.leu.2402890.
73. Lutterbuese R, Raum T, Kischel R, Lutterbuese P, Schlereth B, Schaller E, Mangold S, et al. Potent control of tumor growth by CEA/CD3-bispecific single-chain antibody constructs that are not competitively inhibited by soluble CEA. J Immunother. 2009;32(4). 10.1097/CJI.0b013e31819b7c70.
74. Lutterbuese R, Raum T, Kischel R, Hoffmann P, Mangold S, Rattel B, Friedrich M, et al. T cell-engaging BiTE antibodies specific for EGFR potently eliminate KRAS- and BRAF-mutated colorectal cancer cells. Proc Natl Acad Sci U S A. 2010;107(28):1–6. doi:10.1073/pnas.1000976107.
75. Mack M, Riethmüller G, Kufer P. A small bispecific antibody construct expressed as a functional single-chain molecule with high tumor cell cytotoxicity. Proc Natl Acad Sci U S A. 1995;92(15):1–5.
76. Maletz K, Kufer P, Mack M, Raum T, Pantel K, Riethmüller G, Gruber R. Bispecific single-chain antibodies as effective tools for eliminating epithelial cancer cells from human stem cell preparations by redirected cell cytotoxicity. Int J Cancer. 2001;93(3):1–8.
77. Marmé A, Strauss G, Bastert G, Grischke E-M, Moldenhauer G. Intraperitoneal bispecific antibody (HEA125xOKT3) therapy inhibits malignant ascites production in advanced ovarian carcinoma. Int J Cancer. 2002;101(2):183–9. doi:10.1002/ijc.10562.
78. McBride WJ, Zanzonico P, Sharkey RM, Norén C, Karacay H, Rossi EA, Losman MJ, et al. Bispecific antibody pretargeting PET (immunoPET) with an 124I-labeled hapten-peptide. J Nucl Med. 2006;47(10):1–11.

79. McCall AM, Adams GP, Amoroso AR, Nielsen UB, Zhang L, Horak E, Simmons H, Schier R, Marks JD, Weiner LM. Isolation and characterization of an anti-CD16 single-chain Fv fragment and construction of an anti-HER2/Neu/anti-CD16 bispecific scFv that triggers CD16-dependent tumor cytolysis. Mol Immunol. 1999;36(7):433–45.
80. McDonagh CF, Huhalov A, Harms BD, Adams S, Paragas V, Oyama S, Zhang B, et al. Antitumor activity of a novel bispecific antibody that targets the ErbB2/ErbB3 oncogenic unit and inhibits heregulin-induced activation of ErbB3. Mol Cancer Ther. 2012;11(3):582–93. doi:10.1158/1535-7163.MCT-11-0820.
81. Mellman I, Coukos G, Dranoff G. Cancer immunotherapy comes of age. Nature. 2011; 480(7378):480–9. doi:10.1038/nature10673.
82. Milstein C, Cuello AC. Hybrid hybridomas and their use in immunohistochemistry. Nature. 1983;305(5934):537–40. doi:10.1038/305537a0.
83. Moldenhauer G, Momburg F, Möller P, Schwartz R, Hämmerling GJ. Epithelium-specific surface glycoprotein of Mr 34,000 is a widely distributed human carcinoma marker. Br J Cancer. 1987;56(6):714–21.
84. Mølhøj M, Crommer S, Brischwein K, Rau D, Sriskandarajah M, Hoffmann P, Kufer P, Hofmeister R, Baeuerle PA. CD19-/CD3-bispecific antibody of the BiTE class is far superior to tandem diabody with respect to redirected tumor cell lysis. Mol Immunol. 2007;44(8):1–9. doi:10.1016/j.molimm.2006.09.032.
85. Moore GL, Bautista C, Pong E, Nguyen D-HT, Jacinto J, Eivazi A, Muchhal US, Karki S, Chu SY, Lazar GA. A novel bispecific antibody format enables simultaneous bivalent and monovalent co-engagement of distinct target antigens. mAbs. 2011;3(6):546–57. doi:10.4161/mabs.3.6.18123.
86. Munz M, Baeuerle PA, Gires O. The emerging role of EpCAM in cancer and stem cell signaling. Cancer Res. 2009;69(14):5627–9. doi:10.1158/0008-5472.CAN-09-0654.
87. Offner S, Hofmeister R, Romaniuk A, Kufer P, Baeuerle PA. Induction of regular cytolytic T cell synapses by bispecific single-chain antibody constructs on MHC class I-negative tumor cells. Mol Immunol. 2006;43(6):1–9. doi:10.1016/j.molimm.2005.03.007.
88. Osada T, Hsu D, Hammond S, Hobeika A, Devi G, Clay TM, Lyerly HK, Morse MA. Metastatic colorectal cancer cells from patients previously treated with chemotherapy are sensitive to T-Cell killing mediated by CEA/CD3-bispecific T-cell-engaging BiTE antibody. Br J Cancer. 2010;102(1):124–33. doi:10.1038/sj.bjc.6605364.
89. Ott MG, Marmé F, Moldenhauer G, Lindhofer H, Hennig M, Spannagl R, Essing MM, Linke R, Seimetz D. Humoral response to catumaxomab correlates with clinical outcome: results of the pivotal phase II/III study in patients with malignant ascites. Int J Cancer. 2012;130(9): 2195–203. doi:10.1002/ijc.26258.
90. Otz T, Grosse-Hovest L, Hofmann M, Rammensee H-G, Jung G. A bispecific single-chain antibody that mediates target cell-restricted, supra-agonistic CD28 stimulation and killing of lymphoma cells. Leukemia. 2009;23(1):71–7. doi:10.1038/leu.2008.271.
91. Petsch S, Gires O, Rüttinger D, Denzel S, Lippold S, Baeuerle PA, Wolf A. Concentrations of EpCAM ectodomain as found in sera of cancer patients do not significantly impact redirected lysis and T-cell activation by EpCAM/CD3-bispecific BiTE antibody MT110. mAbs. 2011;3(1):1–7.
92. Pullarkat V, Deo Y, Link J, Spears L, Marty V, Curnow R, Groshen S, Gee C, Weber JS. A phase I study of a HER2/Neu bispecific antibody with granulocyte-colony-stimulating factor in patients with metastatic breast cancer that overexpresses HER2/Neu. Cancer Immunol Immunother. 1999;48(1).
93. Ren-Heidenreich L, Davol PA, Kouttab NM, Elfenbein GJ, Lum LG. Redirected T-cell cytotoxicity to epithelial cell adhesion molecule-overexpressing adenocarcinomas by a novel recombinant antibody, E3Bi, in Vitro and in an animal model. Cancer. 2004;100(5):1095–103. doi:10.1002/cncr.20060.
94. Repp R, van Ojik HH, Valerius T, Groenewegen G, Wieland G, Oetzel C, Stockmeyer B, et al. Phase I clinical trial of the bispecific antibody MDX-H210 (anti-FcgammaRI X

Anti-HER-2/Neu) in combination with filgrastim (G-CSF) for treatment of advanced breast cancer. Br J Cancer. 2003;89(12):1–10. doi:10.1038/sj.bjc.6601367.

95. Ridgway JB, Presta LG, Carter P. 'Knobs-Into-Holes' engineering of antibody CH3 domains for heavy chain heterodimerization. Protein Eng. 1996;9(7):617–21.
96. Riesenberg R, Buchner A, Pohla H, Lindhofer H. Lysis of prostate carcinoma cells by trifunctional bispecific antibodies (alpha EpCAM X alpha CD3). J Histochem Cytochem. 2001;49(7):911–7.
97. Rossi EA, Goldenberg DM, Cardillo TM, McBride WJ, Sharkey RM, Chang C-H. Stably tethered multifunctional structures of defined composition made by the dock and lock method for use in cancer targeting. Proc Natl Acad Sci U S A. 2006;103(18):1–6. doi:10.1073/pnas.0600982103.
98. Ruf P, Lindhofer H. Induction of a long-lasting antitumor immunity by a trifunctional bispecific antibody. Blood. 2001;98(8):1–10.
99. Ruf P, Jäger M, Ellwart J, Wosch S, Kusterer E, Lindhofer H. Two new trifunctional antibodies for the therapy of human malignant melanoma. Int J Cancer. 2004;108(5):1–8. doi:10.1002/ijc.11630.
100. Ruf P, Kluge M, Jäger M, Burges A, Volovat C, Heiss MM, Hess J, Wimberger P, Brandt B, Lindhofer H. Pharmacokinetics, immunogenicity and bioactivity of the therapeutic antibody catumaxomab intraperitoneally administered to cancer patients. Br J Clin Pharmacol. 2010;69(6):1–9. doi:10.1111/j.1365-2125.2010.03635.x.
101. Schaefer G, Haber L, Crocker LM, Shia S, Shao L, Dowbenko D, Totpal K, et al. A two-in-one antibody against HER3 and EGFR has superior inhibitory activity compared with monospecific antibodies. Cancer Cell. 2011;20(4):472–86. doi:10.1016/j.ccr.2011.09.003.
102. Schaefer W, Regula JT, Bähner M, Schanzer J, Croasdale R, Dürr H, Gassner C, et al. Immunoglobulin domain crossover as a generic approach for the production of bispecific IgG antibodies. Proc Natl Acad Sci U S A. 2011;108(27):1–6. doi:10.1073/pnas.1019002108.
103. Schlereth B, Fichtner I, Lorenczewski G, Kleindienst P, Brischwein K, Da Silva A, Kufer P, et al. Eradication of tumors from a human colon cancer cell line and from ovarian cancer metastases in immunodeficient mice by a single-chain Ep-CAM-/CD3-bispecific antibody construct. Cancer Res. 2005;65(7):1–9. doi:10.1158/0008-5472.CAN-04-2637.
104. Schlereth B, Quadt C, Dreier T, Kufer P, Lorenczewski G, Prang N, Brandl C, et al. T-cell activation and B-cell depletion in chimpanzees treated with a bispecific anti-CD19/anti-CD3 single-chain antibody construct. Cancer Immunol Immunother. 2006;55(5):1–12. doi:10.1007/s00262-005-0001-1.
105. Schubert I, Kellner C, Stein C, Kügler M, Schwenkert M, Saul D, Mentz K, et al. A single-chain triplebody with specificity for CD19 and CD33 mediates effective lysis of mixed lineage leukemia cells by dual targeting. mAbs. 2011;3(1):21–30.
106. Sebastian M, Passlick B, Friccius-Quecke H, Jäger M, Lindhofer H, Kanniess F, Wiewrodt R, Thiel E, Buhl R, Schmittel A. Treatment of non-small cell lung cancer patients with the trifunctional monoclonal antibody catumaxomab (anti-EpCAM X Anti-CD3): a phase I study. Cancer Immunol Immunother. 2007;56(10):1–8. doi:10.1007/s00262-007-0310-7.
107. Sebastian M, Kiewe P, Schuette W, Brust D, Peschel C, Schneller F, Rühle K-H, et al. Treatment of malignant pleural effusion with the trifunctional antibody catumaxomab (removab) (anti-EpCAM X anti-CD3): results of a phase 1/2 study. J Immunother. 2009;32(2). 10.1097/CJI.0b013e318195b5bb.
108. Sharkey RM, Karacay H, Litwin S, Rossi EA, McBride WJ, Chang C-H, Goldenberg DM. Improved therapeutic results by pretargeted radioimmunotherapy of non-Hodgkin's lymphoma with a new recombinant, trivalent, anti-CD20, bispecific antibody. Cancer Res. 2008;68(13):1–10. doi:10.1158/0008-5472.CAN-08-0037.
109. Spizzo G, Fong D, Wurm M, Ensinger C, Obrist P, Hofer C, Mazzoleni G, Gastl G, Went P. EpCAM expression in primary tumour tissues and metastases: an immunohistochemical analysis. J Clin Pathol. 2011;64(5):415–20. doi:10.1136/jcp.2011.090274.
110. Stanglmaier M, Faltin M, Ruf P, Bodenhausen A, Schröder P, Lindhofer H. Bi20 (fBTA05), a novel trifunctional bispecific antibody (anti-CD20 X anti-CD3), mediates efficient killing

of B-cell lymphoma cells even with very low CD20 expression levels. Int J Cancer. 2008;123(5):1–9. doi:10.1002/ijc.23626.

111. Stein H, Mason DY, Gerdes J, O'Connor N, Wainscoat J, Pallesen G, Gatter K et al. The expression of the Hodgkin's disease associated antigen Ki-1 in reactive and neoplastic lymphoid tissue: evidence that reed-sternberg cells and histiocytic malignancies are derived from activated lymphoid cells. 1985.
112. Strop P, Ho W-H, Boustany LM, Abdiche YN, Lindquist KC, Farias SE, Rickert M, et al. Generating bispecific human IgG1 and IgG2 antibodies from any antibody pair. J Mol Biol. 2012;420:204–19. doi:10.1016/j.jmb.2012.04.020.
113. Suntharalingam G, Perry MR, Ward S, Brett SJ, Castello-Cortes A, Brunner MD, Panoskaltsis N. Cytokine storm in a phase 1 trial of the anti-CD28 monoclonal antibody TGN1412. N Engl J Med. 2006;355(10):1018–28. 10.1056/NEJMoa063842.
114. Topp MS, Kufer P, Gökbuget N, Goebeler M, Klinger M, Neumann S, Horst H-A, et al. Targeted therapy with the T-cell-engaging antibody blinatumomab of chemotherapy-refractory minimal residual disease in B-lineage acute lymphoblastic leukemia patients results in high response rate and prolonged leukemia-free survival. J Clin Oncol. 2011;29(18):1–6. 10.1200/JCO.2010.32.7270.
115. Torisu-Itakura H, Schoellhammer HF, Sim M-S, Irie RF, Hausmann S, Raum T, Baeuerle PA, Morton DL. Redirected lysis of human melanoma cells by a MCSP/CD3-bispecific BiTE antibody that engages patient-derived T cells. J Immunother. 2011;34(8). 10.1097/CJI.0b013e3182307fd8.
116. Valone FH, Kaufman PA, Guyre PM, Lewis LD, Memoli V, Deo Y, Graziano R, Fisher JL, Meyer L, Mrozek-Orlowski M. Phase Ia/Ib trial of bispecific antibody MDX-210 in patients with advanced breast or ovarian cancer that overexpresses the proto-oncogene HER-2/Neu. J Clin Oncol. 1995;13(9):1–12.
117. Weiner LM, Holmes M, Richeson A, Godwin A, Adams GP, Hsieh-Ma ST, Ring DB, Alpaugh RK. Binding and cytotoxicity characteristics of the bispecific murine monoclonal antibody 2B1. 1993.
118. Weiner LM, Holmes M, Adams GP, LaCreta F. A human tumor xenograft model of therapy with a bispecific monoclonal antibody targeting C-erbB-2 and CD16. Cancer Res. 1993.
119. Weiner LM, Clark JI, Davey M, Li WS. Phase I trial of 2B1, a bispecific monoclonal antibody targeting C-erbB-2 and FcγRIII. Cancer Res. 1995.
120. Wimberger P, Xiang W, Mayr D, Diebold J, Dreier T, Baeuerle PA, Kimmig R. Efficient tumor cell lysis by autologous, tumor-resident T lymphocytes in primary ovarian cancer samples by an EP-CAM-/CD3-bispecific antibody. Int J Cancer. 2003;105(2):241–8. 10.1002/ijc.11056.
121. Wolf E, Hofmeister R, Kufer P, Schlereth B, Baeuerle PA. BiTEs: bispecific antibody constructs with unique anti-tumor activity. Drug Discov Today. 2005;10(18):1–8. doi:10.1016/S1359-6446(05)03554-3.
122. Zeidler R, Reisbach G, Wollenberg B, Lang S, Chaubal S, Schmitt B, Lindhofer H. Simultaneous activation of T cells and accessory cells by a new class of intact bispecific antibody results in efficient tumor cell killing. J Immunol. 1999;163(3):1–8.
123. Zeidler R, Mysliwietz J, Csánady M, Walz A, Ziegler I, Schmitt B, Wollenberg B, Lindhofer H. The Fc-region of a new class of intact bispecific antibody mediates activation of accessory cells and NK cells and induces direct phagocytosis of tumour cells. Br J Cancer. 2000;83(2):1–6. doi:10.1054/bjoc.2000.1237.

Clinical Development of Antibody-Fusion Proteins for Cancer Therapy

Kory L. Alderson, Amy K. Erbe, Margaret Boyden, and Paul M. Sondel

Abstract Antibody-fusion proteins are new, promising derivatives of monoclonal antibodies (mAbs), and some are being used for cancer therapy. Ongoing research efforts are increasing the repertoire and efficacy of mAbs and mAb-based molecules for the treatment of cancer. Antibody-fusion proteins use the antigen recognition capabilities of the mAb to target a tumor antigen, bringing the fusion protein into the tumor microenvironment. Depending upon what other molecule is fused to the mAb component of the molecule (such as other mAbs, cytokines, chemokines, and toxins), a variety of molecular and cellular activities can thereby be localized to the sites of tumor cells. In this review, we discuss different types of antibody-fusion proteins either in clinical trials or in development for multiple malignancies. We also discuss patient-intrinsic factors that affect therapeutic efficacy, including the inhibitory KIR repertoire of a patient's NK cells and the affinity of a patient's Fc receptors for the Fc portion of the mAb molecule. The level of sophistication of antibody-fusion proteins continues to increase with our understanding of patient-intrinsic factors that affect individualized responses to therapy. New and promising fusion proteins that overcome patient-intrinsic limitations are an exciting application of this technology.

K.L. Alderson • A.K. Erbe
Department of Human Oncology, Madison School of Medicine and Public Health,
University of Wisconsin, Madison, WI 53705, USA

M. Boyden
Department of Pediatrics, Madison School of Medicine and Public Health,
University of Wisconsin, Madison, WI 53705, USA

P.M. Sondel (✉)
Department of Human Oncology, Madison School of Medicine and Public Health,
University of Wisconsin, Madison, WI 53705, USA

Department of Pediatrics, Madison School of Medicine and Public Health,
University of Wisconsin, Madison, WI 53705, USA
e-mail: pmsondel@humonc.wisc.edu

J.D. Rosenblatt et al. (eds.), *Advances in Tumor Immunology and Immunotherapy*, Current Cancer Research, DOI 10.1007/978-1-4614-8809-5_11,

© Springer Science+Business Media New York 2014

Keywords Monoclonal antibody • Immunocytokine • Antibody-drug conjugates • Antibody-fusion proteins • Cancer • Antibody-dependent cell-mediated cytotoxicity (ADCC) • NK cell • Disialoganglioside

1 Introduction

The tumor selective recognition provided by monoclonal antibodies (mAb) has enabled a different approach towards the treatment of certain cancers without the spectrum of clinical toxicities associated with conventional cytotoxic anti-neoplastic therapeutics. With the ability to specifically recognize antigens presented primarily on malignant cells, these tumor-reactive mAbs bind to cancer cells and then induce cancer cell death by a number of pathways. While some antibodies can block stimulatory signals required for tumor cell survival, some can transmit direct apoptotic signals, and others induce tumor cell death via complement-dependent cytotoxicity (CDC). Additionally, many antibodies work by eliciting antibody-dependent cellular cytotoxicity (ADCC) [42, 65]. Stimulation of the immune system with cytokines, such as IL2, in combination with mAb results in increased ADCC [34, 82, 87].

In order to improve ADCC, fusion proteins created either by directly linking a tumor-specific antibody to a cytokine [21, 23, 24, 37, 50] or linking two antibodies (or their antigen recognizing components) with differing specificity have been developed to target tumor cells while simultaneously stimulating the immune system. Such an approach to deliver cytokines or direct effector responses to the tumor likely represents the next generation of antibody-directed tumor-specific immunotherapy.

The following sections will discuss modifications made to mAbs to improve their effects on immune cells, decrease toxicity and immunogenicity, increase systemic half life and account for patient-intrinsic factors that can be used to determine optimal treatment on a per patient basis. The complex considerations involved in engineering improved antitumor mAb-based therapeutics range from antigen binding and immune system stimulation considerations to effector cells' receptor glycosylation requirements [23, 24]. Additionally, genotypic variations will be discussed that can further influence antibody-fusion protein efficacy. This chapter highlights fusion protein advances and their potential as cancer therapeutics.

2 Immunoadhesins

Immunoadhesin is a generic term used to describe antibody-like chimeric molecules consisting of human immunoglobulin linked to a human protein with binding specificity for a molecule of interest [4]. One advantage of an immunoadhesin over that

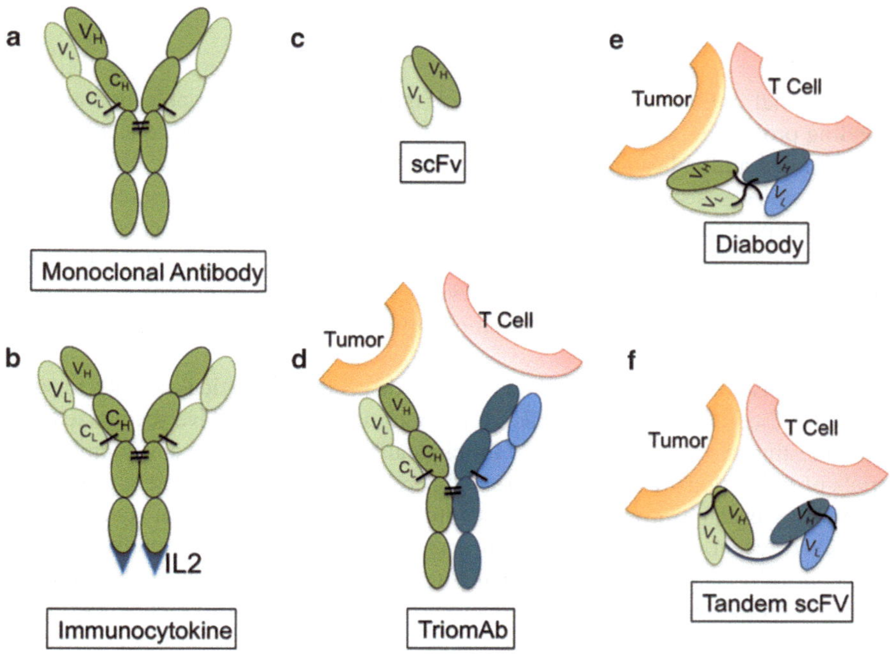

Fig. 1 Illustrated examples of antibody-fusion proteins. (**a**) A monoclonal antibody of an IgG isotype, *light color* denotes light chain and *dark colors* denote heavy chain. Disulfide bonds are shown as *black lines*. (**b**) An immunocytokine comprised of a monoclonal antibody genetically linked to two IL2 proteins in the Fc end. (**c**) A single-chain variable fragment (scFv). (**d**) A triomab comprised of a rat IgG2b immunoglobulin (*green*) targeting a tumor antigen and a mouse IgG2a immunoglobulin (*blue*) portion activating a T cell. (**e**) A diabody, linking the heavy and light chain of opposing Fv regions with a peptide linker that holds the two variable regions in close proximity. (**f**) A tandem scFv fragment, each scFv is held together with a peptide linker, can link multiple scFv together to create a chain of fusion proteins

of a monoclonal antibody is that the binding portion of an immunoadhesin need not be of immunoglobulin origin and can be insoluble, such as a cell surface receptor, or soluble such as a cytokine. Immunoadhesins were developed as an alternative to monoclonal antibodies as a simpler method for targeting human antigens with human reagents. There are many different conceptual applications for immunoadhesins, resulting in products patented for a variety of conditions [76].

Numerous immunoadhesins exist on the market for patients with autoimmunity, including Enteracept®, Arcalyst®, and Amevive® [76]. While immmunoadhesins designed for use as cancer therapeutics have been slower to appear on the market, some recent clinical data suggest that immunoadhesins may be powerful tools in cancer immunotherapy. Because immunoadhesin is a generic term, it can be used to describe most of the products that would be considered antibody-fusion proteins, including immunocytokines and bifunctional antibodies (Fig. 1), which have each shown promise in recent clinical testing.

3 Bifunctional Antibodies

Bifunctional antibodies are a group of reagents that share variable domain-like binding properties, but are otherwise not necessarily similar. Some cancer-directed bifunctional antibodies are designed to tether tumor cells to immune effector cells and in some cases simultaneously activate the effector cells. Because both NK cells and macrophages bear Fc receptors, and can mediate an antibody-dependent cytolytic/effector response, most traditional mAb therapies rely heavily on NK cell and/or macrophage effector functions. However, because tumors often have a large population of infiltrating T lymphocytes, most bifunctional antibodies have been developed to act on T cells.

Initial bispecific antibodies showed some detectable biological activity in vivo, inducing T cells to kill tumor cells they would not otherwise have recognized; but initial testing showed little evidence for clinical benefit [11]. Early development and trials of bifunctional antibodies were hampered by relatively inefficient production techniques, causing difficulties with both purity and quantity of clinical grade reagent. However, recent advances in antibody engineering have improved production and some bifunctional antibodies are proving to be successful in clinical applications.

Early bifunctional antibodies were produced in one of two ways, chemical cross-linking of antibody proteins, or fusion of two hybridomas to produce a hybrid-hybridoma or a quadroma ([60], also reviewed in [11, 58]). A major boost to the field of bifunctional antibodies came in 1995 with the first report of Triomabs. The triomab approach combines immunoglobulin subclasses from two separate species, using rat/mouse quadromas that produced mouse IgG2a and rat IgG2b. Preferential species restricted pairing limits random association of heavy and light chains [60]. Species restricted pairing reduces the number of different antibody combinations made by the quadroma, increasing the production of molecules that are one-half rat, targeting one antigen, and one-half mouse, targeting another (Fig. 1d). Importantly, mouse/rat hybrid bispecific antibodies maintain functional ability to interact with activating human FcR, and therefore maintain their ability to elicit the effector functions of NK cells and other cells bearing FcRs.

The first Triomab produced was a bispecific antibody with reactivity to T cells (anti-CD3) and to Epithelial cancers [anti-epithelial cell adhesion molecule (EpCAM)]. Catumaxomab (anti-CD3 X anti-EpCAM) has received market approval in the European Union as a therapeutic for malignant ascites, particularly for women with ovarian cancer [61]. Engagement of T cells via αCD3 and tumor specificity via αEpCAM, in addition to Fcγ receptor (FcR) engagement through the intact Fc region gives this molecule its "tri-functionality". Namely, this agent can bind to tumor cells (via EpCAM), bind to and activate T cells (via-CD3), and bind to and activate cells that mediate ADCC (through FcRs). Preclinical studies show that Catumaxomab elicits multiple effector pathways simultaneously; including T cell-mediated lysis, cytokine production, ADCC, and antibody-dependent phagocytosis ADCP [90]. The third functional binding site for Catumaxomab, the mouse/rat hybrid Fc region, can elicit effector cells through activating FcγR, CD32 (FcγRII), CD16 (FcγRIII), and CD64 (FcγRI) but not inhibitory FcγR (reviewed in [61]).

Catumaxomab has completed phase I/II testing for intraperitoneal treatment of malignant ascites secondary to epithelial cancers [38]. Heiss et al. treated 258 patients with four increasing doses of catumaxomab (10, 20, 50, and 150 μg) on days 0, 3, 7, and 10, respectively, and followed puncture-free survival (survival time from last clinically required peritoneal aspiration procedure) and time to next paracentesis. While frequent adverse events related to immune activation were reported, patients in the catumaxomab arm had a longer puncture-free survival time (11 days for control paracentesis vs. 46 days with Triomab treatment) and longer median time to next paracentesis. Multiple courses of Catomaxomab have been attempted in one patient and were reasonably well tolerated (i.e., this one patient did not develop any unexpected adverse events) and potentially effective. Despite a rapid human anti-drug antibody (HADA) response, a decrease in EpCAM-positive cells, and increase in CD45-positive cells (leukocytes) in ascites fluid was observed after a second course of therapy [77]. More research is needed to determine the efficacy and toxicity of TriomAb antibodies given systemically rather than "intra-tumorally" such as the case with intraperitoneal administration to patients with ascites.

Bi20 is a trifunctional antibody with specificity for the CD20 target prevalent on CLL and other B cell malignancies. Buhmann et al. treated six B cell lymphoma patients that were refractory to standard therapy with an anti-CD3 X anti-CD20 TriomAb, Bi20, and followed Bi20 infusion with donor lymphocyte infusion (DLI) or hematopoietic stem cell transplant (HSCT) [8]. The side effects were relatively tolerable and they did not observe an HADA response or graft versus host disease. They reported a rapid, but transient, clinical response to therapy. This study may suggest that Bi20, when combined with DLI or HSCT, could be given repeatedly to augment antitumor activity. The efficacy of Bi20 given alone has not been established.

Recombinant antibody technology spurred the invention of multiple bispecific antibody-like products that lack Fc regions after it was hypothesized that the Fc portion of a bifunctional molecule may lead to toxicity [83]. Single-chain variable fragments (scFv fragments), tandem scFv fragments, and diabodies (Fig. 1) were each developed in an attempt to maintain bifunctional binding capabilities while reducing potential Fc-mediated toxicity. Several of these reagents showed promising results in preclinical studies. Some studies have suggested that enhanced antitumor efficacy and minimal activation of peripheral T cells can be achieved by ex vivo pre-arming of T cells with bifunctional antibodies prior to infusion. This has led to a series of studies evaluating the effectiveness of "arming" of T cells with bispecific antibodies. One study that preloaded activated T cells with an anti-Her2 bispecific, Her2Bi (OKT3 X trastuzumab) observed persistence of activated T cells in patients for 14 days and correlated their persistence with an increase in pro-inflammatory cytokines and heightened bispecific Ab-mediated ADCC by peripheral blood mononuclear cells [30]. Since this report, two phase II trials have opened evaluating the role of Her2Bi armed T cells in breast cancer patients (NCT01022138 and NCT01147016).

Bispecific T cell engagers (BiTEs) are tandem scFv fragments (Fig. 1) that target CD3 through one variable fragment and a tumor-specific antigen through the other fragment. A few BiTEs have already been produced despite being relatively new technology. Approval followed exciting clinical data with low dose constant infusion of an anti-CD19-x-anti-CD3 BiTE, blinatumomab [55, 99]. Twenty-one patients with minimal residual acute lymphoblastic leukemia were administered blinatumomab in a portable mini-pump and port system for a 4-week cycle. Sixteen of twenty-one patients responded to therapy reaching a status of minimal residual disease (MRD) negative; twelve of these sixteen patients had previously been refractory to chemotherapy [99]. Within 2 days after starting blinatumomab, B cell counts dropped to borderline undetectable limits and remained low for the entire treatment period. T cells were initially reduced, but quickly rebounded and showed phenotypic signs of activation [55]. While BiTE technology is new, the early clinical data available look very promising and it remains to be seen how BiTEs will enhance the exciting field of bispecific tumor therapy.

4 Tumor-Specific Immunocytokines

Immunocytokines (IC) consist of tumor-reactive monoclonal antibodies (mAb) that have been attached to an activating cytokine. When the mAb portion binds to its particular target cell, the cytokine is then able to activate nearby immune cells, enhancing their ability to effectively kill their target. Current development of these molecules has primarily involved linking existing therapeutic mAbs to cytokines such as IL-2, to allow localized activation of the effector cells of the immune system.

Many mAbs have been shown in preclinical studies to cause in vitro tumor destruction via ADCC [5, 73, 78]. When the Fab portion binds to the antigens on the tumor cell, effector cells carrying Fc receptors (FcRs) are then able to bind to the Fc components of the bound mAb and be activated. Activated effector cells release additional cytokines and chemokines that can recruit and activate other immune cells [79], as well as mediate ADCC via the release of cytotoxic granules and apoptotic signaling pathways [49, 100]. In support of the role of FcRs, in vivo studies have shown that mAbs with antitumor activity lose their killing potential when administered to mice that lack FcRs [69] or when mAbs lack the Fc region [5].

With the addition of IL-2 in vitro, NK cells demonstrate increased levels of ADCC [32]. Following in vivo IL-2 administration in patients, their NK cells have demonstrated increased levels of ADCC when assayed in vitro [33]. In considering these findings, Sosman et al. proposed combining IL-2 therapy with mAb therapy with the goal of boosting the ability of NK cells to perform ADCC [93]. One such antibody involved an mAb against the GD2 disialoganglioside present on melanoma and neuroblastoma cells. Initially, pilot and phase I/II trials involving the 14.G2a murine antibody and its chimeric form (ch14.18) were conducted, including a Children's Oncology Group (COG) phase 1 trial treating pediatric patients with high-risk neuroblastoma in remission after autologous stem cell transplant (ASCT) [1, 20, 28]. IL-2 was incorporated into the treatment regimens, to provide an activating stimulus to the NK cells, and in Gilman et al., GM-CSF was also incorporated to stimulate neutrophils/macrophages [28] to also mediate ADCC. This regimen was reasonably tolerated, with improved clinical outcomes compared to historical controls [28]. This treatment strategy was then employed in a phase III COG trial for pediatric neuroblastoma patients in remission following autologous (hematopoietic) stem cell transplant (ASCT). Interim analysis of the patients in this trial, before the trial had reached its expected patient accrual, revealed statistically better responses by patients enrolled in the immunotherapy arm as compared to standard treatment [108]. Immunotherapy-treated patients demonstrated an average overall survival rate of 86 % (compared to 75 % for the standard arm, $p=0.02$) and an average event-free survival rate of 66 % (compared to 46 %, $p=0.01$). These differences in response led to closure of the standard treatment arm of the study [108]. In contrast, a German study using ch14.18 mAb alone on a similar dosing regimen did not initially see similar results [91], suggesting that the addition of the IL2 and GM-CSF may be responsible for the clinical improvement that was seen.

Following the studies of ch14.18 with IL2 and GM-CSF, the next step was to try to further optimize ADCC by fusing the mAb to the cytokine IL-2, to create immunocytokines (ICs) (Fig. 1b). Through linking the two molecules, the IC would be able to facilitate additional mechanisms of ADCC. An anti-GD2 IC was formed by genetically linking human IL2 to the carboxy terminus of the IgG heavy chain for the chimeric and humanized antiGD2 mAbs, ch14.18, and hu14.18. Initial in vitro studies showed that ICs could trigger NK cells as well as T cells bearing IL2 receptors (IL2R), to mediate GD2-specific lysis [23, 24, 35]. Subsequent animal models of $GD2^+$ neuroblastoma and melanoma cell lines demonstrated that ch14.18-IL2 could mediate more effective killing than ch14.18 and IL2 administered in combination. Similar results were seen in human neuroblastoma cell lines tested in SCID mice [80], a GD2-expressing murine melanoma cell line (B78) tested in immunocompetent syngeneic mice [6, 7], and a neuroblastoma cell line NXS2 in syngeneic immunocompetent mice [62, 63].

Additional IC development has revealed other possible mechanisms of IC-triggered activity [26] tested a deimmunized (DI) form of murine mAb Leu16, linking DI-Leu16 to IL2 in a SCID model of B cell lymphoma. Mice receiving the DI-Leu16-IL2 IC demonstrated higher antitumor activity than those receiving rituximab or rituximab plus IL2 in combination. In this system, DI-Leu16-IL2 was also assayed in parallel with a deglycosylated form of the IC—the latter form was unable to bind to FcRs yet maintained its antitumor activity, suggesting potential non-FcR-dependent mechanisms of immunocytokines.

A subsequent study [31] investigated non-FcR-dependent mechanisms further, by looking both at hu14.18-IL2 and another IC, huKS-IL2, which targets the EpCAM molecule present on ovarian cancer. In vitro assays using an NK cell line with low expression of FcγR and high CD25 (IL-2Rα chain) showed that immunocytokines could aid the conjugation of tumor and effector cells. The polarization of CD25 to the immunological synapse between NKL cells and M21 tumor cells suggested immunocytokines could facilitate cell–cell interactions through IL-2 receptors (Fig. 2) [9, 31]. Although normal peripheral NK cells lack appreciable expression of CD25, the engagement of other IL-2R in addition to FcγR may be a unique functional advantage of immunocytokines.

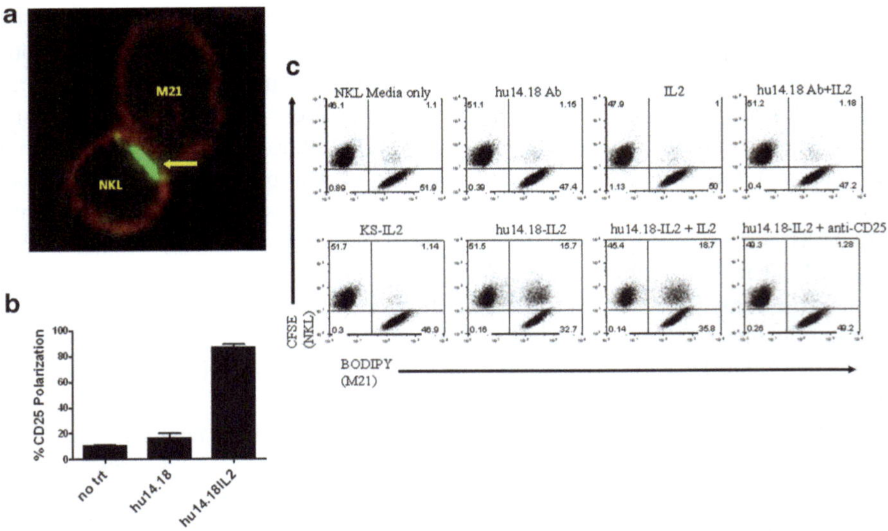

Fig. 2 IL-2 receptors are involved in the conjugation between tumor cells and natural killer cells. (**a**) A natural killer cell line originally derived from NK cell lymphoma (NKL) which has high expression of the IL-2Rα chain (CD25) was cocultured in with M21 melanoma tumor cells ($GD2^+$) and hu14.18-IL2 immunocytokine (anti-GD2 mAb linked to IL2). After incubation, the cells were fixed to a glass coverslip and stained for CD25 (*green*). (**b**) Quantification of percent of NKL cells conjugated with M21 that polarized CD25 to the immunological synapse in the presence of hu14.18 or hu14.18-IL2. (**c**) NKL cells and M21 tumor cells were labeled with CFSE (NKL) or BODIPY (M21), cells were co-incubated in the presence of various tumor-specific antibodies and fusion proteins and visualized by flow cytometry for conjugate formation. The above figure has been reprinted with kind permission from Springer Science+Business Media from: Cancer Immunology Immunotherapy, Ab-IL2 fusion proteins mediate NK cell immune synapse formation by polarizing CD25 to the target cell–effector cell interface, Vol. 60, 2010, pp 1789–1800, Gubbels, JA. Gadbaw, B. Buhtoiarov, IN. et al. Fig. 2a, and Fig. 4b

Phase 1 trials were initially conducted to evaluate the maximum tolerated dose and immune effects of hu14.18-IL2 in both melanoma [54] and neuroblastoma patients [72]. Each patient received three daily IV doses of hu14.18-IL2 (over 4 h), after which they were evaluated for evidence of disease response or progression. The half-life of the hu14.18-IL2 in both studies was approximately 4 h. King et al. reported that 28 patients with measurable melanoma showed no response to hu14.18-IL2 therapy [54]. Five patients entered the study with no evidence of disease, of which three showed disease recurrence at 1, 6, and 92 months, and two patients remained in remission at >74 and >117 months after receiving therapy [54].

In the Osenga et al. study, 28 patients enrolled with measurable neuroblastoma, three patients demonstrated isolated marrow improvement, and one achieved complete remission shortly after completing IC treatment. However, the one patient that achieved complete remission underwent fenretinide therapy shortly after treatment with hu14.18-IL2, therefore it was unclear if remission was the result of hu14.18-IL2 alone or a combination-like effect due to the similar timing of fenretinide and hu14.18-IL2 [72]. These initial trials of hu14.18-IL2 immunocytokine in patients with melanoma and neuroblastoma showed little activity for patients with measurable-bulky refractory tumor; these clinical data were consistent with preclinical data that indicate the amount of measurable tumor at the time of therapy inversely correlates with the likelihood of in vivo antitumor efficacy [67, 106].

A phase II clinical trial of hu14.18-IL2 was then conducted through COG for patients with refractory or recurrent neuroblastoma. Patients were categorized as having radiographically measurable disease (stratum 1), or nonmeasurable yet evaluable disease, detected only by Radio-MIBG scintigraphy or by histological analysis of bone marrow aspirates/biopsies (stratum 2). Hu14.18-IL2 was administered daily for 3 days, at a dose of 12 mg/m^2/day in 28-day cycles. Initial therapy included four cycles. However, if patients had PR or CR, as determined by radiographic imaging and bone marrow testing, they could go on to receive two additional courses [89].

The Shusterman et al. study enrolled 39 patients, 15 in stratum 1 (bulky disease), and 24 in stratum 2 (less-bulky disease). Of the patients in stratum 1, one did not receive therapy due to parental refusal, and a second patient only received one dose of IC due to toxicities—the remaining 13 showed no detectable response (with ten demonstrating progressive disease). Of the 24 patients in stratum 2, one was taken off study and not evaluable for disease state. Evaluation of the remaining 23 patients in stratum 2 showed that five subjects achieved CR status. Four of these five patients relapsed in the long-term (at 9, 13, 20, and 30 months post-therapy), while one patient remained in CR at >35 months. Two other patients also showed some clinical improvement, but their improvement did not meet criteria for PR or CR; one patient achieved CR of the bone marrow and improvement on MIBG scan that was not sufficient to be called PR on independent review, and a second patient cleared MIBG-positive disease while only showing partial bone marrow clearance [89]. Ten patients only received one cycle of therapy, with two patients stopping therapy due to dose-limiting toxicities, seven due to progressive disease, and one due to parental choice [89]. Significant toxicities seen in this study were largely due to the IL2 component of the immunocytokine, with 2 of 39 patients experiencing unacceptable dose-limiting toxicity related to capillary leakage (one patient requiring vasopressor support and another requiring transient ventillatory support for hypoxia).

While the study itself was not designed nor powered to correlate disease status at time of entry with outcome measures, the portion of patients with clinical response in stratum 2 (vs. stratum-1) continue to fit with previous data suggesting that IC activity is most effective in the setting of minimal disease burden [68, 89]. Due to the observable differences between stratum 1 and stratum 2 patients, there is an ongoing COG phase II feasibility study combining hu14.18-IL2 with GM-CSF and retinoic acid as a treatment regimen for stratum 2 patients. The goal of this feasibility study will be to determine if hu14.18-IL2 may be appropriate for "front-line" Phase III testing in patients in first remission. Such a Phase III study would allow a comparison in the clinical activity of hu14.18-IL2+GM-CSF with that of the chimeric antiGD2 mAb (ch14.18) in combination with IL2 and GM-CSF [108].

In addition to the ongoing development of the hu14.18-IL2 IC, other ICs have been tested in preclinical and clinical studies. HuKS-IL2, an IC against the EpCAM

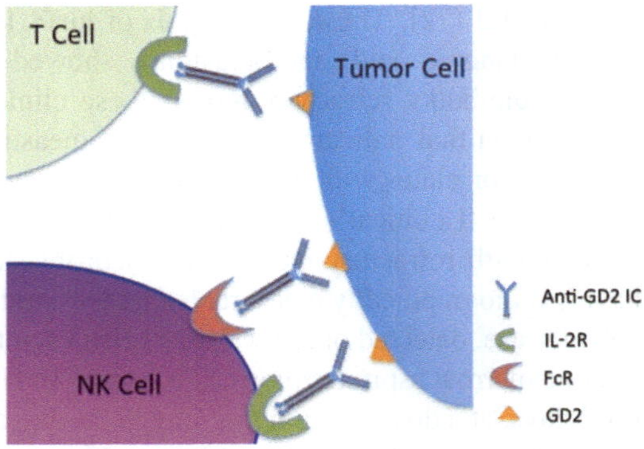

Fig. 3 A schematic representation of the how immunocytokines can act upon cytokine receptors to facilitate the conjugation of tumor cells to either NK cells (utilizing both FcγR and IL-2R) or T cells (utilizing the IL2-R)

molecule on epithelial-derived cancers such as prostate, breast, lung, colon, and ovarian cancer has been studied primarily in the preclinical setting, both in vitro and in murine models [13, 31, 39, 45]. A phase I trial of huKS-IL2 was conducted in patients with prostate cancer, which showed that the IC was relatively well tolerated [56]. DI-Leu16-IL2, that targets CD20, is also being investigated for use against various CD20-expressing cancers [26]. The creators of DI-leu-16 used computer modeling to identify potential T cell epitopes and subsequently remove them from the Fc portion of the antibody [26]. Furthermore, modifications at the intersection between the Fc of the antibody and the IL-2 protein reduce intracellular proteolysis, leading to increased half-life and reduced immunogenicity [25, 26].

Immunocytokines containing modified cytokines are early in development. Alteration of the IL2 molecule at position D20T retains its high level of affinity for high affinity IL-2Rs involving CD25 and limits its interaction with intermediate affinity IL-2Rs [27]. Furthermore, immunocytokine with the D20T mutation was less toxic in SCID mice, suggesting that innate immune cells bearing intermediate affinity IL-2 receptors, and not high affinity IL-2 receptors, may be responsible for inducing vascular toxicity [27]. Therefore, it is hypothesized that patients will better tolerate immunocytokines that selectively activate high affinity receptors. An immunocytokine composed of the NHS76 antibody that targets areas of tumor necrosis in conjunction with a modified interleukin-2 (NHS76-IL2T, Selectikine, or EMD 521873) has been studied for its ability to penetrate, and localize IL-2 to areas of the tumor that would normally have minimal exposure to circulating IC [27]. NHS76-IL2T retains the ability to activate human T cells in vitro, and preclinical murine models suggest that it is better tolerated than NHS76 immunocytokine with unaltered interleukin-2 [27].

Immunocytokines that capitalize on the specificity of monoclonal antibodies and combine it with immune-activation capabilities of cytokines are relatively early in development. The therapeutic benefits of immunocytokines and other antibody-fusion proteins are starting to be realized in clinical trials. The overall goal is based on the ability of the mAb component of the immunocytokine to selectively recognize the tumor and to then have both the Fc end of the immunocytokine, and its cytokine component engage activating receptors on effector cells (Fig. 3).

Factors intrinsic to the fusion protein can greatly affect function and efficacy; namely targeted mutagenesis of the cytokine to intentionally alter its receptor specificity may potentially improve its clinical utility.

5 Drug-Intrinsic Factors Affecting Efficacy

Antibody-fusion proteins have improved the potential therapeutic mechanisms for applications involving monoclonal antibodies by allowing more effector cell types to be directed to the tumor (i.e., T cells) and/or by locally activating effector cells (i.e., IL-2 attached to the end of an antibody). Immunocytokines target the tumor through antigen specificity, thereby allowing effector cell localization and activation via the Fc component of the antibody, as well as simultaneous immune cell stimulation via the cytokine portion of the immunocytokine. This local activation in concert with Fc recognition results not only in increased ADCC, but can potentially reduce unwanted toxicities. Soluble cytokines, such as systemic IL2, are being given in combination with monoclonal antibody therapies to activate effector cells [108]; however immunocytokines use their mAb component to localize the effector cell activation to the site of the tumor, potentially reducing toxicity by decreasing the systemically circulating amount of cytokine required to activate effector cells, which should reduce bystander cell activation at sites distant from tumor.

Eliciting ADCC and CDC are important mechanisms by which many therapeutic antibodies function. For some mAbs, such as the anti-GD2 antibodies, an anti-idiotype network, and cell death through apoptosis are also involved in antitumor action [2, 12, 107]. Certain host responses can interfere with the action of mAbs. The generation of human anti-mouse antibody (HAMA) responses, human anti-chimeric antibody (HACA), and anti-idiotypic antibody (anti-id) responses can at times interfere with the pharmacokinetics or molecular actions of the mAbs [14, 65, 81, 84, 98]. Additionally, some clinical evidence of anti-idiotypic antibodies exists with the anti-GD2 immunocytokine, hu14.18-IL2 [36, 54]. In an effort to decrease the immunogenicity of mAbs, improve recruitment of immune effector cells and increase the antibody half-life, chimeric antibodies, containing both human and mouse components were created, as well as humanized antibodies (~97 % human components) have been successfully developed and used clinically [29, 95].

Specific point mutations in the Fc end of an IgG1 disrupt complement activation, which can be beneficial for some therapeutic antibodies, if it appears that CDC is leading to toxicity rather than antitumor efficacy. Activation of the complement cascade through CDC leads to allodynia, or generalized pain, in patients receiving anti-GD2 antibodies. This allodynia is the result of complement fixation by antibodies on normal neuronal tissue, a site of minimal GD2 expression by normal cells. Complement fixation, or the activation of the complement cascade, occurs after binding of the complement protein C1q to the Fc domain of IgG or IgM [40]. The basic residues in the Fc domain E318, K320, and K322 are designated as the C1q binding motif [17]. By changing a single amino acid at position 322 from lysine (K) to alanine (A), complement activation is disrupted but FcR binding is retained. Preclinical studies with hu14.18K322A, an anti-GD2 mAb with a K322A substitution is better tolerated in preclinical studies [92]. Hu14.18K322A is currently undergoing testing in a phase I clinical trial in pediatric patients with neuroblastoma or melanoma to determine if signs of allodynia are reduced (NCT00743496).

The IgG subclass of Fc receptors is potent at activating cell-killing mechanisms [44]. Therefore most therapeutic antibodies using human immunoglobulin heavy chains are of an IgG1 subclass. Manipulations of antibodies are being pursued in order to have better interaction with the FcγR and enhance ADCC activity. Human IgG1 interacts with both FcγRIIa and FcγRIIIa, expressed on monocytic lineage cells and NK cells, respectively [22]. Furthermore, several groups have found that patients containing FcγRIIIa alleles that have higher binding affinity for IgG show augmented in vivo efficacy following clinical mAb treatment [10, 66, 102, 103]. Antibody binding capacity to FcγRs is heavily influenced by the glycosylation patterns located on the Fc region of the antibody. Manipulations of the carbohydrate moieties on the Fc portion of the antibody revealed sugar side chains that influence the binding affinities to FcγRIIIa. In particular, the removal of fucose from the Fc portion increases the binding affinity to FcγRIIIa, leading to increased ADCC in vitro and in vivo [41, 43, 64, 70, 85, 86, 88, 94]. This increased affinity has been attributed to a subtle conformational change in the antibody allowing for increased interaction with an oligosaccharide at the Asn-162 site on FcγRIIIa, which is more readily accessible when the antibodies are afucosylated. Because of this improvement of interaction between FcγRIIIa and antibody, use of hypofucosylated mAbs in cancer treatment could allow for enhanced antitumor effects [88].

Cell lines used to produce antibody-fusion proteins can affect their therapeutic efficacy due to differences in glycosylation of the Fc end [44]. Currently, most antibodies that are used therapeutically are produced in Chinese hamster ovary (CHO) cells, mouse NSO cells, or in mouse Sp2/0 cells [44]. Mammalian cell lines typically produce heavily fucosylated (>80 %) antibodies [47]. Several cell lines have been identified that can be used to produce antibodies with reduced fucosylation. One cell line able to produce low-fucosylated antibody is a CHO variant with the fucosyltransferase gene, *FUT8*, knocked-out [105]. The importance of glycosylation patterns in the creation of reagents with greater therapeutic efficacy is likely to become even more apparent as demand for therapeutic mAb and mAb-fusion proteins continue to increase.

6 Patient-Intrinsic Factors Affecting Efficacy: KIR

NK cell-mediated ADCC is an important mechanism of action for immunocytokines [68] and ADCC can be partially inhibited by HLA ligation of inhibitory Killer immunoglobulin-like receptors (KIRs) on the surface of human NK cells, and in mice by H-2 ligation of inhibitory Ly49 receptors on the surface of mouse NK cells. MAb and immunocytokine-based therapies have been evaluated in people who have KIR genes for which they do not have the corresponding HLA ligand genes. This "missing ligand" scenario occurs because KIR and HLA genes are inherited independently and are often not present in matched pairs within the same person [74]. Missing an autologous KIR ligand for an expressed KIR has been described as a strong correlate of antitumor responses after ASCT [59], for neuroblastoma patients being treated with fully murine anti-GD2 mAb 3 F8 [101], and more recently in patients receiving hu14.18-IL2 immunocytokines [15, 16].

The primary immunological difference between individuals that are missing a KIR ligand from those that are fully KIR ligated is the presence of so-called "unlicensed" NK cells in the mismatched individuals. Thus, the clinical benefit in the mismatched patients may be the result of unlicensed NK cells. If correct, this observation would potentially appear to be in conflict with the currently understood licensing hypothesis regarding NK cell development. This hypothesis accounts for hyporesponsiveness of NK cells from MHC^{null} individuals by stating that NK cell education must occur through inhibitory receptors by their MHC ligands during early NK cell development [51].

The complexity of NK cell education is a rapidly expanding field and mounting preclinical evidence suggests that all or nothing "gain of function" during development does not apply to NK cells [18, 46].

Early reports on the importance of KIR–HLA interaction for NK cell-mediated ADCC using healthy donor NK cells were contradictory [3, 51]. It was later shown that different assay systems commonly used to evaluate CD16-mediated responses can produce contradictory results, and that plate-bound anti-CD16 mAb is not sufficient to obviate differences between "missing ligand" and "fully KIR ligated" NK cells, whereas differences become clear when using target cells coated with antibody. A recent report from Memorial Sloan Kettering has shown that clinical efficacy of a separate anti-GD2 mAb (3 F8) is also associated with KIR/KIR-L mismatch, in the absence of hematopoietic stem cell transplantation [96, 97]. This important report presents data consistent with the conclusion that the unlicensed NK cells in these patients are playing a critical role in facilitating clinically meaningful ADCC. Despite preclinical data suggesting both that NK cell licensing is required for ADCC [3, 75], or has no effect on ADCC [53, 71], multiple clinical trials have demonstrated a correlation between a patients missing a KIR ligand and a better antitumor immune response, including those elicited by antibody-fusion proteins.

The pairing of KIRs and HLA ligands is an important factor in the response to tumor-targeted immunocytokine, hu14.18-IL2 [89]. Delgado et al. genotyped 38 patients treated as part of a phase II trial of hu14.18-IL2 to retrospectively determine if KIR/HLA status correlated with clinical responses. Seven of the thirty-eight patients that had received hu14.18-IL2 immunocytokine had measureable improvement (five with complete responses and two showing clinical benefit not categorized as a response). In this small analysis (Table 1a), all seven improving patients were in the "missing ligand" category ($P=0.03$), meaning they expressed at least one KIR for which they did not express the corresponding HLA [15, 16].

Table 1 "Missing KIR-L" and FcγR2a genotype are potential prognostic indicators of response to hu14.18-IL2 immunocytokine

(a) Autologous KIR/KIR-ligand (HLA) mismatch vs. response/improvement

	KIR mismatch	KIR match	Total
Response/improvement	7 (29 %)	0 (0 %)	7
No response/no improvement	17 (71 %)	14 (100 %)	31
Total	24	14	38
$P=0.03$			

(b) FcγR2a

	HH	HR+RR	Total
Response/improvement	4 (40 %)	3 (11 %)	7
Nonresponse/non-improvement	6 (60 %)	25 (89 %)	31
Total	10	28	38
$P=0.06$			

(a) Response/improvement for neuroblastoma patients in a phase II clinical trial of hu14.18-IL2 immunocytokine showing an association between an autologous KIR/KIR-Ligand (HLA) mismatch and improvement after immunotherapy ($P=0.03$). (b) Trend towards correlation of response/improvement to hu14.18-IL2 and FcγR2a genotype ($P=0.06$). Both (a) and (b) present data originally published in [15, 16]

To our knowledge, this report was the first, and currently the only study to have examined autologous KIR/HLA matching as a factor for response to tumor-targeted immunocytokine. Larger immunocytokine studies are planned and will be important to confirm the Delgado et al. findings.

7 Patient-Intrinsic Factors Affecting Efficacy: FcR

Much like mAbs, many antibody-fusion proteins stimulate FcγR-mediated effector function as part of their mechanism of action. Three classes of Fcγ receptors are found on human leukocytes (FcγI, FcγII, and FcγIII), which can further be broken down into subclasses [10]. NK cells uniquely express only activating FcγRs (FcγRIIIa and FcγRIIc) without co-expressing inhibitory FcγRs, and are therefore potent mediators of ADCC. Single nucleotide polymorphisms (SNPs) in human FcγR may predict ADCC responses to tumor-targeted mAbs and immunocytokines. SNPs resulting in a higher affinity FcR for human IgGI were initially described in autoimmune patients [57, 104]. FcγRIIa (CD32, expressed on myeloid cells) and FcγRIIIa (CD16, expressed on NK cells, macrophages, monocytes) are activating receptors [69]. SNPs found in the FcγRIIa locus corresponding to amino acid position 131 yield allelotypes with different binding affinities for IgG1. Two allelotypes have been described for FcγRIIa, FcγRIIa-131-H (histidine) has a higher binding affinity than does FcγRIIa-131-R (arginine). SNPs have similarly been identified for FcγRIIIa. FcγRIIIa associated SNPs found at amino acid position 158 that also

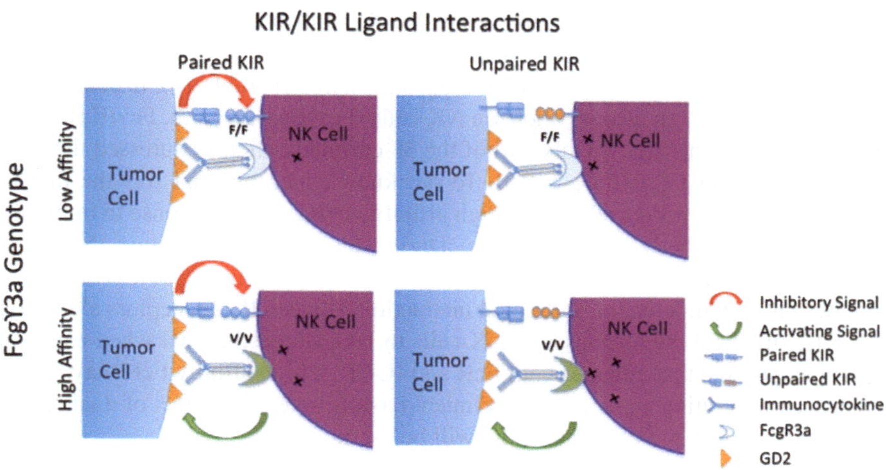

Fig. 4 KIR/KIR-L pairing and FcγR affinity are both likely important factors in the immune magnitude of response to immunocytokines. A schematic representation of the affect of FcγR affinity and KIR/KIR-L pairing on the activation potential of immunocytokine. Increasing magnitude of response is hypothesized to follow a gradation as shown: (**a**) Individuals with "paired KIR" (i.e., KIR/KIR Ligand match) and low affinity FcγR3a (FF) would be expected to have the lowest benefit from immunocytokine-based therapy (*top left*); (**b**, **c**) individuals with unpaired KIR and low affinity FcγR3a (FF) (*upper right*) or with paired KIR and high affinity FcγR3a (VV) (*lower left*) would be expected to have intermediate benefit; (**d**) individuals with unpaired KIR and high affinity FcγR3a (VV) would be expected to benefit the most from immunocytokine-based therapies

affect the binding affinity for the Fc portion found on IgG1 antibodies, such that FcγRIIIa-158-V (valine) has a higher affinity for IgG1-based antibodies than does FcγRIIIa-158-F (phenylalanine) [57]. As our understanding of Fc receptor polymorphic variations increases, many associations between high affinity Fc receptors and clinical responses have been observed. KIR status or FcγR affinity correlate with efficacy of mAb-based therapy in pediatric neuroblastoma patients and adult non-Hodgkin's lymphoma patients [10, 96, 97, 101]. Similarly, we observed a correlation between KIR status and FcγR affinity and response to immunocytokine in a phase II study of hu14.18-IL2 in high-risk neuroblastoma patients [15, 16]. From these observations, we concluded that both KIR status and FcγR affinity could collaborate to affect response to therapeutic immunocytokines as presented in Fig. 4, and such collaboration may also apply to mAb-based therapy.

In 87 follicular lymphoma patients treated with rituximab, Weng and Levy found that both FcγRIIa-H/H and FcγRIIIa-V/V were independently associated with progression-free survival [102]. Furthermore this study, as well as other similar studies, found that homozygosity for FcγRIIIa-V correlates with better response to mAb, such as rituximab, [10, 52, 102]. Delgado et al. evaluated Fcγ receptor polymorphisms in high-risk neuroblastoma patients enrolled in a phase II trial for hu14.18-IL2 immunocytokine [15, 16, 89]. These analyses showed a trend towards a correlation between the high affinity FcγRIIa on myeloid cells and response to therapy; 40 % of the individuals that expressed the high affinity allele FcγIIa-131-H responded to treatment compared to 11 % of individuals who expressed the lower affinity allele, FcγIIa-131-A ($p=0.06$, suggesting a trend) (Table 1b). In contrast, an advantage of the high affinity allele on NK cells (FcγIIIa-158-V vs. FcγIIIa-F) was not observed in this study. Only two of the 38 enrolled patients expressed the high affinity allele for FcγRIIIa [15, 16]. To our knowledge, this trial was the first to show a trend towards correlation of high affinity FcγR2a with response to immunocytokines or antibody-fusion proteins. During target cell recognition, NK cells localize interleukin-2 receptors to the site of the immune synapse [31]. While it has not been tested directly, the additional interaction between IL-2 receptors alongside FcγRIIIa may aid the responses of NK cells to IgG, suggesting that when using an immunocytokine that engages both FcR and IL-2R, a high affinity FcR may not be critical in generating a response. Preclinical models to test the affect of dual receptor engagement (i.e., FcγR and IL2R) will be useful.

Antibody manipulation may also help overcome weaker ADCC for individuals with less favorable FcγR alleles. For example, removing fucose side chains from the Fc portion of the antibody increases its affinity for the low affinity FcγRIIIa-F allele. Since the lower affinity FcγRIIIa-158-F allele is the more commonly expressed variant, optimizing antibody interactions via fucose removal would potentially improve the clinical outlook for individuals with this variant [19, 48, 70]. These observations have, in some models, highlighted the importance for FcR-bearing myeloid derived cells as well as NK cells in the clinical efficacy of therapeutic antibody-fusion proteins as well as some monoclonal antibodies.

8 Conclusions

Monoclonal antibodies have been successfully used as therapeutic agents for some cancers. In recent years, advances in antibody engineering have expanded the uses of monoclonal antibody-based therapeutics by giving researchers the tools to create therapeutic grade antibody-fusion proteins in sufficient quantities to be used clinically.

Many of the new promising antibody-fusion proteins are designed to engage multiple cell surface receptors simultaneously. Bifunctional T cell engagers (BiTEs) and the majority of bispecific trifunctional antibodies (Triomabs) are specifically designed to engage and elicit effector functions by T cells, via recognition and activation of the CD3 molecule on T cells. Immunocytokines, such as hu14.18-IL2, localize activating cytokines, such as IL2 to the tumor cell surface leading to antitumor responses.

With the expansion of antibody-fusion proteins in preclinical development and in clinical trials, it is important to understand both patient-intrinsic and drug-intrinsic factors that affect antitumor responses. The balance of activating and inhibitory receptors in each patient's repertoire and the affinity for which their FcγR bind IgG are important factors in the efficacy of antibody-fusion proteins. Understanding the differences in affinity between Fc region sugar side chains and FcγR may allow for the potential to select customized antibodies that will react with maximal affinity for the individual's FcγR. While many of these observations were made with mAbs, it will be important to determine how these observations may differ when antibody-fusion proteins are simultaneously engaging multiple activating receptors on the effector cells.

References

1. Albertini MR, Hank JA, Schiller JH, Khorsand M, Borchert AA, Gan J, Bechhofer R, Storer B, Reisfeld RA, Sondel PM. Phase IB trial of chimeric antidisialoganglioside antibody plus interleukin 2 for melanoma patients. Clin Cancer Res. 1997;3(8):1277–88.
2. Alvarez-Rueda N, Leprieur S, Clemenceau B, Supiot S, Sebille-Rivain V, Faivre-Chauvet A, Davodeau F, Paris F, Barbet J, Aubry J, Birkle S. Binding activities and antitumor properties of a new mouse/human chimeric antibody specific for GD2 ganglioside antigen. Clin Cancer Res. 2007;13(18 Pt 2):5613s–20.
3. Anfossi N, Andre P, Guia S, Falk CS, Roetynck S, Stewart CA, Breso V, Frassati C, Reviron D, Middleton D, Romagne F, Ugolini S, Vivier E. Human NK cell education by inhibitory receptors for MHC class I. Immunity. 2006;25(2):331–42.
4. Ashkenazi C. Immunoadhesins: an alternative to human monoclonal antibodies. Methods. 1995;8.
5. Basham TY, Palladino MA, Badger CC, Bernstein ID, Levy R, Merigan TC. Comparison of combinations of interferons with tumor specific and nonspecific monoclonal antibodies as therapy for murine B- and T-cell lymphomas. Cancer Res. 1988;48(15):4196–200.
6. Becker JC, Pancook JD, Gillies SD, Furukawa K, Reisfeld RA. T cell-mediated eradication of murine metastatic melanoma induced by targeted interleukin 2 therapy. J Exp Med. 1996;183(5):2361–6.
7. Becker JC, Varki N, Gillies SD, Furukawa K, Reisfeld RA. Long-lived and transferable tumor immunity in mice after targeted interleukin-2 therapy. J Clin Invest. 1996;98(12):2801–4.
8. Buhmann R, Simoes B, Stanglmaier M, Yang T, Faltin M, Bund D, Lindhofer H, Kolb HJ. Immunotherapy of recurrent B-cell malignancies after allo-SCT with Bi20 (FBTA05), a tri-functional anti-CD3 x anti-CD20 antibody and donor lymphocyte infusion. Bone Marrow Transplant. 2009;43(5):383–97.
9. Buhtoiarov IN, Sondel PM, Wigginton JM, Buhtoiarova TN, Yanke EM, Mahvi DA, Rakhmilevich AL. Anti-tumour synergy of cytotoxic chemotherapy and anti-CD40 plus CpG-ODN immunotherapy through repolarization of tumour-associated macrophages. Immunology. 2011;132(2):226–39.
10. Cartron G, Dacheux L, Salles G, Solal-Celigny P, Bardos P, Colombat P, Watier H. Therapeutic activity of humanized anti-CD20 monoclonal antibody and polymorphism in IgG Fc receptor FcgammaRIIIa gene. Blood. 2002;99(3):754–8.
11. Chames P, Baty D. Bispecific antibodies for cancer therapy: the light at the end of the tunnel? MAbs. 2009;1(6):539–47.
12. Cheung NK, Guo HF, Heller G, Cheung IY. Induction of Ab3 and Ab3′ antibody was associated with long-term survival after anti-G(D2) antibody therapy of stage 4 neuroblastoma. Clin Cancer Res. 2000;6(7):2653–60.
13. Connor JP, Felder M, Hank J, Harter J, Gan J, Gillies SD, Sondel P. Ex vivo evaluation of anti-EpCAM immunocytokine huKS-IL2 in ovarian cancer. J Immunother. 2004;27(3):211–9.
14. Courtenay-Luck NS, Epenetos AA, Moore R, Larche M, Pectasides D, Dhokia B, Ritter MA. Development of primary and secondary immune responses to mouse monoclonal antibodies

used in the diagnosis and therapy of malignant neoplasms. Cancer Res. 1986;46(12 Pt 1):6489–93.
15. Delgado DC, Hank JA, Kolesar J, Lorentzen D, Gan J, Seo S, Kim K, Shusterman S, Gillies SD, Reisfeld RA, Yang R, Gadbaw B, DeSantes KB, London WB, Seeger RC, Maris JM, Sondel PM. Genotypes of NK cell KIR receptors, their ligands, and Fcgamma receptors in the response of neuroblastoma patients to Hu14.18-IL2 immunotherapy. Cancer Res. 2010;70(23):9554–61.
16. Delgado DC, Hank JA, Kolesar J, Lorentzen D, Gan J, Seo S, Kim K, Shusterman S, Gillies SD, Reisfeld RA, Yang R, Gadbaw B, DeSantes KB, London WB, Seeger RC, Maris JM, Sondel PM. Genotypes of NK cell KIR receptors, their ligands, and Fcgamma receptors in the response of neuroblastoma patients to Hu14.18-IL2 immunotherapy. Cancer Res. 2010;70(23):9554–61.
17. Duncan AR, Winter G. The binding site for C1q on IgG. Nature. 1988;332(6166):738–40.
18. Elliott JM, Wahle JA, Yokoyama WM. MHC class I-deficient natural killer cells acquire a licensed phenotype after transfer into an MHC class I-sufficient environment. J Exp Med. 2010;207(10):2073–9.
19. Ferrara C, Stuart F, Sondermann P, Brunker P, Umana P. The carbohydrate at FcgammaRIIIa Asn-162. An element required for high affinity binding to non-fucosylated IgG glycoforms. J Biol Chem. 2006;281(8):5032–6.
20. Frost JD, Hank JA, Reaman GH, Frierdich S, Seeger RC, Gan J, Anderson PM, Ettinger LJ, Cairo MS, Blazar BR, Krailo MD, Matthay KK, Reisfeld RA, Sondel PM. A phase I/IB trial of murine monoclonal anti-GD2 antibody 14.G2a plus interleukin-2 in children with refractory neuroblastoma: a report of the Children's Cancer Group. Cancer. 1997;80(2):317–33.
21. Gan J, Kendra K, Ricci M, Hank JA, Gillies SD, Sondel PM. Specific enzyme-linked immunosorbent assays for quantitation of antibody-cytokine fusion proteins. Clin Diagn Lab Immunol. 1999;6(2):236–42.
22. Gessner JE, Grussenmeyer T, Schmidt RE. Differentially regulated expression of human IgG Fc receptor class III genes. Immunobiology. 1995;193(2–4):341–55.
23. Gillies SD, Reilly EB, Lo KM, Reisfeld RA. Antibody-targeted interleukin 2 stimulates T-cell killing of autologous tumor cells. Proc Natl Acad Sci U S A. 1992;89(4):1428–32.
24. Gillies SD, Reilly EB, Lo KM, Reisfeld RA. Antibody-targeted interleukin 2 stimulates T-cell killing of autologous tumor cells. Proc Natl Acad Sci U S A. 1992;89(4):1428–32.
25. Gillies SD, Lo KM, Burger C, Lan Y, Dahl T, Wong WK. Improved circulating half-life and efficacy of an antibody-interleukin 2 immunocytokine based on reduced intracellular proteolysis. Clin Cancer Res. 2002;8(1):210–6.
26. Gillies SD, Lan Y, Williams S, Carr F, Forman S, Raubitschek A, Lo KM. An anti-CD20-IL-2 immunocytokine is highly efficacious in a SCID mouse model of established human B lymphoma. Blood. 2005;105(10):3972–8.
27. Gillies SD, Lan Y, Hettmann T, Brunkhorst B, Sun Y, Mueller SO, Lo KM. A low-toxicity IL-2-based immunocytokine retains antitumor activity despite its high degree of IL-2 receptor selectivity. Clin Cancer Res. 2011;17(11):3673–85.
28. Gilman AL, Ozkaynak MF, Matthay KK, Krailo M, Yu AL, Gan J, Sternberg A, Hank JA, Seeger R, Reaman GH, Sondel PM. Phase I study of ch14.18 with granulocyte-macrophage colony-stimulating factor and interleukin-2 in children with neuroblastoma after autologous bone marrow transplantation or stem-cell rescue: a report from the Children's Oncology Group. J Clin Oncol. 2009;27(1):85–91.
29. Glennie MJ, Johnson PW. Clinical trials of antibody therapy. Immunol Today. 2000;21(8):403–10.
30. Grabert RC, Cousens LP, Smith JA, Olson S, Gall J, Young WB, Davol PA, Lum LG. Human T cells armed with Her2/neu bispecific antibodies divide, are cytotoxic, and secrete cytokines with repeated stimulation. Clin Cancer Res. 2006;12(2):569–76.
31. Gubbels JA, Gadbaw B, Buhtoiarov IN, Horibata S, Kapur AK, Patel D, Hank JA, Gillies SD, Sondel PM, Patankar MS, Connor J. Ab-IL2 fusion proteins mediate NK cell immune

synapse formation by polarizing CD25 to the target cell-effector cell interface. Cancer Immunol Immunother. 2011;60(12):1789–800.
32. Hank JA, Kohler PC, Weil-Hillman G, Rosenthal N, Moore KH, Storer B, Minkoff D, Bradshaw J, Bechhofer R, Sondel PM. In vivo induction of the lymphokine-activated killer phenomenon: interleukin 2-dependent human non-major histocompatibility complex-restricted cytotoxicity generated in vivo during administration of human recombinant interleukin 2. Cancer Res. 1988;48(7):1965–71.
33. Hank JA, Weil-Hillman G, Surfus JE, Sosman JA, Sondel PM. Addition of interleukin-2 in vitro augments detection of lymphokine-activated killer activity generated in vivo. Cancer Immunol Immunother. 1990;31(1):53–9.
34. Hank JA, Albertini MR, Schiller J, Sondel PM. Activation of multiple effector mechanisms to enhance tumor immunotherapy. J Immunother Emphasis Tumor Immunol. 1993;14(4): 329–35.
35. Hank JA, Surfus JE, Gan J, Jaeger P, Gillies SD, Reisfeld RA, Sondel PM. Activation of human effector cells by a tumor reactive recombinant anti-ganglioside GD2 interleukin-2 fusion protein (ch14.18-IL2). Clin Cancer Res. 1996;2(12):1951–9.
36. Hank JA, Gan J, Ryu H, Ostendorf A, Stauder MC, Sternberg A, Albertini M, Lo KM, Gillies SD, Eickhoff J, Sondel PM. Immunogenicity of the hu14.18-IL2 immunocytokine molecule in adults with melanoma and children with neuroblastoma. Clin Cancer Res. 2009;15(18): 5923–30.
37. Harvill ET, Morrison SL. An IgG3-IL-2 fusion protein has higher affinity than hrIL-2 for the IL-2R alpha subunit: real time measurement of ligand binding. Mol Immunol. 1996; 33(11–12):1007–14.
38. Heiss MM, Murawa P, Koralewski P, Kutarska E, Kolesnik OO, Ivanchenko VV, Dudnichenko AS, Aleknaviciene B, Razbadauskas A, Gore M, Ganea-Motan E, Ciuleanu T, Wimberger P, Schmittel A, Schmalfeldt B, Burges A, Bokemeyer C, Lindhofer H, Lahr A, Parsons SL. The trifunctional antibody catumaxomab for the treatment of malignant ascites due to epithelial cancer: results of a prospective randomized phase II/III trial. Int J Cancer. 2010;127(9): 2209–21.
39. Holden SA, Lan Y, Pardo AM, Wesolowski JS, Gillies SD. Augmentation of antitumor activity of an antibody-interleukin 2 immunocytokine with chemotherapeutic agents. Clin Cancer Res. 2001;7(9):2862–9.
40. Hughes-Jones NC, Gardner B. Reaction between the isolated globular sub-units of the complement component C1q and IgG-complexes. Mol Immunol. 1979;16(9):697–701.
41. Iida S, Kuni-Kamochi R, Mori K, Misaka H, Inoue M, Okazaki A, Shitara K, Satoh M. Two mechanisms of the enhanced antibody-dependent cellular cytotoxicity (ADCC) efficacy of non-fucosylated therapeutic antibodies in human blood. BMC Cancer. 2009;9:58.
42. Imai M, Landen C, Ohta R, Cheung NK, Tomlinson S. Complement-mediated mechanisms in anti-GD2 monoclonal antibody therapy of murine metastatic cancer. Cancer Res. 2005;65(22):10562–8.
43. Ito A, Ishida T, Utsunomiya A, Sato F, Mori F, Yano H, Inagaki A, Suzuki S, Takino H, Ri M, Kusumoto S, Komatsu H, Iida S, Inagaki H, Ueda R. Defucosylated anti-CCR4 monoclonal antibody exerts potent ADCC against primary ATLL cells mediated by autologous human immune cells in NOD/Shi-scid, IL-2R gamma(null) mice in vivo. J Immunol. 2009;183(7): 4782–91.
44. Jefferis R. Antibody therapeutics: isotype and glycoform selection. Expert Opin Biol Ther. 2007;7(9):1401–13.
45. Johnson EE, Yamane BH, Buhtoiarov IN, Lum HD, Rakhmilevich AL, Mahvi DM, Gillies SD, Sondel PM. Radiofrequency ablation combined with KS-IL2 immunocytokine (EMD 273066) results in an enhanced antitumor effect against murine colon adenocarcinoma. Clin Cancer Res. 2009;15(15):4875–84.
46. Joncker NT, Shifrin N, Delebecque F, Raulet DH. Mature natural killer cells reset their responsiveness when exposed to an altered MHC environment. J Exp Med. 2010;207(10): 2065–72.

47. Kanda Y, Yamane-Ohnuki N, Sakai N, Yamano K, Nakano R, Inoue M, Misaka H, Iida S, Wakitani M, Konno Y, Yano K, Shitara K, Hosoi S, Satoh M. Comparison of cell lines for stable production of fucose-negative antibodies with enhanced ADCC. Biotechnol Bioeng. 2006;94(4):680–8.
48. Kanda Y, Yamada T, Mori K, Okazaki A, Inoue M, Kitajima-Miyama K, Kuni-Kamochi R, Nakano R, Yano K, Kakita S, Shitara K, Satoh M. Comparison of biological activity among nonfucosylated therapeutic IgG1 antibodies with three different N-linked Fc oligosaccharides: the high-mannose, hybrid, and complex types. Glycobiology. 2007;17(1):104–18.
49. Kausalya S, Hegde SP, Bright JJ, Khar A. Mechanism of antibody-dependent natural killer cell-mediated AK-5 tumor cell death. Exp Cell Res. 1994;212(2):285–90.
50. Kendra K, Gan J, Ricci M, Surfus J, Shaker A, Super M, Frost JD, Rakhmilevich A, Hank JA, Gillies SD, Sondel PM. Pharmacokinetics and stability of the ch14.18-interleukin-2 fusion protein in mice. Cancer Immunol Immunother. 1999;48(5):219–29.
51. Kim S, Poursine-Laurent J, Truscott SM, Lybarger L, Song YJ, Yang L, French AR, Sunwoo JB, Lemieux S, Hansen TH, Yokoyama WM. Licensing of natural killer cells by host major histocompatibility complex class I molecules. Nature. 2005;436(7051):709–13.
52. Kim DH, Jung HD, Kim JG, Lee JJ, Yang DH, Park YH, Do YR, Shin HJ, Kim MK, Hyun MS, Sohn SK. FCGR3A gene polymorphisms may correlate with response to frontline R-CHOP therapy for diffuse large B-cell lymphoma. Blood. 2006;108(8):2720–5.
53. Kim S, Sunwoo JB, Yang L, Choi T, Song YJ, French AR, Vlahiotis A, Piccirillo JF, Cella M, Colonna M, Mohanakumar T, Hsu KC, Dupont B, Yokoyama WM. HLA alleles determine differences in human natural killer cell responsiveness and potency. Proc Natl Acad Sci U S A. 2008;105(8):3053–8.
54. King DM, Albertini MR, Schalch H, Hank JA, Gan J, Surfus J, Mahvi D, Schiller JH, Warner T, Kim K, Eickhoff J, Kendra K, Reisfeld R, Gillies SD, Sondel P. Phase I clinical trial of the immunocytokine EMD 273063 in melanoma patients. J Clin Oncol. 2004;22(22):4463–73.
55. Klinger M, Brandl C, Zugmaier G, Hijazi Y, Bargou RC, Topp MS, Gokbuget N, Neumann S, Goebeler M, Viardot A, Stelljes M, Bruggemann M, Hoelzer D, Degenhard E, Nagorsen D, Baeuerle PA, Wolf A, Kufer P. Immunopharmacologic response of patients with B-lineage acute lymphoblastic leukemia to continuous infusion of T cell-engaging CD19/CD3-bispecific BiTE antibody blinatumomab. Blood. 2012;119(26):6226–33.
56. Ko YJ, Bubley GJ, Weber R, Redfern C, Gold DP, Finke L, Kovar A, Dahl T, Gillies SD. Safety, pharmacokinetics, and biological pharmacodynamics of the immunocytokine EMD 273066 (huKS-IL2): results of a phase I trial in patients with prostate cancer. J Immunother. 2004;27(3):232–9.
57. Koene HR, Kleijer M, Algra J, Roos D, von dem Borne AE, de Haas M. Fc gammaRIIIa-158V/F polymorphism influences the binding of IgG by natural killer cell Fc gammaRIIIa, independently of the Fc gammaRIIIa-48L/R/H phenotype. Blood. 1997;90(3):1109–14.
58. Kontermann RE. Recombinant bispecific antibodies for cancer therapy. Acta Pharmacol Sin. 2005;26(1):1–9.
59. Leung W, Handgretinger R, Iyengar R, Turner V, Holladay MS, Hale GA. Inhibitory KIR-HLA receptor-ligand mismatch in autologous haematopoietic stem cell transplantation for solid tumour and lymphoma. Br J Cancer. 2007;97(4):539–42.
60. Lindhofer H, Mocikat R, Steipe B, Thierfelder S. Preferential species-restricted heavy/light chain pairing in rat/mouse quadromas. Implications for a single-step purification of bispecific antibodies. J Immunol. 1995;155(1):219–25.
61. Linke R, Klein A, Seimetz D. Catumaxomab: clinical development and future directions. MAbs. 2010;2(2):129–36.
62. Lode HN, Xiang R, Varki NM, Dolman CS, Gillies SD, Reisfeld RA. Targeted interleukin-2 therapy for spontaneous neuroblastoma metastases to bone marrow. J Natl Cancer Inst. 1997;89(21):1586–94.
63. Lode HN, Xiang R, Dreier T, Varki NM, Gillies SD, Reisfeld RA. Natural killer cell-mediated eradication of neuroblastoma metastases to bone marrow by targeted interleukin-2 therapy. Blood. 1998;91(5):1706–15.

64. Masuda K, Kubota T, Kaneko E, Iida S, Wakitani M, Kobayashi-Natsume Y, Kubota A, Shitara K, Nakamura K. Enhanced binding affinity for FcgammaRIIIa of fucose-negative antibody is sufficient to induce maximal antibody-dependent cellular cytotoxicity. Mol Immunol. 2007;44(12):3122–31.
65. Mueller BM, Romerdahl CA, Gillies SD, Reisfeld RA. Enhancement of antibody-dependent cytotoxicity with a chimeric anti-GD2 antibody. J Immunol. 1990;144(4):1382–6.
66. Musolino A, Naldi N, Bortesi B, Pezzuolo D, Capelletti M, Missale G, Laccabue D, Zerbini A, Camisa R, Bisagni G, Neri TM, Ardizzoni A. Immunoglobulin G fragment C receptor polymorphisms and clinical efficacy of trastuzumab-based therapy in patients with HER-2/neu-positive metastatic breast cancer. J Clin Oncol. 2008;26(11):1789–96.
67. Neal ZC, Imboden M, Rakhmilevich AL, Kim KM, Hank JA, Surfus J, Dixon JR, Lode HN, Reisfeld RA, Gillies SD, Sondel PM. NXS2 murine neuroblastomas express increased levels of MHC class I antigens upon recurrence following NK-dependent immunotherapy. Cancer Immunol Immunother. 2004;53(1):41–52.
68. Neal ZC, Yang JC, Rakhmilevich AL, Buhtoiarov IN, Lum HE, Imboden M, Hank JA, Lode HN, Reisfeld RA, Gillies SD, Sondel PM. Enhanced activity of hu14.18-IL2 immunocytokine against murine NXS2 neuroblastoma when combined with interleukin 2 therapy. Clin Cancer Res. 2004;10(14):4839–47.
69. Nimmerjahn F, Ravetch JV. Fcgamma receptors as regulators of immune responses. Nat Rev Immunol. 2008;8(1):34–47.
70. Niwa R, Shoji-Hosaka E, Sakurada M, Shinkawa T, Uchida K, Nakamura K, Matsushima K, Ueda R, Hanai N, Shitara K. Defucosylated chimeric anti-CC chemokine receptor 4 IgG1 with enhanced antibody-dependent cellular cytotoxicity shows potent therapeutic activity to T-cell leukemia and lymphoma. Cancer Res. 2004;64(6):2127–33.
71. Orr MT, Murphy WJ, Lanier LL. 'Unlicensed' natural killer cells dominate the response to cytomegalovirus infection. Nat Immunol. 2010;11(4):321–7.
72. Osenga KL, Hank JA, Albertini MR, Gan J, Sternberg AG, Eickhoff J, Seeger RC, Matthay KK, Reynolds CP, Twist C, Krailo M, Adamson PC, Reisfeld RA, Gillies SD, Sondel PM. A phase I clinical trial of the hu14.18-IL2 (EMD 273063) as a treatment for children with refractory or recurrent neuroblastoma and melanoma: a study of the Children's Oncology Group. Clin Cancer Res. 2006;12(6):1750–9.
73. Overdijk MB, Verploegen S, van den Brakel JH, Lammerts van Bueren JJ, Vink T, van de Winkel JG, Parren PW, Bleeker WK. Epidermal growth factor receptor (EGFR) antibody-induced antibody-dependent cellular cytotoxicity plays a prominent role in inhibiting tumorigenesis, even of tumor cells insensitive to EGFR signaling inhibition. J Immunol. 2011;187(6):3383–90.
74. Parham P. MHC class I molecules and KIRs in human history, health and survival. Nat Rev Immunol. 2005;5(3):201–14.
75. Parsons MS, Zipperlen K, Gallant M, Grant M. Killer cell immunoglobulin-like receptor 3DL1 licenses CD16-mediated effector functions of natural killer cells. J Leukoc Biol. 2010;88(5):905–12.
76. Perez de la Lastra JM, Kremer L, de la Fuente J. Recent advances in the development of immunoadhesins for immune therapy and as anti-infective agents. Recent Pat Antiinfect Drug Discov. 2009;4(3):183–9.
77. Pietzner K, Jager M, Schoberth A, Oskay-Ozcelik G, Kuhberg M, Lindhofer H, Sehouli J. First patient treated with a re-challenge of catumaxomab in recurrent malignant ascites: a case report. Med Oncol. 2012;29(2):1391–6.
78. Primus FJ, Finch MD, Wetzel SA, Masci AM, Schlom J, Kashmiri SV. Monoclonal antibody gene transfer. Implications for tumor-specific cell-mediated cytotoxicity. Ann N Y Acad Sci. 1994;716:154–65. discussion 165–6.
79. Roda JM, Parihar R, Lehman A, Mani A, Tridandapani S, Carson 3rd WE. Interleukin-21 enhances NK cell activation in response to antibody-coated targets. J Immunol. 2006;177(1):120–9.

80. Sabzevari H, Gillies SD, Mueller BM, Pancook JD, Reisfeld RA. A recombinant antibody-interleukin 2 fusion protein suppresses growth of hepatic human neuroblastoma metastases in severe combined immunodeficiency mice. Proc Natl Acad Sci U S A. 1994;91(20):9626–30.
81. Schroff RW, Foon KA, Beatty SM, Oldham RK, Morgan Jr AC. Human anti-murine immunoglobulin responses in patients receiving monoclonal antibody therapy. Cancer Res. 1985;45(2):879–85.
82. Schultz KR, Klarnet JP, Peace DJ, Cheever MA, Badger CC, Bernstein ID, Greenberg PD. Monoclonal antibody therapy of murine lymphoma: enhanced efficacy by concurrent administration of interleukin 2 or lymphokine-activated killer cells. Cancer Res. 1990;50(17):5421–5.
83. Segal DM, Weiner GJ, Weiner LM. Bispecific antibodies in cancer therapy. Curr Opin Immunol. 1999;11(5):558–62.
84. Shawler DL, Bartholomew RM, Smith LM, Dillman RO. Human immune response to multiple injections of murine monoclonal IgG. J Immunol. 1985;135(2):1530–5.
85. Shibata-Koyama M, Iida S, Misaka H, Mori K, Yano K, Shitara K, Satoh M. Nonfucosylated rituximab potentiates human neutrophil phagocytosis through its high binding for FcgammaRIIIb and MHC class II expression on the phagocytotic neutrophils. Exp Hematol. 2009;37(3):309–21.
86. Shields RL, Lai J, Keck R, O'Connell LY, Hong K, Meng YG, Weikert SH, Presta LG. Lack of fucose on human IgG1 N-linked oligosaccharide improves binding to human Fcgamma RIII and antibody-dependent cellular toxicity. J Biol Chem. 2002;277(30):26733–40.
87. Shiloni E, Eisenthal A, Sachs D, Rosenberg SA. Antibody-dependent cellular cytotoxicity mediated by murine lymphocytes activated in recombinant interleukin 2. J Immunol. 1987;138(6):1992–8.
88. Shinkawa T, Nakamura K, Yamane N, Shoji-Hosaka E, Kanda Y, Sakurada M, Uchida K, Anazawa H, Satoh M, Yamasaki M, Hanai N, Shitara K. The absence of fucose but not the presence of galactose or bisecting N-acetylglucosamine of human IgG1 complex-type oligosaccharides shows the critical role of enhancing antibody-dependent cellular cytotoxicity. J Biol Chem. 2003;278(5):3466–73.
89. Shusterman S, London WB, Gillies SD, Hank JA, Voss SD, Seeger RC, Reynolds CP, Kimball J, Albertini MR, Wagner B, Gan J, Eickhoff J, DeSantes KB, Cohn SL, Hecht T, Gadbaw B, Reisfeld RA, Maris JM, Sondel PM. Antitumor activity of hu14.18-IL2 in patients with relapsed/refractory neuroblastoma: a Children's Oncology Group (COG) phase II study. J Clin Oncol. 2010;28(33):4969–75.
90. Siberil S, Dutertre CA, Fridman WH, Teillaud JL. FcgammaR: the key to optimize therapeutic antibodies? Crit Rev Oncol Hematol. 2007;62(1):26–33.
91. Simon T, Hero B, Faldum A, Handgretinger R, Schrappe M, Niethammer D, Berthold F. Consolidation treatment with chimeric anti-GD2-antibody ch14.18 in children older than 1 year with metastatic neuroblastoma. J Clin Oncol. 2004;22(17):3549–57.
92. Sorkin LS, Otto M, Baldwin 3rd WM, Vail E, Gillies SD, Handgretinger R, Barfield RC, Ming Yu H, Yu AL. Anti-GD(2) with an FC point mutation reduces complement fixation and decreases antibody-induced allodynia. Pain. 2010;149(1):135–42.
93. Sosman JA, Hank JA, Sondel PM. In vivo activation of lymphokine-activated killer activity with interleukin-2: prospects for combination therapies. Semin Oncol. 1990;17(1 Suppl 1):22–30. discussion 38–41.
94. Suzuki E, Niwa R, Saji S, Muta M, Hirose M, Iida S, Shiotsu Y, Satoh M, Shitara K, Kondo M, Toi M. A nonfucosylated anti-HER2 antibody augments antibody-dependent cellular cytotoxicity in breast cancer patients. Clin Cancer Res. 2007;13(6):1875–82.
95. Swann PG, Shapiro MA. Regulatory considerations for development of bioanalytical assays for biotechnology products. Bioanalysis. 2011;3(6):597–603.
96. Tarek N, Le Luduec JB, Gallagher MM, Zheng J, Venstrom JM, Chamberlain E, Modak S, Heller G, Dupont B, Cheung NK, Hsu KC. Unlicensed NK cells target neuroblastoma following anti-GD2 antibody treatment. J Clin Invest. 2012;122(9):3260–70.

97. Tarek N, Le Luduec JB, Gallagher MM, Zheng J, Venstrom JM, Chamberlain E, Modak S, Heller G, Dupont B, Cheung NK, Hsu KC. Unlicensed NK cells target neuroblastoma following anti-GD2 antibody treatment. J Clin Invest. 2012;122(9):3260–70.
98. Tjandra JJ, Ramadi L, McKenzie IF. Development of human anti-murine antibody (HAMA) response in patients. Immunol Cell Biol. 1990;68(Pt 6):367–76.
99. Topp MS, Kufer P, Gokbuget N, Goebeler M, Klinger M, Neumann S, Horst HA, Raff T, Viardot A, Schmid M, Stelljes M, Schaich M, Degenhard E, Kohne-Volland R, Bruggemann M, Ottmann O, Pfeifer H, Burmeister T, Nagorsen D, Schmidt M, Lutterbuese R, Reinhardt C, Baeuerle PA, Kneba M, Einsele H, Riethmuller G, Hoelzer D, Zugmaier G, Bargou RC. Targeted therapy with the T-cell-engaging antibody blinatumomab of chemotherapy-refractory minimal residual disease in B-lineage acute lymphoblastic leukemia patients results in high response rate and prolonged leukemia-free survival. J Clin Oncol. 2011; 29(18):2493–8.
100. Trapani JA, Browne KA, Dawson M, Smyth MJ. Immunopurification of functional Asp-ase (natural killer cell granzyme B) using a monoclonal antibody. Biochem Biophys Res Commun. 1993;195(2):910–20.
101. Venstrom JM, Zheng J, Noor N, Danis KE, Yeh AW, Cheung IY, Dupont B, O'Reilly RJ, Cheung NK, Hsu KC. KIR and HLA genotypes are associated with disease progression and survival following autologous hematopoietic stem cell transplantation for high-risk neuroblastoma. Clin Cancer Res. 2009;15(23):7330–4.
102. Weng WK, Levy R. Two immunoglobulin G fragment C receptor polymorphisms independently predict response to rituximab in patients with follicular lymphoma. J Clin Oncol. 2003;21(21):3940–7.
103. Weng WK, Czerwinski D, Timmerman J, Hsu FJ, Levy R. Clinical outcome of lymphoma patients after idiotype vaccination is correlated with humoral immune response and immunoglobulin G Fc receptor genotype. J Clin Oncol. 2004;22(23):4717–24.
104. Wu J, Edberg JC, Redecha PB, Bansal V, Guyre PM, Coleman K, Salmon JE, Kimberly RP. A novel polymorphism of FcgammaRIIIa (CD16) alters receptor function and predisposes to autoimmune disease. J Clin Invest. 1997;100(5):1059–70.
105. Yamane-Ohnuki N, Satoh M. Production of therapeutic antibodies with controlled fucosylation. MAbs. 2009;1(3):230–6.
106. Yang RK, Kalogriopoulos NA, Rakhmilevich AL, Ranheim EA, Seo S, Kim K, Alderson KL, Gan J, Reisfeld RA, Gillies SD, Hank JA, Sondel PM. Intratumoral hu14.18-IL-2 (IC) induces local and systemic antitumor effects that involve both activated T and NK cells as well as enhanced ic retention. J Immunol. 2012;189(5):2656–64.
107. Yoshida S, Kawaguchi H, Sato S, Ueda R, Furukawa K. An anti-GD2 monoclonal antibody enhances apoptotic effects of anti-cancer drugs against small cell lung cancer cells via JNK (c-Jun terminal kinase) activation. Jap J Cancer Res. 2002;93(7):816–24.
108. Yu AL, Gilman AL, Ozkaynak MF, London WB, Kreissman SG, Chen HX, Smith M, Anderson B, Villablanca JG, Matthay KK, Shimada H, Grupp SA, Seeger R, Reynolds CP, Buxton A, Reisfeld RA, Gillies SD, Cohn SL, Maris JM, Sondel PM. Anti-GD2 antibody with GM-CSF, interleukin-2, and isotretinoin for neuroblastoma. N Engl J Med. 2010; 363(14):1324–34.

Immunologic Outcomes of Allogeneic Stem Cell Transplantation: Graft-Versus-Host and Graft-Versus-Leukemia Responses and Implications for Future Therapy

Lazaros J. Lekakis and Krishna V. Komanduri

Abstract Allogeneic stem cell transplantation (allo-HCT) is a procedure with the potential to cure many malignant and nonmalignant diseases. The adoptive transfer of a donor immune system into a transplant recipient can result in allorecognition and reactivity of donor immune cells against host target tissues. This can lead to an immune attack against normal tissues in the recipient (graft-versus-host disease, GVHD) but also against the neoplastic cells themselves (graft-versus-tumor effect, GVT). While GVHD has long been recognized as a significant cause of morbidity and mortality after allo-HCT, there has been little progress in advancing the standards of care for GVHD prophylaxis and therapy, which have remain unchanged for more than two decades. Given the more recent recognition that much of the curative benefit of allo-HCT results from the GVT effect, rather than from the cytoreductive effects of conditioning chemotherapy, multiple strategies to take advantage of the GVT effect that aim to limit morbidity and mortality due to GVHD are under investigation, including cellular therapies employing the use of native or engineered graft populations enriched for antitumor responses, and employing donor lymphocyte infusions. Another critical question is how strategies to prevent and/or treat GVHD may be designed to limit the suppression of beneficial T cell responses against pathogens critical to limiting infections in the post-HCT setting. Research in murine models and human subjects has uncovered a great deal regarding the mechanisms of GVHD initiation and persistence, including clinical factors and graft constituents responsible for the acute and chronic forms of GVHD. A variety of cellular mediators, from antigen-presenting cells to effectors, including alloreactive T cells and B cells, have been characterized. Regulatory populations, including CD4+ regulatory T cells and invariant NKT cells, have also been shown to be capable of ameliorating GVHD intensity and survival in model systems. Given this clearer

L.J. Lekakis • K.V. Komanduri (✉)
Adult Stem Cell Transplant Program, University of Miami Sylvester
Cancer Center, Miami, FL, USA
e-mail: kkomanduri@med.miami.edu

J.D. Rosenblatt et al. (eds.), *Advances in Tumor Immunology and Immunotherapy*, Current Cancer Research, DOI 10.1007/978-1-4614-8809-5_12,

© Springer Science+Business Media New York 2014

understanding of GVHD pathophysiology, a variety of novel clinical strategies are in development, from those utilizing classical inhibitors of T cell reactivity, to monoclonal antibody therapies to more novel approaches targeting specific signaling pathways in T cells and other mediators of inflammation. Recent meaningful progress has also been made in approaches using adoptive cellular therapies to decrease GVHD while maintaining or specifically augmenting GVT responses. These strategies bring promise for a future wherein more patients can receive allo-HCT for both malignant and nonmalignant diseases, with reduced rates of complications and improved overall survival.

1 Introduction

1.1 Hematopoietic Stem Cell Transplantation

The recognition that relatively small numbers of hematopoietic stem cells (HSCs) can regenerate the bone marrow function facilitated the use of high doses of chemotherapy and/or radiation [1] for the treatment of human malignancies and other diseases such as bone marrow failure syndromes, primary immune deficiencies, enzymopathies, and hemoglobinopathies [2]. Initially the procedure consisted of high-dose therapy (HDT, chemotherapy or radiation) followed by bone marrow transplantation (BMT). Later it was realized that HSCs are contained in umbilical cord blood and can also be mobilized and collected from the peripheral blood with apheresis. The donor of stem cells can be the patient (autologous hematopoietic stem cell transplantation, auto-HCT) or someone else (allogeneic hematopoietic stem cell transplantation, allo-HCT). This can be either an HLA-matched sibling donor (MSD allo-HCT), a haploidentical relative (haplo-HCT), or someone unrelated but HLA-matched with the patient (matched unrelated donor or MUD allo-HCT). In umbilical cord blood stem cell transplantation (UCB-HCT) the donor is usually unrelated.

1.2 Graft-Versus-Host Disease and Graft-Versus-Tumor Effect

Early in the HCT era, it was apparent that a subset of patients developed a declining course with evidence of inflammation in various organ systems, which in some cases could be lethal. These patients frequently did not have relapse of their malignancy or obvious infection and a term "secondary disease" and later "graft-versus-host disease" (GVHD) (reviewed in [3–5]) was coined to define this process. It became apparent from animal models and in the human clinical setting that GVHD was mediated mainly by alloreactive T cells, since the incidence of GVHD was low in the setting of syngeneic (i.e., identical twin), autologous or T cell-depleted HCT (TCD allo-HCT).

However, it was also recognized that the relapse rates of malignancies were lower after allo-HCT than after auto-HCT. Moreover, relapses were higher after TCD allo-HCT but lower in patients with GVHD (especially chronic GVHD), implying that not only the HDT but also the donor immune system was critical to keep recipients in remission. Subsequently, it was shown that for patients relapsing without GVHD following allo-HCT, the infusion of donor lymphocytes (DLI) could make the malignancy regress or enter another remission, in some cases without the development of GVHD following DLI. The terms graft-versus-leukemia (GVL) or graft-versus-tumor (GVT) have been used to describe this donor immune reactivity against the recipient malignancy [6]. Since the recognition of GVL in allo-HCT, many transplanters have decreased the intensity of HDT, especially for slow-growing malignancies (e.g., follicular lymphomas). We call these attenuated therapies reduced-intensity conditioning (RIC) [7]. An extreme extension of this approach is to rely almost exclusively on GVL and to give only modest doses of immunosuppressive therapy (to avoid graft rejection, mediated by residual host immunity) and then to allow the donor immune system fight the neoplasm (non-myeloablative conditioning, NMA). The introduction of RIC and NMA conditioning regimens allowed the application of HCT to older patients or those with comorbid conditions, which is critical given that most diseases curable by HCT increase in incidence with age. Given the significant morbidity and mortality associated with GVHD and the curative potential of GVT, a critical problem faced by transplant immunologists has been the dissociation of these two phenomena.

1.3 Acute GVHD

Understanding the pathogenesis of GVHD (and of GVL) is essential to facilitate the selective manipulation of these clinical events after HCT. However, a critical problem is that GVHD is an extremely pleomorphic entity. There is an acute and a chronic form (aGVHD and cGVHD, respectively) and also an overlap syndrome that can combine features of both. Initially defined by the time of their onset (day +100 after HCT being the date that separated the two forms), aGVHD and cGVHD are now more appropriately distinguished by their clinical manifestations. aGVHD usually affects the skin, the gastrointestinal (GI) tract and the liver, whereas cGVHD typically involves mucosal surfaces, the eyes and the skin (but can involve nearly any organ system). More severe manifestations of aGVHD may include GI disease (e.g., diarrhea, nausea, emesis, abdominal pain, or failure to thrive, depending on the segment of the GI tract that is targeted), and signs of severe hepatic dysfunction (jaundice, encephalopathy, bleeding, hypoalbuminemia) and severe skin involvement (e.g., generalized maculopapular rash that can progress to erythroderma and exfoliation) [8]. If aGVHD happens before day +14 (usually before engraftment), this is called hyper-acute GVHD and is associated with an adverse prognosis [9]. We now also recognize that a late-onset form of aGVHD may occur even well beyond post-transplant day +100 (delayed-onset aGVHD), in some cases due to the tapering of immunosuppression.

1.4 Chronic GVHD

Chronic GVHD also manifests quite variably [10]. Patients may have sicca symptoms (xeropthalmia, xerostomia) with or without arthralgias/arthritis, oral lichenoid changes, skin rash, poikiloderma, skin lichenification, and/or systemic sclerosis (scleroderma), eosinophilic fasciitis or polymyositis. They can also develop liver dysfunction and cholestasis, anorexia, nausea, emesis, weight loss, malnutrition, bronchiolitis obliterans (BO), or cryptogenic organizing pneumonia (COP, formerly BOOP). Other less common manifestations include glomerulonephritis with or without nephrotic syndrome, hypogonadism, and other hormonal deficiencies. Serosal inflammation with pleural effusions or ascites and nervous system involvement are very rare.

2 Pathobiology of aGVHD (Fig. 1)

2.1 Effector Cells

Classically, the pathogenesis of aGVHD has been defined by three phases: Initiation, effector, and augmentation phase. The main effectors in aGVHD are the donor T cells, given the established preventive effects of TCD and T cell-directed immunosuppressive agents. Both αβ T cells and γδ donor T cells contribute to aGVHD. Either CD4+ or CD8+ T cells are *sufficient* to induce aGVHD. Of the CD4+ T cell subsets, naïve donor T cells seem to be the main effectors [11]. In contrast, central memory CD4+ cells have less ability to induce aGVHD [12], while effector memory CD4 cells seem to be incapable of GVHD induction [13]. It is interesting that both central memory and effector memory T cells have been shown to mediate GvL. Although helper T cell polarization is less clear in humans than in murine models, evidence suggests that both T_H1 and T_H17 subsets may contribute to aGVHD [14], while T_H2 cells have a more controversial, but probably detrimental, role. The main population of human regulatory T cells (T_{REG}) (delineated by the CD4+CD25^{hi}Foxp3+ phenotype) appears to be protective for GVHD and may relatively spare GVL responses [15].

Another population of "regulatory cells", the invariant NKT (iNKT) cells can act prophylactically early on by expanding CD4^{+}CD25^{hi}FoxP3 T_{REG} in a IL-4 dependent fashion [16], but the role of iNKT cells can vary depending on the way they have been activated and polarized.

B cells can also augment aGVHD by promoting alloantigen presentation. However, it appears that some B cell subsets can have a protective role in the effector phase by producing IL-10 [17]. B cells that produce high quantities of IL-10 and co-express Foxp3 (regulatory B cells, B_{REG}) have been described, although their importance in GVHD is uncertain [18].

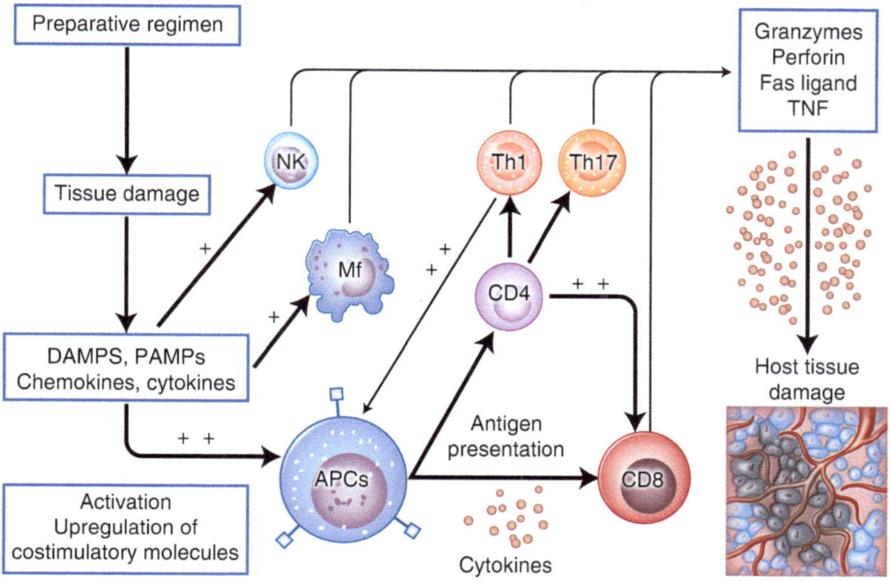

Fig. 1 PATHOBIOLOGY OF ACUTE GVHD: Professional antigen presenting cells (APCs), mainly recipient dendritic cells, become activated under the influence of danger signals that are produced by damaged tissues and microbes. Donor T cells recognize recipient antigens with their T cell receptor and are costimulated by the activated APCs. They are polarized to Th1 or Th17 under the influence of cytokines produced by APCs and monocytes. T cells become activated and produce cytokines, cytotoxic and pro-apoptotic molecules that mediate target-cell damage

2.2 *Tissue Damage: Cytokines, Perforin, and FasL*

The damage to target organs by T cells is mediated by both cell–cell contact and cytokines. Both FasL and perforin mediate apoptosis through cell–cell contact [19]. FasL-mediated apoptosis may be important in hepatic and cutaneous GVHD, while TNFα operates mainly in intestinal GVHD. Both IFNγ and IL-2 perpetuate aGVHD-induced inflammation and tissue damage, but in experimental systems, administration of these cytokines immediately after allo-HCT appears to *prevent* severe GVHD. The protective effect of IL-2 may be mediated by expansion of T_{REG} [20]. T_H17 cells play a significant role in GI aGVHD via IL-17 and IL-21 production [21]. T_H17 cells are induced by IL-6 and TGFβ and their survival and proliferation are supported by IL-23. High levels of IL-6 increase the T_H17/T_{REG} ratio, which may potentiate GVHD, especially in the GI tract.

2.3 T Cell Priming by Antigen-Presenting Cells

The classic teaching is that intrinsic antigens are degraded in proteasomes and presented through MHC class I to CD8+ cells, whereas exogenous phagocytosed antigens are presented after endosomal degradation to CD4+ cells through MHC class II. It has however been recognized that exogenous antigens can be presented directly to CD8 through MHC class I molecules, a phenomenon known as *cross-priming* or *cross-presentation*. This helps donor antigen-presenting cells (donor APCs) to prime donor CD8+ cells directly (without interference of CD4+ cells) against recipient antigens (for example minor histocompatibility antigens, miHA) [22]. After priming, T cells require costimulation (signal two) or otherwise become anergic. The classic second signal is provided by the B7 molecules (CD80 and CD86) of APCs via the CD28 receptor on T cells. Subsequently, cytokines produced by APCs (signal three, e.g., IL-12 and TNFα) further activate T cells and skew their polarization (T_H1 vs. T_H2). Ligation of CD40 on APCs by CD40L (on activated T cells) helps the APC produce the third signal and to upregulate their co-stimulatory molecules [23].

2.4 T Cell Priming: Are Professional APCs Really Required?

Classically, it was demonstrated that in CD8-mediated aGVHD in MHC-matched pairs, recipient (host) APCs of hematopoietic origin are *required* [24] to present antigens to donor (naïve) T cells to initiate GVHD. These APCs can be professional myeloid dendritic cells (mDCs) or "less professional" APCs of hematopoietic origin (macrophages or B cells). Subsequently, it was shown that in CD4-mediated GVHD in MHC-matched pairs, both *recipient and donor hematopoietic APCs* [25, 26] are *sufficient* to prime donor T cells. Lately, this dogma has been called into question following the observation that plasmacytoid dendritic cells can also induce aGVHD [27]. Subsequently, it was shown that recipient non-hematopoietic tissues can actually present the antigens to previously activated (in an antigen-independent fashion) donor CD4 cells, resulting in lethal aGVHD. These non-hematopoietic APCs express vimentin and α-smooth muscle actin and are probably *myofibroblasts*. They express MHC class II and co-stimulatory molecules as well. The *intestinal epithelial cells* themselves, under inflammatory conditions and in the presence of IFNγ, can also express MHC class II and present antigens [28]. It has even been shown that the collective depletion of B cells, mDCs, and pDCs was insufficient to inhibit aGVHD [29].

2.5 Co-stimulatory Molecules

Blockade of CD80 and CD86 either by antibodies or by CTLA4-Ig was shown to ameliorate aGVHD [30]. Similar attenuation of GVHD resulted from targeting of the OX40L–OX40 system, the CD137 (4-1BB), the ICOS, the CD153-CD30 axis, and the LIGHT-HVEM pathway. Targeting of the CD40 pathway may induce tolerance [31]. CTLA-4 seems also to play a role in tolerance, while blocking the co-inhibitory molecule PD-1 appears to aggravate aGVHD. Co-blockade of CD28 and ICOS has an additive effect in GVHD prevention [32] as does blocking anti-CD40L in CD28-knockout animals. Both soluble and membrane-bound CD30 in CD8 central memory and in CD8 effector cells are increased in aGVHD patients, while CD30+ cells were increased in the gut of patients with GVHD [33]. Nevertheless, none of these co-stimulatory axes seem to be independently essential for aGVHD induction.

2.6 Innate Immunity Receptors

Irrespectively of which cell presents the alloantigens to donor T cell, that "antigen-presenting cell" has to be stimulated or activated (whether it is a host tissue cell or a professional APC). It is well known that immature DCs can actually be tolerogenic [34] and increase T_{REG}. APCs seem to be activated through a variety of mechanisms including toll-like receptors (TLRs), NOD-like receptors (NLRs), receptors for damage-associated molecular patterns (DAMPs), CD40, and cytokines. In GVHD mice models, the activation of TLR4 by bacterial lipopolysaccharide (LPS) potentiated GVHD [35]. Similarly deleterious in mice models was the activation of TLR9 [36] by CpG repeats and of TLR7 (the receptor for single-stranded RNA) by a strong agonist (R-848). Activation of TLR5 by flagellin decreases GVHD [37]. NOD2 (an intracellular receptor of muramyl dipeptide, a component of bacterial cell walls) seems to be protective [38]. P2X7 is a DAMP receptor for ATP and it also seems to potentiate GVHD [39], while P2X7 blockade has a protective effect. Strategies of gut decontamination with antibiotics (to reduce APC activation) are actively being investigated.

2.7 Target Antigens

In MHC-matched allo-HCT, donor T cells can recognize as foreign MHC-epitope complexes on the surface of recipient cells if the epitope source is a protein that differs between the donor and the recipient. *Gene polymorphisms* are responsible for the generation of different epitopes on the recipient that are not present on the donor. These antigens are frequently called minor histocompatibility antigens (miHA) [40]. Examples include the male-specific H-Y antigens and the antigens HA-1, HA-2, HPA-3, PECAM (CD31), and PANE-1. Some of these antigens have tissue-dependent expression patterns that could be responsible for *tissue-specific aGVHD*. Some miHA can induce very strong allo-immune reactions [41].

2.8 *Trafficking*

L-selectin (CD62L) is important for homing of naïve T cells to lymphoid structures. P-selectin is expressed on the endothelium and is important for T cell–endothelium interaction, while its ligand (PSGL1) is upregulated during GVHD. The integrin $\alpha4\beta7$ is essential for recruitment of T cells back to the intestines [42]. Multiple chemokine receptors affect T cell trafficking in GVHD including CXCR3, CCR4, and CCR5. The sphingosine-1 receptor FTY720 in experimental GVHD seems to maintain alloreactive T cells in the lymph nodes preventing them from migrating to the inflammatory site [43].

3 Strategies to Prevent aGVHD

3.1 *Find the Best Compatible Donor*

Matched sibling donors are preferred. A high-resolution match between donor and recipient at HLA-A, B, C, and DR is usually required for MUD allo-HCT in Western world countries. National Marrow Donor Program (NMDP) data initially showed that HLA-DQ and HLA-DP mismatches did not have a significant impact on GVHD [44]. Later, an analysis of 8500 transplant pairs demonstrated permissive and nonpermissive HLA-DP mismatches and that nonpermissive mismatches were associated with higher rates of severe aGVHD, non-relapse and overall mortality, but lower incidence of relapse, relative to HLA-DP-matched pairs [45]. Similarly, a mismatch at the minor histocompatibility locus coding for HA-1 increases the risk for GVHD. KIR/KIR ligand mismatch in the haploidentical setting seems to prevent relapses of myeloid malignancies through NK cell-mediated lysis of leukemia after conditioning with TBI and T cell depletion (and without post-transplant immunosuppression) [46]. Furthermore, NMDP data showed that KIR genotyping could identify that donors with high content of the so called "B-motifs" conferred lower relapse risk to recipients with AML but not ALL [47].

MHC haplotype match implies identical genetic material in the entire MHC coding region that seems to encode multiple other genes that affect transplant outcome. MHC haplotype match decreases significantly the GVHD risk. The high-resolution HLA typing that is performed routinely does not guarantee MHC haplotype match. Since 22 % of the high-resolution HLA-identical (allelic match) unrelated donor-recipient pairs do not share identical MHC haplotypes, novel array methodology has been developed to improve matching [48].

The source of stem cells (bone marrow or peripheral blood) also affects the risk of cGVHD with PBSCs conferring higher risk than bone marrow. In the setting of nonmalignant disease (e.g., aplastic anemia) the lack of a GVL-associated benefit has been shown to favor marrow transplantation, due to the excess morbidity and mortality associated with cGVHD.

3.2 Other Factors Affecting GVHD Incidence

Other donor factors that have been suggested to affect the incidence of GVHD are age, gender, and parity and, more recently, the possible use of statins [49]. Older donor age has been associated with an increased incidence of both severe aGVHD and cGVHD and decreased overall survival after allo-HCT. Male recipients who have female multiparous donors (especially mothers of multiple sons) have higher incidence of cGVHD.

3.3 Standard Prevention

So far, the standard of care for GVHD prevention has been the use of low-dose methotrexate (given repeatedly in low doses) plus long-term therapy using a calcineurin inhibitor (CNI, cyclosporine or tacrolimus). The addition of corticosteroids as a third medication, even in a delayed fashion (e.g., starting 2 weeks after transplant) is not beneficial. In UCBT, methotrexate is often replaced by mycophenolate mofetil (MMF) to limit the duration of post-transplant cytopenias.

In most centers some degree of in vivo T cell depletion (ATG or alemtuzumab, which depletes both B and T cells) is applied in the MUD setting. Some centers routinely utilize ex vivo lymphocyte depletion for MUD or even MSD allo-HCT. In allo-HCT for benign diseases the use of ATG is more common even in the MSD setting to reduce GVHD. A recent retrospective analysis compared the outcomes with ATG, alemtuzumab or no TCD after reduced-intensity allo-HCT in patients with hematologic malignancies. The use of ATG compared to no TCD was associated with less GVHD, higher relapse rate and lower 3-year overall survival [50]. The use of alemtuzumab decreased GVHD further but disease relapse and infections were more common.

For decades, some degree of bacterial decontamination of the bouel has been applied at most centers, and it is possible that reducing bacterial load at the time of intestinal mucosal injury may limit danger signals that result in APC activation. Most centers use an oral fluoroquinolone, although in the MSD setting, lower incidence of aGVHD was observed in patients who received ciprofloxacin and metronidazole compared to ciprofloxacin alone.

3.4 Novel Pharmacological Approaches

To improve historical results with CNI-based therapy, recent studies have combined tacrolimus with the mTOR inhibitor sirolimus [51], which allows earlier engraftment and decreases mucositis at the expense of higher risk for thrombotic microangiopathy and sinusoidal obstruction syndrome (SOS), especially when myeloablative doses of busulfan are used. A phase III trial is prospectively comparing the combination tacrolimus-methotrexate with tacrolimus-sirolimus across BMT Clinical Trials Network (CTN) institutions. CNI use is associated with nephrotoxicity, may inhibit T_{REG}, and may harm thymic stroma, potentially impairing immune reconstitution. Sirolimus relatively spares T_{REG}, so attempts to combine sirolimus to improve the ratios of T_{REG}/T_{CON} are under exploration. In one small study, the combination of sirolimus with MMF after busulfan-based conditioning increased the incidence of SOS. In another pilot study, pre-transplant alemtuzumab was given in combination with post-transplant sirolimus in adults with hemoglobinopathies with promising results [52].

In a mouse model, the post-transplant use of IL-2 with sirolimus [20] expanded natural T_{REG} and increased the induction of T_{REG} from CD4+CD25-T_{CON}, increasing the T_{REG}/T_{CON} ratio, and decreasing GVHD incidence. In humans low-dose IL-2 (1 $MU/m^2/day \times 8$ weeks) has been tried in a population of patients with steroid-refractory chronic GVHD (cGVHD) with a remarkable 52 % response rate, facilitating steroid tapering [53].

3.5 Total Lymphoid Irradiation/ATG

In an attempt to increase T_{REG} in the setting of NMA conditioning, low-dose total lymphoid irradiation (TLI) (total of 8 Gy in ten fractions) was combined with ATG (thymoglobulin, total dose = 7.5 mg/kg). The risk of both acute and chronic GVHD were very low, an effect postulated to be caused by radioresistance of iNKT and IL-4 dependent expansion of T_{REG} [54].

3.6 Post-transplant Cyclophosphamide

Another intriguing recent approach to decrease GVHD incidence is the use of post-transplant cyclophosphamide (50 mg/kg × 2 doses on days +3 and +4). At the expense of delayed engraftment, the rates of aGVHD, and especially cGVHD, are remarkably low despite only limited use of other post-transplant immunosuppressive medications [55]. It is believed that cyclophosphamide kills proliferative alloreactive donor T cells that have been primed at this early interval.

3.7 Cytokine-Directed Antibody Therapies

The addition of the 2A3 monoclonal antibody against IL-2Rα (CD25) or the addition of human recombinant IL-1R antagonist (Anakinra) to cyclosporine and methotrexate did not further prevent GVHD. TNFα seems to play a role in the pathogenesis of GVHD and the Michigan group has shown that day +7 TNFR1 (compared to the pre-transplant level) is predictive of occurrence of severe GVHD [56]. Etanercept (soluble TNF-receptor) was tested in a phase II trial in high risk for GVHD patients and decreased the d +7 TNFR1 levels but only in the non-TBI setting (compared to historic controls). That group of patients sustained only a 14 % grade III–IV aGVHD and the 1-year overall survival was 69 % [57]. Infliximab an antibody against TNFα failed to decrease the expected incidence of a GVHD when it was added to cyclosporine-methotrexate.

3.8 *Pentostatin*

A phase I/II study in MUD or mismatched related allo-HCT sought to evaluate the effect of omission of day +11 methotrexate and addition of pentostatin (1.5 mg/m^2 on days +8, +15, +22, and +30) to tacrolimus and ATG. This strategy decreased severe aGVHD but also increased the graft failure rate [58]. The study met its statistical endpoint for success.

3.9 *Maraviroc*

Maraviroc (Selzentry) is a CCR5 oral antagonist which inhibits the RANTES-CCR5 interaction and is FDA-approved for AIDS. In a recent phase I/II trial, maraviroc at a dose of 300 mg twice a day on days −2 to +30 decreased the incidence of severe aGVHD (d +180 cumulative grade III–IV aGVHD of 6 %) without increasing NRM or reducing GVL [59].

4 Treatment of aGVHD

4.1 *Initial Therapy*

Low-grade skin aGVHD can be treated with topical corticosteroids (e.g., triamcinolone), but higher grade aGVHD is treated with systemic glucocorticoids. Most centers start methylprednisolone (MP) at 2 mg/kg/day in divided doses. The calcineurin inhibitor that was used for prophylaxis is typically continued when steroids are added. Strong antimicrobial prophylaxis is started against bacteria, herpesviruses, fungi, and against *Pneumocystis jiroveci*. Close monitoring for reactivation of chronic viral infections (e.g., CMV and EBV) is essential, as high rates of reactivation are common during steroid therapy.

Several studies have assessed outcomes with combination therapies, relative to initial therapy with steroids alone. Indeed, the upfront use of daclizumab (anti-CD25) in combination with steroids increased early mortality. The combination of infliximab+MP was not superior to MP alone [60]. Similarly a combination of ATG+prednisone was not better than prednisone alone. However, a phase II trial of initial etanercept+MP compared favorably to contemporary patients with GVHD treated with MP alone [61]. A randomized phase II study for initial treatment of aGVHD started patients on MP and maintained CNI and randomized them to either MMF, pentostatin, denileukin diflitox, or etanercept [62]. The combination of MMF and MP was the winner, yielding a CR rate of 60 % and improved overall survival at 9 months. A confirmatory phase III trial is needed.

If aGVHD is controlled, steroids are tapered relatively rapidly (e.g., 0.2 mg/kg every 5 days until a dose of 1 mg/kg is reached). Then the dose is tapered more gradually (e.g., a 10–15 % reduction weekly). Nevertheless, a lot of these patients will develop extensive chronic GVHD. For patients who do not respond well to steroids (steroid-refractory) or in whom steroids cannot be tapered (steroid-dependent) the prognosis is very poor.

4.2 *Studies of Immunosuppressive Therapies for Steroid-Refractory GVHD*

Multiple studies have been conducted in the setting of steroid-refractory aGVHD (SR-GVHD) [63]. Although multiple therapies have demonstrated efficacy, all effective therapies increase the rates of opportunistic infections and/or disease relapse. Most of these patients experience a significant decrease in performance status and experience direct and indirect (e.g., infection-related) complications.

Daclizumab is a monoclonal antibody against CD25. It is usually given at a dose of 1.0 mg/kg iv on days 1, 4, 8, 15, 22 and is associated with very good control of aGVHD in at least half of patients with SR-GVHD. Unfortunately the results are temporary in most cases and many patients develop extensive cGVHD.

Infliximab is a monoclonal anti-TNFα antibody which is usually given iv at a dose of 10 mg/kg on days 1, 8, 15, 22. Although very good responses at the range of 60 % have been described especially for GI SR-GVHD, such responses are usually short-lived. The medication is associated with high rates of opportunistic infections including mycobacterial infections.

Etanercept which is soluble TNFα receptor is usually given subcutaneously at a dose of 25 mg twice a week for 4 weeks and then once a week for 4 additional weeks (12 total doses). It has demonstrated encouraging activity in about half of patients with SR-GVHD (mainly GI aGVHD).

The combination of etanercept and daclizumab has demonstrated responses in more than 50 % of patients but the long-term effects of the combination were disappointing with most patients succumbing to infection or GVHD. Similarly the combination of infliximab–daclizumab resulted in a 47 % response rate, although all patients eventually died. However, the same combination was more efficacious in a pediatric population with SR-GVHD, with 68 % of children alive 31 months later [64].

Horse ATG (ATGAM), once a standard treatment for SR-GVHD, was more recently shown to have limited efficacy, with only 5 % of 69 patients surviving long-term. Similarly another study of rabbit ATG (Thymoglobulin) resulted in only 2/36 (6 %) evaluable patients with SR-GVHD being long-term survivors. ATG, however, has been used in combination with etanercept with or without MMF while maintaining MP and CNI. The response rate was high (80 %) with a median survival of 224 days. From the 16 patients on the study, five died from infection, two from GVHD and one from relapse of the underlying malignancy [65].

Alemtuzumab is a very immunosuppressive medication and should be used carefully. Early administration (second line) and low doses (10 mg iv weekly) was more effective than late administration (third line after salvage with ATG/etanercept) and higher doses (10 mg iv daily for 5 days). The former mode of administration gave a 70 % response rate in 20 evaluable patients. Half of the responses were complete and the median survival was 280 days.

The Dana-Farber group reported on the use of denileukin diflitox, which is a conjugate of IL-2 with diphtheria toxin. Hepatotoxicity was the dose-limiting toxicity but the response rate was high with 50 % CR, 21 % PR, and 1/3 of patients surviving at least 6 months [66].

MMF (1,000 mg orally twice daily) yielded a response rate of 42 % but with very few long-term survivors (16 %). Pentostatin at a dose of 1.5 mg/m^2 iv daily for 3 days gave an impressive 64 % CR rate with 26 % of patients with SR-GVHD surviving at 1 year [67]. Sirolimus at relatively high doses benefited 57 % of patients, although only one patient survived more than a year. Other studies have shown better results with sirolimus, either as salvage or as a frontline treatment of aGVHD, in patients in whom steroids could not be used [68, 69].

Another approach to treat acute SR-GVHD is extracorporeal photopheresis (ECP) in which peripheral blood lymphocytes are separated and incubated with 8-methoxypsoralen and then irradiated with ultraviolet A (UVA) before they are returned back to the patient. ECP requires a central catheter and frequent treatments. ECP may result in apoptosis of cells taken up by APCs that become tolerogenic and increase the number of T_{REG}. In the first pilot Austrian study, 21 patients with SR-GVHD grades II–IV were treated with ECP. 57 % of patients were alive after a median follow-up of 25 months. The response rates were very high for grade II–III GVHD, but only 12 % of patients with grade IV aGVHD responded to the treatment. Most other studies have consistently showed encouraging activity for grade II–III with lower efficacy in more severe GVHD [70].

The use of mesenchymal stem cells (MSCs) initially yielded great enthusiasm. Early reports and a phase II study were promising, though a phase III trial failed to demonstrate a statistically significant improvement over placebo in initial aGVHD and SR-GVHD [71].

5 Selected Novel Approaches/Proposals for Prevention and Treatment of Acute GVHD (Table 1)

- Tocilizumab, an anti-IL-6 monoclonal antibody. Besides its inflammatory properties, IL-6 participates in the T_H17 cell differentiation. Absence of IL-6 can skew T cell differentiation to induced regulatory cells (iT_{REG}). In a pilot study [72] four of six patients with acute SR-GVHD responded to this agent.
- Low-dose IL-2 followed by sirolimus. IL-2 has to be given right away after stem cell infusion (before priming of potentially alloreactive T cells). The intent is to expand donor natural T_{REG} and to utilize sirolimus to selectively limit the function/proliferation of alloreactive T_{CON}. This strategy is being investigated in the setting of both initial prophylaxis and steroid-refractory GVHD therapy.

Table 1 Selected novel immune manipulations for prevention or treatment of GVHD

Target	Method	Aim
↑Treg	Infusion of CD4+CD25+CD127(−) cells (before HCT)	Prevent aGVHD
	Low-dose IL-2 post-HCT	Prevent aGVHD or treat cGVHD
	Photopheresis (preferential expansion of Treg)	Treatment of cGVHD
↑iNKT	Total lymphoid irradiation (0.8 Gy × 10) before HCT	Prevention of aGVHD
	Liposomal a-galactosylceramide (REG-2001) after HCT	
↑Th17	Ustekinumab (anti-IL-12 and -IL-23)	Prevent or treat aGVHD by preventing expansion of Th17
	Tocilizumab (anti-IL-6)	
↑Tnaive	Anti-CD45RA before HCT	Prevention of aGVHD through depletion of naïve CD4 cells
Gut flora	Rifaximin, metronidazole peritransplant	Prevention of a GVHD through decreasing TLR stimulation
CD80 CD86	CTLA-4 Ig (Abatacept, Belatacept)	Prevent aGVHD by blocking co-stimulation and inducing anergy
α4β7	MLN-002 (monoclonal antibody)	Prevent homing of T cells to gut
CCR5	Maravicor (oral drug inhibiting RANTES-CCR5 interaction)	Prevent homing of T cells
CD30	Brentuximab vedotin	Kills alloreactive T cells
Proteasome	Bortezomib, Carfilzomib	Prevent cGVHD Prevent aGVHD
BAFF	Belimumab	Prevent, treat cGVHD
HDAC	Vorinostat, romidepsin, panobinostat	Prevent aGVHD. HDAC inhibitors decrease the efficiency of antigen presentation

Abbreviations: *aGVHD* acute graft-versus-host disease, *cGVHD* chronic graft-versus-host disease, *HDAC* histone deacetylase, *BAFF* B-cell activating factor, *Treg* regulatory T cells, *iNKT* invariant natural killer T cells, *TLR* toll-like receptor, *IL* interleukin, *HCT* hematopoietic stem cell transplantation

- Ustekinumab: This represents an antibody against p40, which is shared by the cytokines IL-12 and IL-23. IL-12 has been proposed as a third signal for polarization of T cells to T_H1, while IL-23 facilitates T_H17 differentiation. This has to be given for prevention before T cell polarization happens. A patient with SR-GVHD having failed multiple treatments received this agent and responded completely, but later died of bacterial sepsis [73].
- CD45RA-depleted grafts: CD45RA is expressed on naïve T cells primarily responsible for GVHD induction, and therefore might selectively deplete alloreactivity without compromising GVL and immune reconstitution.
- Bortezomib: By giving bortezomib during conditioning, there is a possibility of sensitization of tumor stem cells to chemotherapy. Also, bortezomib, when is given before and just after allo-HCT, may be able to decrease antigen presentation by MHC class I, impair the maturation of dendritic cells and reduce donor GVHD-mediating T cells [74, 75]. Bortezomib may also be used later in an attempt to decrease cGVHD, through its effect on post-germinal center B cells and plasma cells. Multiple studies are ongoing [76].
- Statins: Use of statins by the donor before stem cell collection and by the recipients before and after transplant may decrease GVHD through direct effects on T cells as well as inhibition of activation of APCs. Retrospective studies of outcomes in donors taking statins and prospective studies of recipients are underway.
- Liposomal a-galactosylceramide (RGI-2001, Regimmune, Inc.) is a molecule that if presented through CD1d to invariant NKT cells, increases the T_{REG}/T_{CON} ratio via iNKT-T_{REG} crosstalk and decreases GVHD. Animal models have shown promising results [77] and the molecule is being tested in a multicenter phase I clinical trial, given immediately post-HCT.
- Inhibition of α4 or α4β7 integrins: If this is done early, it can inhibit migration of potentially alloreactive T cells to the gut. Natalizumab is a α4-specific antibody approved for multiple sclerosis and Crohn disease as a monthly infusion. It is associated with opportunistic infections, including JC-associated progressive multifocal leukoencephalopathy (PML). Novel therapies (e.g., vedolizumab) have demonstrated encouraging results in inflammatory diseases of the gut [78] with the potential to be less immunosuppressive than natalizumab.
- Histone diacetylase inhibitors (HDACi): Vorinostat/panobinostat/romidepsin: In animal models, HDACi reduce GVHD by inhibiting upregulation of costimulatory molecules and secretion of inflammatory cytokines by APC. Their effect seems to be mediated by upregulation of IDO [79]. HDACi also promote the generation and function of T_{REG} [80]. HDACi are being investigated in the setting of GVHD prophylaxis.
- Infusion of T_{REG}. These cells have been reported to decrease GVHD while preserving GVL. Their immunophenotype is CD4+ CD25+ CD127− CD62L+ FoxP3+. Ex vivo expansion and infusion has allowed subsequent low-dose donor T_{CON} infusion in haploidentical allo-HCT in an Italian study [81]. Multiple studies are underway in the setting of conventional and UCB-HCT.

- Brentuximab vedotin: It has been shown that CD30+ T cells number is high in situ in patients with gut aGVHD. Treatment with the anti-CD30 immunotoxin brentuximab vedotin maybe helpful in patients with steroid-refractory or steroid-dependent gut aGVHD, although initial data have shown significant myelosuppression.
- PKCθ inhibitors: In an animal model PKCθ inhibition attenuated T_H1 responses and accentuated T_{REG} function, thereby selectively inhibiting GVHD while preserves GvL and antiviral responses [82]. Sotrastaurin (AEB071), although inferior than tacrolimus in the human renal transplant setting, increased the survival of primates with a renal allograft in combination with a CNI. Its efficacy is currently studied in the solid organ transplant setting in combination with tacrolimus (vs. tacrolimus + MMF).

6 Chronic Graft Versus Disease

6.1 Pathogenesis and Translational Implications

cGVHD is a very frequent complication after allo-HCT with an incidence rate up to 70 %. It is a major determinant of disability and most patients with extensive disease require long-term immunosuppression to control the disease. Its incidence increases with mismatch donor–recipient pairs and with MUD allo-HCT compared to matched MRD allo-HCT. The use of a female donor (especially multiparous) in a male recipient also increases GVHD incidence. cGVHD incidence also increases in the setting of PBSCT vs. BMT and with increasing donor and recipient age. Conversely, ex vivo TCD, ATG [83], or alemtuzumab given before allo-HCT are protective, implying that T cells play a significant role at least in the initiation phase.

6.2 B Cells and cGVHD

Recently it has been appreciated that B cells contribute to cGVHD pathogenesis since many of its manifestations resemble auto-immune diseases (e.g., systemic sclerosis). Anti-host antibodies (e.g., the anti-H-Y anti-male antibodies in cases of gender disparity) [84] and also the agonistic antibodies against the PDGFR have been implicated in the pathogenesis of sclerodermatous cGVHD, which may respond to PDGFR inhibitors like imatinib [85]. Rituximab (an anti-CD20 Ab) may have efficacy in established cGVHD [86] and may prevent cGVHD development [87].

6.3 BAFF and B Cell Homeostasis in cGVHD

Patients with cGVHD have elevated levels of B-cell activating factor (BAFF) and decreased numbers of naïve B cells (B cell dysregulation) [87]. Experiments in mouse models of arthritis have shown that BAFF promotes T_H17 differentiation [88]. BAFF is also important for the survival of plasma cells and its level is high in patients with myeloma. Belimumab [89] is a monoclonal Ab against BAFF, which has been approved for advanced SLE. Its use could possibly affect B cell dysregulation, plasma cell proliferation, and T_H17 polarization in cGVHD. If plasma cells play a role in cGVHD then targeting them with bortezomib may be beneficial. At least one study is evaluating bortezomib in chronic pulmonary cGVHD, with the intent of decreasing the signaling of pro-fibrotic TGF-β1 signaling.

6.4 Direct and Indirect Targeting of Regulatory T Cells

T_{REG} are thought to be beneficial in cGVHD and since they are dependent on IL-2, a Dana-Farber study of low-dose IL-2 in steroid-refractory cGVHD gave very good results [53]. For the same reason, sirolimus is increasingly used in cGVHD [90] instead of calcineurin inhibitors, since it is thought that mTOR inhibitors respect T_{REG}. Extracorporeal photophoresis (ECP) is commonly used successfully in cGVHD and one of its mechanisms of action is thought to be related to T_{REG} upregulation [91].

6.5 First-Line Treatment of cGVHD

Initial therapy of cGVHD is becoming increasingly standardized. If the patient has limited skin involvement or mild involvement of two organs (e.g., sicca symptoms and limited skin involvement) without lung involvement and without thrombocytopenia (PLT < 100,000) or hyperbilirubinemia (total bilirubin > 2 mg/dL), then topical (skin, mouth, eyes) steroids or topical calcineurin inhibitors or oral ursodiol (for isolated elevation of alkaline phosphatase) can be tried with close follow-up. Otherwise the patient should be started on prednisone at 1 mg/kg/day. The combination of oral prednisone and a CNI was not superior to prednisone alone in recipients of bone marrow with moderate cGVHD and without thrombocytopenia [92]. Many physicians, however, prefer such a combination in severe forms of extensive cGVHD or for cGVHD and concurrent thrombocytopenia or when fast tapering of steroids is needed [93–96]. CNI addition is also favored if cGVHD onset concurred with withdrawal of previous prophylactic CNI.

6.6 mTOR Inhibition

Many theorize that mTOR inhibitors are better steroid partners because they are more favorable to T_{REG}. For that reason, the current BMT-CTN trial 0801 randomizes patients to either prednisone-sirolimus or to prednisone-sirolimus plus a calcineurin inhibitor. Irrespectively of the initial treatment, responders stay on an initial high steroid dose initially, with only gradual taper thereafter. Flares of cGVHD can happen with faster tapering. The partner drug of prednisone should be maintained at therapeutic plasma levels during the entire period. Ursodiol for liver disease, topical steroids and minimally absorbable steroids like oral budesonide and oral beclomethasone can be used in combination during this period. The role of extracorporeal photopheresis as an addition to a steroid-based initial treatment of cGVHD is an objective of an ongoing clinical trial. When cGVHD develops during treatment of aGVHD (progressive onset cGVHD) the prognosis is more likely to be adverse.

6.7 Second-Line Treatment of cGVHD

Patients with cGVHD who do not respond to steroid-based treatment (steroid-refractory) or in whom the dose of prednisone can't be tapered below 1 mg/kg/day after 3 months (or fail tapering below 0.5 mg/kg/day) require additional systemic treatment. Agents that have shown efficacy and used frequently include ECP, rituximab, sirolimus, imatinib (for sclerodermatous and pulmonary GVHD), pentostatin, and mycophenolate. Other approaches less commonly employed include switching to the alternative calcineurin inhibitor, pulses of methylprednisolone, methotrexate, infliximab, thalidomide [97], clofazimine, hydroxychloroquine, cyclophosphamide, etanercept [98], oral retinoids, PUVA, alemtuzumab, low dose of thoracoabdominal irradiation [99], and infusion of mesenchymal stem cells. There is a paucity of randomized trials and durable complete responses are only occasionally seen. The use of immunosuppression is associated with many side effects including opportunistic infections and secondary malignancies.

6.8 cGVHD: Organ-Specific Interventions

Organ-specific management of cGVHD can sometimes decrease the needs for potent systemic immunosuppression and improve results [93, 100, 101]. For cutaneous cGVHD topical medium to high potency steroids like triamcinolone or clobetasol are used except from the face and the flexural areas where only mild potency steroids are allowed. Use of topical calcineurin inhibitors like tacrolimus or pimecrolimus can help and is associated with less skin atrophy. Emollients help pruritus and xerosis. Oral anti-histamines, gabapentin, or doxepin are used for intense pruritus. The risk for skin infections (viral, fungal, and bacterial) and malignancies with both steroids and CNI is increased. Sunscreen use is very important. For sclerodermatous cGVHD, physiotherapy should be employed to avoid contractures. ECP can be used as second-line steroid-sparing treatment. UVB and PUVA may be helpful, especially when there is no access to ECP.

In ocular GVHD, artificial tears, and cyclosporine drops help. For severe xerophthalmia, plugging the lacrimal ducts has been tried successfully. Patients with acute/subacute onset of impaired vision and ocular pain should be referred to an ophthalmologist to diagnose and treat disorders like uveitis, retinal problems, herpetic infections, and cataracts. Oral cGVHD is very common and oral solutions of dexamethasone, budesonide, or betamethasone have been used successfully. For significant xerostomia, pilocarpine is used in a similar fashion to patients with Sjogren's syndrome.

All patients with cGVHD are at increased risk of infection, and prophylaxis is required against pneumococcus, viruses, PCP, and fungi (posaconazole preferred for patients on high-dose immunosuppression). Immunoglobulin deficiency should be corrected, and pneumococcal, influenza, and Hemophilus influenza vaccines should be given. Screening for CMV is required.

Pulmonary cGVHD should be confirmed by biopsy and infections must be ruled out. BOOP is usually responsive to steroids, but bronchiolitis obliterans (BO) is problematic. Inhaled corticosteroids in addition to systemic immunosuppression may help. Monthly pulses of steroids have been used. Imatinib and ECP can be beneficial. Oral azithromycin and oral montelukast are often prescribed. Infections are frequent and vaccines, antimicrobial prophylaxis and Ig replenishment are all employed [102]. Long-term prognosis of BO is dismal. All patients with cGVHD on steroids should be monitored and treated for osteoporosis and hormonal (thyroid, gonadal, adrenals') deficiencies.

7 Antitumor Post-transplant Immune Manipulation (Table 2)

Relapse following allo-HCT carries a relatively ominous prognosis. There are three approaches against post-transplant neoplastic relapse: (a) Prevention, (b) Preemptive therapy of minimal residual disease, and (c) Treatment of clinical relapse. The following sections review selected strategies that may be employed against post-HCT relapse.

7.1 Immunomodulatory Molecules

One of the best examples of preventive immunotherapy post-transplant is the use of the immunomodulatory molecules, thalidomide [103], and lenalidomide, for

Table 2 Selected approaches to decrease relapse after allogeneic HCT

Approach	Rationale	Potential problems
Lenalidomide	Augment NK and T cell attack against myeloma MRD	Myelosuppression, GVHD
Abl-TKIs (imatinib, dasatinib, nilotinib, bosutinib, ponatinib)	Target MRD in CML and Ph + ALL	Myelosuppression, immunosuppression
Ibrutinib	Minimize MRD in CLL and B-NHL by targeting Btk	GI symptoms, fatigue, hypogammaglobulinemia
5-Azacytidine	Decrease relapse of myeloid malignancies	Myelosuppression
Rituximab	Decrease relapse of CD20+ malignancies may reduce cGVHD	Hypogammaglobulinemia, myelosuppression
Ipilimumab	Inhibit immunologic tolerance by inhibiting CTLA-4	Aggravation of GVHD, immune endocrinopathies
CT-011	Inhibit anergy by blocking PD1	GVHD?
IL-2, IL-7, IL-21	Boost T cell function	Capillary leak syndrome, fever, arthralgia, GVHD?
Peptide vaccines (WT-1, PR1)	Educate the immune system to attack antigens over-expressed in malignant cells	Low immunogenicity
Dendritic cell vaccines ± TLR7/TLR9 agonists	Enhance cancer cell antigen presentation	Complicated production of the vaccine
CARs	Join an immunoglobulin recognizing a cancer antigen to the TCR signaling cascade	Difficult production, decreased survival of engineered T cells, requires costimulatory receptors and a virus as a vehicle of the genes
NK cell infusion	Augment innate immunity	May need cytokine treatment for enhanced efficacy
Preemptive DLI	Augment GvL	GVHD
Donor with KIR ligand mismatch and/or donor with activating KIR receptors (e.g., KIR2DS1)	Increase NK activity against mainly myeloid malignancies	Difficult to find such donors

Abbreviations: *NK* natural killer cells, *MRD* minimal residual disease, *GVHD* graft-versus-host disease, *TKI* tyrosine kinase inhibitor, *CML* chronic myeloid leukemia, *ALL* acute lymphoblastic leukemia, *NHL* non-hodgkin lymphoma, *CLL* chronic lymphocytic leukemia, *Btk* bruton kinase, *Ph* Philadelphia, *GI* gastrointestinal, *PD1* programmed death-1, *TLR* toll-like receptor, *TCR* T cell receptor, *CAR* chimeric antigen receptor, *GvL* graft versus leukemia, *KIR* killer-immunoglobulin-like receptor, *WT-1* Wilms tumor antigen 1, *Abl* Abelson kinase

prevention of myeloma relapse after auto-HCT. Both have been associated with improved progression-free survival (PFS) and lenalidomide use has been correlated with improved OS as well [104]. It is interesting that the doses used are lower than the conventional anti-myeloma doses and it has been theorized that is not only the anti-myeloma effect but the immune-stimulatory effect of lenalidomide which is responsible for the improved outcome. Lenalidomide increases NK cell cytotoxic function mainly through NKG2D upregulation. It also increases ADCC function of NK cells. In fact lenalidomide has been successfully used with DLI post-allo-HCT in myeloma and trials are being conducted using lenalidomide after allo-HCT for high-risk MDS and AML, especially those with 5q- known to respond to lenalidomide.

7.2 *Tyrosine Kinase Inhibitors*

Although imatinib, dasatinib, and nilotinib have been used both prophylactically and therapeutically for CML relapse post-HCT [105], this is not considered an immune manipulation by itself, although these agents may also influence immune function. Similar post-transplant maintenance may be seen in the future in CLL using agents like PI3Kδ inhibitors or Btk inhibitors. Interestingly, Btk inhibition reduces GVHD in murine models [106] suggesting a role for B cells in pathogenesis.

7.3 *Hypomethylating Agents*

Hypomethylating agents like 5-azacytidine are being used post-allo-HCT to decrease the relapse rate of AML. It may be possible that 5-azacytidine enhances GvL (upregulates the expression of leukemia antigens) without exacerbating GVHD (increases Tregs). Recent encouraging data have emerged from studies treating high-risk patients with myeloid malignancies with post-HCT therapy [107].

7.4 *Anti-Lymphoma Antibodies*

Rituximab was tested successfully as a strategy to prevent relapses of aggressive B cell lymphomas after auto-HCT [108]. After allo-HCT the use of antibody therapy can buy time for an effective GVL to develop and may also facilitate phagocytosis of the targeted cells and tumor antigen cross-priming. Recently it has been shown clearly in preclinical models that both the agonistic anti-CD137 [109] and the antagonistic anti-CD47 can potentiate the effect of monoclonal antibodies including rituximab in preclinical models [110]. Both of these strategies may prove beneficial to prevent and treat post-transplant relapse; however, the use of agonistic CD137 post-allo-HCT must be viewed with caution, given GVHD exacerbation in murine models.

7.5 Fighting Tolerance

CTLA-4 and PD-1 are two very important mediators of post-transplant immune tolerance. Positive clinical trials with antibodies against CTLA-4 and PD-1 have been reported in melanoma and other solid tumors and the anti-CTLA-4 antibody, and ipilimumab has already been granted FDA approval for the treatment of melanoma. Ipilimumab has generated responses in relapsed lymphoma after allo-HCT without inducing GVHD [111]. CT-011 is an anti-PD1 monoclonal being studied in myeloma patients in the post-auto-HCT setting, alone and in combination with a dendritic-myeloma fussion cell vaccine. Another approach to release the brakes of immune response is to inhibit MDSCs. 1-methyl-D-tryptophan is an oral IDO inhibitor and is being tried in solid tumors.

7.6 Cytokines as a Boost

Enhancement of antitumor T cell responses can be tried with cytokines. The selection and dose of cytokine(s) are critical since for example high doses of IL-2 or IFNγ can lead to activation-induced cell death (AICD) and T cell exhaustion. IL-21 is not associated with CD8 exhaustion or AICD and in viral illnesses decreases the percentage of exhausted CD43++/PD-1++ CD8 cells [112]. IL-21 has been tried in metastatic renal cell carcinoma and melanoma and induced responses [113]. IL-15 has been shown to be critical for memory T cells and for optimal NK function and is not associated with T cell exhaustion or AICD. It has been studied in immunotherapy trials of NK cell infusion in AML (University of Minnesota) and in melanoma after lymphodepleting chemotherapy and adoptive transfer of tumor infiltrating lymphocytes (TILs) at NCI. IL-7 plays a role in T cell homeostasis and broadens TCR repertoire and may decrease the frequency of natural T_{REG} which usually do not express CD127. IL-7 facilitates immune reconstitution and may increase GVHD but may also potentiate GVL. It is possible that a combination of such cytokines might be most beneficial. However optimal dosing combinations and schedules have not been determined.

Despite the concerns of T cell exhaustion and AICD, IL-2 has been given in solid tumors post-transplant. In melanoma, clinical trials demonstrated the utility of a non-myeloablative regimen of fludarabine and cyclophosphamide for T cell depletion followed by infusion of autologous stem cells and ex vivo expanded anti-melanoma T cells. These cells were either tumor infiltrating T cells or cells with an engineered anti-melanoma TCR. In the post-transplant environment of lymphopenia, T cells expanded rapidly via lymphopenia-induced proliferation and were activated by exogenously given IL-2. Durable responses were seen [114, 115].

7.7 Antitumor Vaccines

Another approach to prevent and treat post-transplant relapses is the administration of cancer peptide vaccines. Proteins that can be used for that purpose are minor histocompatibility antigens expressed in hematopoietic tissues like HA-1, HA-2, and HB-1. Other antigens include the WT-1 and the PR1 peptides alone or in combination. Both WT1 and PR1 peptide vaccines have induced immunologic and clinical responses [116, 117] with responses appearing improved with minimal disease burden. Other antigens that have been used as peptide vaccines include CD168 and a modified b3a2 fusion peptide in patients with CML. There are more questions than answers regarding the use of leukemia vaccines. What is the optimal antigen? What combination of antigens should be used? When and how often leukemia vaccines should be given? What is the optimal route of administration (intramedullary, intradermally, subcutaneously), and what is the optimal adjuvant? Should they be combined with molecules for breaking tolerance (e.g., anti-CTLA-4 antibodies) or with immune-stimulatory molecules (e.g., IFN, IL-2, IL-7, or IL-21)? Should chemotherapy be given first to debulk the tumor and create a lymphopenic environment to facilitate homeostatic expansion? What is the optimal combination of vaccines with cellular therapy (e.g., DLI)?

Besides peptide vaccines, investigators have tried to create immune responses with DC vaccines or with genetically modified leukemic cells (e.g., leukemic cells modified to secrete GM-CSF) [118]. DCs are often manipulated (e.g., by loading of mRNA via electroporation). Others have used fusion of dendritic cells with tumor cells (with myeloma or leukemia cells) [119] [120, 121]. Other studies are combining DC vaccines with TLR7 or TLR9 stimulation [122].

7.8 T Cell Engineering

A very promising strategy to treat post-transplant relapse is to use engineered T cells. These cells have been transduced with either a TCR specific for a tumor antigen of interest or a chimeric antigen receptor (CAR), which is a fusion immunoglobulin-like molecule able to recognize the target antigen. Recent attempts have combined transduction of CARs with other co-stimulatory molecules (e.g., a fusion of an immunoglobulin-like receptor with CD3ζ, CD28, and CD137). CARs used thus far in clinical trials include a CD19-specific CAR for recognition of precursor B-ALL and mature B cell neoplasms, a κ-light chain-specific CAR to target myeloma cells, and a CD30-specific CAR to recognize Hodgkin and anaplastic large cell lymphoma [123–127] One unresolved question is what cell should be the target for transfection. Options include naïve T cells, central memory cells, and EBV-specific effector

T cells. After infusion, expansion may be optimal in the setting of a lymphopenic environment, potentially yielding a benefit for chemotherapy administration. Recently, a partial response in a patient with indolent lymphoma who received a "third generation" CD20-specific CAR expressing CD28 and CD137 domains was reported [123]. Another study reported that six of eight patients with B-cell malignancies responded to an anti-CD19-CAR-transduced T cell infusion after lymphodepleting chemotherapy [127]. The T cell infusion was followed by IL-2. Patients with advanced neuroblastoma responded to anti-GD2-CAR-transfected T cells, with long-term persistence of transfected T cells [125, 128]. Complete remissions have been reported in two patients with advanced CLL by June and coworkers using CAR-T cells with investigators reporting significant CAR-T expansion and persistence, as well as profound B-cell depletion. A tumor-lysis syndrome was reported in a patient with CLL who received an anti-CD19/CD137 CAR-transduced T cell infusion. The patient stayed in remission, and there was a long-term persistence of transduced T cells which was attributed to the co-transfected CD137 [128]. More encouraging results are expected in the near future with CARs used either before or after HCT. Use of CAR may allow for increasing selective GVL responses, relative to currently employed nonspecific transfer of T cells such as DLI.

7.9 Natural Killer Cell and Cytotoxic Lymphocyte Infusions

Haploidentical NK cell infusion after high-dose fludarabine and cyclophosphamide lymphodepletion-induced complete remissions in five of 19 patients with poor-prognosis leukemia when NK cell infusions were followed by administration of IL-2 [129]. These results were not reproduced in patients with ovarian or breast cancer [130]. Disease-specific cytotoxic lymphocytes (CTLs) have been generated ex vivo and transfused. Clear responses following EBV-CTL infusions have been seen in EBV-related nasopharyngeal carcinomas [131, 132]. Similarly, responses have been obtained in melanoma patients treated with Melan-A-specific CTLs [133]. Transient responses of leukemias that relapsed post-transplant were elicited with miHA-specific CTLs at the expense of pulmonary toxicity [134].

7.10 Donor Lymphocyte Infusions

Despite encouraging results infusing antigen-specific T cells, the most common method of adoptive immunotherapy for post-transplant relapse is the infusion of non-specific donor lymphocytes (DLI) following withdrawal of immunosuppression.

In the last two decades since the original description of anti-leukemic effects of "buffy coat infusions" [135] we have enriched our knowledge about the sensitivity of different diseases to DLI and we have a better idea about the dose and the frequency of DLI in different settings [6]. Diseases like CML and indolent lymphomas respond very well to DLI. Myeloma, Hodgkin, and CLL are also sensitive but not as much as CML. Aggressive lymphomas are less sensitive and AML typically responds best when chemotherapy has decreased the tumor burden. ALL is much less responsive to DLI [136–139].

The dose of DLI used is typically one log higher when the donor is a sibling, relative to that in unrelated transplants, because of the higher incidence of GVHD in the MUD setting. Escalating doses are typically given after 4–8 weeks, if no GVHD is seen and if responses are not optimal. The onset of a DLI response can be delayed and may take 2 months or more. The pace of disease growth and degree of donor–recipient mismatch usually determine the dose and timing of initial and subsequent DLI. Even with initial doses of 20 million CD3+ cells/kg in matched siblings, the treatment-related mortality is typically less than 5 % [140].

7.11 DLI in Chronic Myeloid Leukemia

The response rate of CML to DLI depends on the disease status. It is 90 % for cytogenetic relapses and even higher for molecular relapses. The response of chronic phase CML is 70 % but is lower than 35 % in accelerated phase and even lower in blast phase. Responses in chronic phase are usually durable. Adjuvant cytokines (IFNα, GM-CSF, etc.) may be helpful in conjunction with DLI for CML [141]. A TKI inhibitor can be tried before or concurrently with DLI depending on the previous patient exposure. One recent report examined CML patients who relapsed after allo-HCT who were treated with imatinib, DLI, or the combination [142]. Patients who received the combination did much better with the majority of them achieving durable CRs.

7.12 DLI in Multiple Myeloma

Patients with myeloma frequently respond to DLI but higher doses are usually needed (100 million CD3+ cells/kg). The same recommendations for dose escalation as for CML patients apply because of the high chance of severe GVHD with higher CD3 doses. About 45 % respond and 25 % get a CR, but responses frequently are temporary, so that consolidation DLI should be considered in most cases [143–145]. In one study of 18 relapsed myeloma patients who received DLI in combination with thalidomide, the rate of CR was 22 % and ORR was 67 % with acceptable toxicity [146, 147]. In another study, DLI administered after following two cycles of lenalidomide in relapsed myeloma yielded a 2-year PFS of 50 % [148].

7.13 DLI in Acute Myeloid Leukemia

In AML, while complete responses to DLI are relatively low, DLI has shown to confer a survival benefit in relapsed AML patients, compared to chemotherapy alone (21 % vs. 9 %) [149]. Patients who received DLI with minimal disease burden fared better compared than AML patients who received DLI with active disease. Frequently, relapses happen in sanctuary sites like CNS and the gonads and consideration should be given to screen and treat these areas. Results of DLI for relapsed AML are better if the relapse happens later than 6 months after allo-HCT [150]. In a study of low-dose cytarabine followed by infusion of G-CSF mobilized donor PBSCs and subsequent treatment with GM-CSF in relapsed AML, ten of 36 patients survived for more than 5 years and fared better compared to those treated with DLI alone [151]. Some encouraging results have been obtained with lymphodepleting chemotherapy or low-dose 5-azacytidine before DLI, but it is uncertain if these approaches are better than traditional AML chemotherapy followed by DLI. Preliminary results of DLI after each second cycle of azacytidine showed sustained remission in five of 30 patients [152]. A second allo-HCT may be considered for young patients with relatively long disease-free interval since a CIBMTR report showed a 28 % survival at 5-years for patients with acute or chronic leukemias who underwent a second allo-HCT [153]. Schmid et al. reported on prophylactic DLI in AML patients. In this trial, high-risk AML patients received fludarabine–cytarabine–amsacrine, followed few days later by high-dose cyclophosphamide, low-dose TBI, and ATG. Patients without GVHD who were off immunosuppression started receiving prophylactic DLI on day +120. This yielded a remarkable 2-year leukemia-free survival of 40 %. A similar approach yielded 4-year survival of 61 % with upfront allo-HCT in complex cytogenetics AML [154–156]. In pediatric patients with incomplete donor chimerism, patients receiving prophylactic DLI achieved a much better event-free survival compared to others [157].

7.14 DLI in Lymphomas

Following DLI in relapsed follicular lymphoma after RIC allo-HCT, nine of 13 patients attained a sustained complete remission [158]. In 15 patients with mantle cell lymphoma who relapsed after RIC allo-HCT and received either DLI ($N=14$) or second allo-HCT ($N=1$) [159], 11 of 15 patients achieved a sustained remission. In 15 patients with DLBCL who had active disease after allo-HCT and were treated with different modalities including withdrawal of immunosuppression and/or DLI, six of 15 patients attained a sustained remission [160]. In patients with Hodgkin's lymphoma who had failed auto-HCT and then underwent a RIC allo-HCT, five of 15 patients who relapsed after allo-HCT and received DLI were in CR after a median of 45 months [161]. In a study of DLI outcomes in 17 patients with B-cell lymphoproliferative diseases, CRs were attained in all four patients with mantle cell lymphoma, three of four patients with follicular lymphoma, three of four patients with CLL but none of five patients with DLBCL or Richter transformation [162].

7.15 DLI in Acute Lymphoblastic Leukemia

Results in ALL are disappointing despite the fact that the first patient who survived long after DLI was a male with B-ALL who had a florid relapse after allo-HCT from a female donor [163]. In a study of ten patients with relapsed ALL post-allo-HCT who received chemotherapy (idarubicin + cytarabine + etoposide) followed by DLI, only one patient remained alive in CR, 900 days after DLI. The fact that patients received chemotherapy for disease control before DLI implies that probably not only the disease pace but an inherent ALL resistance to DLI may underlie these failures [164]. The poor outcomes of relapsed ALL after allo-HCT are confirmed by another report, wherein 44 patients with relapsed ALL received DLI with or without preceding chemotherapy and where 3-year survival was only 13 % [165].

7.16 Evolving Strategies for DLI

Potential strategies to enhance the efficacy of DLI in lymphoproliferative disorders include the use of disease-specific antibodies (e.g., rituximab, ofatumumab, or blinatumomab) before DLI and the use of engineered T cells as part of DLI. Another approach is to use preemptive DLI when MRD is detected or in cases of incomplete donor chimerism, especially after RIC allo-HCT for diseases that have a known poor prognosis following florid post-transplant relapse.

DLI infusions are associated with an approximately 35 % risk of GVHD [6]. While higher CD3+ cell dose is associated with increased GVHD risk, the incidence of GVHD remains lower after DLI than after ablative conditioning followed by T-replete grafts, perhaps since some host APC have been replaced by donor APCs or are suppressed by donor T_{REG} [166]. Prior host lymphodepletion (e.g., with fludarabine) [139] or concurrent use of IFNα and DLI increases the risk of GVHD. DLI after previous T cell-depleted transplant is also associated with higher rates of GVHD, perhaps due to a lack of donor T_{REG} [167]. If GVHD occurs, it is often responsive to treatment and many investigators give suboptimal immunosuppression or even tolerate lower degrees of GVHD until they see an improvement of the underlying malignancy [168, 169]. However, DLI may result in overt cytopenias and in extreme cases with marrow aplasia [170], especially if the recipient has completely lost donor chimerism. In such cases administration of a T cell replete stem cell product, rather than DLI alone, may prevent aplasia and restore donor chimerism.

8 Conclusions

Dramatic improvements in HCT, especially the widespread adoption of reduced-intensity conditioning regimens (given our understanding of the importance of GVL responses) have substantially expanded transplant utilization with reduced treatment-related morbidity and mortality. However, five decades into the HCT era, GVHD, and relapse continue to remain vexing problems, resulting in symptom burden and mortality even when the transplant outcome is otherwise successful. The dissection of GVHD from effective GVL and pathogen-specific T cell responses remains a central intellectual challenge and may provide genuine hope for improved transplant approaches. Until then, the focus of clinical trials should be the prevention of GVHD, both the acute and the chronic forms, and on improved studies of initial therapy in both the acute and chronic settings. Adoptive cellular therapies (e.g., using $T_{REG,}$ transduced T cells, or innate immune cells including NK and iNKT cells) are also promising, although pharmacologic interventions that selectively inhibit alloreactivity, while sparing GVL-inducing cells and T_{REG} are also highly desirable strategies. Promotion of tolerance is another mechanism that may reduce GVHD, especially cGVHD. All of these strategies will benefit from an improved understanding of GVHD biomarkers (e.g., promising candidates including TNFR1, HGF, soluble CD25, BAFF, and others) that may facilitate preemptive treatment and early dose escalation or de-escalation of immunosuppression [56, 171–174]. Development of improved animal models that better replicate the human condition, and facilitate a better understanding of cGVHD, will also provide great benefit.

While this review has focused on immunotherapeutic strategies, optimization of conditioning regimens continues to be a priority. Incorporation of agents including gemcitabine [175–177], bendamustine [178] for lymphomas or novel agents like proteasome inhibitors; HDAC inhibitors in myelomas; or Btk or PI3Kδ inhibitors in lymphoid malignancies may also improve outcomes. Antibodies or immunotoxins (brentuximab, anti-CD22 immunotoxins, etc.) are also likely to be increasingly utilized in pre- and post-transplant conditioning and maintenance therapies. Additionally, targeting of putative cancer stem cell pathways (Notch, Hedgehog, β-catenin, etc.) during conditioning may also improve outcomes. Post-transplant maintenance/consolidation treatments have already given good results (e.g., lenalidomide, imatinib) and other promising strategies (e.g., hypomethylating agents in leukemias) are also being developed. Many of these strategies may have intended or unintended immunologic consequences, which should be assessed systematically when clinical trials of these agents are conducted.

In many settings, detection of early relapse before overt clinical signs are evident (e.g., by chimerism or by MRD evaluation) may allow us to more successfully modify the immune environment or apply novel agents. Overall, it is expected that a combination of these diverse new approaches in the next decade will substantially improve post-HCT disease control while decreasing early mortality and late effects of HCT, which may impair immune function and quality of life. To accomplish these aims, thoughtful and systematic basic, translational and clinical studies will be needed. These studies will require the careful cooperation of academic institutions, industry partners and regulatory agencies, but will yield a promising future for the rapidly growing field of HCT.

References

1. Thomas ED et al. Intravenous infusion of bone marrow in patients receiving radiation and chemotherapy. N Engl J Med. 1957;257(11):491–6.
2. Copelan EA. Hematopoietic stem-cell transplantation. N Engl J Med. 2006;354(17): 1813–26.
3. Blazar BR, Murphy WJ, Abedi M. Advances in graft-versus-host disease biology and therapy. Nat Rev Immunol. 2012;12(6):443–58.
4. Ferrara JL et al. Graft-versus-host disease. Lancet. 2009;373(9674):1550–61.
5. Shlomchik WD. Graft-versus-host disease. Nat Rev Immunol. 2007;7(5):340–52.
6. Kolb HJ. Graft-versus-leukemia effects of transplantation and donor lymphocytes. Blood. 2008;112(12):4371–83.
7. Antin JH. Reduced-intensity stem cell transplantation: "...whereof a little More than a little is by much too much." King Henry IV, part 1, I, 2. Hematology Am Soc Hematol Educ Program. 2007: 47–54.
8. Deeg HJ, Antin JH. The clinical spectrum of acute graft-versus-host disease. Semin Hematol. 2006;43(1):24–31.
9. Saliba RM et al. Hyperacute GVHD: risk factors, outcomes, and clinical implications. Blood. 2007;109(7):2751–8.
10. Filipovich AH. Diagnosis and manifestations of chronic graft-versus-host disease. Best Pract Res Clin Haematol. 2008;21(2):251–7.
11. Anderson BE et al. Memory CD4+ T cells do not induce graft-versus-host disease. J Clin Invest. 2003;112(1):101–8.
12. Zheng H et al. Central memory CD8+ T cells induce graft-versus-host disease and mediate graft-versus-leukemia. J Immunol. 2009;182(10):5938–48.
13. Juchem KW et al. A repertoire-independent and cell-intrinsic defect in murine GVHD induction by effector memory T cells. Blood. 2011;118(23):6209–19.
14. Iclozan C et al. T helper17 cells are sufficient but not necessary to induce acute graft-versus-host disease. Biol Blood Marrow Transplant. 2010;16(2):170–8.
15. Hoffmann P et al. Donor-type CD4(+)CD25(+) regulatory T cells suppress lethal acute graft-versus-host disease after allogeneic bone marrow transplantation. J Exp Med. 2002;196(3): 389–99.
16. Pillai AB et al. Host natural killer T cells induce an interleukin-4-dependent expansion of donor CD4+CD25+Foxp3+ T regulatory cells that protects against graft-versus-host disease. Blood. 2009;113(18):4458–67.
17. Shimabukuro-Vornhagen A et al. The role of B cells in the pathogenesis of graft-versus-host disease. Blood. 2009;114(24):4919–27.
18. Kessel A et al. Human CD19(+)CD25(high) B regulatory cells suppress proliferation of CD4(+) T cells and enhance Foxp3 and CTLA-4 expression in T-regulatory cells. Autoimmun Rev. 2012;11(9):670–7.
19. Maeda Y et al. Both perforin and Fas ligand are required for the regulation of alloreactive CD8+ T cells during acute graft-versus-host disease. Blood. 2005;105(5):2023–7.
20. Shin HJ et al. Rapamycin and IL-2 reduce lethal acute graft-versus-host disease associated with increased expansion of donor type CD4+CD25+Foxp3+ regulatory T cells. Blood. 2011;118(8):2342–50.
21. Hanash AM et al. Abrogation of donor T-cell IL-21 signaling leads to tissue-specific modulation of immunity and separation of GVHD from GVL. Blood. 2011;118(2):446–55.
22. Wang X et al. Mechanisms of antigen presentation to T cells in murine graft-versus-host disease: cross-presentation and the appearance of cross-presentation. Blood. 2011;118(24): 6426–37.
23. Saito K et al. Involvement of CD40 ligand-CD40 and CTLA4-B7 pathways in murine acute graft-versus-host disease induced by allogeneic T cells lacking CD28. J Immunol. 1998; 160(9):4225–31.

24. Shlomchik WD et al. Prevention of graft versus host disease by inactivation of host antigen-presenting cells. Science. 1999;285(5426):412–5.
25. Anderson BE et al. Distinct roles for donor- and host-derived antigen-presenting cells and costimulatory molecules in murine chronic graft-versus-host disease: requirements depend on target organ. Blood. 2005;105(5):2227–34.
26. Matte CC et al. Donor APCs are required for maximal GVHD but not for GVL. Nat Med. 2004;10(9):987–92.
27. Koyama M et al. Plasmacytoid dendritic cells prime alloreactive T cells to mediate graft-versus-host disease as antigen-presenting cells. Blood. 2009;113(9):2088–95.
28. Koyama M et al. Recipient nonhematopoietic antigen-presenting cells are sufficient to induce lethal acute graft-versus-host disease. Nat Med. 2012;18(1):135–42.
29. Li H et al. Profound depletion of host conventional dendritic cells, plasmacytoid dendritic cells, and B cells does not prevent graft-versus-host disease induction. J Immunol. 2012; 188(8):3804–11.
30. Guinan EC et al. Transplantation of anergic histoincompatible bone marrow allografts. N Engl J Med. 1999;340(22):1704–14.
31. Prigozhina TB et al. CD40 ligand-specific antibodies synergize with cyclophosphamide to promote long-term transplantation tolerance across MHC barriers but inhibit graft-vs-leukemia effects of transplanted cells. Exp Hematol. 2003;31(1):81–8.
32. Li J et al. Roles of CD28, CTLA4, and inducible costimulator in acute graft-versus-host disease in mice. Biol Blood Marrow Transplant. 2011;17(7):962–9.
33. Chen YB et al. Expression of CD30 in patients with acute graft-vs.-host disease. Blood. 2012;120(3):691–6.
34. Stenger EO et al. Dendritic cells and regulation of graft-versus-host disease and graft-versus-leukemia activity. Blood. 2012;119(22):5088–103.
35. Cooke KR et al. LPS antagonism reduces graft-versus-host disease and preserves graft-versus-leukemia activity after experimental bone marrow transplantation. J Clin Invest. 2001;107(12):1581–9.
36. Calcaterra C et al. Critical role of TLR9 in acute graft-versus-host disease. J Immunol. 2008;181(9):6132–9.
37. Hossain MS et al. Flagellin, a TLR5 agonist, reduces graft-versus-host disease in allogeneic hematopoietic stem cell transplantation recipients while enhancing antiviral immunity. J Immunol. 2011;187(10):5130–40.
38. Penack O et al. NOD2 regulates hematopoietic cell function during graft-versus-host disease. J Exp Med. 2009;206(10):2101–10.
39. Wilhelm K et al. Graft-versus-host disease is enhanced by extracellular ATP activating P2X7R. Nat Med. 2010;16(12):1434–8.
40. Maier T, Holda JH, Claman HN. Graft-vs-host reactions (GVHR) across minor murine histocompatibility barriers. II. Development of natural suppressor cell activity. J Immunol. 1985;135(3):1644–51.
41. Meunier MC et al. T cells targeted against a single minor histocompatibility antigen can cure solid tumors. Nat Med. 2005;11(11):1222–9.
42. Zhou S et al. Predominant donor CD103+CD8+ T cell infiltration into the gut epithelium during acute GvHD: a role of gut lymph nodes. Int Immunol. 2008;20(3):385–94.
43. Kim YM et al. Graft-versus-host disease can be separated from graft-versus-lymphoma effects by control of lymphocyte trafficking with FTY720. J Clin Invest. 2003;111(5): 659–69.
44. Flomenberg N et al. Impact of HLA class I and class II high-resolution matching on outcomes of unrelated donor bone marrow transplantation: HLA-C mismatching is associated with a strong adverse effect on transplantation outcome. Blood. 2004;104(7):1923–30.
45. Fleischhauer K et al. Effect of T-cell-epitope matching at HLA-DPB1 in recipients of unrelated-donor haemopoietic-cell transplantation: a retrospective study. Lancet Oncol. 2012;13(4):366–74.

46. Aversa F et al. Treatment of high-risk acute leukemia with T-cell-depleted stem cells from related donors with one fully mismatched HLA haplotype. N Engl J Med. 1998;339(17): 1186–93.
47. Cooley S et al. Donor selection for natural killer cell receptor genes leads to superior survival after unrelated transplantation for acute myelogenous leukemia. Blood. 2010;116(14): 2411–9.
48. Petersdorf EW et al. MHC haplotype matching for unrelated hematopoietic cell transplantation. PLoS Med. 2007;4(1):e8.
49. Flowers ME et al. Comparative analysis of risk factors for acute graft-versus-host disease and for chronic graft-versus-host disease according to National Institutes of Health consensus criteria. Blood. 2011;117(11):3214–9.
50. Soiffer RJ et al. Impact of immune modulation with anti-T-cell antibodies on the outcome of reduced-intensity allogeneic hematopoietic stem cell transplantation for hematologic malignancies. Blood. 2011;117(25):6963–70.
51. Ho VT et al. Comparison of Tacrolimus and Sirolimus (Tac/Sir) versus Tacrolimus, Sirolimus, and mini-methotrexate (Tac/Sir/MTX) as acute graft-versus-host disease prophylaxis after reduced-intensity conditioning allogeneic peripheral blood stem cell transplantation. Biol Blood Marrow Transplant. 2009;15(7):844–50.
52. Hsieh MM et al. Allogeneic hematopoietic stem-cell transplantation for sickle cell disease. N Engl J Med. 2009;361(24):2309–17.
53. Koreth J et al. Interleukin-2 and regulatory T cells in graft-versus-host disease. N Engl J Med. 2011;365(22):2055–66.
54. Lowsky R et al. Protective conditioning for acute graft-versus-host disease. N Engl J Med. 2005;353(13):1321–31.
55. Luznik L et al. High-dose cyclophosphamide as single-agent, short-course prophylaxis of graft-versus-host disease. Blood. 2010;115(16):3224–30.
56. Paczesny S et al. A biomarker panel for acute graft-versus-host disease. Blood. 2009;113(2): 273–8.
57. Choi SW et al. TNF-inhibition with etanercept for graft-versus-host disease prevention in high-risk HCT: lower TNFR1 levels correlate with better outcomes. Biol Blood Marrow Transplant. 2012;18(10):1525–32.
58. Parmar S et al. Prophylaxis of graft-versus-host disease in unrelated donor transplantation with pentostatin, tacrolimus, and mini-methotrexate: a phase I/II controlled, adaptively randomized study. J Clin Oncol. 2011;29(3):294–302.
59. Reshef R et al. Blockade of lymphocyte chemotaxis in visceral graft-versus-host disease. N Engl J Med. 2012;367(2):135–45.
60. Couriel DR et al. A phase III study of infliximab and corticosteroids for the initial treatment of acute graft-versus-host disease. Biol Blood Marrow Transplant. 2009;15(12):1555–62.
61. Levine JE et al. Etanercept plus methylprednisolone as initial therapy for acute graft-versus-host disease. Blood. 2008;111(4):2470–5.
62. Alousi AM et al. Etanercept, mycophenolate, denileukin, or pentostatin plus corticosteroids for acute graft-versus-host disease: a randomized phase 2 trial from the Blood and Marrow Transplant Clinical Trials Network. Blood. 2009;114(3):511–7.
63. Martin PJ et al. First- and second-line systemic treatment of acute graft-versus-host disease: recommendations of the American Society of Blood and Marrow Transplantation. Biol Blood Marrow Transplant. 2012;18(8):1150–63.
64. Rao K et al. Improved survival and preserved antiviral responses after combination therapy with daclizumab and infliximab in steroid-refractory graft-versus-host disease. J Pediatr Hematol Oncol. 2009;31(6):456–61.
65. Kennedy GA et al. Combination antithymocyte globulin and soluble TNFalpha inhibitor (etanercept) +/– mycophenolate mofetil for treatment of steroid refractory acute graft-versus-host disease. Bone Marrow Transplant. 2006;37(12):1143–7.

66. Ho VT et al. Safety and efficacy of denileukin diftitox in patients with steroid-refractory acute graft-versus-host disease after allogeneic hematopoietic stem cell transplantation. Blood. 2004;104(4):1224–6.
67. Pidala J et al. Pentostatin as rescue therapy for glucocorticoid-refractory acute and chronic graft-versus-host disease. Ann Transplant. 2010;15(4):21–9.
68. Hoda D et al. Sirolimus for treatment of steroid-refractory acute graft-versus-host disease. Bone Marrow Transplant. 2010;45(8):1347–51.
69. Pidala J, Kim J, Anasetti C. Sirolimus as primary treatment of acute graft-versus-host disease following allogeneic hematopoietic cell transplantation. Biol Blood Marrow Transplant. 2009;15(7):881–5.
70. Greinix HT et al. Extracorporeal photochemotherapy in the treatment of severe steroid-refractory acute graft-versus-host disease: a pilot study. Blood. 2000;96(7):2426–31.
71. Le Blanc K et al. Mesenchymal stem cells for treatment of steroid-resistant, severe, acute graft-versus-host disease: a phase II study. Lancet. 2008;371(9624):1579–86.
72. Drobyski WR et al. Tocilizumab for the treatment of steroid refractory graft-versus-host disease. Biol Blood Marrow Transplant. 2011;17(12):1862–8.
73. Pidala J et al. Ustekinumab demonstrates activity in glucocorticoid-refractory acute GVHD. Bone Marrow Transplant. 2012;47(5):747–8.
74. Sun K et al. Differential effects of proteasome inhibition by bortezomib on murine acute graft-versus-host disease (GVHD): delayed administration of bortezomib results in increased GVHD-dependent gastrointestinal toxicity. Blood. 2005;106(9):3293–9.
75. Sun K et al. Inhibition of acute graft-versus-host disease with retention of graft-versus-tumor effects by the proteasome inhibitor bortezomib. Proc Natl Acad Sci U S A. 2004;101(21): 8120–5.
76. Koreth J et al. Bortezomib, tacrolimus, and methotrexate for prophylaxis of graft-versus-host disease after reduced-intensity conditioning allogeneic stem cell transplantation from HLA-mismatched unrelated donors. Blood. 2009;114(18):3956–9.
77. Duramad O et al. Pharmacologic expansion of donor-derived, naturally occurring CD4(+) Foxp3(+) regulatory T cells reduces acute graft-versus-host disease lethality without abrogating the graft-versus-leukemia effect in murine models. Biol Blood Marrow Transplant. 2011;17(8):1154–68.
78. Feagan BG et al. Treatment of ulcerative colitis with a humanized antibody to the alpha-4beta7 integrin. N Engl J Med. 2005;352(24):2499–507.
79. Reddy P et al. Histone deacetylase inhibition modulates indoleamine 2,3-dioxygenase-dependent DC functions and regulates experimental graft-versus-host disease in mice. J Clin Invest. 2008;118(7):2562–73.
80. Tao R et al. Deacetylase inhibition promotes the generation and function of regulatory T cells. Nat Med. 2007;13(11):1299–307.
81. Di Ianni M et al. Tregs prevent GVHD and promote immune reconstitution in HLA-haploidentical transplantation. Blood. 2011;117(14):3921–8.
82. Valenzuela JO et al. PKCtheta is required for alloreactivity and GVHD but not for immune responses toward leukemia and infection in mice. J Clin Invest. 2009;119(12):3774–86.
83. Socie G et al. Chronic graft-versus-host disease: long-term results from a randomized trial on graft-versus-host disease prophylaxis with or without anti-T-cell globulin ATG-Fresenius. Blood. 2011;117(23):6375–82.
84. Miklos DB et al. Antibody responses to H-Y minor histocompatibility antigens correlate with chronic graft-versus-host disease and disease remission. Blood. 2005;105(7):2973–8.
85. Magro L et al. Efficacy of imatinib mesylate in the treatment of refractory sclerodermatous chronic GVHD. Bone Marrow Transplant. 2008;42(11):757–60.
86. Cutler C et al. Rituximab for steroid-refractory chronic graft-versus-host disease. Blood. 2006;108(2):756–62.
87. Arai S et al. Prophylactic rituximab after allogeneic transplantation decreases B-cell alloimmunity with low chronic GVHD incidence. Blood. 2012;119(25):6145–54.
88. Zhou X et al. BAFF promotes Th17 cells and aggravates experimental autoimmune encephalomyelitis. PLoS One. 2011;6(8):e23629.

89. Jacobi AM et al. Effect of long-term belimumab treatment on B cells in systemic lupus erythematosus: extension of a phase II, double-blind, placebo-controlled, dose-ranging study. Arthritis Rheum. 2010;62(1):201–10.
90. Jedlickova Z et al. Therapy of sclerodermatous chronic graft-versus-host disease with mammalian target of rapamycin inhibitors. Biol Blood Marrow Transplant. 2011;17(5):657–63.
91. Biagi E et al. Extracorporeal photochemotherapy is accompanied by increasing levels of circulating CD4+CD25+GITR+Foxp3+CD62L+functional regulatory T-cells in patients with graft-versus-host disease. Transplantation. 2007;84(1):31–9.
92. Koc S et al. Therapy for chronic graft-versus-host disease: a randomized trial comparing cyclosporine plus prednisone versus prednisone alone. Blood. 2002;100(1):48–51.
93. Dignan FL et al. Organ-specific management and supportive care in chronic graft-versus-host disease. Br J Haematol. 2012;158(1):62–78.
94. Dignan FL et al. Diagnosis and management of chronic graft-versus-host disease. Br J Haematol. 2012;158(1):46–61.
95. Inamoto Y, Flowers ME. Treatment of chronic graft-versus-host disease in 2011. Curr Opin Hematol. 2011;18(6):414–20.
96. Wolff D et al. Consensus conference on clinical practice in chronic graft-versus-host disease (GVHD): first-line and topical treatment of chronic GVHD. Biol Blood Marrow Transplant. 2010;16(12):1611–28.
97. Vogelsang GB et al. Thalidomide for the treatment of chronic graft-versus-host disease. N Engl J Med. 1992;326(16):1055–8.
98. Chiang KY et al. Recombinant human tumor necrosis factor receptor fusion protein as complementary treatment for chronic graft-versus-host disease. Transplantation. 2002;73(4):665–7.
99. Robin M et al. Low-dose thoracoabdominal irradiation for the treatment of refractory chronic graft-versus-host disease. Transplantation. 2005;80(5):634–42.
100. Lawitschka A, Ball L, Peters C. Nonpharmacologic treatment of chronic graft-versus-host disease in children and adolescents. Biol Blood Marrow Transplant. 2012;18(1 Suppl):S74–81.
101. Couriel D et al. Ancillary therapy and supportive care of chronic graft-versus-host disease: national institutes of health consensus development project on criteria for clinical trials in chronic graft-versus-host disease: V. Ancillary Therapy and Supportive Care Working Group report. Biol Blood Marrow Transplant. 2006;12(4):375–96.
102. Hildebrandt GC et al. Diagnosis and treatment of pulmonary chronic GVHD: report from the consensus conference on clinical practice in chronic GVHD. Bone Marrow Transplant. 2011;46(10):1283–95.
103. Attal M et al. Maintenance therapy with thalidomide improves survival in patients with multiple myeloma. Blood. 2006;108(10):3289–94.
104. Badros AZ. Lenalidomide in myeloma–a high-maintenance friend. N Engl J Med. 2012;366(19):1836–8.
105. Klyuchnikov E et al. Current status and perspectives of tyrosine kinase inhibitor treatment in the posttransplant period in patients with chronic myelogenous leukemia (CML). Biol Blood Marrow Transplant. 2010;16(3):301–10.
106. Cetkovic-Cvrlje M, Uckun FM. Dual targeting of Bruton's tyrosine kinase and Janus kinase 3 with rationally designed inhibitors prevents graft-versus-host disease (GVHD) in a murine allogeneic bone marrow transplantation model. Br J Haematol. 2004;126(6):821–7.
107. de Lima M et al. Maintenance therapy with low-dose azacitidine after allogeneic hematopoietic stem cell transplantation for recurrent acute myelogenous leukemia or myelodysplastic syndrome: a dose and schedule finding study. Cancer. 2010;116(23):5420–31.
108. Tsirigotis P et al. Post-autologous stem cell transplantation administration of rituximab improves the outcome of patients with aggressive B cell non-Hodgkin's lymphoma. Ann Hematol. 2010;89(3):263–72.
109. Kohrt HE et al. CD137 stimulation enhances the antilymphoma activity of anti-CD20 antibodies. Blood. 2011;117(8):2423–32.

110. Chao MP et al. Anti-CD47 antibody synergizes with rituximab to promote phagocytosis and eradicate non-Hodgkin lymphoma. Cell. 2010;142(5):699–713.
111. Bashey A et al. CTLA4 blockade with ipilimumab to treat relapse of malignancy after allogeneic hematopoietic cell transplantation. Blood. 2009;113(7):1581–8.
112. Yi JS, Du M, Zajac AJ. A vital role for interleukin-21 in the control of a chronic viral infection. Science. 2009;324(5934):1572–6.
113. Schmidt H et al. Safety and clinical effect of subcutaneous human interleukin-21 in patients with metastatic melanoma or renal cell carcinoma: a phase I trial. Clin Cancer Res. 2010;16(21):5312–9.
114. Morgan RA et al. Cancer regression in patients after transfer of genetically engineered lymphocytes. Science. 2006;314(5796):126–9.
115. Dudley ME et al. Cancer regression and autoimmunity in patients after clonal repopulation with antitumor lymphocytes. Science. 2002;298(5594):850–4.
116. Rezvani K et al. Leukemia-associated antigen-specific T-cell responses following combined PR1 and WT1 peptide vaccination in patients with myeloid malignancies. Blood. 2008;111(1):236–42.
117. Van Tendeloo VF et al. Induction of complete and molecular remissions in acute myeloid leukemia by Wilms' tumor 1 antigen-targeted dendritic cell vaccination. Proc Natl Acad Sci U S A. 2010;107(31):13824–9.
118. Zilberberg J et al. Treatment with GM-CSF secreting myeloid leukemia cell vaccine prior to autologous-BMT improves the survival of leukemia-challenged mice. Biol Blood Marrow Transplant. 2011;17(3):330–40.
119. Klammer M et al. Fusion hybrids of dendritic cells and autologous myeloid blasts as a potential cellular vaccine for acute myeloid leukaemia. Br J Haematol. 2005;129(3):340–9.
120. Rosenblatt J et al. Vaccination with dendritic cell/tumor fusion cells results in cellular and humoral antitumor immune responses in patients with multiple myeloma. Blood. 2011; 117(2):393–402.
121. Vasir B et al. Fusion of dendritic cells with multiple myeloma cells results in maturation and enhanced antigen presentation. Br J Haematol. 2005;129(5):687–700.
122. Kasturi SP et al. Programming the magnitude and persistence of antibody responses with innate immunity. Nature. 2011;470(7335):543–7.
123. Till BG et al. CD20-specific adoptive immunotherapy for lymphoma using a chimeric antigen receptor with both CD28 and 4-1BB domains: pilot clinical trial results. Blood. 2012;119(17):3940–50.
124. Kochenderfer JN et al. B-cell depletion and remissions of malignancy along with cytokine-associated toxicity in a clinical trial of anti-CD19 chimeric-antigen-receptor-transduced T cells. Blood. 2012;119(12):2709–20.
125. Louis CU et al. Antitumor activity and long-term fate of chimeric antigen receptor-positive T cells in patients with neuroblastoma. Blood. 2011;118(23):6050–6.
126. Kochenderfer JN et al. Eradication of B-lineage cells and regression of lymphoma in a patient treated with autologous T cells genetically engineered to recognize CD19. Blood. 2010;116(20):4099–102.
127. Kochenderfer JN, Rosenberg SA. Chimeric antigen receptor-modified T cells in CLL. N Engl J Med. 2011;365(20):1937–8. author reply 1938.
128. Porter DL et al. Chimeric antigen receptor-modified T cells in chronic lymphoid leukemia. N Engl J Med. 2011;365(8):725–33.
129. Miller JS et al. Successful adoptive transfer and in vivo expansion of human haploidentical NK cells in patients with cancer. Blood. 2005;105(8):3051–7.
130. Geller MA et al. A phase II study of allogeneic natural killer cell therapy to treat patients with recurrent ovarian and breast cancer. Cytotherapy. 2011;13(1):98–107.
131. Louis CU et al. Enhancing the in vivo expansion of adoptively transferred EBV-specific CTL with lymphodepleting CD45 monoclonal antibodies in NPC patients. Blood. 2009; 113(11):2442–50.

132. Straathof KC et al. Treatment of nasopharyngeal carcinoma with Epstein-Barr virus–specific T lymphocytes. Blood. 2005;105(5):1898–904.
133. Mackensen A et al. Phase I study of adoptive T-cell therapy using antigen-specific CD8+ T cells for the treatment of patients with metastatic melanoma. J Clin Oncol. 2006;24(31): 5060–9.
134. Warren EH et al. Therapy of relapsed leukemia after allogeneic hematopoietic cell transplantation with T cells specific for minor histocompatibility antigens. Blood. 2010;115(19): 3869–78.
135. Kolb HJ et al. Donor leukocyte transfusions for treatment of recurrent chronic myelogenous leukemia in marrow transplant patients. Blood. 1990;76(12):2462–5.
136. Porter DL, Antin JH. Donor leukocyte infusions in myeloid malignancies: new strategies. Best Pract Res Clin Haematol. 2006;19(4):737–55.
137. Warlick ED et al. Successful remission rates and survival after lymphodepleting chemotherapy and donor lymphocyte infusion for relapsed hematologic malignancies postallogeneic hematopoietic cell transplantation. Biol Blood Marrow Transplant. 2012;18(3):480–6.
138. Mielcarek M et al. Outcomes among patients with recurrent high-risk hematologic malignancies after allogeneic hematopoietic cell transplantation. Biol Blood Marrow Transplant. 2007;13(10):1160–8.
139. Miller JS et al. Lymphodepletion followed by donor lymphocyte infusion (DLI) causes significantly more acute graft-versus-host disease than DLI alone. Blood. 2007;110(7):2761–3.
140. Guglielmi C et al. Donor lymphocyte infusion for relapsed chronic myelogenous leukemia: prognostic relevance of the initial cell dose. Blood. 2002;100(2):397–405.
141. Chen X et al. Interferon alpha in combination with GM-CSF induces the differentiation of leukaemic antigen-presenting cells that have the capacity to stimulate a specific anti-leukaemic cytotoxic T-cell response from patients with chronic myeloid leukaemia. Br J Haematol. 2000;111(2):596–607.
142. Savani BN et al. Imatinib synergizes with donor lymphocyte infusions to achieve rapid molecular remission of CML relapsing after allogeneic stem cell transplantation. Bone Marrow Transplant. 2005;36(11):1009–15.
143. Levenga H et al. Multiple myeloma patients receiving pre-emptive donor lymphocyte infusion after partial T-cell-depleted allogeneic stem cell transplantation show a long progression-free survival. Bone Marrow Transplant. 2007;40(4):355–9.
144. Bellucci R et al. Graft-versus-tumor response in patients with multiple myeloma is associated with antibody response to BCMA, a plasma-cell membrane receptor. Blood. 2005;105(10): 3945–50.
145. Zeiser R et al. Donor lymphocyte infusions for multiple myeloma: clinical results and novel perspectives. Bone Marrow Transplant. 2004;34(11):923–8.
146. Kroger N et al. Post-transplant immunotherapy with donor-lymphocyte infusion and novel agents to upgrade partial into complete and molecular remission in allografted patients with multiple myeloma. Exp Hematol. 2009;37(7):791–8.
147. Kroger N et al. Low-dose thalidomide and donor lymphocyte infusion as adoptive immunotherapy after allogeneic stem cell transplantation in patients with multiple myeloma. Blood. 2004;104(10):3361–3.
148. El-Cheikh J et al. Lenalidomide plus donor-lymphocytes infusion after allogeneic stem-cell transplantation with reduced-intensity conditioning in patients with high-risk multiple myeloma. Exp Hematol. 2012;40(7):521–7.
149. Schmid C et al. Donor lymphocyte infusion in the treatment of first hematological relapse after allogeneic stem-cell transplantation in adults with acute myeloid leukemia: a retrospective risk factors analysis and comparison with other strategies by the EBMT Acute Leukemia Working Party. J Clin Oncol. 2007;25(31):4938–45.
150. Levine JE et al. Prospective trial of chemotherapy and donor leukocyte infusions for relapse of advanced myeloid malignancies after allogeneic stem-cell transplantation. J Clin Oncol. 2002;20(2):405–12.

151. Schmid C et al. Low-dose ARAC, donor cells, and GM-CSF for treatment of recurrent acute myeloid leukemia after allogeneic stem cell transplantation. Leukemia. 2004;18(8):1430–3.
152. Lubbert M et al. Efficacy of a 3-day, low-dose treatment with 5-azacytidine followed by donor lymphocyte infusions in older patients with acute myeloid leukemia or chronic myelomonocytic leukemia relapsed after allografting. Bone Marrow Transplant. 2010;45(4): 627–32.
153. Eapen M et al. Second transplant for acute and chronic leukemia relapsing after first HLA-identical sibling transplant. Bone Marrow Transplant. 2004;34(8):721–7.
154. Schmid C et al. Early allo-SCT for AML with a complex aberrant karyotype–results from a prospective pilot study. Bone Marrow Transplant. 2012;47(1):46–53.
155. Schmid C et al. Long-term survival in refractory acute myeloid leukemia after sequential treatment with chemotherapy and reduced-intensity conditioning for allogeneic stem cell transplantation. Blood. 2006;108(3):1092–9.
156. Schmid C et al. Sequential regimen of chemotherapy, reduced-intensity conditioning for allogeneic stem-cell transplantation, and prophylactic donor lymphocyte transfusion in high-risk acute myeloid leukemia and myelodysplastic syndrome. J Clin Oncol. 2005;23(24): 5675–87.
157. Beck JF et al. Relapse of childhood ALL, AML and MDS after allogeneic stem cell transplantation can be prevented by donor lymphocyte infusion in a critical stage of increasing mixed chimerism. Klin Padiatr. 2002;214(4):201–5.
158. Thomson KJ et al. T-cell-depleted reduced-intensity transplantation followed by donor leukocyte infusions to promote graft-versus-lymphoma activity results in excellent long-term survival in patients with multiply relapsed follicular lymphoma. J Clin Oncol. 2010;28(23): 3695–700.
159. Cook G et al. Outcome following reduced-intensity allogeneic stem cell transplantation (RIC AlloSCT) for relapsed and refractory mantle cell lymphoma (MCL): a study of the British Society for Blood and Marrow Transplantation. Biol Blood Marrow Transplant. 2010;16(10):1419–27.
160. Bishop MR et al. Clinical evidence of a graft-versus-lymphoma effect against relapsed diffuse large B-cell lymphoma after allogeneic hematopoietic stem-cell transplantation. Ann Oncol. 2008;19(11):1935–40.
161. Thomson KJ et al. Superiority of reduced-intensity allogeneic transplantation over conventional treatment for relapse of Hodgkin's lymphoma following autologous stem cell transplantation. Bone Marrow Transplant. 2008;41(9):765–70.
162. Russell NH et al. Donor lymphocyte infusions can result in sustained remissions in patients with residual or relapsed lymphoid malignancy following allogeneic haemopoietic stem cell transplantation. Bone Marrow Transplant. 2005;36(5):437–41.
163. Slavin S et al. Allogeneic cell therapy with donor peripheral blood cells and recombinant human interleukin-2 to treat leukemia relapse after allogeneic bone marrow transplantation. Blood. 1996;87(6):2195–204.
164. Choi SJ et al. Treatment of relapsed acute lymphoblastic leukemia after allogeneic bone marrow transplantation with chemotherapy followed by G-CSF-primed donor leukocyte infusion: a prospective study. Bone Marrow Transplant. 2005;36(2):163–9.
165. Collins Jr RH et al. Donor leukocyte infusions in acute lymphocytic leukemia. Bone Marrow Transplant. 2000;26(5):511–6.
166. Johnson BD et al. Role of immunoregulatory donor T cells in suppression of graft-versus-host disease following donor leukocyte infusion therapy. J Immunol. 1999;163(12): 6479–87.
167. Kolb HJ et al. Graft-versus-leukemia effect of donor lymphocyte transfusions in marrow grafted patients. Blood. 1995;86(5):2041–50.
168. Miller JS et al. NCI first international workshop on the biology, prevention, and treatment of relapse after allogeneic hematopoietic stem cell transplantation: Report from the Committee

on the Biology Underlying Recurrence of Malignant Disease following allogeneic HSCT: graft-versus-tumor/leukemia reaction. Biol Blood Marrow Transplant. 2010;16(5):565–86.
169. van den Brink MR et al. Relapse after allogeneic hematopoietic cell therapy. Biol Blood Marrow Transplant. 2010;16(1 Suppl):S138–45.
170. Garicochea B et al. Aplasia after donor lymphocyte infusion (DLI) for CML in relapse after sex-mismatched BMT: recovery of donor-type haemopoiesis predicted by non-isotopic in situ hybridization (ISH). Br J Haematol. 1994;88(2):400–2.
171. Levine JE et al. Acute graft-versus-host disease biomarkers measured during therapy can predict treatment outcomes: a Blood and Marrow Transplant Clinical Trials Network study. Blood. 2012;119(16):3854–60.
172. Harris AC et al. Plasma biomarkers of lower gastrointestinal and liver acute GVHD. Blood. 2012;119(12):2960–3.
173. Clark WB et al. Genetic variation in recipient B-cell activating factor modulates phenotype of GVHD. Blood. 2011;118(4):1140–4.
174. Sarantopoulos S et al. High levels of B-cell activating factor in patients with active chronic graft-versus-host disease. Clin Cancer Res. 2007;13(20):6107–14.
175. Nieto Y et al. High-dose infusional gemcitabine combined with busulfan and melphalan with autologous stem-cell transplant in patients with refractory lymphoid malignancies. Biol Blood Marrow Transplant. 2012;18(8):1150–63.
176. Anderlini P et al. Gemcitabine, fludarabine and melphalan as a reduced-intensity conditioning regimen for allogeneic stem cell transplant in relapsed and refractory Hodgkin lymphoma: preliminary results. Leuk Lymphoma. 2012;53(3):499–502.
177. Oki Y et al. Phase 2 study of gemcitabine in combination with rituximab in patients with recurrent or refractory Hodgkin lymphoma. Cancer. 2008;112(4):831–6.
178. Visani G et al. BeEAM (bendamustine, etoposide, cytarabine, melphalan) before autologous stem cell transplantation is safe and effective for resistant/relapsed lymphoma patients. Blood. 2011;118(12):3419–25.

The Immune System in Head and Neck Squamous Cell Carcinoma: Interactions and Therapeutic Opportunities

Paolo Serafini and Donald T. Weed

Abstract Squamous cell carcinomas of the upper aerodigestive tract exhibit complex interactions with the host immune system that may simultaneously explain resistance to various therapeutic modalities and that may also provide opportunities for therapeutic intervention. The interplay between developing or established malignancy and the host immune system is best understood through a careful analysis of the key components and effector arms of the immune system. These include the complex cellular network of immune modulation as well as tumor-derived factors such as chemokines and cytokines. While the host response to the developing tumor may successfully curtail tumor growth in some cases (immunosurveillance), squamous cell carcinomas of the head and neck are characterized by their ability to create an immunosuppressive environment powerful enough to evade the immune response. It is increasingly apparent that efforts to stimulate a therapeutically effective immune response against established tumors must be coupled with strategies to abrogate this immune-suppressive environment. Preclinical studies and clinical trials have yielded promising results and provide the foundation for further refinements in a broad variety of immunotherapeutic strategies targeting all components of the immune system. Combining such approaches with the established treatment options of surgical resection, radiotherapy, and chemotherapy may ultimately yield substantive improvements in overall survival that to date have been lacking and simultaneously reduce disease-related and treatment-related morbidities for this debilitating and deadly disease.

P. Serafini (✉)
Department of Microbiology and Immunology, Sylvester Comprehensive Cancer Center, Miller School of Medicine, University of Miami, Miami, FL, USA
e-mail: pserafini@med.miami.edu

D.T. Weed (✉)
Department of Otolaryngology, Sylvester Comprehensive Cancer Center, Miller School of Medicine, University of Miami, Miami, FL, USA
e-mail: dweed@med.miami.edu

J.D. Rosenblatt et al. (eds.), *Advances in Tumor Immunology and Immunotherapy*, Current Cancer Research, DOI 10.1007/978-1-4614-8809-5_13,
© Springer Science+Business Media New York 2014

Keywords Squamous cell carcinoma • Immunosurveillance • Immunosuppression • Immunotherapy • Cytokines • T regulatory cells • Myeloid derived suppressor cells • Tumor vaccines • Antibody therapies • Adoptive cell transfer

1 Introduction

The vast majority of tumors (95 %) that arise in the head and neck region are squamous cell carcinomas arising from the epithelium of the upper aerodigestive tract. Head and neck squamous cell carcinomas (HNSCCs) infringe on the highly critical functions of speech, swallowing, and respiration. Current therapies, surgery alone, radio- or chemo-radiotherapy, or combinations of these modalities, leave many of these patients with significant functional deficits that exact a unique physical and social toll. Although significant advances in the areas of reconstructive surgery, minimally invasive surgery, precisely targeted radiotherapy, chemotherapy, and monoclonal antibody therapy have been achieved in the last three decades, the overall survival rates for patients with these cancers have been modestly affected. HNSCC accounts for approximately 2.5 % of all newly diagnosed cancer cases in the United States, with 40,250 new cases estimated in 2012 [1]. Globally, HNSCC (including the oral cavity, oro/hypo/nasopharynx, and larynx) represents the sixth most common malignancy encountered [2] with a high case fatality (ratio of mortality to incidence of 0.53) and with more than 644,000 new cases reported in 2002 worldwide [3]. Although the cause of HNSCC is multifactorial, its risk has been historically associated with tobacco and alcohol use, especially those who use both. Processed tobacco, in fact, contains more than 3,000 chemical compounds, including at least 30 known carcinogens, while cigarette smoke contains approximately 50 known carcinogens and pro-carcinogens [4]. The epidemiology of HNSCC has dramatically changed over the past two decades, however, particularly as this relates to oropharyngeal SCC. As tobacco use, traditionally the most important risk factor for HNSCC, has decreased in the USA, the incidence of tobacco-associated human papillomavirus (HPV)-negative HNSCC has also decreased [5, 6]. Instead, the incidence of HPV-associated oropharyngeal cancers overall is increasing worldwide [7, 8]. The incidence of tonsillar cancer in the USA, especially among men under age 60, increased by 2–3 % each year between 1973 and 1995; however this incidence has increased more rapidly in the last decade [9]. Indeed, while only 16 % of the US oropharyngeal cases were HPV positive in 1984–1989, 73 % of tumors were positive for this virus in 2000–2004 [10]. Interestingly, survival of HPV-positive HNSCC patients is notably better than survival of HPV-negative HNSCC patients (3-year survival of 84 % vs. 57 %, respectively) [11]. Recent analysis of oropharyngeal cancer patient survival among cases from 1984 to 2004 in SEER suggested that median survival was fourfold higher among HPV-positive than HPV-negative oropharyngeal cases (131 vs. 20 months) in the USA during the past two decades. In addition, while survival increased significantly for HPV-positive oropharyngeal cases between 1984 and 2004 ($p=0.003$) survival did not improve for HPV-negative cases ($p=0.18$) [12]. The effect of tobacco remains powerful, however, as patients with HPV-positive tumors who smoke have a prognosis intermediate between smokers whose tumors are HPV negative and nonsmokers with HPV-positive tumors [11].

The better survival and lower rate of recurrence observed in HPV-positive HNSCC highlight the importance that the immune system plays in this malignancy. Indeed, despite the best efforts of the virus to evade host defenses, most HPV infections resolve with time as a result of a successful cell-mediated immune response [13] directed against the early HPV proteins (i.e., E2 and E6) [14, 15]. Furthermore, even in the absence of viral induced cytolysis and cell death, the HPV-infected cells can activate the production of type 1 interferons and evoke a powerful, generic, antiviral, and innate immune system response. The type 1 interferons (IFN-α and IFN-β) have antiviral, antiproliferative, anti-angiogenic, and immunostimulatory properties that act as a bridge between innate and adaptive immunity, activating immature dendritic cells and thus facilitating antigen processing and generation of antiviral immunity [16]. The possible role of the immune system is further suggested in an HPV-positive and HPV-negative preclinical model of tonsil squamous cell carcinoma [17]. While in immune-deficient mice no differences in tumor growth were observed between HPV^+ and HPV^- tumors, in immune-competent mice a significant delay in tumor progression was observed in the group bearing the HPV^+ carcinoma with 20–30 % of animals able to completely clear the tumor [17]. Tumor rejection was dependent on both $CD4^+$ and $CD8^+$ T cells that are spontaneously primed and expanded in the mice bearing the HPV^+ tumor [17]. However, it is important to remember that significant differences exist between the murine transplantable model and spontaneously arising tumors. While transplantable tumors derived from immortalized cell lines grew and developed rapidly when injected in the mice, spontaneous tumors developed slowly through a long interaction with the host. Indeed, while strong evidence exists that specific immune surveillance operates at early stages of tumorigenesis, causing inflammation and neoplastic stabilization, established tumors appear to be able to induce immune tolerance [18] and T cell anergy that allow tumor growth. In the presence of this tumor-driven tolerogenic environment, immune surveillance is restrained and immune interventions, such as vaccination or adoptive cell transfer, are likely to be much less effective. The presence of these suppressive mechanisms generated by growing tumor can explain the low clinical success rates obtained by immunotherapy in the last decades [19].

2 Interaction Between HNSCC and the Immune System

As in many other cancers, the interaction between the immune system and the transformed epithelial cells plays a critical role in the genesis and in the progression of HNSCC. In this malignancy the concept of immune surveillance [20] and tumor–host immune system interaction is sustained by both clinical and experimental observations. For example, one clear indication of the contribution of the immune system in controlling HNSCC is the relative increase in its incidence in the context of pharmaceutical immunosuppression or acquired immunodeficiency. Premalignant leukoplakia is identified in 13 % of renal transplant patients as compared to 0.6 % of control age- and sex-matched individuals [21, 22]. In the majority of these patients leukoplakia evolves into dysplasia, and 10 % develop frank SCC [21, 22]. Similar results are observed in patients who have undergone bone marrow transplantation [23–25] and/or are receiving chronic treatment for GVHD [26]. In these latter cases, the major risk factors for the development of SCC were long duration of chronic GVHD therapy and the use of azathioprine, particularly when combined with cyclosporine and steroids [26]. Although HNSCC is not an AIDS-defining illness, the appearance of this malignancy is seen in excess among HIV-infected individuals [27]. HNSCC patients infected with HIV are significantly younger than non-infected patients, and while there are no differences in tumor location, HIV-infected patients generally present with larger and more advanced tumors and significantly poorer prognosis [28]. Interestingly, despite the fact that HPV is a causative agent of HNSCC and opportunistic infection in HIV patients, a large study in AIDS patients with laryngeal squamous cell carcinoma proved the lack of association with HPV infection. However, it is important to remember that this subsite is not typically associated with HPV-associated malignancy in immunocompetent individuals, suggesting that the increased tumor frequency in this cohort of patients could be primarily due to a defective immune surveillance even in the absence of tumor-promoting HPV infection [29].

Although acquired or iatrogenic immune suppression increases the risk of HNSCC and seems to worsen the prognosis, this malignancy most commonly arises in individuals with a normal and healthy immune system. Indeed, immune surveillance is suggested to clear most preclinical lesions, while immunoediting [30] is the process that characterizes all clinically relevant lesions. This process is thought to play a key role during malignant progression, promoting a selective pressure in the tumor microenvironment that leads to the growth of extremely aggressive neoplastic clones capable of escaping tumor immunity. Indeed, it has long been thought that the immune system functions during tumor formation to select for tumor variants that are better suited to survive in an immunologically intact environment, very much like it does with viruses, bacteria, and parasites [30]. Many studies demonstrate that the repassage of transplantable tumors through immunocompetent hosts generates tumor variants with reduced immunogenicity. Cancer immunoediting is composed of three processes: elimination, equilibrium, and escape. Immunosurveillance occurs during the elimination process, whereas the Darwinian selection of tumor variants occurs during the equilibrium process. This, in turn, can ultimately lead to escape and the appearance of clinically apparent tumors [30]. Indeed, these three processes are not necessarily temporally separated but rather they can coexist.

Although initially immune editing was thought to allow the growth of only those neoplastic clones able to escape immune recognition by losing particular immune-dominant epitopes, by down-regulating the major histocompatibility complex (MHC), or by affecting the antigen processing machinery, it is now clear that the selection of malignant cells with intrinsic immunosuppressive activity is particularly common. Indeed, like many other solid malignancies, almost all HNSCC tumors express or secrete factors that are able to prevent immunological recognition or that can promote apoptosis of tumor-specific T cells. These factors can be expressed on the membrane of neoplastic cells such as in the case of B7-H1 (PDL-1) that is found in the tonsillar crypts, the site of initial HPV infection. In HPV^+ HNSCCs, PD-L1 expression on both tumor cells and $CD68^+$ tumor-associated macrophages (TAMs) is geographically localized to sites of lymphocyte fronts [31]. Despite the strong immunogenicity driven by HPV protein, the majority of $CD8^+$ tumor-infiltrating lymphocytes (TILs) express high levels of PD-1 that upon binding to PDL-1 promote T cell anergy, exhaustion, or apoptosis [32]. These findings support a role for the PD-1:PD-L1 interaction in creating an "immune-privileged" site for initial viral infection and subsequent adaptive immune resistance once tumors are established. In addition to PDL-1, HNSCC tumors can also express other molecules that promote tumoricidal T cell apoptosis. For example, these tumors can express FAS-L [33, 34] or TRAIL [35] that, upon engagement with the cognate receptors on T cells, induces the apoptosis of tumor-specific lymphocytes [35].

Membrane expression of molecules able to promote T cell apoptosis is not the only immunosuppressive mechanism that is exploited by HNSCC as a result of the immunoediting pressure. Indeed, it is now evident that tumors can secrete different factors able to alter normal hematopoiesis and to induce the appearance and the recruitment of cells from the innate and adaptive immune system with an intrinsic immunosuppressive and pro-tumoral phenotype (Fig. 1). For example, the vast majority of HNSCC tumors secrete interleukin (IL)-4, IL-6, IL-8, IL-10, granulocytes macrophage-colony stimulating factor (GM-CSF), granulocytes-colony stimulating factor (G-CSF), vascular endothelial growth factor (VEGF), prostaglandin E2 (PGE2), basic fibroblast growth factor (bFGF), and chemokines that are able to shape not only the tumor microenvironment but also distal sites creating de facto a tumor macro-environment that predisposes the host to the neoplastic growth and to metastatic dissemination of tumor cells.

3 Tumor-Derived Factors in HNSCC

Numerous findings indicate that tumor-derived factors (TDFs) greatly influence the interaction between tumor and the host and can orchestrate important changes in the hematopoietic differentiation generating a tumor macro-environment that facilitates the malignant progression and metastasis (Fig. 1). For example, conditioned media from tumor cell lines can inhibit the in vitro differentiation of dendritic cells from their precursors [36]. Normal bone marrow cells could give rise to immunosuppressive elements simply by culturing them for a few days with supernatants from a highly metastatic Lewis lung carcinoma variant [37]. For more than 25 years efforts have been made to identify and understand the role of these TDFs in tumor progression [38–44]. Tumors secrete a large panel of cytokines, chemokines, or other diffusible molecules that, alone or in combination, can induce myeloid derived suppressor cells (MDSC) recruitment and increase their maturation into fully suppressive cells. To date, a number of candidate proteins (discussed below) have been identified in HNSCC.

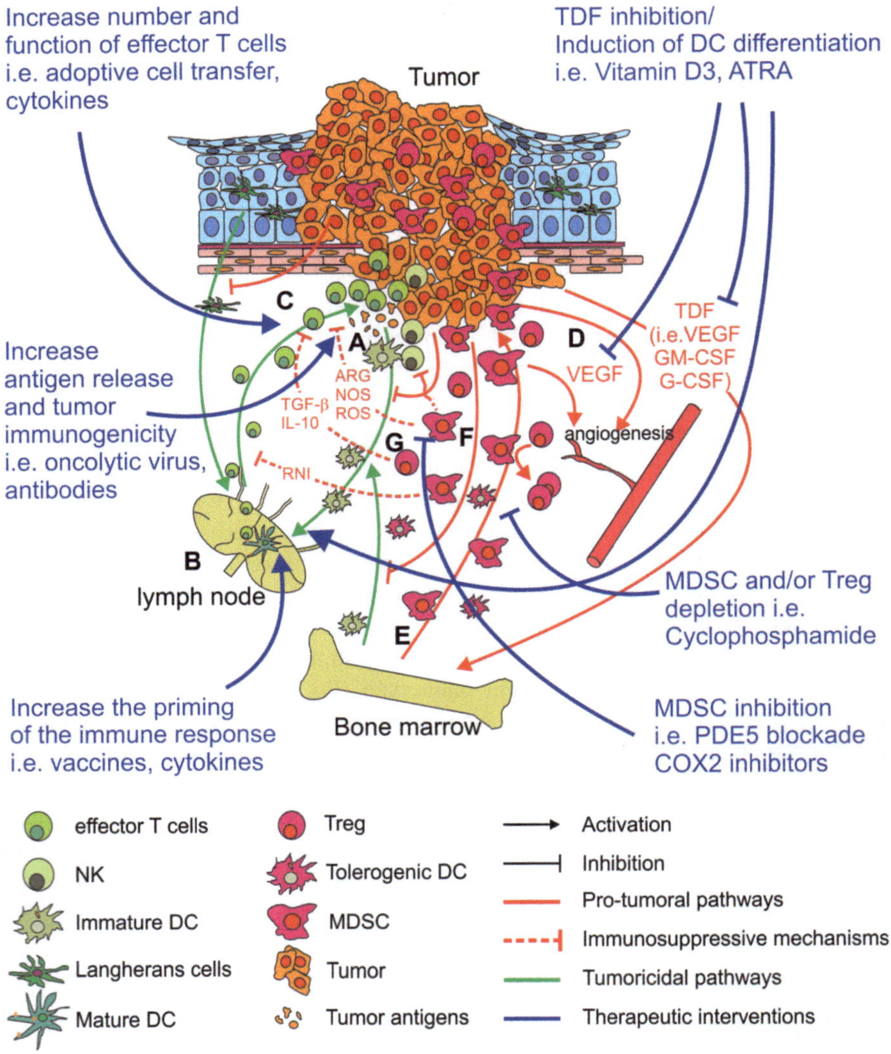

Fig. 1 HNSSC–immune system interactions and current immune therapeutic interventions. (**A**) Tumor antigens released by apoptotic cells are uptaken by immature DC that, after migration to the lymph nodes, (**B**) mature and cross-present the antigens and expand the tumor-specific effector T cells. Driven by the release of inflammatory molecules (i.e., CCL2), effector T cells migrate to the tumor site where they exert their tumoricidal action. (**C**) Immunoediting promotes the selection of neoplastic clones able to secrete (**D**) tumor-derived factors (TDF, i.e., GM-CSF, VEGF) that alter normal myelopoiesis (**E**) arresting DC differentiation while promoting MDSC and tolerogenic DC accumulation. (**F**) MDSCs and tolerogenic DCs can inhibit effector T cells directly or indirectly. The direct mechanisms of immunosuppression include the secretion of ROS, nitric oxide, and TGF-β; the depletion of semi-essential amino acids (i.e., L-Arg, Trp); or the inhibition of T cell trafficking by, for example, chemokine nitration. The indirect mechanisms of immunosuppression mediate the expansion of Tregs that further block effector cell function and DC maturation (**G**) by the secretion of TGF-β and/or IL-10. Additionally, MDSCs promote tumor progression by immune-independent mechanisms such as the promotion of tumor angiogenesis and metastasis by the secretion of metalloproteinases that regulate VEGF bioavailability and tissue modifications. Different therapeutic strategies (in *blue*) have been developed and are currently being tested in ongoing clinical trials to either restrain tumor immunosuppression or promote tumor immunity

3.1 Granulocyte Macrophage-Colony Stimulating Factor

Even though GM-CSF has long been considered an immune adjuvant, different evidence has uncovered its dual role in stimulating as well as suppressing the immune system: First, almost 31 % of tested human tumor cell lines (including HNSCC [45]) secreted this cytokine [46]. GM-CSF is also secreted by many mouse cell lines such as squamous cell carcinoma [47], colon and mammary adenocarcinoma [46], and plasmacytoma [48]. Second, its secretion by HNSCC is associated with a negative prognosis [45]. Third, tumor-transduced GM-CSF, administration of recombinant GM-CSF protein, or use of high doses of GM-CSF vaccines are sufficient to recruit MDSCs into the secondary lymphoid organs to suppress antigen-specific $CD8^+$ T cells and promote tolerance [46, 49, 50]. Fourth, the ability of different tumor-conditioned media to promote MDSC differentiation is inhibited by the use of a GM-CSF-neutralizing antibody, and, conversely, MDSCs can be generated in vitro from BM precursors by the use of either GM-CSF and G-CSF or GM-CSF and IL-6 [51, 52]. Fifth, GM-CSF promotes HNSCC cell invasiveness and malignant phenotype in nude mice [53].

GM-CSF has also been shown to elicit powerful immune responses when combined with γ-irradiated tumor cell vaccines, in various mouse models and in the clinical setting [54, 55], which has led to its widespread use as an immune adjuvant to augment antitumor immunity. In the therapy of HNSCC, oropharyngeal mucositis is a painful, often dose-limiting side effect of radiotherapy and chemotherapy [56, 57]. G-CSF and GM-CSF decrease the incidence of mucositis, and GM-CSF directly promotes wound healing of the mucosa [58]. In addition, G-CSF and GM-CSF are used to prevent potentially life-threatening febrile neutropenia. Nevertheless, the survival benefit for patients under adjuvant therapy with G-CSF and GM-CSF is a matter of controversial discussion. While the beneficial effect on neutropenia and mucositis is shown in several clinical trials [59], a large randomized clinical trial in advanced HNSCC even identified adjuvant G-CSF treatment as a poor prognostic factor with reduced locoregional control [60], others have not shown any significant effect of G-CSF and GM-CSF on overall survival or disease-free survival [61] or a beneficial action when GM-CSF was used in conjunction with radiotherapy and an oncolytic virus [62].

To better understand this dual role of GM-CSF, we used a bystander vaccine strategy in which the antigen dose and steric hindrance could be maintained constant while altering the GM-CSF dose to assess the impact of high vs. low concentrations of GM-CSF. While we confirmed the efficacy of low doses of GM-CSF-secreting vaccine, we also defined a threshold above which the vaccine not only lost its efficacy but also resulted in significant in vivo immunosuppression mediated by MDSC recruitment [50]. A systematic analysis of different clinical trials performed with this cytokine suggests that the same phenomenon can take place in humans. Although in some of these studies GM-CSF appeared to help the generation of an immune response, in others no effect or even a suppressive effect was reported. GM-CSF may increase the vaccine-induced immune response when administered repeatedly at relatively low doses (range 40–80 μg for 1–5 days), whereas an opposite effect was often reported at dosages between 100 and 500 μg [63]. These findings support the dual role of GM-CSF on the immune response and highlight several critical parameters such as dose, systemic concentration, and duration of exposure as key factors for GM-CSF effect on the immune system, all of which need to be considered when utilizing GM-CSF as a vaccine adjuvant.

3.2 *Prostaglandins (PGEs)*

The overexpression of cyclooxygenase (COX)-2 is a frequent event in squamous cell carcinomas of the head and neck [64, 65], and nonsteroidal anti-inflammatory drugs, which are potent inhibitors of COX-1 and COX-2, exert chemopreventive effects on HNSCC cancer development [66]. COX-2 promotes the release of the pro-inflammatory mediator prostaglandin E2 (PGE2), which acts on its cell surface G protein-coupled receptors EP1, EP2, EP3, and EP4. The products of COX2 enzyme activity, prostaglandins and mainly PGE2, have been implicated in tumor-associated subversion of immune functions, since inhibitors of prostaglandin synthesis typically enhanced antitumor immunity. PGE2 is one of the best-characterized and -studied isoform of eicosanoids that possesses both pro-inflammatory and immunosuppressive properties and that is produced during the course of inflammation following cellular stresses, and in response to growth factors, hormones, endotoxin, and inflammatory cytokines, or by growing tumors. Freshly excised solid human tumor cells produce substantially more PGE than established tumor cell lines [67]: interestingly, while primary tumor cell-conditioned media profoundly hampered the in vitro DC differentiation from $CD14^+$ monocytes or $CD34^+$ myeloid precursors, the effects of supernatants derived from established tumor cell lines were minor [67]. Both tumors and MDSCs can actively produce and secrete PGE2. This production and secretion correlate with arginase overexpression, STAT3 and STAT1 phosphorylation, and IL-10 and MIP-2 production, a phenotype typically associated with MDSC suppressive activity [68].

3.3 *Interleukin-4 and -13*

IL-13 and IL-4 are central T helper 2 (Th2) anti-inflammatory and immunomodulatory cytokines with close structural and biological homology. Both are produced mainly by T and B cells, mast cells, and basophils. In HNSCC these cytokines are produced in the tumor microenvironment by the infiltrating leukocytes [69] and by the tumor itself [70, 71]. The promiscuous receptor for IL-4 and IL-13 (alias IL4R type II) is composed of the IL4Rα chain and IL13Rα1 chain [72], while IL4Rα and the gamma chain (γc), common to the receptors for different members of the cytokine family comprising IL-2, IL-4, IL-7, IL-9, IL-15, and IL-21, associate to compose the IL-4 receptor (alias IL4R type I). Since the IL4Rα chain is the only component that possesses kinase-sensitive tyrosine residues in the cytoplasmic domain, signals from both type I and type II IL4R are transduced by the IL4Rα chain [73]. IL4Rα phosphorylation, upon engagement and dimerization, recruits and phosphorylates STAT6 that dimerizes and migrates to the nucleus to activate the transcription of several proteins including arginase 1 [74]. Interestingly, IL4Rα and IL13Rα are constitutively over-expressed in several HNSCC cell lines and, upon engagement with their cognate ligand, were shown to promote neoplastic cell proliferation [75] suggesting a pleiotropic function of these cytokines in this disease.

IL4Rα expression on MDSCs and monocytes is required for their suppressive phenotype [76] and survival [77], and genetic ablation of this receptor on monocytes and granulocytes is sufficient to revert MDSC-mediated immune suppression in vivo whereas its aptamer-mediated blockade is sufficient to promote MDSCs and TAM apoptosis [77]. MDSC and TAM produce IL-13 and IFN-γ and integrate the downstream signals of these cytokines to trigger the molecular pathways suppressing antigen-activated $CD8^+$ T lymphocytes [76].

3.4 *Interleukin-6*

High levels of IL-6 have been detected in leukemia, lymphoma, multiple myeloma, melanoma, as well as breast, lung, ovarian, renal cell, and pancreatic cancers [78] and are associated with a poor prognosis. Elevated IL-6 serum levels are found in the majority of HNSCC cancer patients, and its concentration correlates with tumor stage and lymph node status [79]. Because of the role of IL-6 in the acute-phase response in the liver and in the regulation of the systemic immune response, it is believed that high serum levels of the cytokine contribute to weight loss, night sweats, fever, and other systemic symptoms [80].

The physiological activity of IL-6 is complex, producing both pro-inflammatory and anti-inflammatory effects. In addition, IL-6 affects the differentiation of myeloid lineages, including macrophages and DCs, both in vitro and in vivo [81] through the activation of the transcription factor STAT3, which exerts a negative regulatory function on the adaptive and innate immune system during tumor development. Indeed, treatment in vitro with combinations of GM-CSF, G-CSF, IL-6, and IL-13 induces the rapid differentiation of human and mouse bone marrow precursor cells into cells that resemble suppressive MDSC [82, 83].

Beside its role on MDSC differentiation, IL-6 has an important function on dendritic cell differentiation. Indeed, tumor-derived factors can inhibit the generation of DC [84]. Dendritic cell differentiation can be restored by the use of VEGF- and/or IL-6-specific antibodies that neutralize this inhibitory effect [85].

3.5 Vascular Endothelial Growth Factor

Increased expression of VEGF and its receptors in HNSCCs underscores the importance of the VEGF pathway in angiogenesis and survival of tumor cells under hypoxic conditions [86]. VEGF expression is regulated by hypoxia-inducible factor-1α (HIF-1α)-dependent and -independent processes, both of which involve PI3-K and AKT [87]. VEGF plays an important role in the formation of blood vessels during embryogenesis, hematopoiesis, and tumor neovascularization [88]. It is secreted by most tumors, and high levels correlate with a poor prognosis [89]. Neutralizing antibodies against VEGF restored DC differentiation from hematopoietic precursors blocked by tumor-conditioned media [90]. VEGF has been directly linked with the systemic MDSC expansion. The administration of recombinant VEGF to tumor-free mice, in fact, resulted in inhibition of DC development and was associated with an increase in the number of MDSCs in the spleen [90]. Besides playing a direct role in tumor angiogenesis, this factor promotes cross talk between tumor and tumor-associated MDSCs [91]. By expressing high levels of matrix metalloproteinase 9, tumor-associated MDSCs regulate the bioavailability of VEGF by releasing it from the extracellular matrix [92], suggesting the presence of a positive feedback loop by which MDSCs increase VEGF release that in turn promotes MDSC differentiation and expansion. MMP9 inhibition by amino-biphosphonates significantly decreased MMP-9 expression and the number of macrophages in tumor stroma and reduced MDSC expansion both in bone marrow and peripheral blood [93]. In HNSCC, VEGF-A expression correlated with microvessel density, disease progression, a reduced number of mature DCs, and an increased number of immature DCs and MDSC, confirming the importance of this factor in the progression of this malignancy [94]. These findings underlie the importance of the VEGF–MDSC connection in HNSCC and suggest that treatments aimed to block MDSC or VEGF should have an effect on both tumor immunosuppression and angiogenesis.

3.6 Chemokines

Chemokines are leukocyte chemoattractants that are usually classified into two main subgroups: the inflammatory and the homeostatic. While the first group promotes leukocyte infiltration at the inflammation site and is inducible by proinflammatory cytokines, the homeostatic chemokines are constitutively expressed and regulate hematopoiesis and lymphoid organ development [95]. Both classes of chemokines can play a role in various aspects of malignancies. Because of the importance of leukocytes in HNSCC outcome, it is not surprising that CCL-3, CCL-4, and CCL-5 [96] are expressed by HNSCC tumors and that CCL-2 [97] and its receptor have been proposed as genetic markers for oral squamous cell carcinoma [98]. Similarly, the expression of CXC chemokine receptor 2 (CXCR2) is increased in the laryngeal squamous cell carcinoma, and its expression correlates with the lymph node metastases, with the histological grade, and with 5-year survival [99]. Additionally, CXCR4 was shown to be important in HNSCC tumor progression and organ-specific metastasis [100, 101] and could be used as a prognostic marker [102].

Approximately 50 chemokines and 20 receptors have been identified to date, and they can interact in a complex network in which the signal can be differentially integrated in each target cell (depending on the particular chemokine receptor profile). Each chemokine can bind multiple receptors, and a receptor can be activated by different chemokines, allowing chemokine redundancy [103], robustness [103], integration [104], and synergy [105]. While the initially attributed importance of redundancy was challenged by subsequent studies [106], the significance of signal integration, robustness, and synergy are being confirmed and explored by numerous studies. Chemokines can form homo- and hetero-dimers, integrating or modulating their own signal and the one from the dimeric partner [107, 108]. For example, CXCL4 can form a heterodimer with CCL5 that promotes monocyte arrest [109], while each chemokine alone is chemotactic. Chemokine integration and synergy can also involve the binding of different chemokines in the same cell that can result not only in the activation of the different individual pathways mediated by each chemokine but also in the integration of both transduced signals [110–113]. In human monocytes, CCL21 engagement of chemokine receptor (CCR)-7 dramatically amplifies the effect of CCL2 binding to CCR2 [114]. Because of the signal complexity and the different effects on the target cell population, it is not surprising that individual chemokines are reported to have opposite effects on tumor outcome. For example CCL5 in Ewing sarcoma [115] can promote tumor immunity by recruiting T cells at the tumor site, whereas in other cancers it is thought to inhibit tumor immunity and promote tumor angiogenesis and metastasis through MDSC and macrophage (tumor-educated myeloid cells (TEMCs)) recruitment [116, 117]. Interestingly, the antitumor effect of adoptively transferred T cells is increased by CCL5 but only when intratumoral $CD11c^{+}$ cells are depleted [118]. Similarly, CCL21 was shown to induce Th1 polarization [119], boost the efficacy of DNA vaccine [120], and promote the antitumor immunity [121]. Nevertheless the very same chemokine is secreted by many human tumors [122], and the expression of its receptor (CCR7) correlates with the metastatic activity in HNSCC [123] and is necessary for the formation of a tolerogenic lymphoid-like organ within the tumor [124]. Although the examples of contradictory roles of the same chemokines are too numerous to be listed here, it is noteworthy to report the opposite roles of CCL2. CCL2 secreted by the majority of solid tumors [125, 126] is able to attract both TEMCs and T cells in the tumor microenvironment and plays an important role in the proper homing into the tumor of adoptively transferred tumor-specific T cells [127]. Nevertheless, CCL2 mediates the recruitment of TEMC to the primary and secondary tumor sites, promoting tumor progression and metastasis [128–131]. Several studies have demonstrated that, contrary to TEMCs, T cells do not freely travel within the tumor but rather they remain trapped in the stroma surrounding the cancer cells [132]. The explanation of this phenomenon was recently clarified: reactive nitrogen species produced by TEMCs and neoplastic cells induce the nitration/nitrosilation of CCL2 that, once nitrosilated, can no longer attract cytotoxic T cells but can still recruit myeloid cells to the tumor [133]. These findings implicate the existence of a protumoral positive feedback mechanism by which TAM and MDSC promote the recruitment of new protumoral myeloid cells while hindering T cell infiltration.

4 Cellular Network of Immune Modulation in HNSCC

It is increasingly clear that tumors enforce strict connections with the surrounding environment creating a "microenvironment" that supports tumor progression. Moreover, by releasing soluble factors and exosomes, neoplastic cells can also condition distant sites, such as bone marrow, to sustain the demand of myeloid cells and precursors necessary for tumor neovascularization and spreading to local and distant anatomical sites. This creates de facto a complex interplay that can be viewed as a tumor-driven "macro-environment." The recognition that tumor macro- and microenvironments play pivotal roles in tumor progression suggests that innovative attempts should be made to block tumor/environment interactions that facilitate tumor progression and to enhance those counteracting malignancy.

Cancers are not only a mass of neoplastic cells; instead, they contain several noncancerous stromal cells. In many cases tumor stromal cells, which include TAMs, MDSCs, granulocytes, endothelial cells, fibroblasts, and T cells, may outnumber the malignant cells (Fig. 1) [134]. These accessory cells, most of which are leukocytes, are not innocent bystanders, but, rather, they interact with the malignant cells and play a key role in the disease outcome [135]. Depending on the composition and activation status of the immune infiltrate, the net effect can be either favorable or detrimental to tumor progression and metastasis. While effector T cells (quality and quantity) infiltrating the tumor correlate with a better survival in HNSCC patients [136–138] by either destroying or inducing dormancy in neoplastic cells, the infiltration of tumor-educated myeloid cells is associated with a higher mortality [45, 139].

4.1 Effector T Cells

Effector $CD4^+$ and $CD8^+$ T cells are considered the most important immune cells acting against cancer promotion and progression, as discussed elsewhere in this book. Although patients with HNSCC have reduced number of lymphocytes in their blood compared with healthy individuals [140], a significant shift from naive to effector memory T cells is observed in patients with oropharynx or larynx squamous cell carcinomas with an increased number of effector memory T cells in HPV^+ oropharyngeal squamous cell carcinomas [141], suggesting that a strong immune response against the tumor can be generated. Indeed, in recent years extraordinary progress has been made in the identification of tumor-associated antigens (TAA) in HNSCC. For example an analysis of the TILs in HNSCC revealed the prevalence of effector lymphocytes against the TAA cyclin B1 and NY ESO-1 that can be expanded in vitro and potentially used as a treatment modality [138]. Additionally, HNSCCs were found to express melanoma-associated antigens (i.e., MAGE 1 and MAGE 3) [142, 143] and, because of the changes in the epidemiology of this malignancy, viral antigens such as HPV E6 and E7 [144, 145]. Despite the presence of effector/memory tumor-specific T cells, these cells are unable to either reach the tumor or fully perform their tumoricidal action most likely because of the presence of a suppressive network orchestrated by the tumor. This hypothesis is supported by the finding that the functional impairment of T cells from HNSCC conferred by intrinsic molecular defects that have been demonstrated in this cell population can be reversed by removal of immune suppression by a pharmacologic treatment (Serafini, Weed unpublished data) or by radio- or chemotherapy [146]. This reversal is sufficient to reestablish T cell functionality in these tumors.

4.2 Dendritic Cells

Dendritic cells (DCs) are a family of specialized APCs and are essential mediators of immunity and tolerance [147]. DC may derive from the lymphoid (i.e., plasmacytoid DC) or myeloid precursors. While plasmacytoid DCs are mainly found in the blood and in the secondary lymphoid organs, myeloid DCs can infiltrate the dermis (dermal/interstitial myeloid dendritic cells) or the epidermis (Langerhans cells) of the mucosa of the upper aerodigestive tract [148] where they show an immature phenotype and a great capacity to uptake antigens. Upon encountering inflammatory signals (i.e., IL-1, TNF-α) or microbial products (i.e., TLR ligands) they migrate to the secondary lymphoid organs, assuming a mature phenotype and the capacity to cross-present the captured antigens, promoting the priming and the expansion of effector T cells. Because of their immunological role and their localization, myeloid DCs and Langerhans are particularly important in orchestrating the interaction between the immune system and HNSCC. Interestingly, tobacco and alcohol consumption, two main risk factors in HNSCC, are associated with an increased number of oral mucosal Langerhans cells that could suggest an active role of these cells in the initial phase of immunosurveillance [149, 150]. Indeed, their number seems to be higher in benign lesions than in normal mucosa or in neoplastic lesions [151]. Furthermore, their number seems to decrease with tumor grade [152], and, in laryngeal and nasopharyngeal carcinomas, a strong infiltration of Langerhans cells has been associated with longer disease-free survival, less locoregional recurrence [153], and a better prognosis [154]. Similarly, a larger number of DCs was found to be present in nonmetastatic lymph nodes than in metastatic lymph nodes in a series of hypopharyngeal and laryngeal carcinomas [155]. However, molecular defects, an inability to mature, and a reduced number of circulating myeloid DCs are found in patients with HNSCC (discussed in more detail below). The fact that surgical removal of the tumor is sufficient to restore the number and the function of DC [156] highlights that this reduction is due to the presence of tumor, is reversible, and is most likely one of the mechanisms of immune escape in HNSCC patients.

4.3 *Myeloid Derived Suppressor Cells and Tumor-Associated Macrophages*

MDSCs have been described in patients affected by different tumors. In HNSCC, for example, the release of GM-CSF and the tumor infiltration with $CD34^+$ MDSCs were determined to be negative prognostic factors and were associated with an increased rate of tumor metastasis and recurrence [157]. The increased frequency of $CD34^+$ cells in the PBMCs was also correlated with the suppression of the anamnestic responses to recall antigens, a frequent finding in HNSCC patients [158]. A more extensive study of the peripheral blood of patients with HNSSC, breast cancer, and non-small-cell lung cancer better characterized the phenotype of MDSCs that were described as immature cells positive for the markers CD34, CD33, and CD13 but negative for the myelomonocytic marker CD15. We recently confirmed these markers as associated with MDSCs in HNSCC and determined also that $IL4R\alpha^+$ $CD33^+$ cells are the most immunosuppressive myeloid cell subsets in these patients (Serafini, Weed, unpublished data). Although the murine counterpart of MDSC is characterized by the expression of the markers CD11b and Gr1, murine MDSCs share many functional features with human MDSC (such as the expression of the functional marker IL4Rα, the immature phenotype, and the molecular mechanisms of immunosuppression) and have allowed the dissection of the molecular mechanisms employed to restrain the immune response. These mechanisms were shown to utilize either the metabolism of L-arginine (L-Arg) or TGF-β production to render lymphocytes unresponsive to antigen stimulation. L-Arg is metabolized in myeloid cells (macrophages, granulocytes, and DCs) by two enzymes: (1) nitric oxide synthase (NOS), which oxidizes L-Arg in two steps that generate NO and citrulline, and (2) arginase (ARG), which converts L-Arg into urea and L-ornithine [159, 160]. By up-regulating Arg1 and consuming L-Arg in the surrounding microenvironment MDSC inhibited re-expression of the ζ-chain of CD3 complex in T lymphocytes, thereby impairing their function [161]. Alternatively, by NOS2 up-regulation, MDSC can S-nitrosilate, on T cells, crucial cysteine residues of important signaling proteins in the IL-2-receptor pathway including JAK1, JAK3, STAT5, ERK, and AKT [162]. S-nitrosilation makes T cells unresponsive to IL-2 inhibiting their proliferation and effector function [162]. Furthermore MDSC can express both Arg1 and NOS2. In these conditions MDSCs produce high quantities of peroxynitrite [163] that can induce either apoptosis [163] or anergy [164] in activated T cells and promote the nitration of particular chemokines affecting T cell infiltration into the tumor [133]. This hypothesis is further confirmed by the presence of NOS [165] and peroxynitrate metabolites [166] in the tumor bed of HNSSC patients. These observations are of clinical importance, because a reduced T cell proliferative capability to mitogenic stimulation has been associated with a poorer outcome for patients with HNSCC [167]. Moreover, the maturation of dendritic cells in patients with HNSCC is impaired [168] and associated with an increase of immature $CD34^+$ MDSC in the blood and in the tumor bed [169]. These observations are supported by murine data in which inhibition of DC maturation correlates with MDSC accumulation in the blood [170]. Attempts to overcome the immune dysfunction of patients with HNSCC have included combining in vivo immunization with autologous, irradiated HNSCC plus GM-CSF [171, 172]. Such treatments of patients with recurrent and metastatic HNSCC disease have shown the capacity to stimulate in vitro antitumor immune reactivity. However, in most cases the in vitro antitumoral activities of these T cells do not translate with a tumoricidal activity in vivo. These paradoxical results can be explained by the immunosuppressive network generated by the tumor that prevents CTL activities in vivo. These considerations are consistent with the preclinical data demonstrating that tumor-associated MDSC can induce anergy or apoptosis in tumor-specific T cells [173–175]. Similar inhibitory $CD34^+$ cells are also present within the cancer mass of patients with HNSCC where they can inhibit the activity of intratumoral T cells [157, 176–178].

The pro-tumoral activity of MDSCs and TAMs is not limited to their immunosuppressive role. Upon activation, these leukocytes secrete matrix-remodeling proteases and serine proteases that are associated with more advanced tumor grade and metastasis [179–181]. Additionally, following IL4Rα engagement, TAMs and MDSCs express elevated levels of the cysteine protease cathepsin B and expression of this protease is found within macrophages at the invasive edge of pancreatic cancers [179–181]. Metalloproteinase (MMP) and cathepsin B secretion by TAMs and MDSCs are partially regulated by IL-6 [182]. It is important to note that this cytokine, in concert with GM-CSF, is one of the key elements that regulate MDSC differentiation [52] and levels of both are particularly elevated in the sera of HNSCC [183]. In particular, GM-CSF, G-CSF, and IL-6 allowed a rapid generation of MDSCs from precursors present in mouse and human bone marrow (BM). These cytokines induce the activation of C/EBPβ in the myeloid lineage, a transcription factor necessary for MDSC differentiation. Genetic inactivation of this factor in the myeloid lineage blocked MDSC differentiation and reestablished the efficacy of antitumor immune interventions [52].

4.4 Regulatory T Cells

Tregs share the capacity to induce antigen-specific T cell tolerance and play an important role in preventing the development of autoimmune responses [184]. The very same cells are recruited by growing tumors to protect themselves from the immunological assault. In fact, the in vivo depletion of $CD4^+CD25^+$ T cells by anti-CD25 antibody (PC61), prior to tumor challenge, enhances tumor immunosurveillance and induces the rejection of multiple immunogenic tumors in different mouse strains [185]. Phenotypically, Treg cells express CD4 and CD25 and the functional marker forkhead/winged helix transcription factor (FoxP3) [186, 187]. Functionally, Treg cells inhibit T cell activity through their production of soluble inhibitory mediators such as TGF-β and IL-10 [187, 188]. Increased levels of $CD4^+CD25^+FoxP3^+$ Treg have been shown in the peripheral blood of patients with HNSCC [186] and have been associated with poor prognosis [189–191]. Tregs localizing to tumor tissue in HNSCC comprise a unique subset of $CD4^+CD25^{high}$ $Foxp3^+$ T cells, which secrete IL-10 and TGF-β1 and mediate a strong suppressor function [192]. Studies with patients with hepatocellular carcinoma showed increased levels of Treg within tumor tissue compared with normal tissue and increased levels of TGF-β expression in the peripheral blood of these patients compared with controls [193, 194]. The presence at the tumor site of these $CD4^+CD25^{high}FOXP3^+$ T cells seems to be a characteristic feature of T3/T4-stage HNSCC tumors and can be associated with a poor prognosis [192]. Nevertheless, the extent to which Treg cells contribute to the immune depression of patients with HNSCC is still unclear. Indeed, contradictory reports exist on the role of Treg in patients with oral cavity carcinoma: while initial studies associate the tumor infiltration of $FOXP3^+$ T cell with a worse prognosis [195, 196], other reports associate the infiltration of $FOXP3^+$ T cells with a better survival [197] or with better locoregional control of the tumor [198]. No significant associations were found in other studies [199]. Although technical differences in the Treg quantification (i.e., the antibody used, scoring system, number of markers) may explain these contradictory reports, the role of biological components also needs to be considered. Indeed, it is known that, contrary to murine Treg, human T cells may transiently express FOXP3 upon activation [200]. In this case, FOXP3 expression is not indicative of a regulatory function but, instead, of either incompletely activated effector cells [201, 202] or activated memory effector T cells [202]. Thus, although the effect of FOXP3 on activated T cells may be to down-regulate some of their effector functions, its expression could identify two distinct subsets of TILs with opposite effects on tumor outcome. An important breakthrough can derive from the work of Magg et al. [203] demonstrating that activated human effector T cells express FOXP3 mainly in the cytoplasm whereas Tregs are characterized mostly by a nuclear localization of this important transcription factor [203]. In accordance with this observation we recently found in patients with oral tongue SCC that the presence of $CD4^+$ cells expressing FOXP3 in the cytoplasm is associated with a favorable prognosis whereas its nuclear localization correlates with the risk of recurrence [204].

5 Immunologic Defects in HNSCC Patients

The impact of HNSCC on immune function is underscored by numerous molecular defects and alteration induced by the tumor in the immune system of the patients. The impact of HNSCC on immune function is underscored by the reduced number of $CD3^+$, $CD4^+$, and $CD8^+$ T cells (with $CD3^+CD4^+$ cell levels being more prominently reduced in patients with active disease) in the peripheral blood [205]. Even after curative surgery these levels remain low for several years further highlighting the profound consequences of this tumor on the immune system. The mechanisms by which HNSCC reduce T cell number seem to be multiple and complex. The induction of apoptosis can explain a reduction in the number of tumor-specific T cells. Indeed, neoplastic and stromal cells can trigger different pro-apoptotic signaling on T cells by the engagement of FAS by FAS-L or of DR4 and 5 by TRAIL [2]. Alternatively MDSCs and TAMs were shown to promote T cell apoptosis by different mechanisms that include nitration, deprivation of semi-essential amino acids, or production of reactive oxygen species [83]. Nevertheless additional mechanisms mediated by the tumor macro-environment also seem to affect the T cells with a specificity different from the tumor. Indeed, an increase in the ratio between the pro-apoptotic protein BAX and the anti-apoptotic factor Bcl-2 is found in most of the CD8 T cells of HNSCC patients [34], suggesting that apoptosis is induced in T cells regardless of the specificity. The defects associated with T cells in HNSCC regardless of their intrinsic specificity can be also partially explained by the changes in the cytokine macro-environment induced by the tumor. Indeed, compared with plasma cytokine levels of age-matched controls, cytokine levels in HNSCC patients demonstrated a shift to a Th2 bias with an increase of IL-4, IL-6, and IL-10 and a reduction of IFN-γ [69]. IFN-γ, besides being extremely important for many immunological processes (i.e., increasing antigen presentation, promotion of Th1 and CTL activity, induction of MHC class I), can inhibit the expression of BAX in T cells upon engagement of the beta chain of its receptor [206]. Thus, a significant and prolonged reduction of this cytokine could increase BAX expression, promoting T cell apoptosis. Interestingly, although the number of IL-2$^+$CD4$^+$ and CD8$^+$ T cells seems to be reduced in HNSCC patients [207], the serological level of IL-2 seems to be higher in this cohort of patients [69], partially excluding a role for IL-2 deprivation in T cell apoptosis.

Besides the reduced number of T cells, intrinsic molecular defects are detectable in the T cells of HNSCC patients. For example, lymphocytes of HNSCC patients show a profound down-regulation of the ζ-chain of the CD3 complex, a low responsiveness to IL-2 [208], and a reduced proliferative capability to mitogenic stimulation. The degree of reduction to the mitogenic stimula correlates with a poorer outcome for patients with HNSCC [167]. Considering that both CD3 ζ-chain down-regulation (by L-Arg deprivation) and IL-2 unresponsiveness (by STAT5 nitration) are two of the mechanisms by which MDSCs control the immune response [209], these observations can highlight the role of MDSC accumulation in the immunological defects observed in HNSCC.

HNSCC not only alters T cells but, as mentioned above, also has important consequences on the DC and myelopoiesis. Indeed, defects in DC function are considered a hallmark of immune system dysfunction in HNSCC [210]. For example, the accumulation of histiocytes/DCs in the distended sinuses of lymph nodes is a reflection of DC defects and is present in the lymph nodes of HNSCC patients. The buildup of these cells in the nodal sinuses prevents their entry into the node parenchyma, and maturation is, therefore, impaired, preventing optimal T cell stimulation [211]. A drastic reduction of circulating DC is also observed in HNSCC: while patients with early disease show a twofold decrease in circulating DC, patients with advanced disease show a fourfold reduction [168]. The decreased number of circulating DC seems to be confined to the myeloid subset, whereas the number of lymphoid DC is not affected [156]. The reduction of DC seems to be dependent on the release of GM-CSF and VEGF by the tumor that hijacks the physiological hematopoietic differentiation, promoting the accumulation of MDSCs and immature DCs in the lymphoid organs and at the tumor site [91]. The accumulation at the tumor site can be explained by the impaired migratory function of DC in hypoxic conditions [212] and by the presence of extracellular adenosine that characterize the tumor microenvironment. Under hypoxic conditions, DC not only failed to migrate in the lymph node but also acquired the chemokine receptor profile necessary for homing to the peripheral tissue. Moreover, hypoxia reduced DC maturation [212] and antigen uptake capability [213]. Finally, the up-regulation of the hypoxia-inducible factor 1α induced the expression of the adenosine receptor A2B that, once engaged, caused the DC to drive $CD4^+$ T cells toward a Th2 phenotype [213], a characteristic of HNSCC.

6 Immunotherapy for HNSCC

Immunotherapeutic strategies for HNSCC can be broadly categorized as antigen specific or antigen nonspecific (Fig. 1). Antigen-nonspecific therapies are designed to broadly enhance the immune response either by the selective addition of various immune stimulatory cytokines or by strategies to reverse or abrogate the immunosuppression mediated by the tumor. Intuitively it would seem that antigen-specific therapies would be the most powerful, and perhaps the least likely to generate systemic toxicity, due to their tumor cell-specific targeting. Yet it is precisely the host's own failure to generate a sufficient immune response against the developing tumor that suggests the importance of therapeutic strategies to nonspecifically enhance the immune response against already established tumor antigens. Clinically evident tumors have already survived the processes of immunosurveillance and immunoediting to be by their nature resistant to the immune response. Overcoming this resistance is essential to the success of immunotherapeutic strategies.

6.1 Antigen-Nonspecific Therapies

Antigen-nonspecific therapies may be used alone or in combination with antigen-specific immunotherapies. For example, IL-2 is often used in conjunction with adoptive cell transfer therapies to sustain the vitality and efficacy of transferred CTLs. Moreover, removal of immunosuppression is thought to be extremely important to potentiate the efficacy of antigen-specific immunotherapeutic intervention.

6.1.1 Cytokine Treatment Approaches

Cytokines have been used therapeutically either alone or in combination with chemotherapy, with varying degrees of success. These represent some of the earliest immunotherapeutic strategies employed against HNSCC. Administration of IL-2 to HNSCC patients has resulted in measurable increases in IL-2 levels, an increase in the number of NK cells within the tumor, and an increase in the overall activity of TIL [215, 216]. In both of these studies the cytokine was delivered locally to the tumor by peritumoral [215] or intranodal injection or intraarterial infusion [216]. Injection of recombinant IL-2 around the cervical lymph node chain for 10 days preoperatively in patients with T3-4, N0-3, M0 SCC of the oral cavity or oropharynx who subsequently underwent surgery for definitive tumor resection and radiotherapy resulted in significant increases in disease-free and overall survival with limited toxicity [217]. Systemic infusion of recombinant IL-2 combined with intramuscular or subcutaneous administration of interferon alpha resulted in an 18 % partial response rate (2/11) with substantial associated toxicity [218]. High doses of IL-2 may result in severe systemic toxicities (hypotension, capillary leak syndrome, and oliguria) [215], while at low doses the therapeutic efficacy might not be reached. Specific delivery of IL-2 at the tumor site is being explored in order to reach the therapeutic concentration locally while maintaining tolerable concentration systemically. For example, ALT-801 [216], a fusion protein composed of IL-2 and a TCR specific for the p53 (aa264-272)/HLA-A*0201 complex, is a new drug that moves toward this direction that targets IL-2 to the tumor cells overexpressing p53. Its use, in patients with different malignancies including head and neck cancer, seems to suggest a higher efficacy and a lower toxicity than high doses of IL-2 [216]. Interferon alpha has been used in combination with cisplatin and 5-fluorouracil in the treatment of advanced esophageal carcinoma (SCC and adenocarcinoma), with an overall response rate of 55 and a response rate of 61 % with esophageal SCC. Significant toxicities were reported [219]. Interferon gamma infused intravenously over a 24-h period once weekly for four infusions resulted in measurable response in three of eight patients with advanced resectable HNSCC with minimal toxicity noted and with histopathologic changes attributed to the therapy noted at the time of resection [220]. Intratumoral administration of recombinant IL-12 in patients with HNSCC resulted in a significant activation of B cells and the B cell compartment, with the presence of tumor-infiltrating B cells correlating with overall survival in 30 patients studied (irrespective of IL-12 treatment) [221]. IL-12 intratumoral administration resulted in an increase in the number of B cells and B cell proliferation in regional lymph nodes, a measurable increase in B cell interferon gamma mRNA expression, and a highly significant IgG subclass switch measured in plasma, indicating a switch to a T helper 1 phenotype [222]. Intratumoral administration of IL-12 resulted in increased number of $CD56^+$ NK cells in the primary tumor with no differences seen in primary tumor infiltration by $CD8^+$ and $CD4^+$ lymphocytes, with increased production of interferon gamma measured in $CD56^+$ NK cells and $CD8^+$ and $CD4^+$ lymphocytes in regional lymph nodes [222]. A more recent strategy undergoing ongoing clinical trials is to employ a cocktail of cytokines administered subcutaneously in preoperative fashion in patients with HNSCC [223–226]. IRX-2 is a primary cell-derived biologic containing physiologic quantities of T helper type 1 cytokines and monokines. Its primary active components are IL-2, IL-1β, IFNγ, and tumor necrosis factor alpha (TNF-alpha), which are combined with zinc (important in the development and function of cellular immunity), indomethacin (activates immune response and reduces immunosuppressive effects of prostaglandins), and low-dose cyclophosphamide (enhances the cell-mediated immune response by depleting and inhibiting immunosuppressive Tregs) as complementary methods to enhance immune responsiveness [225]. Preliminary studies have shown increases in $CD3^+$, $CD20^+$, and $CD68^+$ cells in surgical tumor specimens compared with pre-treatment biopsies, with $CD3^+$ T cells localized to intratumoral regions. $CD4^+$ cells were localized to peritumoral areas, while $CD8^+$ T cells were mainly intratumoral. $CD20^+$ B cells were primarily peritumoral, with $CD68^+$ macrophages localized to intratumoral regions [226]. The treatment was well tolerated, with $CD3^+$ lymphocyte infiltration in the surgical specimen having the strongest association with overall survival (all patients were treated without comparison control group) [225, 226].

6.1.2 Reversal of Immunosuppression

While the above-described nonspecific strategies for immune stimulation have the potential to generate increased quantity and quality of antitumor effector cells, their efficacy can be severely limited by tumor-mediated immunosuppression. Indeed, a tumor-specific immune tolerance and a generalized immunosuppression are the main immunological characteristics of HNSCC. Thus, it is not surprising that different anti-immunosuppressive strategies are being developed now that the multiple mechanisms of immunosuppression in HNSCC are being delineated. These strategies are designed to (1) reestablish a micro- and macro-environment favorable for immune surveillance, (2) deplete the suppressive populations that are recruited by the tumor, or (3) block the molecular mechanisms by which the negative regulators of the immune response shield the tumor from immunological recognition.

In the first class of immune therapeutic intervention, the signaling by which the HNSCC promotes the expansion of immune-modulatory cells (i.e., MDSC, Treg) is targeted. For example, it is known that VEGF, PGE2, GM-CSF, IL-6, and other tumor-derived factors activate aberrant intracellular pathways (i.e., IL6st, STAT3) in the myeloid lineage, expand the pool of MDSCs, and prevent DC maturation. Thus inhibition of these intracellular pathways can be a strategy to revert the suppressive tumor macro-environment and restore effective immune surveillance. Sunitinib for example is a small molecule that inhibits multiple tyrosine kinases (VEGFR-1, VEGFR-2, VEGFR-3, PDGFR, c-kit, ret, and STAT3) and that has shown potent effects against MDSC in both animal models and human studies [227]. Clinical studies in advanced renal cell carcinomas have found reversal of MDSC accumulation in addition to tumor cell apoptosis in sunitinib-treated patients [228]. However, a clinical trial using sunitinib in HNSCC demonstrated important hematological toxicities (i.e., lymphopenia, neutropenia, and thrombocytopenia) or bleeding complications in many patients [229] and poor therapeutic efficacy [230, 231]. Considering the capacity of this molecule to inhibit multiple tyrosine kinases and the fact that some of these pathways need to be transiently activated during normal myelopoiesis and lymphopoiesis, these results are not completely surprising.

Nevertheless positive antitumor results were obtained when sunitinib was administered in conjunction with image-guided radiotherapy for the treatment of patients with oligometastases [232]. Thus, despite the intrinsic toxicity (that could be significantly reduced by a nanotargeted delivery in the future) sunitinib may yet maintain its therapeutic promise as a component of a possible multimodal therapy or in situations of minimal residual disease.

1α,25-dihydroxyvitamin D_3 is another compound that may have important therapeutic potential in the treatment of HNSCC. This well-tolerated vitamin has previously been shown to induce, in vitro, the maturation of immune-suppressive $CD34^+$ MDSC into immune-stimulatory dendritic cells [233, 234]. Further studies demonstrate that patients treated with 1α,25-dihydroxyvitamin D_3 for 21 days before surgery had reduced intratumoral levels of MDSCs, an increased level of mature dendritic cells, and a higher number of effector $CD4^+$ and $CD8^+$ T cells infiltrating the tumor and expressing the early activator marker CD69. More importantly, this short presurgical treatment was sufficient to double the time of HNSCC recurrence in the treated patients [235]. Interestingly, these antitumor effects of 1α,25-dihydroxyvitamin D_3 were characterized by a profound modulation of the cytokine concentration in the plasma and in the tumor specimen [236]. Although induction of MDSC differentiation into immune-stimulatory DC may be one of the mechanisms that promotes the immunomodulatory activity of 1α,25-dihydroxyvitamin D_3, other actions might be involved. Indeed, 1α,25-dihydroxyvitamin D_3 has been shown to inhibit tumor angiogenesis in vivo and the production of VEGF and hypoxia factor 1α in many human tumor cell lines [237]. Since both VEGF and HIF1α are implicated in the induction of MDSCs by the tumor, it is possible that by modulating the transcriptome profile of neoplastic cells, 1α,25-dihydroxyvitamin D_3 deprives tumors of those elements that allow for their escape from immune surveillance.

Another agent that has been used to reverse immune suppression in HNSCC belongs to the class of cyclooxygenase-2 (COX2) inhibitors. As we mentioned above, COX2 is overexpressed in the tumor microenvironment and its expression correlates with a poor prognosis in HNSCC [65]. COX2 expression is localized both in the neoplastic cells and in the surrounding stroma [65], and by producing PGE2 it is able not only to activate the suppressive phenotype in the MDSCs but also to facilitate the differentiation of MDSCs from their hematopoietic precursors [68]. Thus, COX2 inhibition can be seen as an important opportunity to reverse HNSCC-induced immune suppression by blocking both MDSC differentiation and activation (i.e., by inducing arginase 1 and iNOS [238]) at the tumor site. Interestingly, celecoxib (a specific COX2 inhibitor) has demonstrated antitumor activity in advanced HNSCC when used in combination with erlotinib (a specific inhibitor of EGFR) and in combination with radiotherapy. In combination with erlotinib, 25 % of the treated patients with unresectable recurrent locoregional and/or distant metastatic HNSCC show a partial response and a low toxicity profile [239]. Instead, when the same treatment was used in combination with local irradiation on patients with previously irradiated HNSCC, 60 % of the patients showed locoregional control and 37 % progression-free survival at 1 year [240]. Celecoxib unfortunately was also found to be associated with a dose-dependent cardiovascular morbidity, which limited its dosage and prevented its long-term use in reversing tumor-induced immunosuppression [241–243].

In addition to the use of drug to restrain MDSC differentiation, other strategies have been developed targeting specifically the suppressive mechanisms by which these cells inhibit antitumor immunity. We previously demonstrate in preclinical models that PDE5 is a key protein that mediates MDSC suppression [175]. This enzyme, by controlling the intracellular concentration of cGMP, directly controls the expression of iNOS, IL4Rα, and arginase 1 on MDSCs [175], thereby controlling their suppressive action. Indeed, pharmacologic inhibition of PDE5 using sildenafil or tadalafil (FDA-approved drugs for the treatment of erectile dysfunction) was sufficient to restrain tumor-induced immune suppression, prime a spontaneous antitumor immune response, and drastically reduce tumor progression in murine models of breast and colon cancer [175]. Furthermore, in a lymphoma model of tumor-induced tolerance, PDE5 was sufficient to restrain the MDSC-mediated expansion of tumor-specific Treg [244]. Finally, and more importantly, when Sildenafil was added to anti-CD3/anti-CD28-stimulated PBMCs from patients with HNSCC and multiple myeloma, PDE5 blockade was sufficient to restore the otherwise repressed T cell proliferation [244]. Based on these results two independent clinical trials (at Johns Hopkins University and at the University of Miami) were started in HNSCC patients to test the immune modulatory capacity of tadalafil daily administration before surgical resection of the primary tumor. Interim analyses in both clinical trials seem to suggest that PDE5 blockade lowers MDSC and Treg concentrations in the blood and in the tumor tissue, promotes the tumor infiltration of activated ($CD69^+$) $CD4^+$ and $CD8^+$ T cells, and expands the systemic pool of tumor-specific T cells. Only reversible negative side effects (back pain) have been found in a small percentage of treated patients suggesting the possible use of PDE5 inhibitors to down-modulate immune suppression in HNSCC (Weed and Serafini unpublished observation).

It is important to remember that MDSCs are not the only mediator of immunosuppression in HNSCC. As described above Tregs are significantly expanded in HNSCC patients, and this cell population is thought to play an important role in tumor-induced T cell anergy, inhibition of DC maturation, and malignant progression [192]. Despite therapies specifically aimed at depleting or inactivating Tregs in HNSCCs that have not yet been clinically tested (or results are still unavailable) there is the indication that low dosage of cyclophosphamide or ifosfamide can selectively deplete Treg in cancer patients [245]. These alkylating agents have been shown to be effective in the treatment of HNSCC even when used as a single agent [246]. Interestingly ifosfamide's therapeutic efficacy was increased when it was administered in association with cisplatin and 13-*Cis* retinoic acid, with a response rate of 72 % in distant metastatic HNSCC [247]. In this study a restoration of tumor immunity was hypothesized because of the prolonged response observed once the chemotherapeutic regimen was terminated. In light of the new understanding that 13-*Cis* retinoic acid can *trans*-isomerize in vivo to produce all-*trans*-retinoic acid (ATRA) [248] and that ATRA can force MDSC to differentiate into mature DC [249], it is highly possible that at least part of the beneficial effect of this chemotherapeutic combination was due to the restoration of a correct immunological milieu by MDSC conversion and Treg depletion. Because of the possible beneficial role that cyclophosphamide-dependent Treg depletion can act in synergy with other therapies in head and neck cancer, different trials are currently ongoing, but results are still unavailable.

In summary, the better understanding of the cellular and molecular mechanisms that regulate tumor immunosuppression in HNSCC and the technical advances in drug isolation and development are offering many strategies for the immunomodulation of tumor immunity. Nevertheless, many of the identified pathways are implicated in normal physiological activity, and thus their inhibition may lead to extremely serious side effects. A specific targeting using nanoparticle or other similar strategies needs to be developed in order to minimize the negative side effect and maximize antitumor efficacy. It is important to note that despite the coexistence of multiple suppressive pathways, the inhibition of only one is often sufficient to tilt the balance and generate a micro- and macro-environment favorable to an effective immune surveillance.

6.2 *Antigen-Specific Approaches*

Immune-specific therapeutic strategies seek to harness the natural immune response to tumor by virtue of amplifying one or more of the effector arms of the immune system targeting specific tumor antigens. These strategies include antibody therapies, adoptive cell transfer, and various tumor vaccine approaches. The efficacy of these approaches is likely to be substantially improved when combined with nonspecific immunotherapeutic approaches and particularly with strategies designed to reverse tumor-induced immunosuppression. Additionally, the efficacy of combinations of both antigen-specific and -nonspecific immunotherapeutic strategies with conventional chemotherapy, radiation therapy, and surgical protocols is only beginning to be elucidated.

6.2.1 Antibody Therapies

The most widely studied antibody therapy for HNSCC involves the use of antibodies targeting the epidermal growth factor receptor (EGFR). These strategies are summarized in useful reviews by De Costa and Young [250], Ferris et al. [251], and Russell and Colevas [252]. The EGFR is overexpressed in oral premalignant and malignant lesions [253] and is the most common tumor antigen against which antibody therapies are directed in HNSCC. Other antibody targets include HER2/neu and VEGF. Corresponding therapeutic antibodies include cetuximab (EGFR/HER1), panitumimab (EGFR/HER/1), trastuzumab (HER2/neu), and bevacizumab (VEGF).

The tumor antigens mentioned above are cell surface molecules that have functional capabilities as mediators of signaling pathways responsible for cell growth and endothelial cell proliferation as examples. These receptors are found on normal cells as well as tumor, indicating that toxicity to normal tissues can occur with these therapies. Monoclonal antibody-based therapies can therefore have a dual effect on tumor cells bearing increased expression of these receptor antigens. The signaling pathway initiated by the receptor may be inhibited by antibody blockade, typically a preferred outcome for these tumors. Additionally, cell-mediated cytotoxicity may be initiated by the monoclonal antibody bound to the tumor antigen resulting in tumor cell death. Fortunately treatment with these antibodies does not typically result in severe allergic reactions or systemic toxicity [251]. Treatment with these antibodies alone can result in limited responses, even in advanced pretreated disease [254]. Their efficacy is typically increased in combination with chemotherapy and radiation therapy.

The clinical success of cetuximab has been demonstrated in single agent and combinational phase I studies, showing both good patient tolerance and clinical efficacy [255–257]. The most common side effect of treatment is an acneiform rash. A phase III trial of 424 HNSCC patients randomized to radiation alone or cetuximab and radiation resulted in an increase in locoregional control in the cetuximab group (24.4 months vs. 14.9 months, $p=0.005$) [258]. This study, and its relatively limited toxicity, resulted in FDA approval of cetuximab for use in combination with radiation therapy for locally advanced HNSCC in 2006. The longer term follow-up of this trial still showed efficacy of the cetuximab-treated patients, with 45.6 % vs. 36.4 % overall 5-year survival and the notable observation that improved overall survival was seen in patients experiencing at least a grade 2 acneiform rash during treatment [259]. Studies combining cetuximab with both chemotherapy and radiation therapy have noted considerably greater toxicities that become therapy limiting, making demonstration of efficacy difficult over standard platinum-based chemo-radiation strategies [252, 260, 261]. Studies comparing the efficacy of cetuximab combined with radiation therapy vs. cisplatin-based chemoradiation therapy are ongoing [252].

The mechanism of action of monoclonal antibody blockade leading to tumor response and death is likely twofold, as mentioned above. Blockade of signal transduction alone is not likely to yield the clinical benefits described above, with an immunologic mediated cell death being an important component of the success of monoclonal antibody-based therapies as well as a key contributor to the variable responses seen with such therapies [251, 262–264]. In cell culture tumor cell apoptosis does not occur with treatment by monoclonal antibody alone but only when lymphocytes are added to the culture system [251, 265]. Clinical response can be correlated in patients with polymorphisms of monoclonal antibody-binding receptors on NK cells, monocytes, and granulocytes that are known to have lytic activity [251]. Interestingly, the level of EGFR expression, activation, or gene amplification does not correlate with clinical response to monoclonal antibody therapy. This finding suggests that factors other than blockade of signal transduction contribute to the observed clinical effect [251, 266]. Possible explanations for the variability of response are many. The monoclonal antibody isotype subclass plays an important role in the extent of cell-dependent lysis of the target cell. IgG1 and IgG3 subclasses are more efficient than IgG2 and IgG4 subclasses at mediating lysis of target cells [251, 267, 268]. This is clinically relevant as cetuximab is an IgG1 isotype, whereas panitumimab, another monoclonal antibody targeting the EGFR, is an IgG2 isotype and is predicted to have a lower ability to induce cellular immune reactions [251, 265, 269]. Complement-dependent cytotoxicity can be seen with IgG1 isotype monoclonal antibodies, but this mechanism of cell death occurs rapidly and is not consistent with the observed clinical responses seen in cetuximab therapy in HNSCC where tumor shrinkage is noted over weeks. This is also inconsistent with an NK cell-mediated cell death, which should occur over a matter of hours, and is more indicative of a T-lymphocyte-mediated lytic effect [251]. Another factor which may influence clinical response to monoclonal antibody-based therapies includes Fc gamma R polymorphisms, particularly as this relates to the role of NK cell-mediated cytotoxicity, although clinical relevance of such polymorphisms is not well elucidated [251, 267]. It is also possible that an initial antibody-mediated neoplastic cell death and macrophage infiltration result in the release of tumor antigens and increase cross-priming that allows the generation of an adaptive immune response that promotes tumor regression.

Taken together, data regarding antibody-based immunotherapies for HNSCC have clearly demonstrated the greatest clinical efficacy and certainly the most widespread use in clinical practice today. The complexity of interactions that occur at the cellular level with such strategies likely explains the variable responses seen and the lack of clear correlation with antigen (receptor) levels and treatment response. This complexity also argues for further investigation of treatment strategies designed to exploit the immunologic effects of monoclonal antibody-based therapies, in the form of either combined strategies to reverse immunosuppression or perhaps adoptive T cell therapies that may ultimately further strengthen the already established clinical efficacy of these treatments [270].

6.2.2 Adoptive Cell Transfer

Adoptive cell transfer is a therapeutic strategy designed to provide a primed antigen-specific population of effector cells that can result in cell-mediated tumor cytotoxicity. Studies utilizing this method are few, in part due to the technically challenging and cumbersome nature of the therapies. One such trial [171] involved a study of 17 patients with recurrent and metastatic HNSCC who were vaccinated in the thigh with irradiated autologous tumor cells admixed with GM-CSF followed by three additional daily injections of GM-CSF at the vaccination site. Eight to ten days later inguinal lymph nodes draining the vaccine site were resected, and lymphocytes harvested from these nodes were activated with staphylococcal enterotoxin A and expanded in IL-2 in vitro. The cultured cells were then infused back into the patients peripherally as outpatients. 15 patients were successfully infused (2 showed insufficient vaccine response), with the toxic effects of infusion limited to grade 2 reactions in 3 of 16 total treatments. The infused cells were predominately $CD3^+$, a mixture of $CD4^+$ and $CD8^+$ cells. Three patients showed disease stabilization where progression had been evident pre-treatment, with two patients described as having a favorable clinical course [171].

Another adoptive cell strategy [271] was employed utilizing the antibody catumaxomab that binds epithelial cell adhesion molecule (EpCAM) with one arm and CD3⁺ T cells with its other arm. Peripheral blood mononuclear cells (PBMC) of four patients were collected by leukopheresis, then incubated ex vivo with catumaxomab for 24 h, and cleared and released from cytokines. Each patient received an escalated dose of the opsonized PBMC intravenously at bi-weekly intervals. The opsonized PBMC released significant amounts of IFN-γ and TNF-α in vitro, which was removed prior to administration. Catumaxomab up-regulated CD25, CD69, and CD83 on PBMC, and catumaxomab-loaded PBMC released IFN-γ and granzyme B when coincubated with EpCAM(⁺)BHY cells. This suggested cell activation and target-directed biological activity. Adverse events were significant at higher doses, but lower doses were well tolerated and one patient showed stable disease at 6 months and one in complete remission at 27 months [271].

A recent study evaluated a bimodal ex vivo expansion method to harvest tumor-specific T cells [272]. TIL bulk cultures were established from primary and recurrent HNSCC in high-dose IL-2. Next selected bulk cultures were rapidly expanded using anti-CD3 antibody, feeder cells, and high-dose IL-2. T cell subsets were phenotypically characterized using flow cytometry. Interferon gamma detection by Elispot and ^{51}Cr release assay was used to determine the specificity and functional capacity of selected TIL pre- and post-rapid expansion. Bulk TIL cultures were expanded in 80 % of the patients included with tumor specificity demonstrated in 60 %. Rapid expansions generated up to 3,500-fold expansion of selected TIL cultures within 17 days. The cultures consisted primarily of T-effector memory cells, with varying distributions of CD8⁺ and CD4⁺ subtypes. TCR clonotype mapping demonstrated oligoclonal expanded cultures with 10–30 T cell clonotypes. The TIL from large-scale rapid expansions maintained both functional capacity and contained tumor-specific T cells. This study provides the basis for future clinical trials utilizing this method of ex vivo T cell expansion in adoptive cell transfers in HNSCC [272].

Nevertheless adoptive cell transfer strategies are limited by the need to isolate and expand antitumor reactive lymphocytes that preexist in the patient and often are anergic to the in vitro restimulation [273]. Gene modification of T lymphocytes [217, 225] may overcome the requirement for preexisting tumor-specific immunity. With this strategy, PBMCs from patients are retrovirally transduced with TCR specific for the tumor, thus conferring them with additional specificity for the neoplastic cells before reinfusion. Additional genes that protect the lymphocytes from the tumor-suppressive mechanisms can also be added, making this strategy extremely interesting [220]. As a proof of concept for the therapy, PBMCs from melanoma patients were retrovirally transfected with high-affinity TCR specific for p53–HLA-A2 complex and, as anticipated, were shown to be able to recognize different p53-expressing human tumor cell lines [274]. Considering the importance that p53 antigen plays in HNSCC and that this strategy is already being tested in other malignancies, the use of TCR-transduced PBMCs could be rapidly tested in P53⁺ head and neck cancer.

Besides the transfer of CTL, the antitumor efficacy of adoptively transferred effector Vα24 NKT cells has been tested in HNSCC [275]. Since NKT cells have an antitumor effect, Yamasaki et al. evaluated the safety and therapeutic efficacy of ex vivo-expanded NKT cells adoptively transferred to ten locally recurrent and operable HNSCC patients. One course of nasal submucosal administration of αGalCer-pulsed APCs and intra-arterial infusion of activated NKT cells via tumor-feeding arteries was given before salvage surgery. Five patients achieved objective tumor regression. The number of NKT cells increased in cancer tissues in seven cases and was associated with tumor regression [275].

Adoptive cell transfer of HNSCC-reactive cells seems to be a promising therapeutic option that could be used in association with anti-immunosuppressive strategies and/or with other standard therapeutic options.

6.2.3 Antitumor Vaccines

The intrinsic genetic instability and the particular etiology of HNSCC result in the expression of both unique and shared TAA by the malignant cells. These differences provide an important therapeutic opportunity to educate the immune system to recognize and destroy the neoplastic cells while preserving the normal tissues. TAA are presented as epitope by the MHC of the cancerous and precancerous cells, allowing their identification by the cytotoxic T cells. Many HNSCC-associated antigens have been identified and characterized, and vaccine strategies aimed to mount an immune response against these antigens are being developed. For example, 71 % of HNSCC express antigens from at least one of the six melanoma antigen genes (MAGE) [142, 276–278]. Additionally, NY-ESO-1, a testis-specific antigen, is highly expressed in HNSCC [279]. Moreover, mutations of normal protein (i.e., p53) are extremely common in HNSCC because they contribute to the malignant phenotype, and these give rise to tumor-specific antigens [62]. Finally, because of the changes in HNSCC epidemiology, the HPV-associated antigens E6 and E7 can be used as epitopes to target the immune response against the tumor [280].

Different strategies (described elsewhere in this book) can be used to promote an immune response against the tumor; however, the clinical evaluation of these strategies in HNSCC remains in its infancy, with few clinical studies available. Nevertheless several lines of evidence make the development of HNSCC-specific vaccines extremely appealing. For example, p53-specific CTL can be expanded in patients with HNSCC [281]. By using autologous DC pulsed with the HLA-A2.1-restricted wt $p53^{264-272}$ CTL-specific clones could be expanded in vitro and detected in vivo from the PBMCs of many HNSCC patients. Interestingly, while p53-specific T cells could be expanded and detected in vivo from the group of patients whose tumors express low levels of p53, the group of patients whose tumor expresses high levels of p53 showed fewer circulating P53-specific CTLs that only rarely could be expanded in vitro [281]. These data are in line with the hypothesis that immune selection and immune editing might have intervened in the first group selecting those neoplastic clones with a lower p53 expression but also indicate that it might be difficult to raise an immune response in patients in whom immune surveillance has already failed. Nevertheless, in these cases different strategies might be adopted: more immunogenic modified epitope might be used for the immunization or the immunogen can be given with an adequate adjuvant such as on DC co-pulsed with adjuvant helper peptides. Indeed, more immunogenic variants of the $p53^{264-272}$ are able to rescue the expansion even from the PBMCs of patients with high p53-expressing tumor [282]. Furthermore, an appreciable immune response was observed when autologous DC pulsed with the p53 peptide and a tetanus-derived helper peptide were given as a vaccine in stage I–IVa patients (pts) with HNSCC with no active disease [266]. Vaccination was well tolerated by all HNSCC patients. Increased p53-specific T cells were seen in 11/16 patients (69 %) with positive IFN-γ secretion in 4/16 patients (25 %). Frequencies and absolute number of Treg were significantly decreased after vaccination ($p=0.006$). Disease-free survival (85 %) at 24 months of follow-up appeared to be favorable as compared to historical unvaccinated HNSCC patients [283].

6.3 HPV as a Potential Immunological Target

With the recognition of the important role of HPV infection in HNSCC tumorigenesis, particularly in nonsmokers, this expanding subset of patients is a particularly attractive patient population in which to study novel vaccine strategies. One reason for this is that the HPV is an immunoreactive target for which a vaccine has already been established and currently approved for prophylactic use [272]. One strategy for vaccine therapy in HNSCC, therefore, is a preventive one. Vaccination of not just girls but also boys should result in more than an additive effect in the long-term prevention of HPV-related malignancies given that HPV-related malignancies are sexually transmitted diseases [284]. Vaccination programs targeting both boys and girls will likely result in a significant reduction in the overall incidence of HPV-related HNSCC in the future. Nevertheless therapeutic HPV vaccines are also being developed. These vaccines are being designed to target not the HPV capside antigens L1 and L2, that are not expressed once the virus is integrated, but rather E6 and E7 that are constitutively expressed in all levels of epithelium and that are critical for the maintenance of malignant transformation in HPV-infected cells by inactivating the tumor-suppressor protein p53 and retinoblastoma (RB) [280]. Different methods of immunization are currently being tested in cervical and head and neck cancer. These vaccines include the use of HPV-E6 peptides, live attenuated listeria *monocytogenes* bacteria carrying E7 fusion protein, vaccinia-based vaccines, naked DNA vaccines, and DC-based vaccines. Live attenuated listeria *monocytogenes* bacteria encoding E6 and E7 vaccines (ADXS11-001) are a relatively new and interesting method of immunization that takes advantage of capacity of listeria *monocytogenes* to both stimulate the innate immunity and, by naturally infecting the antigen-presenting cells, to promote DC antigen cross-presentation activating both $CD4^+$ and $CD8^+$ T cells [285]. Preclinical data demonstrate that ADXS11-001 vaccine induces the regression of established tumors, by reducing the suppressive activity of Treg and MDSCs at the tumor site, by promoting the chemotaxis and maturation of dendritic cells, and by generating memory effector T cells [286]. An initial phase I clinical trial was performed in a population of refractory cervical cancer patients in which no therapy had been shown to extend survival [287]. Despite the presence of a transient adverse flu-like effect in 100 % of the patients, 73 % of the patients had a performance status ECOG 2–4, 1-year survival increased to 53 % from the historical 5 %, and a significant reduction of tumor size was appreciated in 33 % of the patients [287]. Considering that listeria *monocytogenes* can be killed by the use of antibiotics, this strategy is extremely promising for the treatment of HPV^+ HNSCC. Based on these and other results, a clinical trial started in the UK in which patients with $HPV16^+$ oropharyngeal SCC are being treated with three different doses of ADXS11-001 in addition to the current chemo-, radio-, and/or surgical treatment (T.M. Jones, Liverpool CR-UK Centre, personal communication). Results of this ongoing trial are still unavailable.

Another strategy being explored for inducing a strong immune response against HPV epitope is the use of "Trojan" peptides. Trojan peptide-based vaccines contain a penetrin peptide sequence derived from HIV-TAT which allows the entire peptide to translocate through the cell membrane and penetrate directly into the endoplasmatic reticulum and the Golgi apparatus. There, they can form peptide–HLA complexes without the need of proteosomal processing and TAP transportation. This strategy has been used to vaccinate patients with advanced HNSCC against the TAA MAGE 3 and HPV-16 [288]. In particular the penetrin peptide was fused via furin cleavable linker to MAGE and HPV-16-derived HLA-I- and HLA-II-restricted peptides. Following four immunizations with GM-CSF and Montanide ISA 51 as adjuvant, systemic immune response against the Trojan and the HLA-II-restricted peptides were measurable in most patients whereas the CD8-mediated responses were less pronounced [288]. Interestingly, analysis of the tumor specimen of one patient that underwent surgical resection of the malignancy after treatment revealed great infiltration of MAGE-specific $CD4^+$ and $CD8^+$ T cells (absent in the pretreatment biopsies) and large areas of apoptotic tumor cells [288]. Although this was only a proof-of-concept pilot study, the obtained data strengthen the enthusiasm for the development of tumor vaccines in HNSCC.

6.4 *Whole Tumor Vaccines in HNSCC*

Since the use of a small number of epitopes in a vaccine formulation can result in further immune editing and relevant antigen lost from tumor, other vaccination methods include the use of the whole tumor with the rationale to target the whole repertoire of tumor antigens. As mentioned above, patients have been vaccinated with autologous irradiated tumor cells and then received adoptive transfer of in vitro-expanded $CD4^+$ and $CD8^+$ lymphocytes harvested from lymph nodes draining the vaccination site [171]. This strategy achieved a limited clinical response while being well tolerated and is an example of one way in which two separate but related types of cellular immunotherapies can be combined in an effort to achieve greater efficacy with appropriate toxicity profile [171]. Another example of a vaccine strategy that utilized autologous tumor cells involved modification of autologous tumor cells harvested at the time of tumor resection with Newcastle disease virus [271]. The treated patients were divided into groups receiving IL-2 alone or IL-2 combined with vaccination with virus-modified autologous tumor. The vaccinated group showed increased levels of tumor-reactive T cells, enhanced antitumor delayed-type hypersensitivity responses, and a prolonged long-term survival that was associated with an increase in immune reactivity [271]. Finally, another strategy exploited to prime an HNSCC-specific immune response is based on the use of oncolytic virus encoding for immune-stimulatory cytokines. Indeed, oncolytic virus therapy is a promising approach to cancer treatment, particularly for the locoregional control of solid tumors. The rationale for the use of these viruses is that they selectively replicate in tumor in a way that tumor cells are killed by lytic virus replication while normal cells are spared. Thus, having the virus encoding immune-stimulatory cytokines such as GM-CSF, the tumor mass is reduced not only by the direct viral effect but also by the release of tumor antigens in an immune-stimulatory environment, inducing a tumor-specific immune response that protects the host from local and distant recurrence.

One of the first examples reported in HNSCC was a phase I clinical trial using an oncolytic herpes simplex virus expressing GM-CSF [289]. In this clinical trial, the virus was injected intratumorally in patients with head and neck cancer, breast cancer, and malignant melanoma that had failed previous therapies. The virus was generally well tolerated with local inflammation, erythema, and febrile responses being the main side effects. Nineteen of 26 patient posttreatment biopsies contained residual tumor, of which 14 showed tumor necrosis, which in some cases was extensive, or apoptosis. The overall responses to treatment were that three patients had stable disease, six patients had tumors flattened, and four patients showed inflammation of un-injected as well as the injected tumor, which, in nearly all cases, became inflamed [289]. Interestingly, in some patients both injected and un-injected lesions became inflamed and flattened over time suggesting that either the virus spread to distant metastases or an important immune response was generated. Additional studies were performed in patients with stage III/IVA/IVB HNSCC in conjunction with chemoradiotherapy (cisplatin plus 70 Gy/35 fractions) and underwent neck dissection 6–10 weeks later. 82.3 % of the patients showed tumor response by Response Evaluation Criteria in Solid Tumors, and pathologic complete remission was confirmed in 93 % of patients at neck dissection. HSV was detected in injected and adjacent un-injected tumors at levels higher than the input dose, indicating viral replication. All patients were seropositive at the end of the treatment. No patient developed locoregional recurrence, and disease-specific survival was 82.4 % at a median follow-up of 29 months [290]. Although an extensive analysis of tumor immunity in head and neck cancer patients treated with oncoviral vector has not yet been performed, similar studies performed in melanoma as well as preclinical studies indicate that the therapeutic potential of oncolytic virus is linked to both innate and adaptive immunity [291]. Indeed, in melanoma patients, regression of untreated lesions has been reported after treatment with oncolytic GM-CSF-encoding virus [291, 292]. In a murine model, tumor-bearing mice treated and cured are resistant to subsequent challenge with the same but not an unrelated tumor [292]. In summary, significant progress is being made in promoting an HNSCC-specific antitumor immunity using a variety of strategies in currently ongoing clinical trials.

7 Conclusion

The promise of immunotherapy in HNSCC remains elusive, yet its realization is closer now than ever. Advances in our understanding of the complex interactions of head and neck squamous cell carcinomas and the immune system have led to innovative immunotherapeutic approaches tested in both preclinical and clinical settings. It is increasingly apparent that efforts to stimulate an effective immune response must be coupled with strategies to abrogate the immune-suppressive environment characteristic of these tumors. Preclinical studies and clinical trials have yielded very promising results and provide the foundation for further refinements in a broad variety of immunotherapeutic strategies targeting all components of the immune system. Combining such approaches with the established treatment options of surgical resection, radiotherapy, and chemotherapy may ultimately yield substantive improvements in overall survival that to date have been lacking. Novel combinations of immunotherapies with traditional therapies may further reduce both disease-related and treatment-related morbidities for this debilitating and deadly disease.

References

1. Siegel R, Naishadham D, Jemal A. Cancer statistics, 2012. CA Cancer J Clin. 2012;62(1):10–29. doi:10.3322/caac.20138.
2. Duray A, Demoulin S, Hubert P, Delvenne P, Saussez S. Immune suppression in head and neck cancers: a review. Clin Dev Immunol. 2010;2010:701657. doi:10.1155/2010/701657.
3. Parkin DM, Bray F, Ferlay J, Pisani P. Global cancer statistics, 2002. CA Cancer J Clin. 2005;55(2):74–108.
4. Ho T, Wei Q, Sturgis EM. Epidemiology of carcinogen metabolism genes and risk of squamous cell carcinoma of the head and neck. Head Neck. 2007;29(7):682–99.
5. Chaturvedi AK, Engels EA, Anderson WF, Gillison ML. Incidence trends for human papillomavirus-related and -unrelated oral squamous cell carcinomas in the United States. J Clin Oncol. 2008;26(4):612–9. doi:10.1200/JCO.2007.14.1713.
6. Ryerson AB, Peters ES, Coughlin SS, Chen VW, Gillison ML, Reichman ME, et al. Burden of potentially human papillomavirus-associated cancers of the oropharynx and oral cavity in the US, 1998–2003. Cancer. 2008;113(10 Suppl):2901–9. doi:10.1002/cncr.23745.
7. Auluck A, Hislop G, Bajdik C, Poh C, Zhang L, Rosin M. Trends in oropharyngeal and oral cavity cancer incidence of human papillomavirus (HPV)-related and HPV-unrelated sites in a multicultural population: the British Columbia experience. Cancer. 2010;116(11):2635–44. doi:10.1002/cncr.25087.

8. Hocking JS, Stein A, Conway EL, Regan D, Grulich A, Law M, et al. Head and neck cancer in Australia between 1982 and 2005 show increasing incidence of potentially HPV-associated oropharyngeal cancers. Br J Cancer. 2011;104(5):886–91. doi:10.1038/sj.bjc.6606091.
9. Marur S, D'Souza G, Westra WH, Forastiere AA. HPV-associated head and neck cancer: a virus-related cancer epidemic. Lancet Oncol. 2010;11(8):781–9. doi:10.1016/S1470-2045(10)70017-6.
10. Chaturvedi AK. Epidemiology and clinical aspects of HPV in head and neck cancers. Head Neck Pathol. 2012;6 Suppl 1:S16–24. doi:10.1007/s12105-012-0377-0.
11. Ang KK, Harris J, Wheeler R, Weber R, Rosenthal DI, Nguyen-Tan PF, et al. Human papillomavirus and survival of patients with oropharyngeal cancer. N Engl J Med. 2010;363(1):24–35. doi:10.1056/NEJMoa0912217.
12. Chaturvedi AK, Engels EA, Pfeiffer RM, Hernandez BY, Xiao W, Kim E, et al. Human papillomavirus and rising oropharyngeal cancer incidence in the United States. J Clin Oncol. 2011;29(32):4294–301. doi:10.1200/JCO.2011.36.4596.
13. Coleman N, Birley HD, Renton AM, Hanna NF, Ryait BK, Byrne M, et al. Immunological events in regressing genital warts. Am J Clin Pathol. 1994;102(6):768–74.
14. de Jong A, van der Burg SH, Kwappenberg KM, van der Hulst JM, Franken KL, Geluk A, et al. Frequent detection of human papillomavirus 16 E2-specific T-helper immunity in healthy subjects. Cancer Res. 2002;62(2):472–9.
15. Welters MJ, de Jong A, van den Eeden SJ, van der Hulst JM, Kwappenberg KM, Hassane S, et al. Frequent display of human papillomavirus type 16 E6-specific memory t-Helper cells in the healthy population as witness of previous viral encounter. Cancer Res. 2003;63(3):636–41.
16. Le Bon A, Tough DF. Links between innate and adaptive immunity via type I interferon. Curr Opin Immunol. 2002;14(4):432–6.
17. Williams R, Lee DW, Elzey BD, Anderson ME, Hostager BS, Lee JH. Preclinical models of HPV+ and HPV− HNSCC in mice: an immune clearance of HPV+ HNSCC. Head Neck. 2009;31(7):911–8. doi:10.1002/hed.21040.
18. Pardoll D. Does the immune system see tumors as foreign or self? Annu Rev Immunol. 2003;21:807–39.
19. Rosenberg SA, Yang JC, Restifo NP. Cancer immunotherapy: moving beyond current vaccines. Nat Med. 2004;10(9):909–15.
20. Burnet M. Cancer; a biological approach. I. The processes of control. Br Med J. 1957;1(5022):779–86.
21. King GN, Healy CM, Glover MT, Kwan JT, Williams DM, Leigh IM, et al. Increased prevalence of dysplastic and malignant lip lesions in renal-transplant recipients. N Engl J Med. 1995;332(16):1052–7. doi:10.1056/NEJM199504203321602.
22. Harris JP, Penn I. Immunosuppression and the development of malignancies of the upper airway and related structures. Laryngoscope. 1981;91(4):520–8.
23. Bhatia S, Louie AD, Bhatia R, O'Donnell MR, Fung H, Kashyap A, et al. Solid cancers after bone marrow transplantation. J Clin Oncol. 2001;19(2):464–71.
24. Avital I, Moreira AL, Klimstra DS, Leversha M, Papadopoulos EB, Brennan M, et al. Donor-derived human bone marrow cells contribute to solid organ cancers developing after bone marrow transplantation. Stem Cells. 2007;25(11):2903–9. doi:10.1634/stemcells.2007-0409.
25. Baker KS, DeFor TE, Burns LJ, Ramsay NK, Neglia JP, Robison LL. New malignancies after blood or marrow stem-cell transplantation in children and adults: incidence and risk factors. J Clin Oncol. 2003;21(7):1352–8.
26. Curtis RE, Metayer C, Rizzo JD, Socie G, Sobocinski KA, Flowers ME, et al. Impact of chronic GVHD therapy on the development of squamous-cell cancers after hematopoietic stem-cell transplantation: an international case–control study. Blood. 2005;105(10):3802–11. doi:10.1182/blood-2004-09-3411.
27. Haigentz Jr M. Aerodigestive cancers in HIV infection. Curr Opin Oncol. 2005;17(5):474–8.

28. Singh B, Balwally AN, Shaha AR, Rosenfeld RM, Har-El G, Lucente FE. Upper aerodigestive tract squamous cell carcinoma. The human immunodeficiency virus connection. Arch Otolaryngol Head Neck Surg. 1996;122(6):639–43.
29. Moyano S, Ordi J, Caballero M, Garcia F, Diaz A, de Sanjose S, et al. Laryngeal squamous cell carcinoma in HIV-positive patients: lack of association with human papillomavirus infection. HIV Med. 2009;10(10):634–9. doi:10.1111/j.1468-1293.2009.00737.x.
30. Dunn GP, Bruce AT, Ikeda H, Old LJ, Schreiber RD. Cancer immunoediting: from immunosurveillance to tumor escape. Nat Immunol. 2002;3(11):991–8. doi:10.1038/ni1102-991.
31. Lyford-Pike S, Peng S, Young GD, Taube JM, Westra WH, Akpeng B, et al. Evidence for a role of the PD-1:PD-L1 pathway in immune resistance of HPV-associated head and neck squamous cell carcinoma. Cancer Res. 2013;73:1733–41. doi:10.1158/0008-5472.CAN-12-2384.
32. Zha Y, Blank C, Gajewski TF. Negative regulation of T-cell function by PD-1. Crit Rev Immunol. 2004;24(4):229–37.
33. Gastman BR, Atarshi Y, Reichert TE, Saito T, Balkir L, Rabinowich H, et al. Fas ligand is expressed on human squamous cell carcinomas of the head and neck, and it promotes apoptosis of T lymphocytes. Cancer Res. 1999;59(20):5356–64.
34. Gastman BR, Yin XM, Johnson DE, Wieckowski E, Wang GQ, Watkins SC, et al. Tumor-induced apoptosis of T cells: amplification by a mitochondrial cascade. Cancer Res. 2000;60(24):6811–7.
35. Kassouf N, Thornhill MH. Oral cancer cell lines can use multiple ligands, including Fas-L, TRAIL and TNF-alpha, to induce apoptosis in Jurkat T cells: possible mechanisms for immune escape by head and neck cancers. Oral Oncol. 2008;44(7):672–82. doi:10.1016/j.oraloncology.2007.08.013.
36. Gabrilovich DI, Chen HL, Girgis KR, Cunningham HT, Meny GM, Nadaf S, et al. Production of vascular endothelial growth factor by human tumors inhibits the functional maturation of dendritic cells. Nat Med. 1996;2(10):1096–103.
37. Young MR, Young ME, Wright MA. Myelopoiesis-associated suppressor-cell activity in mice with Lewis lung carcinoma tumors: interferon-gamma plus tumor necrosis factor-alpha synergistically reduce suppressor cell activity. Int J Cancer. 1990;46(2):245–50.
38. Pegoraro L, Fierro MT, Lusso P, Giovinazzo B, Lanino E, Giovarelli M, et al. A novel leukemia T-cell line (PF-382) with phenotypic and functional features of suppressor lymphocytes. J Natl Cancer Inst. 1985;75(2):285–90.
39. Cirillo C, Montaldo P, Lanciotti M, Parodi MT, Castagnola E, Ponzoni M. Immunosuppressive factors produced by a T cell line derived from acute lymphoblastic leukemia. Boll Ist Sieroter Milan. 1988;67(4):295–308.
40. Lim SH, Worman CP, Jewell A, Goldstone AH. Production of tumour-derived suppressor factor in patients with acute myeloid leukaemia. Leuk Res. 1991;15(4):263–8.
41. Kunicka JE, Fox FE, Seki H, Oleszak EL, Platsoucas CD. Hybridoma-derived human suppressor factors: inhibition of growth of tumor cell lines and effect on cytotoxic cells. Hum Antibodies Hybridomas. 1991;2(3):160–9.
42. Young MR, Wright MA, Coogan M, Young ME, Bagash J. Tumor-derived cytokines induce bone marrow suppressor cells that mediate immunosuppression through transforming growth factor beta. Cancer Immunol Immunother. 1992;35(1):14–8.
43. Moore SC, Shaw MA, Soderberg LS. Transforming growth factor-beta is the major mediator of natural suppressor cells derived from normal bone marrow. J Leukoc Biol. 1992;52:596–601.
44. Heldin CH. Development and possible clinical use of antagonists for PDGF and TGF-beta. Ups J Med Sci. 2004;109(3):165–78.
45. Young MR, Wright MA, Lozano Y, Prechel MM, Benefield J, Leonetti JP, et al. Increased recurrence and metastasis in patients whose primary head and neck squamous cell carcinomas secreted granulocyte-macrophage colony-stimulating factor and contained CD34+ natural suppressor cells. Int J Cancer. 1997;74(1):69–74.
46. Bronte V, Chappell DB, Apolloni E, Cabrelle A, Wang M, Hwu P, et al. Unopposed production of granulocyte-macrophage colony-stimulating factor by tumors inhibits CD8+ T cell

responses by dysregulating antigen-presenting cell maturation. J Immunol. 1999;162(10): 5728–37.
47. Smith CW, Chen Z, Dong G, Loukinova E, Pegram MY, Nicholas-Figueroa L, et al. The host environment promotes the development of primary and metastatic squamous cell carcinomas that constitutively express proinflammatory cytokines IL-1alpha, IL-6, GM-CSF, and KC. Clin Exp Metastasis. 1998;16(7):655–64.
48. Merchav S, Apte RN, Tatarsky I, Ber R. Effect of plasmacytoma cells on the production of granulocyte-macrophage colony-stimulating activity (GM-CSA) in the spleen of tumor-bearing mice. Exp Hematol. 1987;15(9):995–1000.
49. Adeegbe D, Serafini P, Bronte V, Zoso A, Ricordi C, Inverardi L. In vivo induction of myeloid suppressor cells and CD4Foxp3 T regulatory cells prolongs skin allograft survival in mice. Cell Transplant. 2011;20:941–54. doi:ct0121adeegbe [pii]10.3727/096368910X540621.
50. Serafini P, Carbley R, Noonan KA, Tan G, Bronte V, Borrello I. High-dose granulocyte-macrophage colony-stimulating factor-producing vaccines impair the immune response through the recruitment of myeloid suppressor cells. Cancer Res. 2004;64(17):6337–43.
51. Young MR, Wright MA, Young ME. Antibodies to colony-stimulating factors block Lewis lung carcinoma cell stimulation of immune-suppressive bone marrow cells. Cancer Immunol Immunother. 1991;33:146–52.
52. Marigo I, Bosio E, Solito S, Mesa C, Fernandez A, Dolcetti L, et al. Tumor-induced tolerance and immune suppression depend on the C/EBPbeta transcription factor. Immunity. 2010;32(6):790–802. doi:S1074-7613(10)00202-5 [pii]10.1016/j.immuni.2010.05.010.
53. Gutschalk CM, Herold-Mende CC, Fusenig NE, Mueller MM. Granulocyte colony-stimulating factor and granulocyte-macrophage colony-stimulating factor promote malignant growth of cells from head and neck squamous cell carcinomas in vivo. Cancer Res. 2006;66(16):8026–36. doi:10.1158/0008-5472.CAN-06-0158.
54. Dranoff G. GM-CSF-based cancer vaccines. Immunol Rev. 2002;188:147–54.
55. Dranoff G. GM-CSF-secreting melanoma vaccines. Oncogene. 2003;22(20):3188–92.
56. American Society of Clinical Oncology. Recommendations for the use of hematopoietic colony-stimulating factors: evidence-based, clinical practice guidelines. J Clin Oncol. 1994;12(11):2471–508.
57. Carl W, Havens J. The cancer patient with severe mucositis. Curr Rev Pain. 2000;4(3): 197–202.
58. Biron P, Sebban C, Gourmet R, Chvetzoff G, Philip I, Blay JY. Research controversies in management of oral mucositis. Support Care Cancer. 2000;8(1):68–71.
59. Palmeri S, Leonardi V, Danova M, Porta C, Ferrari S, Fincato G, et al. Prospective, randomized trial of sequential interleukin-3 and granulocyte- or granulocyte-macrophage colony-stimulating factor after standard-dose chemotherapy in cancer patients. Haematologica. 1999;84(11):1016–23.
60. Staar S, Rudat V, Stuetzer H, Dietz A, Volling P, Schroeder M, et al. Intensified hyperfractionated accelerated radiotherapy limits the additional benefit of simultaneous chemotherapy—results of a multicentric randomized German trial in advanced head-and-neck cancer. Int J Radiat Oncol Biol Phys. 2001;50(5):1161–71.
61. Papaldo P, Lopez M, Cortesi E, Cammilluzzi E, Antimi M, Terzoli E, et al. Addition of either lonidamine or granulocyte colony-stimulating factor does not improve survival in early breast cancer patients treated with high-dose epirubicin and cyclophosphamide. J Clin Oncol. 2003;21(18):3462–8. doi:10.1200/JCO.2003.03.034.
62. Rapidis AD, Wolf GT. Immunotherapy of head and neck cancer: current and future considerations. J Oncol. 2009;2009:346345. doi:10.1155/2009/346345.
63. Parmiani G, Castelli C, Pilla L, Santinami M, Colombo MP, Rivoltini L. Opposite immune functions of GM-CSF administered as vaccine adjuvant in cancer patients. Ann Oncol. 2006;18:226–32.
64. Nathan CO, Leskov IL, Lin M, Abreo FW, Shi R, Hartman GH, et al. COX-2 expression in dysplasia of the head and neck: correlation with elF4E. Cancer. 2001;92(7):1888–95.

65. Itoh S, Matsui K, Furuta I, Takano Y. Immunohistochemical study on overexpression of cyclooxygenase-2 in squamous cell carcinoma of the oral cavity: its importance as a prognostic predictor. Oral Oncol. 2003;39(8):829–35.
66. Hoshikawa H, Goto R, Mori T, Mitani T, Mori N. Expression of prostaglandin E2 receptors in oral squamous cell carcinomas and growth inhibitory effects of an EP3 selective antagonist, ONO-AE3-240. Int J Oncol. 2009;34(3):847–52.
67. Sombroek CC, Stam AG, Masterson AJ, Lougheed SM, Schakel MJ, Meijer CJ, et al. Prostanoids play a major role in the primary tumor-induced inhibition of dendritic cell differentiation. J Immunol. 2002;168(9):4333–43.
68. Serafini P. Editorial: PGE2-producing MDSC: a role in tumor progression? J Leukoc Biol. 2010;88(5):827–9. doi:10.1189/jlb.0510303.
69. Lathers DM, Achille NJ, Young MR. Incomplete Th2 skewing of cytokines in plasma of patients with squamous cell carcinoma of the head and neck. Hum Immunol. 2003;64(12): 1160–6.
70. Pries R, Thiel A, Brocks C, Wollenberg B. Secretion of tumor-promoting and immune suppressive cytokines by cell lines of head and neck squamous cell carcinoma. In Vivo. 2006; 20(1):45–8.
71. Squarize CH, Castilho RM, Sriuranpong V, Pinto Jr DS, Gutkind JS. Molecular cross-talk between the NFkappaB and STAT3 signaling pathways in head and neck squamous cell carcinoma. Neoplasia. 2006;8(9):733–46. doi:10.1593/neo.06274.
72. Terabe M, Park JM, Berzofsky JA. Role of IL-13 in regulation of anti-tumor immunity and tumor growth. Cancer Immunol Immunother. 2004;53(2):79–85.
73. Keegan AD, Nelms K, White M, Wang LM, Pierce JH, Paul WE. An IL-4 receptor region containing an insulin receptor motif is important for IL-4-mediated IRS-1 phosphorylation and cell growth. Cell. 1994;76(5):811–20.
74. Gray MJ, Poljakovic M, Kepka-Lenhart D, Morris Jr SM. Induction of arginase I transcription by IL-4 requires a composite DNA response element for STAT6 and C/EBPbeta. Gene. 2005;353(1):98–106.
75. Kawakami K, Leland P, Puri RK. Structure, function, and targeting of interleukin 4 receptors on human head and neck cancer cells. Cancer Res. 2000;60(11):2981–7.
76. Gallina G, Dolcetti L, Serafini P, Santo CD, Marigo I, Colombo MP, et al. Tumors induce a subset of inflammatory monocytes with immunosuppressive activity on CD8 T cells. J Clin Invest. 2006;116(10):2777–90.
77. Roth F, De La Fuente AC, Vella JL, Zoso A, Inverardi L, Serafini P. Aptamer-mediated blockade of IL4Ralpha triggers apoptosis of MDSCs and limits tumor progression. Cancer Res. 2012;72(6):1373–83. doi:10.1158/0008-5472.CAN-11-2772.
78. Trikha M, Corringham R, Klein B, Rossi JF. Targeted anti-interleukin-6 monoclonal antibody therapy for cancer: a review of the rationale and clinical evidence. Clin Cancer Res. 2003;9(13):4653–65.
79. Riedel F, Zaiss I, Herzog D, Gotte K, Naim R, Hormann K. Serum levels of interleukin-6 in patients with primary head and neck squamous cell carcinoma. Anticancer Res. 2005;25(4): 2761–5.
80. Hong DS, Angelo LS, Kurzrock R. Interleukin-6 and its receptor in cancer: implications for translational therapeutics. Cancer. 2007;110(9):1911–28. doi:10.1002/cncr.22999.
81. Park SJ, Nakagawa T, Kitamura H, Atsumi T, Kamon H, Sawa S, et al. IL-6 regulates in vivo dendritic cell differentiation through STAT3 activation. J Immunol. 2004;173(6):3844–54.
82. Marigo I, Bosio E, Solito S, Mesa C, Fernandez A, Dolcetti L, et al. Tumor-induced tolerance and immune suppression depend on the C/EBPbeta transcription factor. Immunity. 2010;32(6):790–802. doi:S1074-7613(10)00202-5 [pii]10.1016/j.immuni.2010.05.010.
83. Gabrilovich DI, Ostrand-Rosenberg S, Bronte V. Coordinated regulation of myeloid cells by tumours. Nat Rev Immunol. 2012;12(4):253–68. doi:10.1038/nri3175.
84. Ratta M, Fagnoni F, Curti A, Vescovini R, Sansoni P, Oliviero B, et al. Dendritic cells are functionally defective in multiple myeloma: the role of interleukin-6. Blood. 2002;100(1): 230–7.

85. Hayashi T, Hideshima T, Akiyama M, Raje N, Richardson P, Chauhan D, et al. Ex vivo induction of multiple myeloma-specific cytotoxic T lymphocytes. Blood. 2003;102(4):1435–42.
86. Shang ZJ, Li ZB, Li JR. VEGF is up-regulated by hypoxic stimulation and related to tumour angiogenesis and severity of disease in oral squamous cell carcinoma: in vitro and in vivo studies. Int J Oral Maxillofac Surg. 2006;35(6):533–8. doi:10.1016/j.ijom.2005.09.006.
87. Liang X, Yang D, Hu J, Hao X, Gao J, Mao Z. Hypoxia inducible factor-alpha expression correlates with vascular endothelial growth factor-C expression and lymphangiogenesis/angiogenesis in oral squamous cell carcinoma. Anticancer Res. 2008;28(3A):1659–66.
88. Jain RK. Normalization of tumor vasculature: an emerging concept in antiangiogenic therapy. Science. 2005;307(5706):58–62.
89. Toi M, Kondo S, Suzuki H, Yamamoto Y, Inada K, Imazawa T, et al. Quantitative analysis of vascular endothelial growth factor in primary breast cancer. Cancer. 1996;77(6):1101–6.
90. Gabrilovich D, Ishida T, Oyama T, Ran S, Kravtsov V, Nadaf S, et al. Vascular endothelial growth factor inhibits the development of dendritic cells and dramatically affects the differentiation of multiple hematopoietic lineages in vivo. Blood. 1998;92(11):4150–66.
91. Gabrilovich D. Mechanisms and functional significance of tumour-induced dendritic-cell defects. Nat Rev Immunol. 2004;4(12):941–52.
92. Yang L, DeBusk LM, Fukuda K, Fingleton B, Green-Jarvis B, Shyr Y, et al. Expansion of myeloid immune suppressor Gr+CD11b+ cells in tumor-bearing host directly promotes tumor angiogenesis. Cancer Cell. 2004;6(4):409–21.
93. Melani C, Sangaletti S, Barazzetta FM, Werb Z, Colombo MP. Amino-biphosphonate-mediated MMP-9 inhibition breaks the tumor-bone marrow axis responsible for myeloid-derived suppressor cell expansion and macrophage infiltration in tumor stroma. Cancer Res. 2007;67(23):11438–46. doi:10.1158/0008-5472.CAN-07-1882.
94. Strauss L, Volland D, Kunkel M, Reichert TE. Dual role of VEGF family members in the pathogenesis of head and neck cancer (HNSCC): possible link between angiogenesis and immune tolerance. Med Sci Monit. 2005;11(8):BR280–92.
95. Murooka TT, Rahbar R, Fish EN. CCL5 promotes proliferation of MCF-7 cells through mTOR-dependent mRNA translation. Biochem Biophys Res Commun. 2009;387(2):381–6. doi:10.1016/j.bbrc.2009.07.035.
96. Chakraborty K, Bose A, Chakraborty T, Sarkar K, Goswami S, Pal S, et al. Restoration of dysregulated CC chemokine signaling for monocyte/macrophage chemotaxis in head and neck squamous cell carcinoma patients by neem leaf glycoprotein maximizes tumor cell cytotoxicity. Cell Mol Immunol. 2010;7(5):396–408. doi:10.1038/cmi.2010.29.
97. Kross KW, Heimdal JH, Olsnes C, Olofson J, Aarstad HJ. Tumour-associated macrophages secrete IL-6 and MCP-1 in head and neck squamous cell carcinoma tissue. Acta Otolaryngol. 2007;127(5):532–9. doi:10.1080/00016480600951384.
98. Bektas-Kayhan K, Unur M, Boy-Metin Z, Cakmakoglu B. MCP-1 and CCR2 gene variants in oral squamous cell carcinoma. Oral Dis. 2012;18(1):55–9. doi:10.1111/j.1601-0825.2011.01843.x.
99. Han L, Jiang B, Wu H, Wang X, Tang X, Huang J, et al. High expression of CXCR2 is associated with tumorigenesis, progression, and prognosis of laryngeal squamous cell carcinoma. Med Oncol. 2012;29(4):2466–72. doi:10.1007/s12032-011-0152-1.
100. Tan CT, Chu CY, Lu YC, Chang CC, Lin BR, Wu HH, et al. CXCL12/CXCR4 promotes laryngeal and hypopharyngeal squamous cell carcinoma metastasis through MMP-13-dependent invasion via the ERK1/2/AP-1 pathway. Carcinogenesis. 2008;29(8):1519–27. doi:10.1093/carcin/bgn108.
101. Rehman AO, Wang CY. CXCL12/SDF-1 alpha activates NF-kappaB and promotes oral cancer invasion through the Carma3/Bcl10/Malt1 complex. Int J Oral Sci. 2009;1(3):105–18. doi:10.4248/IJOS.09059.
102. Wang N, Wu QL, Fang Y, Mai HQ, Zeng MS, Shen GP, et al. Expression of chemokine receptor CXCR4 in nasopharyngeal carcinoma: pattern of expression and correlation with clinical outcome. J Transl Med. 2005;3:26. doi:10.1186/1479-5876-3-26.

103. Zlotnik A. Involvement of chemokine receptors in organ-specific metastasis. Contrib Microbiol. 2006;13:191–9. doi:10.1159/000092973.
104. Nath A, Chattopadhya S, Chattopadhyay U, Sharma NK. Macrophage inflammatory protein (MIP)1alpha and MIP1beta differentially regulate release of inflammatory cytokines and generation of tumoricidal monocytes in malignancy. Cancer Immunol Immunother. 2006;55(12):1534–41. doi:10.1007/s00262-006-0149-3.
105. Vaday GG, Peehl DM, Kadam PA, Lawrence DM. Expression of CCL5 (RANTES) and CCR5 in prostate cancer. Prostate. 2006;66(2):124–34. doi:10.1002/pros.20306.
106. Cozar JM, Canton J, Tallada M, Concha A, Cabrera T, Garrido F, et al. Analysis of NK cells and chemokine receptors in tumor infiltrating CD4 T lymphocytes in human renal carcinomas. Cancer Immunol Immunother. 2005;54(9):858–66. doi:10.1007/s00262-004-0646-1.
107. Sun Y, Cheng Z, Ma L, Pei G. Beta-arrestin2 is critically involved in CXCR4-mediated chemotaxis, and this is mediated by its enhancement of p38 MAPK activation. J Biol Chem. 2002;277(51):49212–9. doi:10.1074/jbc.M207294200.
108. Azenshtein E, Luboshits G, Shina S, Neumark E, Shahbazian D, Weil M, et al. The CC chemokine RANTES in breast carcinoma progression: regulation of expression and potential mechanisms of promalignant activity. Cancer Res. 2002;62(4):1093–102.
109. Rainwater SM, Wu X, Nduati R, Nedellec R, Mosier D, John-Stewart G, et al. Cloning and characterization of functional subtype A HIV-1 envelope variants transmitted through breastfeeding. Curr HIV Res. 2007;5(2):189–97.
110. Aoki MN, Da Silva do Amaral Herrera AC, Amarante MK, do Carneiro JL, Fungaro MH, Watanabe MA. CCR5 and p53 codon 72 gene polymorphisms: implications in breast cancer development. Int J Mol Med. 2009;23(3):429–35.
111. Davidson B, Dong HP, Holth A, Berner A, Risberg B. The chemokine receptor CXCR4 is more frequently expressed in breast compared to other metastatic adenocarcinomas in effusions. Breast J. 2008;14(5):476–82. doi:10.1111/j.1524-4741.2008.00625.x.
112. Darbon JM. A new model of metastatic dissemination of breast cancer bringing into play mesenchymal stem cells. Bull Cancer. 2007;94(12):1035–6. doi:10.1684/bdc.2007.0523.
113. Walker UA. Antiretroviral therapy-induced liver alterations. Curr Opin HIV AIDS. 2007;2(4):293–8. doi:10.1097/COH.0b013e328122dbaa.
114. Levina V, Nolen BM, Marrangoni AM, Cheng P, Marks JR, Szczepanski MJ, et al. Role of eotaxin-1 signaling in ovarian cancer. Clin Cancer Res. 2009;15(8):2647–56. doi:10.1158/1078-0432.CCR-08-2024.
115. Berghuis D, Santos SJ, Baelde HJ, Taminiau AH, Egeler RM, Schilham MW, et al. Pro-inflammatory chemokine-chemokine receptor interactions within the Ewing sarcoma microenvironment determine CD8(+) T-lymphocyte infiltration and affect tumour progression. J Pathol. 2011;223(3):347–57. doi:10.1002/path.2819.
116. Mi Z, Bhattacharya SD, Kim VM, Guo H, Talbot LJ, Kuo PC. Osteopontin promotes CCL5-mesenchymal stromal cell-mediated breast cancer metastasis. Carcinogenesis. 2011;32(4):477–87. doi:10.1093/carcin/bgr009.
117. Yaal-Hahoshen N, Shina S, Leider-Trejo L, Barnea I, Shabtai EL, Azenshtein E, et al. The chemokine CCL5 as a potential prognostic factor predicting disease progression in stage II breast cancer patients. Clin Cancer Res. 2006;12(15):4474–80. doi:10.1158/1078-0432.CCR-06-0074.
118. Nesbeth Y, Scarlett U, Cubillos-Ruiz J, Martinez D, Engle X, Turk MJ, et al. CCL5-mediated endogenous antitumor immunity elicited by adoptively transferred lymphocytes and dendritic cell depletion. Cancer Res. 2009;69(15):6331–8. doi:10.1158/0008-5472.CAN-08-4329.
119. Flanagan K, Moroziewicz D, Kwak H, Horig H, Kaufman HL. The lymphoid chemokine CCL21 costimulates naive T cell expansion and Th1 polarization of non-regulatory CD4+ T cells. Cell Immunol. 2004;231(1–2):75–84. doi:10.1016/j.cellimm.2004.12.006.
120. Yamano T, Kaneda Y, Hiramatsu SH, Huang S, Tran AN, Giuliano AE, et al. Immunity against breast cancer by TERT DNA vaccine primed with chemokine CCL21. Cancer Gene Ther. 2007;14(5):451–9. doi:10.1038/sj.cgt.7701035.

121. Wu S, Xing W, Peng J, Yuan X, Zhao X, Lei P, et al. Tumor transfected with CCL21 enhanced reactivity and apoptosis resistance of human monocyte-derived dendritic cells. Immunobiology. 2008;213(5):417–26. doi:10.1016/j.imbio.2007.10.003.
122. Shields JD, Fleury ME, Yong C, Tomei AA, Randolph GJ, Swartz MA. Autologous chemotaxis as a mechanism of tumor cell homing to lymphatics via interstitial flow and autocrine CCR7 signaling. Cancer Cell. 2007;11(6):526–38. doi:10.1016/j.ccr.2007.04.020.
123. Wang J, Xi L, Hunt JL, Gooding W, Whiteside TL, Chen Z, et al. Expression pattern of chemokine receptor 6 (CCR6) and CCR7 in squamous cell carcinoma of the head and neck identifies a novel metastatic phenotype. Cancer Res. 2004;64(5):1861–6.
124. Shields JD, Kourtis IC, Tomei AA, Roberts JM, Swartz MA. Induction of lymphoidlike stroma and immune escape by tumors that express the chemokine CCL21. Science. 2010;328(5979):749–52. doi:10.1126/science.1185837.
125. Viola A, Sarukhan A, Bronte V, Molon B. The pros and cons of chemokines in tumor immunology. Trends Immunol. 2012;33:496–504. doi:10.1016/j.it.2012.05.007.
126. Heimdal JH, Olsnes C, Olofsson J, Aarstad HJ. Monocyte and monocyte-derived macrophage secretion of MCP-1 in co-culture with autologous malignant and benign control fragment spheroids. Cancer Immunol Immunother. 2001;50(6):300–6.
127. Brown CE, Vishwanath RP, Aguilar B, Starr R, Najbauer J, Aboody KS, et al. Tumor-derived chemokine MCP-1/CCL2 is sufficient for mediating tumor tropism of adoptively transferred T cells. J Immunol. 2007;179(5):3332–41.
128. Loberg RD, Day LL, Harwood J, Ying C, St John LN, Giles R, et al. CCL2 is a potent regulator of prostate cancer cell migration and proliferation. Neoplasia. 2006;8(7):578–86. doi:10.1593/neo.06280.
129. Bailey C, Negus R, Morris A, Ziprin P, Goldin R, Allavena P, et al. Chemokine expression is associated with the accumulation of tumour associated macrophages (TAMs) and progression in human colorectal cancer. Clin Exp Metastasis. 2007;24(2):121–30. doi:10.1007/s10585-007-9060-3.
130. Ueno T, Toi M, Saji H, Muta M, Bando H, Kuroi K, et al. Significance of macrophage chemoattractant protein-1 in macrophage recruitment, angiogenesis, and survival in human breast cancer. Clin Cancer Res. 2000;6(8):3282–9.
131. Huang B, Lei Z, Zhao J, Gong W, Liu J, Chen Z, et al. CCL2/CCR2 pathway mediates recruitment of myeloid suppressor cells to cancers. Cancer Lett. 2007;252(1):86–92. doi:10.1016/j.canlet.2006.12.012.
132. Molon B, Viola A, Bronte V. Smoothing T cell roads to the tumor: chemokine post-translational regulation. Oncoimmunology. 2012;1(3):390–2. doi:10.4161/onci.19069.
133. Molon B, Ugel S, Del Pozzo F, Soldani C, Zilio S, Avella D, et al. Chemokine nitration prevents intratumoral infiltration of antigen-specific T cells. J Exp Med. 2011;208(10):1949–62. doi:10.1084/jem.20101956.
134. Olkhanud PB, Baatar D, Bodogai M, Hakim F, Gress R, Anderson RL, et al. Breast cancer lung metastasis requires expression of chemokine receptor CCR4 and regulatory T cells. Cancer Res. 2009;69(14):5996–6004. doi:10.1158/0008-5472.CAN-08-4619.
135. Velasco-Velazquez M, Jiao X, De La Fuente M, Pestell TG, Ertel A, Lisanti MP, et al. CCR5 antagonist blocks metastasis of basal breast cancer cells. Cancer Res. 2012;72(15):3839–50. doi:10.1158/0008-5472.CAN-11-3917.
136. Ogino T, Shigyo H, Ishii H, Katayama A, Miyokawa N, Harabuchi Y, et al. HLA class I antigen down-regulation in primary laryngeal squamous cell carcinoma lesions as a poor prognostic marker. Cancer Res. 2006;66(18):9281–9. doi:10.1158/0008-5472.CAN-06-0488.
137. Wolf GT, Hudson JL, Peterson KA, Miller HL, McClatchey KD. Lymphocyte subpopulations infiltrating squamous carcinomas of the head and neck: correlations with extent of tumor and prognosis. Otolaryngol Head Neck Surg. 1986;95(2):142–52.
138. Junker N, Kvistborg P, Kollgaard T, Straten P, Andersen MH, Svane IM. Tumor associated antigen specific T-cell populations identified in ex vivo expanded TIL cultures. Cell Immunol. 2012;273(1):1–9. doi:10.1016/j.cellimm.2011.12.004.

139. Marcus B, Arenberg D, Lee J, Kleer C, Chepeha DB, Schmalbach CE, et al. Prognostic factors in oral cavity and oropharyngeal squamous cell carcinoma. Cancer. 2004;101(12):2779–87. doi:10.1002/cncr.20701.
140. Kuss I, Hathaway B, Ferris RL, Gooding W, Whiteside TL. Decreased absolute counts of T lymphocyte subsets and their relation to disease in squamous cell carcinoma of the head and neck. Clin Cancer Res. 2004;10(11):3755–62. doi:10.1158/1078-0432.CCR-04-0054.
141. Turksma A, Bontkes H, van den Heuvel H, de Gruijl T, von Blomberg B, Braakhuis B, et al. Effector memory T-cell frequencies in relation to tumour stage, location and HPV status in HNSCC patients. Oral Dis. 2012. doi:10.1111/odi.12037.
142. Eura M, Ogi K, Chikamatsu K, Lee KD, Nakano K, Masuyama K, et al. Expression of the MAGE gene family in human head-and-neck squamous-cell carcinomas. Int J Cancer. 1995;64(5):304–8.
143. Kienstra MA, Neel HB, Strome SE, Roche P. Identification of NY-ESO-1, MAGE-1, and MAGE-3 in head and neck squamous cell carcinoma. Head Neck. 2003;25(6):457–63. doi:10.1002/hed.10223.
144. Albers A, Abe K, Hunt J, Wang J, Lopez-Albaitero A, Schaefer C, et al. Antitumor activity of human papillomavirus type 16 E7-specific T cells against virally infected squamous cell carcinoma of the head and neck. Cancer Res. 2005;65(23):11146–55. doi:10.1158/0008-5472.CAN-05-0772.
145. Devaraj K, Gillison ML, Wu TC. Development of HPV vaccines for HPV-associated head and neck squamous cell carcinoma. Crit Rev Oral Biol Med. 2003;14(5):345–62.
146. Gelbard A, Garnett CT, Abrams SI, Patel V, Gutkind JS, Palena C, et al. Combination chemotherapy and radiation of human squamous cell carcinoma of the head and neck augments CTL-mediated lysis. Clin Cancer Res. 2006;12(6):1897–905. doi:10.1158/1078-0432.CCR-05-1761.
147. Liu K, Nussenzweig MC. Origin and development of dendritic cells. Immunol Rev. 2010;234(1):45–54. doi:10.1111/j.0105-2896.2009.00879.x.
148. Valladeau J, Saeland S. Cutaneous dendritic cells. Semin Immunol. 2005;17(4):273–83. doi:10.1016/j.smim.2005.05.009.
149. Cruchley AT, Williams DM, Farthing PM, Speight PM, Lesch CA, Squier CA. Langerhans cell density in normal human oral mucosa and skin: relationship to age, smoking and alcohol consumption. J Oral Pathol Med. 1994;23(2):55–9.
150. Boyle JO, Gumus ZH, Kacker A, Choksi VL, Bocker JM, Zhou XK, et al. Effects of cigarette smoke on the human oral mucosal transcriptome. Cancer Prev Res (Phila). 2010;3(3):266–78. doi:10.1158/1940-6207.CAPR-09-0192.
151. Girod SC, Kuhnast T, Ulrich S, Krueger GR. Langerhans cells in epithelial tumors and benign lesions of the oropharynx. In Vivo. 1994;8(4):543–7.
152. Albuquerque Jr RL, Miguel MC, Costa AL, Souza LB. Correlation of c-erbB-2 and S-100 expression with the malignancy grading and anatomical site in oral squamous cell carcinoma. Int J Exp Pathol. 2003;84(6):259–65.
153. Yilmaz T, Gedikoglu G, Celik A, Onerci M, Turan E. Prognostic significance of Langerhans cell infiltration in cancer of the larynx. Otolaryngol Head Neck Surg. 2005;132(2):309–16. doi:10.1016/j.otohns.2004.04.018.
154. Gallo O, Libonati GA, Gallina E, Fini-Storchi O, Giannini A, Urso C, et al. Langerhans cells related to prognosis in patients with laryngeal carcinoma. Arch Otolaryngol Head Neck Surg. 1991;117(9):1007–10.
155. Li X, Takahashi Y, Sakamoto K, Nakashima T. Expression of dendritic cell phenotypic antigens in cervical lymph nodes of patients with hypopharyngeal and laryngeal carcinoma. J Laryngol Otol Suppl. 2009;31:5–10.
156. Hoffmann TK, Muller-Berghaus J, Ferris RL, Johnson JT, Storkus WJ, Whiteside TL. Alterations in the frequency of dendritic cell subsets in the peripheral circulation of patients with squamous cell carcinomas of the head and neck. Clin Cancer Res. 2002;8(6):1787–93.
157. Young MR, Wright MA, Lozano Y, Prechel MM, Benefield J, Leonetti JP, et al. Increased recurrence and metastasis in patients whose primary head and neck squamous cell carcinomas

secreted granulocyte-macrophage colony- stimulating factor and contained CD34+ natural suppressor cells. Int J Cancer. 1997;74(1):69–74.
158. Pak AS, Wright MA, Matthews JP, Collins SL, Petruzzelli GJ, Young MRI. Mechanisms of immune suppression in patients with head and neck cancer: presence of CD34(+) cells which suppress immune functions within cancers that secrete granulocyte-macrophage colony-stimulating factor. Clin Cancer Res. 1995;1(1):95–103.
159. Wu G, Morris Jr SM. Arginine metabolism: nitric oxide and beyond. Biochem J. 1998;336(Pt 1):1–17.
160. Bogdan C. Nitric oxide and the immune response. Nat Immunol. 2001;2(10):907–16.
161. Rodriguez PC, Quiceno DG, Zabaleta J, Ortiz B, Zea AH, Piazuelo MB, et al. Arginase I production in the tumor microenvironment by mature myeloid cells inhibits T-cell receptor expression and antigen-specific T-cell responses. Cancer Res. 2004;64(16):5839–49.
162. Mazzoni A, Bronte V, Visintin A, Spitzer JH, Apolloni E, Serafini P, et al. Myeloid suppressor lines inhibit T cell responses by an NO-dependent mechanism. J Immunol. 2002;168(2):689–95.
163. Bronte V, Serafini P, De Santo C, Marigo I, Tosello V, Mazzoni A, et al. IL-4-induced arginase 1 suppresses alloreactive T cells in tumor- bearing mice. J Immunol. 2003;170(1):270–8.
164. Nagaraj S, Gupta K, Pisarev V, Kinarsky L, Sherman S, Kang L, et al. Altered recognition of antigen is a mechanism of CD8(+) T cell tolerance in cancer. Nat Med. 2007;13(7):828–35.
165. Rosbe KW, Prazma J, Petrusz P, Mims W, Ball SS, Weissler MC. Immunohistochemical characterization of nitric oxide synthase activity in squamous cell carcinoma of the head and neck. Otolaryngol Head Neck Surg. 1995;113(5):541–9.
166. Bentz BG, Haines 3rd GK, Radosevich JA. Increased protein nitrosylation in head and neck squamous cell carcinogenesis. Head Neck. 2000;22(1):64–70.
167. Heimdal JH, Aarstad HJ, Olofsson J. Peripheral blood T-lymphocyte and monocyte function and survival in patients with head and neck carcinoma. Laryngoscope. 2000;110(3 Pt 1): 402–7.
168. Almand B, Resser JR, Lindman B, Nadaf S, Clark JI, Kwon ED, et al. Clinical significance of defective dendritic cell differentiation in cancer. Clin Cancer Res. 2000;6(5):1755–66.
169. Young MR, Cigal M. Tumor skewing of CD34+ cell differentiation from a dendritic cell pathway into endothelial cells. Cancer Immunol Immunother. 2006;55(5):558–68.
170. Serafini P, De Santo C, Marigo I, Cingarlini S, Dolcetti L, Gallina G, et al. Derangement of immune responses by myeloid suppressor cells. Cancer Immunol Immunother. 2004;53(2): 64–72.
171. To WC, Wood BG, Krauss JC, Strome M, Esclamado RM, Lavertu P, et al. Systemic adoptive T-cell immunotherapy in recurrent and metastatic carcinoma of the head and neck: a phase 1 study. Arch Otolaryngol Head Neck Surg. 2000;126(10):1225–31.
172. Chang AE, Li Q, Jiang G, Teknos TN, Chepeha DB, Bradford CR. Generation of vaccine-primed lymphocytes for the treatment of head and neck cancer. Head Neck. 2003;25(3): 198–209.
173. Kusmartsev S, Nagaraj S, Gabrilovich DI. Tumor-associated CD8+ T cell tolerance induced by bone marrow-derived immature myeloid cells. J Immunol. 2005;175(7):4583–92.
174. Kusmartsev S, Gabrilovich DI. STAT1 signaling regulates tumor-associated macrophage-mediated T cell deletion. J Immunol. 2005;174(8):4880–91.
175. Serafini P, Meckel K, Kelso M, Noonan K, Califano J, Koch W, et al. Phosphodiesterase-5 inhibition augments endogenous antitumor immunity by reducing myeloid-derived suppressor cell function. J Exp Med. 2006;203(12):2691–702.
176. Pandit R, Lathers DM, Beal NM, Garrity T, Young MR. CD34+ immune suppressive cells in the peripheral blood of patients with head and neck cancer. Ann Otol Rhinol Laryngol. 2000;109(8 Pt 1):749–54.
177. Pak AS, Wright MA, Matthews JP, Collins SL, Petruzzelli GJ, Young MR. Mechanisms of immune suppression in patients with head and neck cancer: presence of CD34(+) cells which suppress immune functions within cancers that secrete granulocyte-macrophage colony-stimulating factor. Clin Cancer Res. 1995;1(1):95–103.

178. Wiers K, Wright MA, Vellody K, Young MR. Failure of tumor-reactive lymph node cells to kill tumor in the presence of immune-suppressive CD34+ cells can be overcome with vitamin D3 treatment to diminish CD34+ cell levels. Clin Exp Metastasis. 1998;16(3):275–82.
179. Coussens LM, Tinkle CL, Hanahan D, Werb Z. MMP-9 supplied by bone marrow-derived cells contributes to skin carcinogenesis. Cell. 2000;103(3):481–90.
180. Pahler JC, Tazzyman S, Erez N, Chen YY, Murdoch C, Nozawa H, et al. Plasticity in tumor-promoting inflammation: impairment of macrophage recruitment evokes a compensatory neutrophil response. Neoplasia. 2008;10(4):329–40.
181. Xiang M, Gu Y, Zhao F, Lu H, Chen S, Yin L. Mast cell tryptase promotes breast cancer migration and invasion. Oncol Rep. 2010;23(3):615–9.
182. Mohamed MM, Cavallo-Medved D, Rudy D, Anbalagan A, Moin K, Sloane BF. Interleukin-6 increases expression and secretion of cathepsin B by breast tumor-associated monocytes. Cell Physiol Biochem. 2010;25(2–3):315–24. doi:000276564 [pii]10.1159/000276564.
183. Lathers DM, Young MR. Increased aberrance of cytokine expression in plasma of patients with more advanced squamous cell carcinoma of the head and neck. Cytokine. 2004;25(5):220–8. doi:10.1016/j.cyto.2003.11.005.
184. Jonuleit H, Schmitt E. The regulatory T cell family: distinct subsets and their interrelations. J Immunol. 2003;171(12):6323–7.
185. Terabe M, Berzofsky JA. Immunoregulatory T cells in tumor immunity. Curr Opin Immunol. 2004;16(2):157–62.
186. Schaefer C, Kim GG, Albers A, Hoermann K, Myers EN, Whiteside TL. Characteristics of CD4+CD25+ regulatory T cells in the peripheral circulation of patients with head and neck cancer. Br J Cancer. 2005;92(5):913–20.
187. Zheng SG, Wang JH, Gray JD, Soucier H, Horwitz DA. Natural and induced CD4+CD25+ cells educate CD4+CD25- cells to develop suppressive activity: the role of IL-2, TGF-beta, and IL-10. J Immunol. 2004;172(9):5213–21.
188. Huber S, Schramm C, Lehr HA, Mann A, Schmitt S, Becker C, et al. Cutting edge: TGF-beta signaling is required for the in vivo expansion and immunosuppressive capacity of regulatory CD4+CD25+ T cells. J Immunol. 2004;173(11):6526–31.
189. Liyanage UK, Moore TT, Joo HG, Tanaka Y, Herrmann V, Doherty G, et al. Prevalence of regulatory T cells is increased in peripheral blood and tumor microenvironment of patients with pancreas or breast adenocarcinoma. J Immunol. 2002;169(5):2756–61.
190. Wolf AM, Wolf D, Steurer M, Gastl G, Gunsilius E, Grubeck-Loebenstein B. Increase of regulatory T cells in the peripheral blood of cancer patients. Clin Cancer Res. 2003;9(2):606–12.
191. Okita R, Saeki T, Takashima S, Yamaguchi Y, Toge T. CD4+CD25+ regulatory T cells in the peripheral blood of patients with breast cancer and non-small cell lung cancer. Oncol Rep. 2005;14(5):1269–73.
192. Strauss L, Bergmann C, Szczepanski M, Gooding W, Johnson JT, Whiteside TL. A unique subset of CD4+CD25highFoxp3+ T cells secreting interleukin-10 and transforming growth factor-{beta}1 mediates suppression in the tumor microenvironment. Clin Cancer Res. 2007;13(15):4345–54.
193. Unitt E, Rushbrook SM, Marshall A, Davies S, Gibbs P, Morris LS, et al. Compromised lymphocytes infiltrate hepatocellular carcinoma: the role of T-regulatory cells. Hepatology. 2005;41(4):722–30.
194. Ormandy LA, Hillemann T, Wedemeyer H, Manns MP, Greten TF, Korangy F. Increased populations of regulatory T cells in peripheral blood of patients with hepatocellular carcinoma. Cancer Res. 2005;65(6):2457–64.
195. Zhang YL, Li J, Mo HY, Qiu F, Zheng LM, Qian CN, et al. Different subsets of tumor infiltrating lymphocytes correlate with NPC progression in different ways. Mol Cancer. 2010;9:4. doi:10.1186/1476-4598-9-4.
196. Distel LV, Fickenscher R, Dietel K, Hung A, Iro H, Zenk J, et al. Tumour infiltrating lymphocytes in squamous cell carcinoma of the oro- and hypopharynx: prognostic impact may

depend on type of treatment and stage of disease. Oral Oncol. 2009;45(10):e167–74. doi:10.1016/j.oraloncology.2009.05.640.
197. Pretscher D, Distel LV, Grabenbauer GG, Wittlinger M, Buettner M, Niedobitek G. Distribution of immune cells in head and neck cancer: CD8+ T-cells and CD20+ B-cells in metastatic lymph nodes are associated with favourable outcome in patients with oro- and hypopharyngeal carcinoma. BMC Cancer. 2009;9:292. doi:10.1186/1471-2407-9-292.
198. Badoual C, Hans S, Rodriguez J, Peyrard S, Klein C, Agueznay Nel H, et al. Prognostic value of tumor-infiltrating CD4+ T-cell subpopulations in head and neck cancers. Clin Cancer Res. 2006;12(2):465–72. doi:10.1158/1078-0432.CCR-05-1886.
199. Zingg U, Montani M, Frey DM, Dirnhofer S, Esterman AJ, Went P, et al. Tumour-infiltrating lymphocytes and survival in patients with adenocarcinoma of the oesophagus. Eur J Surg Oncol. 2010;36(7):670–7. doi:10.1016/j.ejso.2010.05.012.
200. Morgan ME, van Bilsen JH, Bakker AM, Heemskerk B, Schilham MW, Hartgers FC, et al. Expression of FOXP3 mRNA is not confined to CD4+CD25+ T regulatory cells in humans. Hum Immunol. 2005;66(1):13–20. doi:10.1016/j.humimm.2004.05.016.
201. Wang J, Ioan-Facsinay A, van der Voort EI, Huizinga TW, Toes RE. Transient expression of FOXP3 in human activated nonregulatory CD4+ T cells. Eur J Immunol. 2007;37(1):129–38. doi:10.1002/eji.200636435.
202. Kmieciak M, Gowda M, Graham L, Godder K, Bear HD, Marincola FM, et al. Human T cells express CD25 and Foxp3 upon activation and exhibit effector/memory phenotypes without any regulatory/suppressor function. J Transl Med. 2009;7:89. doi:10.1186/1479-5876-7-89.
203. Magg T, Mannert J, Ellwart JW, Schmid I, Albert MH. Subcellular localization of FOXP3 in human regulatory and nonregulatory T cells. Eur J Immunol. 2012;42(6):1627–38. doi:10.1002/eji.201141838.
204. Weed DT, Walker G, De La Fuente AC, Nazarian R, Vella JL, et al. FOXP3 Subcellular localization predicts recurrence in oral squamous cell carcinoma. PLoS ONE. 2013;8(8):e71908. doi:10.1371/journal.pone.0071908.
205. Kuss I, Hathaway B, Ferris RL, Gooding W, Whiteside TL. Imbalance in absolute counts of T lymphocyte subsets in patients with head and neck cancer and its relation to disease. Adv Otorhinolaryngol. 2005;62:161–72.
206. Gomez JA, Sun W, Gama V, Hajkova D, Yoshida T, Wu Z, et al. The C-terminus of interferon gamma receptor beta chain (IFNgammaR2) has antiapoptotic activity as a Bax inhibitor. Cancer Biol Ther. 2009;8(18):1771–86.
207. Manchanda P, Sharma SC, Das SN. Differential regulation of IL-2 and IL-4 in patients with tobacco-related oral squamous cell carcinoma. Oral Dis. 2006;12(5):455–62. doi:10.1111/j.1601-0825.2005.01220.x.
208. Farace F, Angevin E, Vanderplancke J, Escudier B, Triebel F. The decreased expression of CD3 zeta chains in cancer patients is not reversed by IL-2 administration. Int J Cancer. 1994;59(6):752–5.
209. Serafini P, Borrello I, Bronte V. Myeloid suppressor cells in cancer: recruitment, phenotype, properties, and mechanisms of immune suppression. Semin Cancer Biol. 2006;16(1):53–65.
210. Dunn G, Oliver KM, Loke D, Stafford ND, Greenman J. Dendritic cells and HNSCC: a potential treatment option? (Review). Oncol Rep. 2005;13(1):3–10.
211. Meneses A, Verastegui E, Barrera JL, de la Garza J, Hadden JW. Lymph node histology in head and neck cancer: impact of immunotherapy with IRX-2. Int Immunopharmacol. 2003;3(8):1083–91. doi:10.1016/S1567-5769(03)00017-1.
212. Mancino A, Schioppa T, Larghi P, Pasqualini F, Nebuloni M, Chen IH, et al. Divergent effects of hypoxia on dendritic cell functions. Blood. 2008;112(9):3723–34. doi:10.1182/blood-2008-02-142091.
213. Elia AR, Cappello P, Puppo M, Fraone T, Vanni C, Eva A, et al. Human dendritic cells differentiated in hypoxia down-modulate antigen uptake and change their chemokine expression profile. J Leukoc Biol. 2008;84(6):1472–82. doi:10.1189/jlb.0208082.
214. Yang M, Ma C, Liu S, Shao Q, Gao W, Song B, et al. HIF-dependent induction of adenosine receptor A2b skews human dendritic cells to a Th2-stimulating phenotype under hypoxia. Immunol Cell Biol. 2010;88(2):165–71. doi:10.1038/icb.2009.77.

215. Rosenberg SA, Lotze MT, Yang JC, Aebersold PM, Linehan WM, Seipp CA, et al. Experience with the use of high-dose interleukin-2 in the treatment of 652 cancer patients. Ann Surg. 1989;210(4):474–84. discussion 484–75.
216. Fishman MN, Thompson JA, Pennock GK, Gonzalez R, Diez LM, Daud AI, et al. Phase I trial of ALT-801, an interleukin-2/T-cell receptor fusion protein targeting p53 (aa264-272)/HLA-A*0201 complex, in patients with advanced malignancies. Clin Cancer Res. 2011;17(24):7765–75. doi:10.1158/1078-0432.CCR-11-1817.
217. Rossig C, Brenner MK. Genetic modification of T lymphocytes for adoptive immunotherapy. Mol Ther. 2004;10(1):5–18. doi:10.1016/j.ymthe.2004.04.014.
218. Shirakura Y, Mizuno Y, Wang L, Imai N, Amaike C, Sato E, et al. T-cell receptor gene therapy targeting melanoma-associated antigen-A4 inhibits human tumor growth in non-obese diabetic/SCID/gammacnull mice. Cancer Sci. 2012;103(1):17–25. doi:10.1111/j.1349-7006.2011.02111.x.
219. Linnemann C, Schumacher TN, Bendle GM. T-cell receptor gene therapy: critical parameters for clinical success. J Invest Dermatol. 2011;131(9):1806–16. doi:10.1038/jid.2011.160.
220. Jorritsma A, Schotte R, Coccoris M, de Witte MA, Schumacher TN. Prospects and limitations of T cell receptor gene therapy. Curr Gene Ther. 2011;11(4):276–87.
221. Davis JL, Theoret MR, Zheng Z, Lamers CH, Rosenberg SA, Morgan RA. Development of human anti-murine T-cell receptor antibodies in both responding and nonresponding patients enrolled in TCR gene therapy trials. Clin Cancer Res. 2010;16(23):5852–61. doi:10.1158/1078-0432.CCR-10-1280.
222. Ochi T, Fujiwara H, Yasukawa M. Application of adoptive T-cell therapy using tumor antigen-specific T-cell receptor gene transfer for the treatment of human leukemia. J Biomed Biotechnol. 2010;2010:521248. doi:10.1155/2010/521248.
223. Bendle GM, Linnemann C, Hooijkaas AI, Bies L, de Witte MA, Jorritsma A, et al. Lethal graft-versus-host disease in mouse models of T cell receptor gene therapy. Nat Med. 2010;16(5):565–70. doi:10.1038/nm.2128. 561–70.
224. Leisegang M, Turqueti-Neves A, Engels B, Blankenstein T, Schendel DJ, Uckert W, et al. T-cell receptor gene-modified T cells with shared renal cell carcinoma specificity for adoptive T-cell therapy. Clin Cancer Res. 2010;16(8):2333–43. doi:10.1158/1078-0432.CCR-09-2897.
225. Govers C, Sebestyen Z, Coccoris M, Willemsen RA, Debets R. T cell receptor gene therapy: strategies for optimizing transgenic TCR pairing. Trends Mol Med. 2010;16(2):77–87. doi:10.1016/j.molmed.2009.12.004.
226. Bendle GM, Haanen JB, Schumacher TN. Preclinical development of T cell receptor gene therapy. Curr Opin Immunol. 2009;21(2):209–14. doi:10.1016/j.coi.2009.02.007.
227. Ozao-Choy J, Ma G, Kao J, Wang GX, Meseck M, Sung M, et al. The novel role of tyrosine kinase inhibitor in the reversal of immune suppression and modulation of tumor microenvironment for immune-based cancer therapies. Cancer Res. 2009;69(6):2514–22. doi:10.1158/0008-5472.CAN-08-4709.
228. Porta C, Paglino C, Imarisio I, Ganini C, Pedrazzoli P. Immunological effects of multikinase inhibitors for kidney cancer: a clue for integration with cellular therapies? J Cancer. 2011;2:333–8.
229. Choong NW, Kozloff M, Taber D, Hu HS, Wade 3rd J, Ivy P, et al. Phase II study of sunitinib malate in head and neck squamous cell carcinoma. Invest New Drugs. 2010;28(5):677–83. doi:10.1007/s10637-009-9296-7.
230. Fountzilas G, Fragkoulidi A, Kalogera-Fountzila A, Nikolaidou M, Bobos M, Calderaro J, et al. A phase II study of sunitinib in patients with recurrent and/or metastatic non-nasopharyngeal head and neck cancer. Cancer Chemother Pharmacol. 2010;65(4):649–60. doi:10.1007/s00280-009-1070-1.
231. Machiels JP, Henry S, Zanetta S, Kaminsky MC, Michoux N, Rommel D, et al. Phase II study of sunitinib in recurrent or metastatic squamous cell carcinoma of the head and neck: GORTEC 2006–01. J Clin Oncol. 2010;28(1):21–8. doi:10.1200/JCO.2009.23.8584.

232. Kao J, Packer S, Vu HL, Schwartz ME, Sung MW, Stock RG, et al. Phase 1 study of concurrent sunitinib and image-guided radiotherapy followed by maintenance sunitinib for patients with oligometastases: acute toxicity and preliminary response. Cancer. 2009;115(15):3571–80. doi:10.1002/cncr.24412.
233. Garrity T, Pandit R, Wright MA, Benefield J, Keni S, Young MR. Increased presence of CD34+ cells in the peripheral blood of head and neck cancer patients and their differentiation into dendritic cells. Int J Cancer. 1997;73(5):663–9.
234. Young MR, Wright MA, Vellody K, Lathers DM. Skewed differentiation of bone marrow CD34+ cells of tumor bearers from dendritic toward monocytic cells, and the redirection of differentiation toward dendritic cells by 1alpha,25-dihydroxyvitamin D3. Int J Immunopharmacol. 1999;21(10):675–88.
235. Walsh JE, Clark AM, Day TA, Gillespie MB, Young MR. Use of alpha,25-dihydroxyvitamin D3 treatment to stimulate immune infiltration into head and neck squamous cell carcinoma. Hum Immunol. 2010;71(7):659–65. doi:10.1016/j.humimm.2010.04.008.
236. Walker DD, Reeves TD, de Costa AM, Schuyler C, Young MR. Immunological modulation by 1alpha,25-dihydroxyvitamin D3 in patients with squamous cell carcinoma of the head and neck. Cytokine. 2012;58(3):448–54. doi:10.1016/j.cyto.2012.03.002.
237. Ben-Shoshan M, Amir S, Dang DT, Dang LH, Weisman Y, Mabjeesh NJ. 1alpha,25-dihydroxyvitamin D3 (Calcitriol) inhibits hypoxia-inducible factor-1/vascular endothelial growth factor pathway in human cancer cells. Mol Cancer Ther. 2007;6(4):1433–9. doi:10.1158/1535-7163.MCT-06-0677.
238. Ochoa AC, Zea AH, Hernandez C, Rodriguez PC. Arginase, prostaglandins, and myeloid-derived suppressor cells in renal cell carcinoma. Clin Cancer Res. 2007;13(2 Pt 2):721s–6. doi:13/2/721s [pii]10.1158/1078-0432.CCR-06-2197.
239. Wirth LJ, Haddad RI, Lindeman NI, Zhao X, Lee JC, Joshi VA, et al. Phase I study of gefitinib plus celecoxib in recurrent or metastatic squamous cell carcinoma of the head and neck. J Clin Oncol. 2005;23(28):6976–81. doi:10.1200/JCO.2005.02.4182.
240. Kao J, Genden EM, Chen CT, Rivera M, Tong CC, Misiukiewicz K, et al. Phase 1 trial of concurrent erlotinib, celecoxib, and reirradiation for recurrent head and neck cancer. Cancer. 2011;117(14):3173–81. doi:10.1002/cncr.25786.
241. Dajani EZ, Islam K. Cardiovascular and gastrointestinal toxicity of selective cyclo-oxygenase-2 inhibitors in man. J Physiol Pharmacol. 2008;59 Suppl 2:117–33.
242. Solomon SD, McMurray JJ, Pfeffer MA, Wittes J, Fowler R, Finn P, et al. Cardiovascular risk associated with celecoxib in a clinical trial for colorectal adenoma prevention. N Engl J Med. 2005;352(11):1071–80. doi:10.1056/NEJMoa050405.
243. Huang WF, Hsiao FY, Wen YW, Tsai YW. Cardiovascular events associated with the use of four nonselective NSAIDs (etodolac, nabumetone, ibuprofen, or naproxen) versus a cyclooxygenase-2 inhibitor (celecoxib): a population-based analysis in Taiwanese adults. Clin Ther. 2006;28(11):1827–36. doi:10.1016/j.clinthera.2006.11.009.
244. Serafini P, Mgebroff S, Noonan K, Borrello I. Myeloid-derived suppressor cells promote cross-tolerance in B-cell lymphoma by expanding regulatory T cells. Cancer Res. 2008; 68(13):5439–49.
245. Ghiringhelli F, Menard C, Puig PE, Ladoire S, Roux S, Martin F, et al. Metronomic cyclophosphamide regimen selectively depletes CD4+CD25+ regulatory T cells and restores T and NK effector functions in end stage cancer patients. Cancer Immunol Immunother. 2007;56(5):641–8. doi:10.1007/s00262-006-0225-8.
246. Airoldi M, Cortesina G, Giordano C, Pedani F, Bumma C. Ifosfamide in the treatment of head and neck cancer. Oncology. 2003;65 Suppl 2:37–43.
247. Recchia F, Lalli A, Lombardo M, De Filippis S, Saggio G, Fabbri F, et al. Ifosfamide, cisplatin, and 13-Cis retinoic acid for patients with advanced or recurrent squamous cell carcinoma of the head and neck: a phase I–II study. Cancer. 2001;92(4):814–21.
248. Schroeder M, Zouboulis CC. All-trans-retinoic acid and 13-cis-retinoic acid: pharmacokinetics and biological activity in different cell culture models of human keratinocytes. Horm Metab Res. 2007;39(2):136–40. doi:10.1055/s-2007-961813.

249. Gabrilovich DI, Nagaraj S. Myeloid-derived suppressor cells as regulators of the immune system. Nat Rev Immunol. 2009;9(3):162–74. doi:10.1038/nri2506.
250. De Costa AM, Young MR. Immunotherapy for head and neck cancer: advances and deficiencies. Anticancer Drugs. 2011;22(7):674–81. doi:10.1097/CAD.0b013e328340fd18.
251. Ferris RL, Jaffee EM, Ferrone S. Tumor antigen-targeted, monoclonal antibody-based immunotherapy: clinical response, cellular immunity, and immunoescape. J Clin Oncol. 2010; 28(28):4390–9. doi:10.1200/JCO.2009.27.6360.
252. Russell JS, Colevas AD. The use of epidermal growth factor receptor monoclonal antibodies in squamous cell carcinoma of the head and neck. Chemother Res Pract. 2012;2012:761518. doi:10.1155/2012/761518.
253. Young MR, Neville BW, Chi AC, Lathers DM, Boyd Gillespie M, Day TA. Oral premalignant lesions induce immune reactivity to both premalignant oral lesions and head and neck squamous cell carcinoma. Cancer Immunol Immunother. 2007;56(7):1077–86. doi:10.1007/s00262-006-0242-7.
254. Adams GP, Weiner LM. Monoclonal antibody therapy of cancer. Nat Biotechnol. 2005;23(9):1147–57. doi:nbt1137 [pii]10.1038/nbt1137.
255. Baselga J, Pfister D, Cooper MR, Cohen R, Burtness B, Bos M, et al. Phase I studies of anti-epidermal growth factor receptor chimeric antibody C225 alone and in combination with cisplatin. J Clin Oncol. 2000;18(4):904–14.
256. Robert F, Ezekiel MP, Spencer SA, Meredith RF, Bonner JA, Khazaeli MB, et al. Phase I study of anti–epidermal growth factor receptor antibody cetuximab in combination with radiation therapy in patients with advanced head and neck cancer. J Clin Oncol. 2001;19(13):3234–43.
257. Shin DM, Donato NJ, Perez-Soler R, Shin HJ, Wu JY, Zhang P, et al. Epidermal growth factor receptor-targeted therapy with C225 and cisplatin in patients with head and neck cancer. Clin Cancer Res. 2001;7(5):1204–13.
258. Bonner JA, Harari PM, Giralt J, Azarnia N, Shin DM, Cohen RB, et al. Radiotherapy plus cetuximab for squamous-cell carcinoma of the head and neck. N Engl J Med. 2006;354(6):567–78. doi:10.1056/NEJMoa053422.
259. Bonner JA, Harari PM, Giralt J, Cohen RB, Jones CU, Sur RK, et al. Radiotherapy plus cetuximab for locoregionally advanced head and neck cancer: 5-year survival data from a phase 3 randomised trial, and relation between cetuximab-induced rash and survival. Lancet Oncol. 2010;11(1):21–8. doi:10.1016/S1470-2045(09)70311-0.
260. Pfister DG, Su YB, Kraus DH, Wolden SL, Lis E, Aliff TB, et al. Concurrent cetuximab, cisplatin, and concomitant boost radiotherapy for locoregionally advanced, squamous cell head and neck cancer: a pilot phase II study of a new combined-modality paradigm. J Clin Oncol. 2006;24(7):1072–8. doi:10.1200/JCO.2004.00.1792.
261. Merlano M, Russi E, Benasso M, Corvo R, Colantonio I, Vigna-Taglianti R, et al. Cisplatin-based chemoradiation plus cetuximab in locally advanced head and neck cancer: a phase II clinical study. Ann Oncol. 2011;22(3):712–7. doi:10.1093/annonc/mdq412.
262. Harari PM, Allen GW, Bonner JA. Biology of interactions: antiepidermal growth factor receptor agents. J Clin Oncol. 2007;25(26):4057–65. doi:10.1200/JCO.2007.11.8984.
263. Harari PM, Huang S. Radiation combined with EGFR signal inhibitors: head and neck cancer focus. Semin Radiat Oncol. 2006;16(1):38–44. doi:10.1016/j.semradonc.2005.08.005.
264. Kim S, Grandis JR, Rinaldo A, Takes RP, Ferlito A. Emerging perspectives in epidermal growth factor receptor targeting in head and neck cancer. Head Neck. 2008;30(5):667–74. doi:10.1002/hed.20859.
265. Lopez-Albaitero A, Ferris RL. Immune activation by epidermal growth factor receptor specific monoclonal antibody therapy for head and neck cancer. Arch Otolaryngol Head Neck Surg. 2007;133(12):1277–81. doi:10.1001/archotol.133.12.1277.
266. Andrade P, Deleo A, Visus C, Butterfield L, Argiris A, Ferris RL. Phase I adjuvant trial of multi-epitope p53 vaccine for patients with squamous cell carcinoma of the head and neck. J Clin Oncol. 2009;27:15s.

267. Lopez-Albaitero A, Lee SC, Morgan S, Grandis JR, Gooding WE, Ferrone S, et al. Role of polymorphic Fc gamma receptor IIIa and EGFR expression level in cetuximab mediated, NK cell dependent in vitro cytotoxicity of head and neck squamous cell carcinoma cells. Cancer Immunol Immunother. 2009;58(11):1853–64. doi:10.1007/s00262-009-0697-4.
268. Kurai J, Chikumi H, Hashimoto K, Yamaguchi K, Yamasaki A, Sako T, et al. Antibody-dependent cellular cytotoxicity mediated by cetuximab against lung cancer cell lines. Clin Cancer Res. 2007;13(5):1552–61. doi:10.1158/1078-0432.CCR-06-1726.
269. Andrade Filho PA, Lopez-Albaitero A, Gooding W, Ferris RL. Novel immunogenic HLA-A*0201-restricted epidermal growth factor receptor-specific T-cell epitope in head and neck cancer patients. J Immunother. 2010;33(1):83–91. doi:10.1097/CJI.0b013e3181b8f421.
270. Dechant M, Weisner W, Berger S, Peipp M, Beyer T, Schneider-Merck T, et al. Complement-dependent tumor cell lysis triggered by combinations of epidermal growth factor receptor antibodies. Cancer Res. 2008;68(13):4998–5003. doi:10.1158/0008-5472.CAN-07-6226.
271. Riechelmann H, Wiesneth M, Schauwecker P, Reinhardt P, Gronau S, Schmitt A, et al. Adoptive therapy of head and neck squamous cell carcinoma with antibody coated immune cells: a pilot clinical trial. Cancer Immunol Immunother. 2007;56(9):1397–406. doi:10.1007/s00262-007-0283-6.
272. Junker N, Andersen MH, Wenandy L, Dombernowsky SL, Kiss K, Sorensen CH, et al. Bimodal ex vivo expansion of T cells from patients with head and neck squamous cell carcinoma: a prerequisite for adoptive cell transfer. Cytotherapy. 2011;13(7):822–34. doi:10.3109/14653249.2011.563291.
273. Dudley ME, Rosenberg SA. Adoptive-cell-transfer therapy for the treatment of patients with cancer. Nat Rev Cancer. 2003;3(9):666–75. doi:10.1038/nrc1167.
274. Cohen CJ, Zheng Z, Bray R, Zhao Y, Sherman LA, Rosenberg SA, et al. Recognition of fresh human tumor by human peripheral blood lymphocytes transduced with a bicistronic retroviral vector encoding a murine anti-p53 TCR. J Immunol. 2005;175(9):5799–808.
275. Yamasaki K, Horiguchi S, Kurosaki M, Kunii N, Nagato K, Hanaoka H, et al. Induction of NKT cell-specific immune responses in cancer tissues after NKT cell-targeted adoptive immunotherapy. Clin Immunol. 2011;138(3):255–65. doi:10.1016/j.clim.2010.11.014.
276. Lee KD, Lee HH, Joo HB, Lee HS, Yu TH, Chang HK, et al. Expression of MAGE A 1–6 mRNA in sputa of head and neck cancer patients–a preliminary report. Anticancer Res. 2006;26(2B):1513–8.
277. Lee KD, Chang HK, Jo YK, Kim BS, Lee BH, Lee YW, et al. Expression of the MAGE 3 gene product in squamous cell carcinomas of the head and neck. Anticancer Res. 1999;19(6B):5037–42.
278. Lee KD, Eura M, Ogi K, Nakano K, Chikamatsu K, Masuyama K, et al. Expression of the MAGE-1, -2, -3, -4, and –6 genes in non-squamous cell carcinoma lesions of the head and neck. Acta Otolaryngol. 1996;116(4):633–9.
279. Clark CE, Vonderheide RH. Cancer-testis antigens in tumor biology and immunotherapy. Cancer Biol Ther. 2006;5(9):1226–7.
280. Ma B, Yijie X, Hung C-F, Wu T-C (2010) HPV and therapeutic vaccines: where we stand in 2010. Curr Cancer Ther Rev 6:81–103
281. Hoffmann TK, Bier H, Donnenberg AD, Whiteside TL, De Leo AB. p53 as an immunotherapeutic target in head and neck cancer. Adv Otorhinolaryngol. 2005;62:151–60. doi:10.1159/000082505.
282. Hoffmann TK, Loftus DJ, Nakano K, Maeurer MJ, Chikamatsu K, Appella E, et al. The ability of variant peptides to reverse the nonresponsiveness of T lymphocytes to the wild-type sequence p53(264–272) epitope. J Immunol. 2002;168(3):1338–47.
283. Schuler PJH, Harasymczuk M, Visus C, Hoffmann TK, Lang S, Argiris A, DeLeo AB, Whiteside TL, Ferris RL (2012) Adjuvant P53 peptide loaded dendritic cell vaccination in patients with head and neck cancer – a phase I/II clinical trial 8th international conference on head and neck cancer. Metro Toronto Convention Centre, 21–25 July 2012. http://ahns.jnabstracts.com/Detail.aspx?ID=0252

284. Marty R, Roze S, Bresse X, Largeron N, Smith-Palmer J. Estimating the clinical benefits of vaccinating boys and girls against HPV-related diseases in Europe. BMC Cancer. 2013;13(1):10. doi:10.1186/1471-2407-13-10.
285. Wallecha A, French C, Petit R, Singh R, Amin A, Rothman J. Lm-LLO-based immunotherapies and HPV-associated disease. J Oncol. 2012;2012:542851. doi:10.1155/2012/542851.
286. Gunn GR, Zubair A, Peters C, Pan ZK, Wu TC, Paterson Y. Two Listeria monocytogenes vaccine vectors that express different molecular forms of human papilloma virus-16 (HPV-16) E7 induce qualitatively different T cell immunity that correlates with their ability to induce regression of established tumors immortalized by HPV-16. J Immunol. 2001;167(11): 6471–9.
287. Maciag PC, Radulovic S, Rothman J. The first clinical use of a live-attenuated Listeria monocytogenes vaccine: a Phase I safety study of Lm-LLO-E7 in patients with advanced carcinoma of the cervix. Vaccine. 2009;27(30):3975–83. doi:10.1016/j.vaccine.2009.04.041.
288. Voskens CJ, Sewell D, Hertzano R, DeSanto J, Rollins S, Lee M, et al. InducTION of mage-A3 and HPV-16 immunity by Trojan vaccines in patients with head and neck carcinoma. Head Neck. 2012;34(12):1734–46. doi:10.1002/hed.22004.
289. Hu JC, Coffin RS, Davis CJ, Graham NJ, Groves N, Guest PJ, et al. A phase I study of OncoVEXGM-CSF, a second-generation oncolytic herpes simplex virus expressing granulocyte macrophage colony-stimulating factor. Clin Cancer Res. 2006;12(22):6737–47. doi:10.1158/1078-0432.CCR-06-0759.
290. Harrington KJ, Hingorani M, Tanay MA, Hickey J, Bhide SA, Clarke PM, et al. Phase I/II study of oncolytic HSV GM-CSF in combination with radiotherapy and cisplatin in untreated stage III/IV squamous cell cancer of the head and neck. Clin Cancer Res. 2010;16(15):4005–15. doi:10.1158/1078-0432.CCR-10-0196.
291. Prestwich RJ, Errington F, Diaz RM, Pandha HS, Harrington KJ, Melcher AA, et al. The case of oncolytic viruses versus the immune system: waiting on the judgment of Solomon. Hum Gene Ther. 2009;20(10):1119–32. doi:10.1089/hum.2009.135.
292. Naik JD, Twelves CJ, Selby PJ, Vile RG, Chester JD. Immune recruitment and therapeutic synergy: keys to optimizing oncolytic viral therapy? Clin Cancer Res. 2011;17(13):4214–24. doi:10.1158/1078-0432.CCR-10-2848.

T Cell Co-regulatory Signals and Their Role in Cancer Therapy

Eitan R. Friedman, Lynn Feun, Pasquale Benedetto, and Joseph D. Rosenblatt

Abstract T cell activation is initiated by signaling through the TCR after binding to MHC-presented antigen. Both positive and negative co-regulatory signaling can modify this original activating signal. T cell co-regulation is provided by receptors on the T cell surface membrane. Inhibitory signals are provided by CTLA4 or PD-1, while co-stimulation is provided by CD28, 4-1BB, OX40, or GITR. These signals are being studied in the laboratory and at the clinical level in order to therapeutically modulate T cell responses to tumor cells. T cells can recognize tumor antigens in the same way that these immune cells recognize bacteria, viral antigens, and other foreign peptides. If appropriately activated by the tumor antigen, the immune system can mediate an antitumor gene response. Unfortunately, immune cells with antitumor specificity are not present in abundance and are often inhibited by tumor expression of CTLA4 or PD-1 ligands. Thus manipulation of co-regulatory signals can be used as a strategy by which to strengthen the immune response, via augmentation of T cell co-stimulation and/or blockade of inhibitory signals, in order to effectively treat cancer. In this chapter we review the basic principles and science as well as the ongoing clinical efforts in this area that have had recent success and offer additional promise.

1 Normal Biology of T Cell Activation and Checkpoint Signaling

T cells have long been a focus of translational oncology research, for in addition to their ability to dispose of foreign viruses, bacteria, and infected tissues, they may possess the ability to recognize cancer cells. Cell-mediated immunity may be

E.R. Friedman (✉) • L. Feun • P. Benedetto • J.D. Rosenblatt (✉)
School of Medicine, University of Miami, Miami, FL, USA
e-mail: EFriedman@med.miami.edu; JRosenblatt@med.miami.edu

J.D. Rosenblatt et al. (eds.), *Advances in Tumor Immunology and Immunotherapy*, Current Cancer Research, DOI 10.1007/978-1-4614-8809-5_14,

© Springer Science+Business Media New York 2014

mediated by cytotoxic, CD8+ effector T lymphocytes, which recognize and kill cells expressing targeted antigens, and by CD4+ helper T cells that can facilitate CD8 T cell activation and induce B cells to mature into antibody-producing plasma cells [1].

The mounting of an immune response by the adaptive immune system involves coordination between several different cell types. This process begins in a lymph node where an antigen-presenting cell (APC), having phagocytized foreign antigen and processed it into smaller peptides intracellularly, presents it on its surface via the major histocompatibility complex (MHC) to a T cell for antigen sampling. CD4 T cells include TH1 cells which amongst their activities secrete cytokines such as interferon γ that activate macrophages and TH2 cells which generally secrete cytokines such as IL-4 to activate the B cells to produce antigen-specific antibodies. Alternatively, a virally infected somatic cell may directly present peptide antigen through MHC-I present on the cell surface. The T cell receptor (TCR), together with CD4 or CD8 co-receptors, recognizes cognate antigen presented on the MHC by the APC. A cognate antigen is an antigen recognized by both the T cell via the TCR complex and the APC or the somatic cell via the MHC complex. This provides the first step towards T cell activation, initiating a signaling cascade within the T cell known as signal 1, causing a naïve T cell, which has never been exposed to antigen, to become primed. However, to become an armed effector T cell and to allow its subsequent expansion, the T cell also requires a second signal. The requisite co-regulatory ligands are provided as surface molecules by the same APC presenting the MHC-bound antigen to the TCR. When cognate receptors are bound by these co-stimulatory ligands, positive signals are imparted to the activated T cell as signal 2.

In addition to these activating, co-stimulatory signals, other co-regulatory signals may dampen the T cell response [1]. Such inhibitory signals provided to the T cell are known as immune checkpoints, as they limit the extent to which an immune response is strengthened and prevent hyperactivity and autoimmunity. Examples of co-inhibitory receptors present on T lymphocytes include CTLA4 and PD-1, and examples of co-stimulatory receptors include CD28, 4-1BB, OX40, and GITR (Fig. 1).

Several of these immune checkpoints are being studied in the laboratory and in the clinical setting as potential targets of immunotherapy, with promising results. Cancer cells express tumor-specific antigens due to mutations that occur in their genome and due to epigenetic changes that alter normal expression of genes, which can theoretically be recognized and targeted by the immune system. Recent studies have shown that targeting T cell co-regulatory signals can slow, halt, or even reverse cancer growth. The hypothesis underlying these efforts is that blocking immune checkpoint inhibitory signals or strengthening T cell co-stimulatory signals with biologic therapeutics will strengthen the immune system's response against tumor antigens. In point of fact, the cancer cells themselves often express T cell inhibitory ligands on their surface that weaken the immune response [2]. Hence, efforts have been directed at blocking inhibitory signals in order to strengthen effector responses.

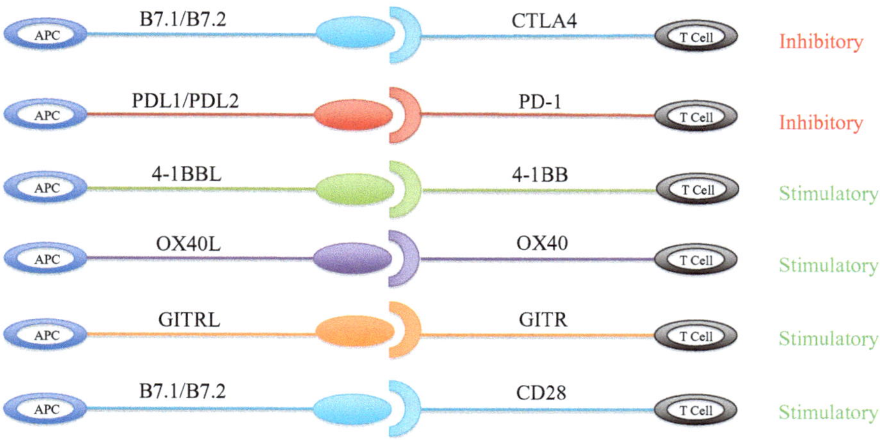

Fig. 1 APC and T cell with their ligands and bound co-regulatory receptors. The ligands on the APC bind to the T cell co-regulatory receptors and can alter the signaling of these receptors. CTLA4 and PD-1 are inhibitory receptors, and positive signals are sent from 4-1BB, OX40, GITR, and CD28

2 CTLA4 and CD28

CTLA4 is one of the better studied and well-defined inhibitory immune checkpoint receptors. It is a member of the immunoglobulin superfamily, and its gene is located on chromosome 2q33. CTLA4 is expressed on the surface membrane of activated T cells and counters the stimulatory effect of the CD28 receptor, which is another member of the immunoglobulin superfamily and is present on naïve CD4 and most naïve CD8 T cells [3]. The CD28 gene is also found on chromosome 2q33, and its protein on the T cell surface membrane binds to its ligands B7.1 (CD80) or B7.2 (CD86) expressed on APCs. The resulting co-stimulatory signals induce T cells to proliferate and differentiate into effector and memory T cells. However, once activated the T cells up-regulate the expression of CTLA4, providing negative feedback to dampen the T cell activation signals [1]. CTLA4 is an alternate receptor for B7, and its amino acid sequence is very similar to that of CD28. In fact, B7 binds CTLA4 with an affinity 20 times stronger than CD28. Once bound, CTLA4 signal transduction activates inhibitory phosphatases, including SHP2 and PP2A, which counter the stimulatory kinase signaling of the B7:CD28 interaction. CTLA4 signaling has an inhibitory effect on CD8 effectors, preventing their cytotoxic effects, and on CD4 helper T cells, preventing these cells from activating B cells. In contrast, CTLA4 activation has been found to have a stimulatory effect on T regulatory cells (Tregs) where it is expressed constitutively, as its signaling causes increased immunosuppressive Treg activity. The mechanism of Treg stimulation by CTLA4 signaling is not known. The normal role of CTLA4 is to keep the immune system from becoming over-activated by preventing the uncontrolled activation of naïve T cells, and CTLA4 knockout mice develop fatal T cell hyperactivity and autoimmunity [2].

CTLA4 has been well studied in the laboratory in preclinical studies. Partial blockade of the CTLA4 receptor with antibodies in mice has demonstrated significant antitumor activity. Researchers predicted that antibody blockade of the CTLA4 receptor would cause increased immune activity and autoimmunity [2]. However, although CTLA4 knockout is lethal in mice, anti-CTLA4 antibodies are better tolerated as they only partially inhibit CTLA4 activity and can be employed following the development of a normal T cell repertoire. Notably, such partial blockade is sufficient for an inhibitory effect on tumor growth [4]. Studies have been done showing no effect on melanoma tumors in mice treated with CTLA4 antibody alone; however, when treated with antibody in addition to a GM-CSF-expressing tumor vaccine, inhibition was observed in 80 % of mice. GM-CSF vaccines consist of cancer cells that secrete GM-CSF, which causes migration and accumulation of APCs at the injection site, allowing increased antigen presentation and thus increased activation of the T cell immune response [5]. In addition, there was rejection of the melanoma following rechallenge, suggesting the establishment of immunological memory.

B7 and CD28 have also been the focus of research efforts. T cells in the tumor microenvironment become anergic secondary to receiving signaling through only the TCR:MHC complex as the co-stimulatory ligands B7.1 and B7.2 are not present on the tumor cells and receipt of signal 1 in the absence of signal 2 induces T cell anergy. In preclinical experiments B7 was shown to be important when its exogenous expression in tumor cells induced a CD8 T cell response allowing for tumor rejection. These experiments were performed in several different tumor models, and rejection was seen primarily with relatively immunogenic tumors [6].

Anti-CD28 agonistic antibodies have been used to expand T cell populations. These antibodies allow for T cell proliferation, survival, and cytokine secretion. In preclinical experiments in which humanized anti-CD28 antibodies were injected into monkeys, peripheral T cells were activated, with secretion of low levels of proinflammatory cytokines. However, in a phase I clinical trial with a super-agonist humanized antibody TGN1412, CD28 resulted in severe cytokine storm which was life threatening for many patients [7]. Subsequent efforts have largely involved use of anti-CD28 antibodies for purposes of ex-vivo T cell expansion.

3 PD-1

PD-1 is another immune checkpoint inhibitory receptor on the T cell surface membrane. The PD-1 receptor is a 50–55 kDa transmembrane glycoprotein receptor of the immunoglobulin superfamily. The ligands for PD-1 are PDL1, also referred to as B7-H1 or CD274, and PDL2, also referred to as B7-DC or CD273. These ligands are up-regulated on APCs during the inflammatory response. PDL1 is up-regulated in response to interferon γ and is expressed on hematopoietic, endothelial, and epithelial cells. PDL2 is expressed on macrophages and dendritic cells in response to IL-4 and other cytokines. The PD-1 receptor is expressed on B cells, NK T cells, and Tregs. PD-1 limits autoimmunity and the T cell response during inflammation and primarily inhibits activated effector T cells. PD-1 dampens the T cell response in the peripheral tissues during inflammation, and it also limits the immune response to prevent autoimmunity. Since its ligands are expressed on peripheral surrounding tissues, these areas are protected from inflammation spreading to areas outside the main focus of inflammation [8]. PD-1 also plays a role in induction of T cell anergy and tolerance [9]. Its expression is increased following T cell activation. Binding of PDL1 or PDL2 to PD-1 results in activation of the inhibitory phosphatase SHP2 and decreased TCR signaling. B7.1 (CD80) on the T cell has also been shown to bind PDL1, sending additional inhibitory signals into the T cell [2]. PD-1 knockout mice also develop significant autoimmunity suggesting that, as with CTLA4, PD-1 prevents the immune system from becoming overactive [8]. Other studies in mice infected with lymphocytic choriomeningitis virus have shown that CD8 T cells in a chronic infectious setting become "exhausted" and less active and that antibody blockade of PD-1 restores the CD8 T cell function and reverses such exhaustion [10]. PD-1 has also been shown to deplete memory B cells, as shown in experiments in which rhesus macaques infected with the SIV virus had rapid depletion of memory B cells that specifically expressed PD-1. The researchers then blocked PD-1 using antibodies in vitro, which prevented the depletion of the memory B cells. Inhibiting PD-1 using antibodies in macaques resulted in increased humoral immunity, presumed to be due to increased survival of memory B cells [11]. PDL1 has also been shown to promote Treg inhibitory functions, as PDL1-coated beads promote Treg proliferation in vitro and Tregs are significantly reduced in number in dual $PDL1^{-/-}/PDL2^{-/-}$ double-knockout mice [12].

Malignant tumors often contain tumor-infiltrating CD8 and Treg lymphocytes that express PD-1, and tumor cells at times express PDL1 or PDL2 leading to T cell anergy. In malignant cells, PDL1 expression increases when the PTEN tumor-suppressor gene is deactivated or when the cells are exposed to interferon γ. Tumor expression of inhibitory T cell checkpoint ligands is an example of the tumor co-opting natural immune functions to protect against immune attack and induce tolerance. Inhibiting PD-1 signaling therefore has the potential to increase immunity against cancer [2].

There have been several preclinical mouse studies showing that antibody blockade of the PD-1 receptor or its ligand inhibits tumor growth. Anti-PDL1 antibodies were administered to mice with myeloma and inhibited cancer cell growth transiently; however, in mice deficient for PD-1, tumor growth was inhibited completely without the addition of anti-PDL1 antibodies [13]. Mice lacking PD-1, PDL1, or PDL2 survive, unlike CTLA4 knockout mice, suggesting that there would be less toxicity associated with its blockade in humans, and this appears to be true in human trials [2]. When over-expressed in mouse tumors, PDL1 promotes tumor-reactive T cell apoptosis and tumor cell proliferation. It has also been shown that human cancers such as lung, ovary, colon, and melanoma express increased PDL1 relative to their normal cell counterparts [14]. Therefore, PD-1 inhibition appears to be a viable strategy by which to augment antitumor response.

4 4-1BB/CD137

Positive, co-stimulatory regulators have also been shown to have potential as therapeutic targets. One such example is 4-1BB, also known as CD137, a 27 kDa member of the TNF receptor superfamily. 4-1BB signaling stimulates survival and proliferation signals and inhibits apoptosis. 4-1BB ligand activates 4-1BB. While CD28 co-stimulation causes expansion of CD4 T cells, CD8 T cells are activated preferentially by 4-1BB. In particular, beads linked to anti-CD28 stimulate CD4 but not CD8 T cells to expand in vitro, while the converse is seen with beads linked to anti-4-1BB antibodies. Prior to activation only a small proportion of resting naïve and memory CD8 T cells express 4-1BB. Furthermore it was found that 4-1BB signaling stimulated the growth and survival of CD8 memory cells while CD28 signaling allowed for proliferation of naïve CD8 cells. This suggests that temporally in CD8 T cell activation, CD28 signaling occurs first, which then leads to up-regulation of 4-1BB, allowing 4-1BB signaling which can then strengthen the positive co-stimulation. Potentially, 4-1BB signaling can be utilized to specifically increase antigen-specific memory CD8 T cells which can then be utilized in adoptive cell transfer to specifically allow proliferation of antigen-specific CD8 T cells [15]. 4-1BB, although mainly expressed on the surface of CD8 T cells, can also be found on CD4, NK, dendritic, and Treg cells. 4-1BB ligand also stimulates release of IL-12 and IL-8 by dendritic cells and macrophages [16].

Preclinical experiments studying 4-1BB show that the immune response is strengthened through increased 4-1BB signaling. 4-1BB can be activated in T cells by antibodies or by soluble 4-1BB ligand [17]. Mittler et al. showed that anti-4-1BB blocking antibodies decrease activation of T cells upon challenge with T cell-dependent antigens and increase the number of anergic CD4 T cells [18]. Similarly, Hong et al. showed that anti-4-1BB blocking antibodies suppress T cell reaction to ovalbumin in monkeys [19].

The first studies to show that 4-1BB antibody has anticancer activity were done using mouse models for sarcoma or mastocytoma. In mice treated with an agonistic anti-4-1BB antibody, cytotoxic T cell activity increased and the tumors regressed [20]; this effect required both CD4 and CD8 T cells [21]. Other experiments in mice have combined anti-4-1BB with other treatments to show anticancer effect; for example, treatment of melanoma cells with IL-12 gene transfer alone or with anti-4-1BB alone was not as effective as when these strategies were combined [2].

5 OX40

OX40 (CD134) is another co-stimulatory regulator present on the surface of activated T cells and like 4-1BB is also a member of the TNF receptor superfamily. OX40 is present mainly on CD4 T cells but is also found on CD8 T cells, DCs, PMNs, and Tregs. OX40 expression and up-regulation on the T cell surface membrane are dependent on naïve T cell activation through CD28 [22]. OX40 is increased 48–72 h after the T cell is activated through CD28, and 120 h later it is down-regulated [23]. Binding of OX40 to its ligand OX40L (CD252), which is present mainly on APCs, stimulates proliferation, function, and survival of T cells [24]. It also stimulates the secretion of IL-2 and IL-2R [23]. Studies show that initial versus delayed OX40 signaling causes antibody class switching which allows different antibody subsets to be secreted. Initial OX40 binding causes interferon γ and IL-4 to be secreted as well as IgG2a and IgG1, while delayed signaling causes a stronger TH2 cell response than that seen in the initial response and facilitates IgG1 production.

Preclinical experiments demonstrated an increase in T cell proliferation with the use of OX40 agonists [24]. One of the initial experiments involved inoculating mice with the MCA 303 methylcholanthrene-induced sarcoma tumor cells and then injecting these mice with an OX40L:Ig fusion protein or saline control; tumor regression occurred in up to 60 % of OX40L:Ig-treated mice compared to controls in which no mice survived. In addition, the mice were resistant to re-challenge, suggesting development of antitumor memory. Similarly, in another experiment mice inoculated with the weakly immunogenic B16/F10 melanoma tumor cell line were treated with OX40L:Ig fusion protein, OX40 receptor agonist antibody, or PBS or IgG controls. Results showed that in both experimental groups 25 % of mice with increased OX40 signaling due to the applied therapy survived, whereas no mice in the control groups survived [25]. It was determined that the above result was dependent on both CD4 and CD8 T cells as their depletion allowed the tumors to grow [26].

6 GITR

The glucocorticoid-induced tumor necrosis factor receptor (GITR) is another co-stimulatory TNF superfamily member found on T cells. GITR binds to its ligand, GITR-L, which is expressed in low levels on antigen-presenting macrophages, B cells, and dendritic cells, where it is up-regulated when these cells are activated. Studies have shown that GITR provides a positive growth signal to CD4 and CD8 naïve T cells allowing for enhanced survival and function. GITR works by signaling through the NF-κB pathway causing up-regulation of IL-2R, IL-2, and interferon γ, and GITR knockout mice have decreased number and reduced survival of CD8 T cells. GITR is also expressed on NK T cells where signaling causes increased cytotoxicity, with increased production of interferon γ and other inflammatory cytokines [27]. GITR is expressed in high concentrations on Treg cells, and its activation decreases Treg function. GITR expression on Tregs is controlled by Foxp3, a potent transcriptional regulator. While GITR reduces Treg function, preventing their suppressive roles, GITR signaling also induces Treg proliferation. Therefore, once transient GITR signaling terminates, the Tregs will regain their suppressive function, and since there is now an expanded population, these suppressive activities are stronger than they were previously. Thus while the immediate function of GITR is to decrease Treg function, GITR stimulation causes a long-term strengthening of Treg suppressive abilities [28].

Studies have shown that agonistic anti-GITR antibodies help overcome self-tolerance and Treg suppression [29]. In other experiments using a mouse model of melanoma it was shown that GITR monoclonal antibody could be used as immunotherapy; the antibody induced suppression of Tregs and tumor challenge was rejected [30]. When dendritic cells engineered to express GITR-L-Fc fusion protein or GITR agonistic antibody were injected into a melanoma mouse model, they decreased tumor survival by about 60 %, compared to 100 % survival in controls [31]. Vaccines that targeted sarcoma antigens combined with GITRL also decreased tumor growth [32]. In vivo studies have shown that anti-GITR antibody causes tumor-infiltrating Tregs to lose suppressive properties because they lose expression of Foxp3—which may move T cells toward effector rather than regulatory function [30].

6.1 Clinical Trials

Table 1 provides a summary of the clinical trials discussed in this review.

7 Targeting CTLA4

One of the first clinical trials, led by Dranoff and co-workers, was a phase I study in which an antagonistic antibody against CTLA4 called MDX-CTLA4, a humanized monoclonal antibody, was injected into nine patients with different types of advanced cancer. MDX-CTLA4 caused tumor necrosis in three of the patients, each of whom had metastatic melanoma and had been previously injected with a GM-CSF-secreting tumor cell vaccine. In addition, anti-CTLA4 antibody treatment reduced or arrested the increase in CA-125 in two patients who had metastatic ovarian cancer that had also been previously treated with a GM-CSF-secreting tumor cell vaccine. However, there was no effect seen in four metastatic melanoma patients treated with a vaccine consisting of melanoma antigens. Several patients developed autoimmune side effects, as predicted by preclinical studies, including grade I reticular and erythematous rash, and T cells appeared to infiltrate into the area of the rash. Patients also had low levels of autoimmune antibodies, including antinuclear, antithyroglobulin, and rheumatoid factor; however, no additional symptoms were manifested. Therefore anti-CTLA4 treatment had an effect on malignancy with acceptable autoimmune side effects [33]. With this initial success, other trials were designed and a phase I trial in advanced stage IV melanoma patients was completed with 14 patients using the human monoclonal anti-CTLA4 antibody, MDX-010, also named ipilimumab. In this study by Seipp et al., ipilimumab was administered in conjunction with peptide vaccines derived from gp100 melanoma-associated antigen. The study achieved two complete remissions and one partial remission. Six of the 14 patients in this trial suffered severe grade 3 and 4 autoimmune side effects

Table 1 Summary of clinical trials

Antibody	Target	Phase	Diseases	Trial	Response	Reference
MDX-CTLA4	CTLA4	I	Melanoma, ovarian	Injected into 9 patients—3 melanoma and 2 ovarian patients previously treated with GM-CSF vaccine, and 4 melanoma patients treated previously with a vaccine consisting of melanoma antigens	Tumor necrosis in 3 melanoma patients treated with GM-CSF vaccine, reduced or stopped the increase of CA-125 in 2 ovarian patients, no response in a vaccine consisting of melanoma antigens	[33]
Ipilimumab	CTLA4	I	Melanoma	Ipilimumab was given to 14 patients with vaccinations of peptides derived from gp100 melanoma-associated antigen	2 CR, 1 PR	[34]
Ipilimumab	CTLA4	II	RCC	Ipilimumab was given to one group of 21 patients as a loading dose at 3 mg/kg and then subsequent dosing at 1 mg/kg every 3 weeks, and the second group of 40 patients was given ipilimumab at 3 mg/kg every 3 weeks	In the first group only 1 PR was seen, and the second group had 5 PRs	[35]
Ipilimumab	CTLA4	III	Melanoma	676 patients given either ipilimumab with or without GP100 and one group of patients given GP100 alone	10-month median survival vs. 6 months in the control group	[37]
Ipilimumab	CTLA4	III	Melanoma	502 patients received a combination of ipilimumab and dacarbazine or dacarbazine alone during weeks 1, 4, 7, and 10, followed by dacarbazine alone every 3 weeks until week 22	11-month median survival vs. 9 months in the control group	[38]
Tremelimumab	CTLA4	I	Melanoma	1-h infusions every 90 days up to four times, in 36 evaluable patients	4 PRs	[39]

(continued)

Table 1 (continued)

Antibody	Target	Phase	Diseases	Trial	Response	Reference
Tremelimumab	CTLA4	II	Melanoma	In this 246-patient study the test drug was given at 15 mg/kg every 90 days and repeated up to four times if the patient had tumor stabilization or response	Response rate of 6.6 %, with 16 partial responses. The duration of response lasted 9 to 30 months	[40]
Tremelimumab	CTLA4	III	Melanoma	655 treatment-naïve, unresectable stage III and IV melanoma patients received tremelimumab or standard chemotherapy	36-month duration of response vs. 14 months in the control group	[41]
MDX-1106	PD-1	I	Several refractory solid tumors including RCC, melanoma, colon cancer, NSCLC	Tested escalating doses of MDX-1106 to a maximum dose of 10 mg/kg in 39 patients with renal cell carcinoma, melanoma, prostate, colon cancer, or NSCLC	1 CR and 2 PRs	[43]
MDX-1106	PD-1	I	Melanoma, NSCLC, prostate cancer, RCC, colorectal cancer	296 patients received treatment with MDX-1106	Response rates were 18 % in NSCLC, 28 % in melanoma, and 27 % in RCC. Also, 20 of 31 patients followed for over a year had responses lasting over a year	[44]
MDX-1106	PD-1	I	Refractory metastatic RCC, prostate cancer, melanoma, NSCLC, and colorectal cancer	126 patients received 1, 3, or 10 mg/kg of the drug administered biweekly	16 RCC patients treated with 10 mg/kg had an overall response rate of 31.2 % with sustained disease of over 4 months in 6 of 16 patients. One of the 2 RCC patients treated with 1 mg/kg had a PR for 12 months, and one had sustained disease for 21 months. Also, one of the 15 evaluable patients with prostate cancer had a PR lasting over 2 months, and 3 of 15 had sustained disease for over 4 months	[46]

CT-011	PD-1	I	Hematologic malignancies	17 patients were given escalating doses of CT-011, to a maximum dose of 6 mg/kg, as a single IV infusion	33 % response rate and 1 CR	[47]
BMS-936559	PDL1	I	Melanoma, colon cancer, RCC pancreatic, gastric, breast, and NSCLC	207 patients were treated with 1-h infusions on days 1, 15, and 29 of 6-week cycles, and they received up to 16 cycles as long as they were able to tolerate the treatments	Overall response rate of 19 % in melanoma patients. An overall response rate of 10 % in NSCLC, 6 % in ovarian cancer, and 12 % of RCC	[48]
BMS-666513	4-1BB	I	Melanoma, renal cell carcinoma, prostate cancer, or ovarian cancer	83 patients studied. The drug, at several dose levels, was given IV every 3 weeks, and response was tested after the fourth dose and then every 2 doses thereafter	9 PRs in 54 melanoma patients tested	[49]
anti-OX40	OX40	I	Variety of refractory solid tumors	30-patient study in which the test drug was infused on days 1, 3, and 5 of each cycle at 0.1, 0.4, or 2 mg/kg, with 10 patients in each dose category	Being assessed	[50]
TRX518	GITR	I	Melanoma	Testing safety of TRX518	In process	[27]

including dermatitis, enterocolitis, hepatitis, and hypophysitis [34]. A phase II clinical trial in metastatic renal cell carcinoma (RCC) was performed by Rosenberg et al. In this study, one group of 21 patients was treated with a loading dose of ipilimumab at 3 mg/kg and then subsequent dosing at 1 mg/kg every 3 weeks, and the second group of 40 patients was treated with ipilimumab at 3 mg/kg every 3 weeks. In the first group only one partial response was seen. In addition, three of the patients suffered enterocolitis, and one of these three also developed a generalized rash and multiarticular arthritis. The second group who received ipilimumab only at 3 mg/kg had five partial responses. Seventeen patients suffered from immune-mediated autoimmune side effects. Thirteen had enteritis, one had hypophysitis, one had both enteritis and hypophysitis, one had primary adrenal insufficiency, and one had aseptic meningitis with cerebral spinal fluid lymphocytosis [35]. Interestingly, most of the patients who had antitumor responses also developed significant autoimmune side effects such that a response rate of 30 % was seen in those patients with autoimmune events and 0 % response rate seen in patients without autoimmune events ($P=0.009$) [36].

A phase III, randomized, double-blinded trial was carried out by Urba et al. and tested ipilimumab in advanced stage III and IV melanoma patients. In this trial ipilimumab was administered with or without GP100, a melanoma tumor antigen, and one group of patients received GP100 peptide alone. The results showed a 10-month median survival in the ipilimumab-administered groups whether or not GP100 was also given, and a 6.4-month median survival in patients only given GP100. Sixty percent of the 676 enrolled patients had severe immune-related side effects when given ipilimumab, including diarrhea, injection-site reactions, vitiligo, and colitis. Fourteen deaths occurred out of the 540 patients who received ipilimumab [37]. In another phase III trial, 502 patients with metastatic melanoma who were treatment naïve received a combination of ipilimumab and dacarbazine or dacarbazine alone during weeks 1, 4, 7, and 10, followed by dacarbazine alone every 3 weeks until week 22. After this time if patients had a response then they received dacarbazine or placebo every 12 weeks as maintenance regardless of their original treatment group. This randomized controlled trial led by Wolchok showed 20.8 % vs. 12.2 % survival, at 3 years in patients who received ipilimumab together with dacarbazine compared with those who received dacarbazine alone. Similar side effects were seen in this trial as in the earlier trial with GP100 randomization; however, no deaths and less severe gastrointestinal side effects were observed. Administering high-dose steroids appears to be effective in reducing grade III–IV diarrhea (colitis) and subsequent drug-induced mortality [38]. As a result, the FDA approved the use of ipilimumab in metastatic melanoma in 2010.

Another monoclonal anti-CTLA4 antibody was developed named tremelimumab, a human IgG2 monoclonal anti-CTLA4 antibody. A phase I trial was conducted by Gonzalez et al. in which stage 3 and 4 melanoma patients received tremelimumab in 1-h infusions every 90 days up to four times. Of 36 patients evaluable for response to therapy, 4 had a partial remission and there were no complete remissions, and the drug was well tolerated without major complications. The side effects included fatigue, diarrhea, and dehydration [39]. In addition, a phase II trial by

Bulanhagui et al. studied the tumor response of tremelimumab when administered to refractory melanoma patients. The drug was given at 15 mg/kg every 90 days. The infusion was repeated up to four times if the patient had tumor stabilization or response. This study involved 246 patients with a response rate of 6.6 %, with 16 partial responses. The duration of response ranged from 9–30 months [40]. The positive results of early trials led to the recent phase III trial by Hauschild et al. In this study 655 treatment-naïve, unresectable stage III and IV melanoma patients received tremelimumab or standard chemotherapy (either temozolomide or dacarbazine, investigators' choice). Results showed no difference between the groups in response rate, which was approximately 10 %; however, duration of response was longer in the tremelimumab group (36 months vs. 14 months, $P<0.0011$). Side effects included rash, pruritis, and diarrhea. In addition, there were 7 deaths due to the tremelimumab, which is 2 % of the 325 patients treated, versus 1 death of the 319 patients in the chemotherapy group, which is <1 % of the patients treated. The authors pointed out that 16 % of the control arm received ipilimumab as salvage therapy and that this may have impacted the difference in survival. Furthermore, this trial excluded patients with lactate dehydrogenase (LDH) more than twice the upper limit of normal, whereas ipilimumab trials did not. Thus, patients on the chemotherapy control arm may have done better than expected and this may have lessened the survival difference. This is suggested by analysis of the forest plot in which there is a trend toward better hazard ratio in patients with more advanced melanoma (e.g., higher LDH baseline levels). Thus, a number of factors may explain why the results of this trial were different from the results of the phase III ipilimumab trials [41]. Although these studies demonstrated little improvement compared to standard chemotherapy, additional clinical trials are ongoing [42].

8 Targeting PD-1

Following the success of CTLA4 monoclonal antibodies, anti-PD-1 therapies have also been developed. There are three PD-1 antagonistic antibodies and one fusion protein currently being tested in the clinic. These are known as MDX-1106, CT-011, MK-3475, and AMP-224, respectively. The first three are monoclonal anti-PD-1 antagonistic antibodies, and the fourth is a B7-DC/IgG1 fusion protein [8]. In addition, trials of antibodies targeting PDL1 are also being conducted, and BMS-936559 is one such antagonistic anti-PDL1 antibody.

9 MDX-1106

A phase I trial conducted by Topalian et al. tested MDX-1106, a human monoclonal IgG4 antagonistic antibody also known as BMS-936558. It was given to patients with several types of metastatic refractory solid tumors including RCC, melanoma, prostate, colon cancer, and non-small-cell lung cancer (NSCLC). The study was designed to test escalating doses to a maximum dose of 10 mg/kg of MDX-1106 and included 39 patients. Results include one complete remission in colon cancer and two partial responses in melanoma and NSCLC. The study also demonstrated durability of the drug's effect and showed that the drug was well tolerated [43].

Another phase I trial reported by Sznol involved patients with advanced melanoma, NSCLC, castration-resistant prostate cancer, RCC, or colorectal cancer and treatment with MDX-1106. Complete or partial responses were seen in NSCLC, melanoma, or RCC. Of the 296 patients included in this study, response rates were 18 % in 76 patients with NSCLC, 28 % in 94 patients with melanoma, and 27 % in 33 patients with RCC. These responses were often durable, with 20 of 31 patient responses lasting over a year in patients that had at least a year of follow-up. Thirty-two of the total 296 patients had severe drug-related events, including pneumonitis, vitiligo, colitis, hepatitis, hypophysitis, and thyroiditis. Intriguingly, PDL1 expression on tumors appears to correlate with response [44]. Also, effective reinduction therapy with anti-PD-1 antibody has been reported [45]. A recent phase I trial by Wigginton et al. tested MDX-1106 in refractory metastatic RCC, prostate cancer, melanoma, NSCLC, and colorectal cancer. The study tested 1, 3, or 10 mg/kg of the drug administered biweekly in 126 patients. Side effects included rash, pruritus, diarrhea, and fatigue. This study included 16 RCC patients treated with 10 mg/kg, and at this dose an overall response rate of 31.2 % (5 of 16 patients) was observed with sustained disease of over 4 months observed in 6 of 16 patients. One of the two RCC patients treated with 1 mg/kg had a partial remission lasting over 12 months, and one had sustained disease lasting over 21 months. One of the 15 evaluable patients with prostate cancer had a partial response lasting over 2 months, and 3 of 15 had stable disease for over 4 months [46].

CT-011 is a humanized monoclonal IgG1 antagonistic antibody against PD-1. CT-011 has also been investigated in a phase I trial by Nagler et al. to identify the maximum tolerated dose. In this study 17 patients were given escalating doses of CT-011, to a maximum dose of 6 mg/kg, as a single IV infusion. The drug was well tolerated with diarrhea being the main side effect, and no maximal tolerated dose was determined. CT-011 showed preliminary antitumor efficacy, with 33 % of patients having a response and one patient having a complete remission. This trial tested the drug in hematologic malignancies including acute myeloid leukemia (AML), chronic lymphocytic leukemia, non-Hodgkin's lymphoma, Hodgkin's lymphoma, or multiple myeloma [47].

A phase I anti-PDL1 antibody trial has also been conducted. BMS-936559 is a humanized IgG4 monoclonal antibody, which prevents PDL1 binding to PD-1. BMS-936559 was tested in patients with several cancers including melanoma, colon, pancreatic, gastric, and breast cancer, RCC, and NSCLC. Patients were treated with 1-h infusions on days 1, 15, and 29 of 6-week cycles, and they received up to 16 cycles as long as they were able to tolerate the treatments. This study, conducted by Wigginton et al., showed durable tumor regression, with an overall response rate of 19 % in melanoma patients with response seen in 9 of 52 patients.

An overall response rate was observed in 10 % or 5 of 49 patients with NSCLC as well as in 6 % or 1 of 17 patients with ovarian cancer and in 12 % of 207 patients with RCC. These data are overall average responses seen in patients treated with 1, 3, or 10 mg/kg BMS-936559; and the highest doses gave the highest response rates when analyzed alone. Immune side effects related to the drug occurred in 81 of the 207 patients and included rash, hypothyroidism, hepatitis, sarcoidosis, endophthalmitis, diabetes, and myasthenia gravis [48].

10 Anti-4-IBB Therapy

There are several anti-4-1BB agonist antibodies under study in the clinical setting. BMS-666513 is a human monoclonal antibody that has been tested in a phase I trial by Logan et al. The study was conducted in 83 patients with melanoma, RCC, prostate cancer, or ovarian cancer. The drug, at several dose levels, was given intravenously every 3 weeks, and response was tested after the fourth dose and then every two doses thereafter. There were partial responses in 9 of 54 melanoma patients. The therapy was well tolerated with a 6–15 % side effect rate including neutropenia, increased liver function tests, fatigue, rash, pruritis, diarrhea, and fever [49].

11 Anti-OX40 Therapy

A phase I trial of anti-OX40 led by Weinberg and Curti using a mouse monoclonal agonist antibody. To determine a safe and effective dose the antibody was infused on days 1, 3, and 5 of each cycle at 0.1, 0.4, or 2 mg/kg. The study involved 30 patients with a variety of refractory solid tumors, with 10 patients in each dose category. It was thought that since there are few T cells that express OX40 the immune response would be efficacious without having the same high side effect profile as agents targeting CTLA4. This turned out to be the case, with mild fatigue and lymphopenia being most common adverse effects. The efficacy of the OX40 antibody in this trial is still being assessed [50], and anti-OX40 antibodies are also being used in other ongoing trials.

12 GITR-Targeted Therapy

Phase I trials targeting GITR are ongoing. One is a trial in melanoma testing the safety of GITR agonistic antibody TRX518. Another is a phase I trial in melanoma patients testing dendritic cells alone or dendritic cells expressing GITRL, anti-CTLA4, or both together [27].

13 Conclusion

There are many other receptor and ligand co-stimulatory or inhibitory pairs that affect T cell activity that are being studied in the laboratory and in the clinic. As we gain knowledge regarding the normal functions of the different T cell co-regulatory receptors, we will be able to better manipulate their functions in hopes of further improving immunotherapy as a standard treatment option for cancer patients, to be used alone or in conjunction with other treatment modalities such as chemotherapy or radiation therapy. Manipulation of co-regulatory receptor signaling has already demonstrated early efficacy and will increasingly be incorporated in combination with additional immune therapy strategies in a variety of human tumors.

References

1. Janeway Jr CA, Travers P, Walport M, Shlomchik MJ. Immunobiology; the immune system in health and disease. 6th ed. New York, NY: Garland Science; 2005. p. 26–31. 327-328.
2. Pardoll DM. The blockade of immune checkpoints in cancer immunotherapy. Nat Rev Cancer. 2012;12:254–62.
3. Sansom DM. CD28, CTLA4, and their ligands: who does what and to whom? Immunology. 2000;101:169–77.
4. Leach DR, Krummel MF, Allison JP. Enhancement of antitumor immunity by CTLA-4 blockade. Science. 1996;271:1734–6.
5. Van Elsas A, Hurwitz AA, Allison JP. Combination immunotherapy of B16 melanoma using anti-cytotoxic T lymphocyte-associated antigen 4 (CTLA-4) and granulocyte/macrophage colony-stimulating factor (GM-CSF)-producing vaccines induces rejection of subcutaneous and metastatic tumors accompanied by autoimmune depigmentation. J Exp Med. 1999;19: 355–66.
6. Capece D, Verzella D, Fischietti M, Zazzeroni F, Alesse E. Targeting costimulatory molecules to improve antitumor immunity. J Biomed Biotechnol. 2012;2011:1–17.
7. Poirier N, Blancho G, Vanhove B. CD28-Specific immunomodulating antibodies: what can be learned from experimental models. Am J Transplant. 2012;7:1682–90.
8. Topalian SL, Drake CG, Pardoll DM. Targetting the PD-1/B7-H1(PD-L1) pathway to activate anti-tumor immunity. Curr Opin Immmunol. 2012;24:207–12.
9. Sharpe AH, Wherry JE, Ahmed R, Freeman GJ. The function of programmed cell death 1 and its ligands in regulating autoimmunity and infection. Nat Immunol. 2007;8:239–45.
10. Barber DL, Wherry EJ, Masopust D, Zhu B, Allison JP, Sharpe AH, Freeman GJ, Ahmed R. Restoring function in exhausted CD8 T cells during chronic viral infection. Nature. 2006;439: 682–7.
11. Titanji K, Velu V, Chennareddi L, Vijay-Kumar M, Gewirtz AT, Freeman GJ, Amara RR. Acute depletion of activated memory B cells involves the PD-1 pathway in rapidly progressing SIV-infected macaques. J Clin Invest. 2010;120:3878–90.
12. Francisco LM, Salinas VH, Brown KE, Vanguri VK, Freeman GJ, Kuchroo VK, Sharpe AH. PD-L1 regulates the development, maintenance, and function of induced regulatory T cells. J Exp Med. 2009;206:3015–29.
13. Iwai Y, Ishida M, Tanaka Y, Okazaki T, Honjo T, Minato N. Involvement of PD-L1 on tumor cells in the escape from host immune system and tumor immunotherapy by PD-L1 blockade. Proc Natl Acad Sci U S A. 2002;99:12293–7.

14. Dong H, Strome SE, Salomao DR, Tamura H, Hirano F, Flies DB, Roche PC, Lu J, Zhu G, Tamada K, Lennon VA, Celis E, Chen L. Tumor-associated B7-H1 promotes T-cell apoptosis: a potential mechanism of immune evasion. Nat Med. 2002;8:793–800.
15. Zhang H, Snyder KM, Suhoski MM, Maus MV, Kapoor V, June CH, Mackall CL. 4-1BB Is superior to CD28 costimulation for generating CD8+ cytotoxic lymphocytes for adoptive immunotherapy. J Immunol. 2007;179:4910–8.
16. Vinay DS, Kwon BS. Immunotherapy of cancer with 4-1BB. Mol Cancer Ther. 2012;11: 1062–70.
17. Croft M. Co-stimulatory members of the TNFR family: keys to effective T-cell immunity. Nat Rev Immunol. 2003;3:609–20.
18. Mittler RS, Bailey TS, Klussman K, Trailsmith MD, Hoffmann MK. Anti-4-1BB monoclonal antibodies abrogate T cell-dependent humoral immune responses in vivo through the induction of helper T cell anergy. J Exp Med. 1999;190:1535–40.
19. Hong HJ, Lee JW, Park SS, Kang YJ, Chang SY, Kim KM, Kim JO, Murthy KK, Payne JS, Yoon SK, Park MJ, Kim IC, Kim JG, Kang CY. A humanized anti-4-1BB monoclonal antibody suppresses antigen-induced humoral immune response in nonhuman primates. J Immunother. 2000;23:613–21.
20. Melero I, Shuford WW, Newby SA, Aruffo A, Ledbetter JA, Hellstrom KE, Mittler RS, Chen L. Monoclonal antibodies against the 4-1BB T-cell activation molecule eradicate established tumors. Nat Med. 1997;3:682–5.
21. Kim JA, Averbook BJ, Chambers K, Rothchild K, Kjaergaard J, Papay R, Shu S. Divergent effects of 4-1BB antibodies on antitumor immunity and on tumor-reactive T-cell generation. Cancer Res. 2001;61:2031–7.
22. Lane P. Role of OX40 signals in coordinating CD4 T cell selection, migration, and cytokine differentiation in T helper Th1 and Th2 cells. J Exp Med. 2000;2:201–6.
23. Redmond WL, Ruby CE, Weinberg AD. The role of OX40-mediated Co-stimulation T cell activation and survival. Crit Rev Immunol. 2009;29:187–201.
24. Weinberg WD, Morris NP, Kovacsovics-Bankowski M, Urba WJ, Curti BD. Science gone translational: the OX40 agonist story. Immunol Rev. 2011;244:218–31.
25. Weinberg AD, Rivera MM, Prell R, Morris A, Ramstad T, Vetto JT, Urba WJ, Alvord G, Bunce C, Shields J. Engagement of the OX-40 receptor in vivo enhances antitumor immunity. J Immunol. 2000;164:2160–9.
26. Kjaergaard J, Tanaka J, Kim JA, Rothchild K, Weinberg A, Shu S. Therapeutic efficacy of OX-40 receptor antibody depends on tumor immunogenicity and anatomic site of tumor growth. Cancer Res. 2000;60:5514–21.
27. Schaer DA, Murphy JT, Wolchok JD. Modulation of GITR for cancer immunotherapy. Curr Opin Immunol. 2012;24:217–24.
28. Nocentini G, Ronchetti S, Cuzzocrea S, Riccardi C. GITR/GITRL: more than an effector T cell co-stimulatory system. Eur J Immunol. 2007;37:1165–9.
29. Shimizu J, Yamazaki S, Takahashi T, Ishida Y, Sakaguchi S. Stimulation of CD25(+)CD4(+) regulatory T cells through GITR breaks immunological self-tolerance. Nat Immunol. 2002;3:135–42.
30. Cohen AD, Schaer DA, Liu C, Li Y, Hirschhorn-Cymmerman D, Kim SC, Diab A, Rizzuto G, Duan F, Perales MA, Merghoub T, Houghton AN, Wolchok JD. Agonist anti-GITR monoclonal antibody induces melanoma tumor immunity in mice by altering regulatory T cell stability and intra-tumor accumulation. PLoS One. 2010;5:1–12.
31. Boczkowski D, Lee J, Pruitt S, Nair S. Dendritic cells engineered to secrete anti-GITR antibodies are effective adjuvants to dendritic cell-based immunotherapy. Cancer Gene Ther. 2009;16:900–11.
32. Nishikawa H, Kato T, Hirayama M, Orito Y, Sato E, Harada N, Gnjatic S, Old LJ, Shiku H. Regulatory T cell-resistant CD8+ T cells induced by glucocorticoid-induced tumor necrosis factor receptor signaling. Cancer Res. 2008;68:5948–54.
33. Hodi FS, Mihm MC, Soiffer RJ, Haluska FG, Butler M, Seiden MV, Davis T, Henry-Spires R, MacRae S, William A, Padera R, Jaklitsch MT, Shanker S, Chen TC, Korman A, Allison JP,

Dranoff G. Biologic activity of cytotoxic T lymphocyte-associated antigen 4 antibody blockade in previously vaccinated metastatic melanoma and ovarian carcinoma patients. Proc Natl Acad Sci U S A. 2003;100:4712–7.
34. Phan GQ, Yang JC, Sherry RM, Hwu P, Topalian SL, Schwartzentruber DJ, Restifo NP, Hawarth LR, Seipp CA, Freezer LJ, Morton KE, Mavroukakis SA, Duray PH, Steinberg SM, Allison JP, Davis TA, Rosenberg SA. Cancer regression and autoimmunity induced by cytotoxic T lymphocyte-associated antigen 4 blockade in patients with metastatic melanoma. Proc Natl Acad Sci U S A. 2003;100:8372–7.
35. Yang JC, Hughes M, Kammula U, Royal R, Sherry R, Topalian SL, Suri KB, Levy C, Allen T, Mavroukakis S, Lowy I, White DE, Rosenberg SA. Ipilimumab (anti-CTLA4 antibody) causes regression of metastatic renal cell cancer associated with enteritis and hypophysitis. J Immunother. 2007;30:825–30.
36. Escudier B. Emerging immunotherapies for renal cell carcinoma. Ann Oncol. 2012;23 Suppl 8:viii35–40.
37. Hodi FS, O'Day SJ, McDermott DF, Weber RW, Sosman JA, Haanen JB, Gonzalez R, Robert C, Schadendorf D, Hassel JC, Akerley W, van den Eertwegh AJ, Lutzky J, Lorigan P, Vaubel JM, Linette GP, Hogg D, Ottensmeier CH, Lebbe C, Peschel C, Quirt I, Clark JI, Wolchok JD, Weber JS, Tian J, Yellin MJ, Nichol GM, Hoos A, Urba WJ. Improved survival with ipilimumab in patients with metastatic melanoma. N Engl J Med. 2010;363:711–23.
38. Robert C, Thomas L, Bondarenko I, O'Day S, M D JW, Garbe C, Lebbe C, Baurain JF, Testori A, Grob JJ, Davidson N, Richards J, Maio M, Hauschild A, Miller Jr WH, Gascon P, Lotem M, Harmankaya K, Ibrahim R, Francis S, Chen TT, Humphrey R, Hoos A, Wolchok JD. Ipilimumab plus dacarbazine for previously untreated metastatic melanoma. N Engl J Med. 2011;364:2517–26.
39. Ribas A, Chesney JA, Gordon MS, Abernethy AP, Logan TF, Lawson DH, Chmielowski B, Glaspy JA, Lewis K, Huang B, Wang E, Hsyu PH, Gomez-Navarro J, Gerhardt D, Marshall MA, Gonzalez R. Safety profile and pharmacokinetic analyses of the anti-CTLA4 antibody tremelimumab administered as a one hour infusion. J Transl Med. 2012;10:1–6.
40. Kirkwood JM, Lorigan P, Hauschild A, Robert C, McDermott D, Marshall MA, Gomez-Navarro J, Liang JQ, Bulanhagui CA. Phase II trial of tremelimumab (CP-675,206) in patients with advanced refractory or relapsed melenoma. Clin Cancer Res. 2010;16:1042–8.
41. Ribas A, Kefford R, Marshall MA, Punt CJ, Haanen JB, Marmol M, Garbe C, Gogas H, Schachter J, Linette G, Lorigan P, Kendra KL, Maio M, Trefzer U, Smylie M, McArthur GA, Dreno B, Nathan PD, Mackiewicz J, Kirkwood JM, Gomez-Navarro J, Huang B, Pavlov D, Hauschild A. Phase III randomized clinical trial comparing tremelimumab with standard-of-care chemotherapy in patients with advanced melanoma. J Clin Oncol. 2013;31(5):616–22.
42. Dolgin E. FDA okays potential blockbuster melanoma drug. Http://blogs.nature.com. N.p., 25 Mar. 2011. Web. 10 Feb. 2013.
43. Brahmer JR, Drake CG, Wollner I, Powderly J, Picus J, Sharfman W, Stankevich E, Pons A, Salay TM, McMiller TL, Gilson MM, Wang C, Selby M, Taube JM, Anders R, Chen L, Korman AJ, Pardoll DM, Lowry I, Topalian SL. Phase I study of single-agent anti-programmed death-1 (MDX-1106) in refractory solid tumors: safety, clinical activity, pharmacodynamics, and immunologic correlates. J Clin Oncol. 2010;28:3167–75.
44. Topalian SL, Hodi FS, Brahmer JR, Gettinger SN, Smith DC, McDermott DF, Powderly JD, Carvajal RD, Sosman JA, Atkins MB, Leming PD, Spigel DR, Antonia SJ, Horn L, Drake CG, Pardoll DM, Chen L, Sharfman WH, Anders RA, Taube JM, McMiller TL, Xu H, Korman AJ, Jure-Kunkel M, Agrawal S, McDonald D, Kollia GD, Gupta A, Wigginton JM, Sznol M. Safety, activity, and immune correlates of anti-PD-1 antibody in cancer. N Engl J Med. 2012;366:2443–54.
45. Lipson EJ, Sharfman WH, Drake CG, Wollner I, Taube JM, Anders RA, Xu H, Yao S, Pons A, Chen L, Pardoll DM, Brahmer JR, Topalian SL. Durable cancer regression off-treatment and effective reinduction therapy with an anti-PD-1 antibody. Clin Cancer Res. 2013;19:462–8.
46. McDermott D, Drake CG, Sznol M, Sosman JA, Smith DC, Powderly JD, Feltquate DM, Kollia G, Gupta KA, Wigginton J. A Phase I study to evaluate safety and antitumor activity of

biweekly BMS-936558 (Anti-PD-1, MDX-1106/ONO-4538) in Patients with RCC and other advanced refractory malignancies. J Clin Oncol 2011;29:7(Suppl): Abstract 331.
47. Berger R, Rotem-Yehudar R, Slama G, Landes S, Kneller A, Leiba M, Koren-Michowitz M, Shimoni A, Nagler A. Phase I safety and pharmacokinetic study of CT-011, a humanized antibody interacting with PD-1, in patients with advanced hematologic malignancies. Clin Cancer Res. 2008;14:3044–51.
48. Brahmer JR, Tykodi SS, Chow LQ, Hwu WJ, Topalian SL, Hwu P, Drake CG, Camacho LH, Kauh J, Odunsi K, Pitot HC, Hamid O, Bhatia S, Martins R, Eaton K, Chen S, Salay TM, Alaparthy S, Grosso JF, Korman AJ, Parker SM, Agrawal S, Goldberg SM, Pardoll DM, Gupta A, Wigginton JM. Safety and activity of anti-PD-L1 antibody in patients with advanced cancer. N Engl J Med. 2012;366:2455–65.
49. Sznol M, Hodi FS, Margolin K, McDermott DF, Ernstoff MS, Kirkwood JM, Wojtaszek C, Feltquate D, Logan T. Phase I Study of BMS-663513, a Fully Human Anti-CD137 Agonist Monoclonal Antibody, in Patients with Advanced Cancer (CA). J Clin Oncol 26: 2008 (May 20 suppl; abstr 3007).
50. Jensen SM, Maston LD, Gough MJ, Ruby CE, Redmond WL, Crittenden M, Li Y, Puri S, Poehlein CH, Morris N, Kovacsovics-Bankowski M, Moudgil T, Twitty C, Walker EB, Hu HM, Urba WJ, Weinberg AD, Curti B, Fox BA. Signaling through OX40 enhances anti-tumor immunity. Semin Oncol. 2010;37:524–32.

Assessment of Immune Response in Biotherapy Trials and Clinical Endpoints

Theresa L. Whiteside

Abstract Today, biological therapies occupy an important place among available clinical modalities for treatment of cancer. Their true impact on the disease cannot be unraveled, however, without an understanding of immune mechanisms that therapies target and possibly alter. Immune monitoring is necessary to help identify and define these mechanisms. Recent introduction of rapid, high-throughput assays based on new insights into molecular pathways and attention to assay standardization has improved the quality of immune monitoring. Multiplex profiling of immune phenotypes, definition of regulatory immune cell subsets, identification of critical signaling molecules, and recognition of biologically relevant targets have all played a major role in defining immune competence of patients enrolled in biotherapy clinical trials. Today, the major objective of immune monitoring, to correlate therapy-induced alterations in immune responses and clinical endpoints, is finally being achieved, and potential immune biomarkers of disease-free or overall survival are being identified. In most cases, validation of these immune biomarkers remains to be performed. There is hope that reliable immune biomarkers of response to biotherapy will soon emerge as a result of expert serial monitoring. Immune monitoring is critical to establishing surrogate biomarkers of outcome in biotherapy clinical trials and thus to a better selection and delivery of biologics to patients with cancer.

Keywords Cancer • Immune biomarkers • Immune signature • Biotherapy • Prognosis • Response to biotherapy

---

Supported in part by the NIH grant PO1-CA109688 to Theresa L. Whiteside.

T.L. Whiteside, Ph.D., A.B.M.L.I. (✉)
University of Pittsburgh Cancer Institute, Hillman Cancer Center,
5117 Centre Avenue, Suite 1.27, Pittsburgh, PA 15213, USA
e-mail: whitesidetl@upmc.edu

J.D. Rosenblatt et al. (eds.), *Advances in Tumor Immunology and Immunotherapy*, Current Cancer Research, DOI 10.1007/978-1-4614-8809-5_15,
© Springer Science+Business Media New York 2014

Abbreviations

CFC	Cytokine flow cytometry
QA/QC	Quality assurance/quality control
GLP	Good laboratory practice
OBD	Optimal biologic dose
MTD	Maximal tolerated dose
PBMC	Peripheral blood mononuclear cells
CRC	Colorectal cancer
ELISA	Enzyme-linked immunosorbent assay
ELISPOT	Enzyme-linked immunospot
HNSCC	Head and neck squamous cell cancer
HPV	Human papilloma virus
IGKC	Immunoglobulin G kappa chain
Treg	Regulatory T cells
MDSC	Myeloid derived suppressor cells
NRL	Neutrophil-to-lymphocyte ratio

1 Introduction

Biotherapy utilizes a variety of biologic agents ranging from bacterial products, soluble factors, cells or cell products, and vaccines to treat cancer. In general, the current interest in clinical applications of biologics to therapy of human cancer reflects the need for more effective, less toxic, and preferably natural ways for treatment of patients, especially those with conditions that are refractory to standard therapies. Biologic agents used as therapeutics are expected to modify clinical responses, often through effects on the host immune system, and to improve the host capability to recover and reacquire normal homeostasis. Because most biologics target molecular and cellular immunologic pathways, there is an obvious requirement for assessments of direct or indirect effects these agents exert in vivo. For this reason, immunologic monitoring has emerged as an advisable and, more recently, as a necessary adjunct to clinical trials with biologic agents. In the past, immunologic monitoring fell under the "correlative studies" category. Today, it is often a protocol-mandated requirement, and an immunologic response to therapy is the primary endpoint. Immune monitoring has become a critically important part of patient assessment because of expectations that it will facilitate relating clinical responses to a specific immune mechanism and to predict responsiveness to therapy or help in estimating survival. The possibility that immune measures could serve as biomarkers or as surrogate endpoints of clinical responses has been intensively investigated in preclinical studies and in biotherapy trials. The recently published recommendations for the development and use of immunotherapy biomarkers by the joint SITC/NCI/FDA Taskforce not only emphasize the existing need for such biomarkers but also offer guidelines for how to establish, standardize, and evaluate immune assays to see whether they meet a biomarker designation [1]. This document makes it clear that in the era of personalized medicine and at the time when biotherapies are gaining place in cancer management, immunologic biomarkers of therapeutic efficacy are required if the field is to move forward.

The purpose of this chapter is to describe performance of selected immune methodologies in estimating clinical responses to biotherapies and to illustrate conceptual, technical, and biostatistical issues that arise in attempts to establish the predictive role of immune measures as intermediate biomarkers of cancer progression or recurrence following biotherapies.

2 Monitoring of Complex Biological Interactions

The immune system is exquisitely well prepared to handle insults by pathogens and is always ready to respond to "danger signals" originating within or outside the body [2, 3]. However, in cancer, the host immune system becomes compromised, unable to stop tumor progression or eliminate malignant growth [4]. This is a result of tumor-induced immune suppression, and many mechanisms used by human tumors to disable the host antitumor immunity have now been identified [5]. Biological therapies used in cancer are expected to restore the integrity of host antitumor immunity by up-regulating immune surveillance, blocking inhibitory signals, and/or removing/silencing suppressor cells [6, 7]. Some biologic therapies target innate or natural immunity, in hope of up-regulating surveillance functions of the immune cells such as monocytes, natural killer (NK) cells, or NKT cells [8]. Other biologic therapies preferentially aim at enhancing adaptive immune responses, to selectively augment functions of T or B lymphocytes that are responsible for protection against antigen-specific insults [6, 9, 10]. Although much has been learned in recent years about dysregulation of the immune system in cancer, the complexity of cellular signals and molecular interactions between innate and adaptive immunity [11] and of the existing cross talk with the neural, endocrine, and hormonal networks [12] complicate the interpretation of effects generated as a result of any particular immune-based therapy. It is, therefore, a foregone conclusion that the interpretation of immune monitoring results will be difficult, often intuitive, and not always informative. It is, therefore, not surprising or unexpected that the interpretation of benefits for any biologic therapy may differ depending on skills of investigators in performing, analyzing, and correlating the monitoring results with clinical outcome. Nevertheless, recent results from a number of biologic therapy trials indicate that beneficial clinical results can be linked to the identifiable changes in immunologic responses to therapy. This, in turn, offers an intriguing possibility of using selected immunologic characteristics as biomarkers of therapeutic responses or even survival. This possibility is explored in this chapter, and examples are provided to illustrate the emerging potential of immunologic markers as intermediate predictors of clinical responses of cancer patients to biotherapies.

In addition to complex biologic interactions of the immune system components, immune monitoring itself has been traditionally viewed as a particularly complex and poorly controlled enterprise relative to conventional biochemical assays used in the clinic. Serial immune assessments undertaken at the population level (i.e., "bulk" assays) were viewed as difficult, laborious, and not adequately informative. These have been largely replaced today by highly sophisticated technologies, many performed at a single-cell level and enabling assessments in situ, i.e., at the tissue site of disease as well as in the lymph nodes or peripheral circulation. Technologies currently available for measuring immune responses of cancer patients enrolled in biotherapy trials are numerous and varied, including high-throughput technologies such as arrays, multiplex formats, proteomics, genomics, high-content screening by flow cytometry, imaging, or tissue microarrays. While these newer "state-of-the-art" technologies offer possibilities for rapid screening of multiple samples and for simultaneous detection of many immunologic biomarkers, few, if any, have been formally validated so far. Most of these technologies have been standardized to meet quality control specifications for reliability and precision that are required for a large-scale monitoring of clinical trials. These technologies will be mentioned but not discussed in detail here, and the reader is referred to the summary of a Workshop on Immunological Molecular Markers in Oncology [13] for an excellent review of their use and potential.

3 Rationale for Immunologic Monitoring of Biotherapy Trials

"Monitoring" refers to serial specimen acquisition and testing. The process of immune monitoring starts with selection of methods that are applicable to reliable serial assessments, continues with their performance under defined QA/QC conditions, and ends with the analysis of results and their interpretation. Its major goal is to establish a correlation between phenotypic and functional changes in immune cells induced by therapy and clinical responses. In practical terms, this involves documenting a significant difference between the baseline and post-therapy immune measures and correlating it to clinical outcome. This entire process requires support that can only be provided in a specialized laboratory operated to handle and reliably test serial specimens and, preferably, functioning as a good laboratory practice (GLP) facility. It also requires appropriate statistical input to determine the significance of a change in immunologic measures from the pre-therapy baseline.

The rationale for immune monitoring rests on the premise that biotherapeutic interventions achieve their effects as a result of modification(s) in one or more components of the patient's immune system. These therapy-induced modifications seem to occur gradually, as beneficial clinical effects are often observed long after biotherapy is terminated. The expectation is that by serially measuring selected immune biomarkers that undergo significant changes relative to their pre-therapy baseline levels, it might be possible to define immunologic mechanisms responsible for biologic and possibly also clinical activity of the therapeutic agent. As biologic agents have a bell-shaped activity curve that shifts depending on the dose and time of their delivery, serial monitoring is necessary to define the optimal biologic dose (OBD) of a therapeutic agent. The OBD is distinct from the maximal tolerated dose (MTD) commonly used to define toxicity of drugs. However, most biologic agents have no or little toxicity, and the OBD is the more appropriate measure of their effects. Since, however, these agents are likely to have multiple biologic (and clinical) effects, the definition of OBD may not be straightforward, depending on more than one immunologic assessment. In designing biotherapy trials, the definition of OBD is critically important, and immunologic assays are likely to be very useful in this respect.

4 Specimen Processing Requirements for Serial Monitoring

To monitor, specimens must be collected from subjects prior to, at defined intervals during, and at the end of as well as after therapy. The origin of immune cells to be tested in the course of serial monitoring is important. Peripheral blood mononuclear cells (PBMC), representing less than 2 % of total body mononuclear cells, are most commonly employed, although it appears that cells derived from the disease site (e.g., the tumor, interstitial tumor fluids collected by cannulation, tumor draining lymph nodes, body fluids) might better reflect the extent of alterations induced by the disease. Thus, whenever available, such specimens should be collected, banked, and evaluated in parallel with peripheral blood.

The specimens harvested for immune monitoring should arrive at the laboratory no later than 24 h after collection. This requires an overnight delivery of specimens originating at distant locations [14]. The specimens are bar-coded and processed immediately upon arrival. The separated immune cells are either cryopreserved at −80 °C in 2 mL cryovials and banked for future testing or are immediately tested in assays which cannot be performed with cryopreserved/thawed cells. The monitoring laboratory is cognizant of assays that have to be performed on fresh as opposed to banked/thawed cells and will handle the specimens accordingly. The monitoring laboratory must have the capability to cryopreserve, bank, and maintain samples at a large scale under GLP conditions for prolonged periods of time [1]. Cryopreservation and recovery of thawed samples with a minimal loss of viability are required for successful monitoring [15]. The correctly performed process of freezing/thawing of immune cells is by far the most crucial determinant for preserving their true functional potential and for "batch" testing of serial specimens.

5 Selection of Assays for Immunological Monitoring

The first decision facing a monitoring laboratory is the selection of assays for "batch testing" that can be performed with banked cells or body fluids without compromising cellular functions or the analyte integrity, respectively. This is because the only reliable way to determine differences between pre-therapy and post-therapy results is to test these samples in the same assay. Specimens "batched" for testing in the same assay represent the entire collection of samples obtained from one subject throughout therapy. However, batching is only possible when the selected assay can be reliably performed with cryopreserved cells, as ascertained a priori through comparisons of fresh and frozen specimens tested in the same assay. Assays with established reliable performance when executed with thawed specimens are the best candidates for serial monitoring. Conversely, assays that must be performed on freshly harvested samples, notably those that measure cellular cytotoxicity [15], require documentation of minimal inter-assay variability so that therapy-induced changes can be reliably and convincingly distinguished from spurious assay-related differences.

Sensitive and reliable monitoring assays are required to measure changes occurring in the immune cell phenotype or function in response to biotherapy. Technical advances and new insights into immunologic mechanisms have led to the development of many new types of immunoassays that perform well in monitoring, as previously reviewed [15]. Today, clinical investigators can choose from a considerable list of cellular vs. molecular, phenotypic vs. functional, specific vs. nonspecific, and direct vs. indirect immune assays. The selected assay should be easily adaptable to serial testing with a minimal loss of accuracy, have a high throughput to accommodate large-volume testing, lend itself to automation, and be cost effective. These requirements are imposed by the need to accommodate batched serial samples from many time points collected from multiple subjects enrolled in a clinical protocol.

The range and sophistication of currently available monitoring assays predicate that careful consideration is required for selection of the "right" assay, i.e., one that best fits with the hypothesis being tested and with the laboratory expertise. As indicated in the schema for immune monitoring in Fig. 1, each biotherapy trial should be designed to test a hypothesis formulated on the basis of immune mechanisms that are most likely to contribute to the expected therapeutic benefits. Results of preclinical studies that are nearly always performed in support of biotherapy clinical trials usually point to mechanisms responsible for immunologic activity. Immune endpoints and assays selected to measure them need to fit with the hypothesis tested and should be based on preclinical data accumulated in support of this hypothesis.

The clinical investigator and the laboratory personnel are generally required to devote much thought and time to selecting monitoring assays, because the decision may determine not only scientific/correlative results of testing but also may have significant financial impact. Ideally, a combination of assays assessing the frequency of immune cells based on the phenotype as well as their functional attributes is selected to measure therapy-induced changes. For example, an excellent summary of cellular and molecular approaches for the characterization of cytotoxic T cells

Hypothesis relevant to a potential immune mechanism(s)

↓

Immune endpoint(s) defined based on pre-clinical data

↓

Assay selection guided by the hypothesis tested
- screening vs. confirmatory
- phenotypic vs. functional
- in situ vs. PBMC
- fresh vs. banked specimens
- cost, turn-around time

↓

Assay standardization (or validation for phase III trials)
- specificity, sensitivity, precision, accuracy, robustness

↓

Protocol schema specifying time points for serial sample collection
- relevance to predicted activity of the agent tested
- biostatistical input

↓

Sample arrival, processing, banking
- monitoring in a laboratory experienced to test serial samples
- GLP facility recommended

↓

Batch-testing of serial specimens
- high-throughput assays preferable
- applicable only to specimens not sensitive to freezing/thawing
- extended storage might interfere with result quality

↓

Assay results
- assay interpretation requires an immunologist
- data analysis requires a clinician-biostatistician partnership

↓

Correlations with clinical endpoints

Fig. 1 Designing immune monitoring for biotherapy clinical trials

following therapeutic vaccinations can be found in a review by Iancu [16]. Functional assays are more difficult to perform, requiring viable cells in numbers that may be difficult to procure. For this reason, the population-based "bulk" assays, such as proliferation or cytotoxicity, have been largely replaced by single-cell assays, allowing for measurements of expression levels of various cell components by highly sensitive technologies such as multiparameter flow cytometry [17]. However, this approach is only justified based on previous evidence confirming that the component expression level is directly related to its biologic function. As cryopreservation of immune cells might selectively impair viability of cell subsets or activity of cellular components, some functional assays have to be performed with freshly processed and not cryopreserved cells, as recently described for the subsets of human myeloid derived suppressor cells [18] and as previously emphasized for T cell and NK cell subsets mediating cytotoxicity [19].

Selection of monitoring immunoassays for a biotherapy protocol is a critically important step with consequences that are likely to affect efforts seeking to establish correlations between immunological results and clinical outcomes.

6 Standardization and Validation of Immunologic Assays

The selection of a "right" assay for immune monitoring is followed by its standardization to ensure that it can accurately measure therapy-induced changes. Assay standardization is performed prior to its acceptance for a routine use and involves repeated testing with cells or body fluids obtained from healthy donors under previously established optimized invariant conditions to establish the mean, median, and 80 % normal range and coefficient of variation. The intra-assay variability is also determined. A set of appropriate controls has to be included. For example, a large lot of cryopreserved PBMC obtained from a normal donor can be prepared, its range of reactivity determined, and thawed cells used in the assay to monitor day-to-day variability. With fresh cells, it is always advisable to include fresh control cells obtained from a healthy volunteer. In this respect, it is necessary to have in place an IRB approval for drawing blood from consented normal donors and to maintain a pool of such donors for QC purposes.

Whatever assay is selected, it should have the following attributes when performed under defined conditions: specificity, sensitivity, precision, accuracy, and robustness. These criteria traditionally used with chemical assays may not be easily applicable to some immunologic assays. Cell-based assays are especially troublesome to standardize and may never be as precise or robust as chemical assays. For example, it is not unusual to see coefficients of variation (CV) greater than 20 % in cellular assays. Functional cellular assays are not only especially difficult to standardize but are also more costly than phenotypic or molecular assays.

Assay "standardization" should not be confused with assay "validation." The former is a requisite part of the QC program, and the latter is a formal evaluation of an assay performed as defined in the Bioanalytical Method Validation issued by FDA in May 2001 (21CFR part 58) and qualifying it to be used in phase III clinical trials as an immunological endpoint. Validation consists of a series of large-scale experiments designed to evaluate accuracy, precision, selectivity, sensitivity, reproducibility, and stability characteristics of the method. Validation of an assay should be performed in prospective clinical trials. Again, while the existing validation criteria are defined for chemical assays, immunologic assays do not always fit into these criteria. Nevertheless, because no separate guidelines exist for immunologic assays, those developed for chemical assays are generally followed. Validation of immunologic assays is expensive, and it also faces a number of problems, especially with cell-based assays, which are typically lacking in precision. Further, no reference standards for cellular assays are currently available. In contrast, validation of immune assays measuring soluble products, such as immunoglobulins or cytokines, can and should follow validation recommendations for the development of chemical assays.

7 Can Immunologic Measures Serve as Intermediate Biomarkers of Clinical Outcome?

In view of the widely entertained hypothesis that the host immune system influences cancer development, progression, and therapy, the search for systemic and local immunologic biomarkers that would facilitate clinical decisions seems reasonable and important. Although studies in animal models of cancer support the role of antitumor immunity in cancer therapy, evidence from human clinical trials is not clear or straightforward. This may be due to profoundly immune-inhibitory effects of factors produced by human tumors [4] with the result that antitumor responses of patients are ineffective in controlling cancer progression. Therefore, it might be possible to evaluate either (a) the degree of tumor-induced suppression or (b) the recovery from this suppression after therapy. In the first instance, the immune evaluation takes place at diagnosis and prior to any therapy; in the second, immune monitoring during and after therapy is required. However, the immune biomarkers that measure immunosuppression levels at diagnosis might not be as informative as biomarkers of response to therapy or of clinical outcome. Hence, in most biotherapy trials, both approaches are used with the hope that intermediate biomarkers of suppression as well as biomarkers of therapy-induced recovery can be identified. The complexity of the host–tumor interactions has made both these approaches difficult to implement despite the availability of expert immunologic monitoring. Nevertheless, current preclinical and clinical data suggest that in a sufficiently large cohort of cancer patients with similar demographic and clinicopathologic features, the disease- or therapy-related immunologic alterations can be detected and measured. Further, in a limited number of cases, such an alteration has been shown to correlate with clinical outcome suggesting that, pending validation, it might serve as a future biomarker of prognosis or response to therapy. To date, only a few robust immune biomarkers predictive of clinical response or outcome have emerged. Still, recent progress in uncovering immune correlates associated with cancer progression or with response to therapy in preclinical and clinical studies provides reassurance that immune measures capable of serving as intermediate biomarkers of clinical outcome will be identified and validated in the near future.

8 "Immune Score" in the Tumor Microenvironment

It is well recognized that the tumor microenvironment has a profound impact on immune cells, and the nature, phenotype, localization, and density of immune cells present in the tumor stroma or parenchyma have long been considered to be critical for tumor progression [20]. Immune cells accumulating in human tumors have been extensively examined and found to have unique phenotypic and functional characteristics (reviewed in [21, 22]).

8.1 *The T Cell Signature*

Initially, it was typing of T lymphocytes by immunohistochemistry (IHC) in human tumors and correlations of CD8+ T cell infiltrates with prognosis that suggested the role of immune cells as predictors of risk [23]. However, TIL isolated from human tumors were found to be functionally impaired relative to T cells in normal donors [21, 22] leading to a debate as to whether TIL were harbingers of poor or good prognosis in cancer. Most of these early studies were retrospective, small, and technically variable and perhaps biased by the use of imperfect manual cell counts for in situ TIL evaluations. Since Rosenberg and others succeeded in expanding TIL for adoptive therapy, it seemed that if TIL were functionally deficient in situ, they clearly regained the ability to eliminate tumor cells upon culture in the presence of IL-2 [24]. The realization that the tumor–host interactions might be critical for the fate of immune cells and ultimately that of cancer patients prompted the reassessment of the role TIL play in cancer progression. The report on TIL in colorectal cancer (CRC) published by Galon and colleagues in 2006 [25] has dramatically and convincingly altered our perception of the prognostic significance of these T cells. Using modern techniques of systems biology and an objective scoring system, these investigators showed that type, density, and location of immune cells within tumors predicted positive clinical outcome [25]. In a series of studies in CRC, Fridman's group has demonstrated by immunostaining of hundreds of tumor specimens that a strong local immune reaction, including CD3+, CD8+, and memory CD45RO+ T cells, correlates with a favorable prognosis regardless of the local extent of the tumor or the regional lymph node involvement [26, 27]. At the same time, a number of reports from various laboratories on the nature and cellular composition of immune infiltrates into human tumors have given support to the role of TIL in estimating clinical outcome in cancer [28]. For example, an independent report by Mahmoud et al. confirmed the prognostic significance of the T cell signature in breast cancer [29]. T cell infiltrates emerged as the stronger independent prognostic factor than the current clinicopathological criteria such as tumor size, depth of infiltration, differentiation, or nodal status [30]. These results have motivated investigators to propose routine evaluations of the tumor microenvironment for density, location, phenotype, and function of T cells in order to define "an immune score" for each tumor as a part of the standard pathologic examination [31]. It has to be determined whether and how soon this practice will be embraced by the pathologists. Of concern are the standardization of methods for routine consumption and requirements for automated image analyses. Nevertheless, globally collected data strongly support the merit of the "immune score," and it makes sense to evaluate its predictive value, especially in the context of ongoing biotherapy clinical trials. Thus, the immune score emerges as the first immunologic marker of risk in cancer with a potential to be incorporated into prognostically relevant immune classification of human cancer equal to or better than the conventional TNM classification [31].

8.2 The Frequency of Tumor-Specific T Cells in the Circulation

In addition to scoring T cells at sites of tumor growth, the frequency and functions of T cells circulating in the peripheral blood have been examined as potential biomarkers in patients with cancer. The availability of standardized single-cell assays able to detect tumor antigen-specific T cells (ELISPOT, cytokine flow cytometry (CFC), and tetramer binding) has facilitated evaluation of epitope-specific T cells as potential biomarkers [32]. These assays, especially ELISPOT, have been standardized for serial monitoring [32] and can be reliably utilized to measure the frequency of epitope-specific T cells in blood or body fluids. Both CFC and tetramer assays require flow cytometry and thus are restricted to facilities equipped with a cytometer operated by a skilled technologist. For this reason and because these assays only measure the frequency of cells expressing a marker, ELISPOT has become the most widely used single-cell assay. ELISPOT defines the frequency of T cells able to respond to the recognized epitope by cytokine production. In a recent ECOG-sponsored 1696 Phase II multicenter trial testing vaccination with melanoma peptides delivered alone, with GM-CSF, IFN-α2b, or both cytokines to HLA-A2+ patients with metastatic melanoma, we serially monitored the frequency of CD8+tetramer+ (tet+) T cells, their differentiation stages, and ELISPOT responses of CD8+ T cells [33]. These immunologic data results were related to patients' clinical responses. Only IFN-γ ELISPOT results correlated with clinical responses, and neither the frequency of CD8+tet+ T cells in the periphery nor their differentiation stage were significant correlates of outcome [33]. These data suggest that only the functional status of tumor peptide-specific CD8+ T cells, and not their phenotype or differentiation, is a relevant biomarker for correlating immune and clinical responses to a peptide-based antitumor vaccine [33].

8.3 CD8+ T Cell Differentiation

In a series of studies measuring the frequency of CD8+CCR7+ T cells in the peripheral circulation of patients with head and neck squamous cell carcinoma (HNSCC), we observed that the low frequency of these cells at diagnosis, as assessed by flow cytometry of PBMC, discriminated HNSCC patients from healthy subjects [34]. We further showed that a low frequency of CD8+CCR7+ circulating T cells at diagnosis (i.e., fewer than 28 %) was a significant risk factor ($p<0.0115$) for disease recurrence. After up to 4 years of follow-up, disease-free survival (DFS) was found to be shorter for patients with fewer than 28 % of circulating CD8+CCR7+ T cells at diagnosis compared to those with higher percentages of these cells [34]. The results suggest that the CD8+CCR7+ cell subset might play a role in cancer control and that a simple blood test at diagnosis could have a prognostic value for predicting disease recurrence in HNSCC. Thus, a single surrogate immune marker measured in the peripheral blood at diagnosis can accurately predict recurrence regardless of the type of definitive therapy the patients receive. While these preclinical data are encouraging, the predictive value of this flow cytometry-based assay needs to be confirmed in additional much larger prospective studies. Nevertheless, the data provide preliminary evidence that immune biomarkers based on T cell differentiation could be useful in predicting recurrence.

8.4 *The B-Cell Signature*

To date, a search for promising immune correlates of cancer diagnosis, prognosis, and survival has been largely limited to adaptive cellular immune responses. In their definition of the immune score, Fridman and colleagues rarely mention B cells or plasma cells. Yet, considerable evidence exists in support of the presence of these cells in tumors, especially in breast cancer [35]. Results recently reported by Schmidt and colleagues provide evidence that validates B-cell signature as the robust prognostic factor in breast cancer [36]. The immunoglobulin kappa chain (IGKC) has been validated as an immunologic biomarker of prognosis and response to chemotherapy in patients with breast cancer, non-small-cell lung cancer, and colorectal carcinoma [36]. The IGKC was microscopically identified as a product of plasma cells present in the tumor stroma and was validated as a prognostic biomarker by the RNA- and protein-based expression studies independently performed in thousands of formalin-fixed, paraffin-embedded specimens at 20 different centers. Expression of the IGKC transcript was the strongest discriminator of patients with breast cancer with and without metastases among the 60 genes found in the B-cell metagene, while transcripts of the T cell metagene had no prognostic significance [35]. Further, the most important feature of IGKC as a biomarker is that it predicts responses to neoadjuvant therapy in breast cancer and as such qualifies as the first immune marker of response to cancer treatment. Because tumor immunologists have an ongoing debate about the role of humoral vs. cellular immunity in tumor development, progression, and therapy, the finding of the B-cell signature as a validated biomarker of prognosis and response to therapy provides a strong support for the view that humoral immunity is as important as T cells in controlling cancer [37].

8.5 *Suppressor Cells*

Accumulations of regulatory T cells (Treg) and myeloid derived suppressor cells (MDSC) in human tumors and their increased frequency in the circulation of cancer patients have been widely reported [38, 39]. Many reports, but not all, link these accumulations of CD4+FOXP3+CD25^{high} Treg to poor prognosis due to suppression of antitumor responses by the accumulating Treg [38]. Notably, in CRC, the presence and density of FOXP3+ Treg have been reported to predict favorable outcome and a better locoregional control of the tumor [40, 41]. These discrepant results are based on the prevalent use of FOXP3 transcription factor expression as a marker of Treg. However, a recent comprehensive review of the prognostic significance of FOXP3+ T cells in 16 non-lymphoid cancers suggested that FOXP3 by itself is not a reliable marker of human Treg and that the tumor site, i.e., the tumor microenvironment, has a major impact on biologic effects of FOXP3+ Treg [38, 42]. Because Treg are heterogeneous, consisting on many subsets of functionally distinct cells and because no universal distinguishing marker for Treg is currently available, their use as a biomarker of prognosis is limited and has to be taken with caution. Furthermore, current attempts to therapeutically deplete Treg might enhance tumor immunity in some patients but be detrimental in others [38, 42]. Overall, the prognostic value of FOXP3+ Treg in cancer is questionable, although it is possible that the introduction of more specific assays for Treg might provide a more discriminating approach for evaluating their prognostic value.

A similar situation exists with respect to MDSC. Their accumulations in the tumor and blood of cancer patients have also been correlated to poor clinical outcome [39, 43]. The problem that confounds their use as biomarkers of outcome is twofold. First, their tremendous phenotypic and functional heterogeneity creates a situation where everyone evaluates a different subset making it impossible to compare results. Specifically, HLA-DR^{neg}Lin^{neg} MDSC present in the human peripheral blood contain cells with monocytic and granulocytic features, which can be subdivided into at least four distinct subsets (CD33+, CD11b+, CD15+, and CD14+) and which differ with respect to mechanisms used for suppression [44]. A recently proposed immunophenotyping schema for MDSC, which utilizes multiparameter flow cytometry, provides a unifying approach to future evaluations of the role these cells play in disease [45]. This, however, does not eliminate the second problem of the sensitivity of CD15+ and CD33+ MDSC subsets to cryopreservation [18]. Only the frequency of CD14+ and CD11b+ subsets was not significantly decreased after PBMC cryopreservation, although their ability to produce ROS after ex vivo stimulation was lost [18]. These findings led to a conclusion that studies of human MDSC should be performed in fresh blood samples [18]. This requirement complicates monitoring of MDSC in clinical trials and thus their evaluation as potential prognostic biomarkers.

While both Treg and MDSC clearly play a major role in cancer progression and perhaps responses to immunotherapy, their usefulness as biomarkers of outcome or response to therapy has to await further development of monitoring assays that better reflect their biologic significance in cancer.

8.6 *The Neutrophil-to-Lymphocyte Ratio*

Chronic inflammation is closely associated with the development of certain human cancers, e.g., inflammatory bowel disease predisposes to CRC or human papilloma virus (HPV) infection to oropharyngeal squamous cell carcinoma. Evidence has accumulated that the total white blood count and especially the elevated neutrophil-to-lymphocyte ratio (NLR) measured prior to oncological therapies predict adverse clinical outcome in patients with lung, breast, renal, ovarian, and head and neck cancers [46]. Further, the high NLR is a significant but not yet validated marker of poor response to chemotherapy [46]. These observations fit well with previously reported low lymphocyte counts in patients with cancer [47]. We have reported spontaneous apoptosis of circulating CD8+ antigen-responding effector T cells leading to rapid lymphocyte turnover and depressed absolute number of T cell subsets in cancer patients tested prior to oncologic therapies [48]. Together, these data identifying the high pretreatment NLR as a significant independent predictor of poor cancer-specific survival compel us to consider a rapid validation of this promising biomarker.

8.7 Cytokine Expression and Levels

Cytokine gene or protein profiling, whether by multiplex immunoassays, microarrays, or proteomics technologies, is especially well suited to evaluations of the tumor microenvironment. The potential for capturing polarization in the cytokine repertoire or differences in patterns of their production by immune or tumor cells and of relating them to a specific clinical response have a tremendous appeal. Systemic and local therapies with cytokines are becoming increasingly common, and there is a need for monitoring cytokine levels in relation to clinical endpoints. Such monitoring has greatly expanded our knowledge of the cytokine biology and has provided clinically useful information about cytokine involvement in human disease. In cancer, considered to be a Th2-dominant disease with excess of IL-4, IL-5, IL-10, and TGF-β production, a therapeutically driven shift back toward the Th1 profile is of interest, as it might correlate with immune and perhaps clinical recovery [49]. Indeed, plasma cytokines have been used as prognostic biomarkers in cancer [50], with individual cytokines emerging as especially promising markers of survival. For example, elevated circulating levels of IL-6 have been associated with decreased survival in patients with cancer [51]. The production of pro-inflammatory cytokines, IL-1β, IL-6, and TNFα, all of which facilitate tumor growth, in the tumor microenvironment might be due to STAT3 hyperactivation in both the tumor and immune cells [52].

While cytokines and chemokines can be measured in the patients' circulation by many different methods, multiplex bead immunoassays designed to work in conjunction with a Luminex-type instrument have all but replaced traditional ELISA. These assays allow for a simultaneous measurement of pro-inflammatory cytokines, Th1- vs. Th2-type cytokines, growth-promoting as opposed to suppressive cytokines, etc., in a small (0.5 mL) sample of a body fluid. The result is a quantitative profile of as many as 20–30 cytokines, and changes in this profile can be sequentially followed in the course of a clinical trial. Usually, such time course analysis is performed with banked serum specimens, and often samples are banked for extended periods of time before being tested. It appears that despite standardized and controlled procedures used for cytokine assessments, the length of storage (months, years) in −80 °C freezer profoundly and significantly alters the measured cytokine levels [53, 54]. While IL-8 values generally increased after prolonged storage, those for other cytokines tended to decrease, for example [53]. This serves as a reminder that retrospective measurements of cytokines are highly prone to errors resulting from handling of samples, as also previously emphasized [55]. To avoid pitfalls due to long-term storage and sample freezing/thawing, biomarker analyses should be performed with fresh, prospectively collected specimens. The utility of any one cytokine as a candidate biomarker of clinical outcome has to be carefully scrutinized for bias, because it is strictly dependent on the sample integrity, rigorous testing, and result interpretation [53].

8.8 Exosomes

Tumor-derived exosomes have recently come into the limelight as potential biomarkers in cancer. These membranous nanovesicles (50–100 nM in diameter) carry a large variety of cellular components, including proteins, mRNA, microRNA, and DNA [56]. Exosome molecular content closely reflects that of tumor cells from which they originate and thus can serve as a sort of "liquid biopsy" in place of a conventional tissue biopsy. For this reason, exosomes are of great current interest, and preliminary studies suggest that their protein levels in the plasma and their molecular content reflect the tumor presence, its progression or regression after therapy, and possibly its recurrence [57]. Exosome fractions obtained from the plasma of melanoma patients with stage 4 disease had the highest protein concentrations relative to exosomes of patients with less advanced disease. Also, stage 4 patients with protein-poor exosomal fractions had a significant survival advantage over those with protein-rich exosomes [58]. These data suggest that exosome protein content alone may be a biomarker of prognosis in cancer. In murine melanoma, tumor-derived exosomes contributed to metastatic invasion by carrying messenger proteins that direct bone marrow-derived cells toward a pro-metastatic phenotype [57, 58]. We recently showed that exosomes isolated from sera of AML patients at diagnosis inhibited functions of NK cells via membrane-tethered TGF-β [59] and observed by using western blots that levels of this exosome-bound cytokine decreased during remission (preliminary results). Exosomes carry and present membrane-bound enzymes, receptors, and cytokines to target cells, serving as message carriers and delivering signals to immune and tissue cells [56]. Because membrane-bound proteins often have greater biological effects than their soluble counterparts, analysis of exosomes might be of greater prognostic value than are measures of serum proteins. Currently, methods for capture of tumor-derived exosomes to separate them from those secreted by normal cells in the plasma of cancer patients are being developed. With this technical improvement, the potential value of exosomes as biomarkers of the tumor fate during and after therapy can be confirmed in future prospective studies.

9 Statistical Analysis to Correlate Immunologic and Clinical Endpoints

Results obtained from immune monitoring require expert statistical analysis to explore their association with clinical outcome. In preparation for such analysis, the monitoring data need to be examined for outliers and corrected for potential errors made during data entry or assay performance. When the statistician is satisfied with the completeness and accuracy of the data set, he/she begins an analysis strategy that has been previously agreed to in consultation with clinical investigators. Ideally, the analysis selection is based on the primary or the secondary clinical trial objectives rather than ad hoc objectives. Usually, the object of the analysis is to establish the importance of immunologic changes with therapy by finding association with clinical outcomes such as clinical response, recurrence, or survival. Several statistical methods are available for this type of analysis as previously described [15, 60]. Nonparametric tests are generally superior in smaller data sets. Differences in posttreatment levels relative to the pretreatment baseline can utilize the Wilcoxon signed rank test for paired data (a single posttreatment observation) or Freidman's test for more than a single posttreatment data point. For larger data sets or for data that have been transformed to meet the assumptions of parametric analysis, a paired t test or a repeated measure analysis of variance may be used.

Comparisons between treatment groups can be accomplished by comparing mean group differences. Repeated-measures analyses are sensitive to occasional extreme data points and to skewed distributions, and suitable data transformations are recommended as are more robust fitting methods, which down-weight the influence of extreme data points. When multiple immunological endpoints are available, newer statistical methods, such as recursive partitioning models, can be applied to patient classification to estimate the classification accuracy of a combination or a "signature" of immune parameters [60]. No matter how extensive the statistical analysis, it is important to remember that the availability of data from adequate number of subjects, demographic and clinical homogeneity of the cohort, and the ability of a selected monitoring assay to discriminate responders from nonresponders are important components of an immunologic investigation. All of these should be thoughtfully planned prior to any data collection. For discovering correlations between immunologic results and clinical outcome reliable, objective, and rigorously collected clinical data with sufficiently long follow-up are essential.

Interpretations of monitoring results require statistical analysis capable of modeling therapy-induced changes in multiple cellular interactions over time. It is expected that when these requirements are adequately addressed and immune monitoring becomes an integral part of all biotherapy trials, the so far tenuous goal of establishing immune correlates of clinical responses will be achieved.

Interpretation of immunologic results is not straightforward however, and expertise may be needed to provide a correct interpretation. The difficulty often arises when counterintuitive results are obtained, for example, when expected immune recovery is camouflaged by a suppressive factor, such as the presence of Treg. The correct interpretation may only emerge upon performing an additional assay which is selected based on potential mechanisms involved. Results derived from a hypothesis-driven study monitored with a standardized assay targeting a specific mechanism is most likely to correlate with clinical outcome. Therefore, close interaction between the biostatistician, clinical investigator, and immunologist is a hallmark of successful immune monitoring and biomarker discovery.

10 Immune Profiling in Cancer

As biotherapy trials, including antitumor vaccines, antitumor antibody therapies, and checkpoint inhibitors, are increasingly often performed, the need for surrogate markers of response has become more urgent. A definition of the immunologic profile predictive or survival or response to therapy would greatly facilitate decisions about the choice of biotherapies and help identify cancer patients likely to respond to selected biotherapies. As genomics- and proteomics-based technologies are gaining increasingly important place in screening for immune alterations, a concept of "immune profiling" has been introduced, referring to measurements of several immune and genetic markers that together establish a characteristic "immune portrait" of cancer [61]. Such a profile would incorporate not just T cells infiltrating the tumor but also other immune cells and their products both in the tumor microenvironment and in the peripheral blood or body fluids [61–63]. An "immune profile" combining immunologic, proteomics, and genomics results would be expected to discriminate cancer patients from healthy controls or distinguish cancer patients who favorably respond to therapy from those who do not. Optimally, an immunologic profile, once defined for a set of immune markers, could broadly serve to predict clinical responses in biotherapy trials. An intensive search for the set of such biomarkers has been ongoing but, so far, has not provided an immunologic profile linked to improved survival in cancer. This is not surprising given the difficulties associated with defining a "normal" immune profile due to extreme interindividual and biological variability in components of the immune system. Immune responses are subject to environmental, hormonal, and neurologic as well as pathologic changes [64, 65]. Therefore, the discrimination of therapy-related alterations from biologically mediated normal responses to infections, stress, or endocrine activity might be very difficult. Perhaps a more realistic approach would be to define a "personal immune profile" for each patient at baseline (i.e., at diagnosis; prior to any therapy) using multiple immune and genetic markers and monitor for alterations in this profile in the course of treatment. The immune markers discussed above and genetic biomarkers (e.g., transcriptional signatures) emerging from many preclinical studies [65–67] have provided a number of candidates for such personalized immune profiling that are currently under scrutiny for their diagnostic or prognostic value.

11 Conclusions

Immune monitoring of clinical trials is complex and requires considerable resources. It is, however, necessary for ensuring that clinical endpoints are correlated to the immunologic mechanisms potentially responsible for therapy-induced changes. Linking correlative immunologic studies with clinical endpoints has been difficult, possibly because of the requirement for extensive laboratory support or because of biological variability inherent to the immune system. Serial studies are especially demanding to perform reliably, and a GLP facility specializing in immune monitoring is an appropriate venue for studies in support of clinical trials. New high-throughput technologies including the genomic and proteomic platforms provide tools necessary for establishing personalized immune profiles for patients receiving biotherapies. Changes in this profile in the course of treatment or as a result of disease progression or regression might serve as intermediate markers of outcome. However, much work remains to first confirm a reliable association of these profile changes with clinical endpoints and then to validate each potential biomarker in the series of prospective clinical trials.

The current expertise in technical and conceptual aspects of immune monitoring of patients undergoing biotherapy is largely a by-product of efforts to centralize monitoring to specialized laboratories and to apply clinical, immunologic, and biostatistics insights into data interpretation. To take advantage of immune monitoring, it is necessary to (a) ensure that it adequately and reliably measures changes induced by administered biotherapy and (b) establish strong and transparent interactions between the clinical investigator, clinical immunologist, and biostatistician assisting in data analysis (Table 1).

Table 1 Technologies available for adaptation to establishing an "immune profile" of patients treated with biotherapies in clinical trials

Genomic analysis: DNA arrays
Transcriptional signature: RT-PCR or qRT-PCR for molecular markers of disease
Proteome signature: Serum/plasma and tissue proteomics, including antibody microarrays and multiplexing for cytokines and chemokines; exosome profiling
Molecular signaling; receptor/ligand interactions
Immune polymorphisms
High-content cell screening by flow cytometry and image analysis
Tissue microarrays and immunocytochemistry
Assessment of immune infiltrates into tissues: "Immune score"
Assessments of cell apoptosis vs. necrosis

References

1. Butterfield LH, et al. Recommendations from the iSBTc-SITC/FDA/NCI Workshop on Immunotherapy Biomarkers. Clin Cancer Res. 2011;17(10):3064–76.
2. Matzinger P. The danger model: a renewed sense of self. Science. 2002;296(5566):301–5.
3. Huang B, et al. TLR signaling by tumor and immune cells: a double-edged sword. Oncogene. 2008;27(2):218–24.
4. Whiteside TL. The tumor microenvironment and its role in promoting tumor growth. Oncogene. 2008;27(45):5904–12.
5. Whiteside TL, et al. Mechanisms of tumor escape from the immune system: adenosine-producing Treg, exosomes and tumor-associated TLRs. Bull Cancer. 2011;98(2):E25–31.
6. Postow MA, Harding J, Wolchok JD. Targeting immune checkpoints: releasing the restraints on anti-tumor immunity for patients with melanoma. Cancer J. 2012;18(2):153–9.
7. Whiteside TL. Inhibiting the inhibitors: evaluating agents targeting cancer immunosuppression. Expert Opin Biol Ther. 2010;10(7):1019–35.
8. Vivier E, et al. Targeting natural killer cells and natural killer T cells in cancer. Nat Rev Immunol. 2012;12(4):239–52.
9. Mellman I, Coukos G, Dranoff G. Cancer immunotherapy comes of age. Nature. 2011; 480(7378):480–9.
10. Restifo NP, Dudley ME, Rosenberg SA. Adoptive immunotherapy for cancer: harnessing the T cell response. Nat Rev Immunol. 2012;12(4):269–81.
11. DeNardo DG, Coussens LM. Inflammation and breast cancer. Balancing immune response: crosstalk between adaptive and innate immune cells during breast cancer progression. Breast Cancer Res. 2007;9(4):212.
12. Eskandari F, Sternberg EM. Neural-immune interactions in health and disease. Ann N Y Acad Sci. 2002;966:20–7.
13. Tahara H, et al. Emerging concepts in biomarker discovery; the US-Japan Workshop on Immunological Molecular Markers in Oncology. J Transl Med. 2009;7:45.
14. Whiteside TL, et al. Shipping of therapeutic somatic cell products. Cytotherapy. 2011;13(2):201–13.
15. Whiteside T. *Monitoring of Immunologic Therapies*. In: Hamilton RG, Detrick B, Folds JD, editors. Manual of molecular and clinical laboratory immunology. Washington, DC: ASM Press; 2006. p. 1171–82.
16. Iancu, EM et al. Profile of a serial killer: cellular and molecuar approaches to study individual cytotoxic t-cells following therapeutic vaccination. J Biomed Biotechnol 2011; p. 21.
17. Nomura L, Maino VC, Maecker HT. Standardization and optimization of multiparameter intracellular cytokine staining. Cytometry A. 2008;73(11):984–91.
18. Kotsakis A, et al. Myeloid-derived suppressor cell measurements in fresh and cryopreserved blood samples. J Immunol Methods. 2012;381(1–2):14–22.
19. Whiteside TL. Immune monitoring of clinical trials with biotherapies. Adv Clin Chem. 2008;45:75–97.
20. Whiteside TL. The role of immune cells in the tumor microenvironment. Cancer Treat Res. 2006;130:103–24.
21. Frey AB, Monu N. Signaling defects in anti-tumor T cells. Immunol Rev. 2008;222: 192–205.
22. Whiteside TL. Immune responses to malignancies. J Allergy Clin Immunol. 2010;125(2 Suppl 2):S272–83.
23. von Kleist S, et al. Immunohistological analysis of lymphocyte subpopulations infiltrating breast carcinomas and benign lesions. Int J Cancer. 1987;40(1):18–23.
24. Dudley ME, et al. Generation of tumor-infiltrating lymphocyte cultures for use in adoptive transfer therapy for melanoma patients. J Immunother. 2003;26(4):332–42.
25. Galon J, et al. Type, density, and location of immune cells within human colorectal tumors predict clinical outcome. Science. 2006;313(5795):1960–4.

26. Fridman WH, et al. Prognostic and predictive impact of intra- and peritumoral immune infiltrates. Cancer Res. 2011;71(17):5601–5.
27. Pages F, et al. Effector memory T cells, early metastasis, and survival in colorectal cancer. N Engl J Med. 2005;353(25):2654–66.
28. Sato E, et al. Intraepithelial CD8+ tumor-infiltrating lymphocytes and a high CD8+/regulatory T cell ratio are associated with favorable prognosis in ovarian cancer. Proc Natl Acad Sci U S A. 2005;102(51):18538–43.
29. Mahmoud SM, et al. Tumor-infiltrating CD8+ lymphocytes predict clinical outcome in breast cancer. J Clin Oncol. 2011;29(15):1949–55.
30. Mlecnik B, et al. Histopathologic-based prognostic factors of colorectal cancers are associated with the state of the local immune reaction. J Clin Oncol. 2011;29(6):610–8.
31. Galon J, et al. The immune score as a new possible approach for the classification of cancer. J Transl Med. 2012;10:1.
32. Britten CM, et al. Minimal information about T cell assays: the process of reaching the community of T cell immunologists in cancer and beyond. Cancer Immunol Immunother. 2011;60(1):15–22.
33. Schaefer C, et al. Function but not phenotype of melanoma peptide-specific CD8(+) T cells correlate with survival in a multiepitope peptide vaccine trial (ECOG 1696). Int J Cancer. 2012;131(4):874–84.
34. Czystowska M, et al. The immune signature of CD8+ CCR7+ T cells in the peripheral circulation assoicates with disease recurrence in patients with HNSCC. Clin Cancer Res. 2013;19(4):889–99.
35. Schmidt M, et al. The humoral immune system has a key prognostic impact in node-negative breast cancer. Cancer Res. 2008;68(13):5405–13.
36. Schmidt M, et al. A comprehensive analysis of human gene expression profiles identifies stromal immunoglobulin kappa C as a compatible prognostic marker in human solid tumors. Clin Cancer Res. 2012;18(9):2695–703.
37. Whiteside TL, Ferrone S. For breast cancer prognosis, immunoglobulin kappa chain surfaces to the top. Clin Cancer Res. 2012;18(9):2417–9.
38. Whiteside TL. What are regulatory T cells (Treg) regulating in cancer and why? Semin Cancer Biol. 2012;22(4):327–34.
39. Marigo I, et al. Tumor-induced tolerance and immune suppression by myeloid derived suppressor cells. Immunol Rev. 2008;222:162–79.
40. Salama P, et al. Tumor-infiltrating FOXP3+ T regulatory cells show strong prognostic significance in colorectal cancer. J Clin Oncol. 2009;27(2):186–92.
41. Badoual C, et al. Prognostic value of tumor-infiltrating CD4+ T-cell subpopulations in head and neck cancers. Clin Cancer Res. 2006;12(2):465–72.
42. deLeeuw RJ, et al. The prognostic value of FoxP3+ tumor-infiltrating lymphocytes in cancer: a critical review of the literature. Clin Cancer Res. 2012;18(11):3022–9.
43. Raychaudhuri B, et al. Myeloid-derived suppressor cell accumulation and function in patients with newly diagnosed glioblastoma. Neuro Oncol. 2011;13(6):591–9.
44. Greten TF, Manns MP, Korangy F. Myeloid derived suppressor cells in human diseases. Int Immunopharmacol. 2011;11(7):802–7.
45. Dumitru CA, et al. Neutrophils and granulocytic myeloid-derived suppressor cells: immunophenotyping, cell biology and clinical relevance in human oncology. Cancer Immunol Immunother. 2012;61(8):1155–67.
46. Perisanidis C, Kornek G, Poschl PW, Holzinger D, Pirklbauer K, Schopper C, Ewers R. High neutrophil-to-lymphocyte ratio is an independent marker of poor disease-specific survival in patients with oral cancer. Med Oncol. 2013;30(1):334.
47. Kuss I, et al. Imbalance in absolute counts of T lymphocyte subsets in patients with head and neck cancer and its relation to disease. Adv Otorhinolaryngol. 2005;62:161–72.
48. Whiteside TL. Lymphocyte homeostasis and the antitumor immune response. Expert Rev Clin Immunol. 2005;1(3):369–78.

49. Lucey DR, Clerici M, Shearer GM. Type 1 and type 2 cytokine dysregulation in human infectious, neoplastic, and inflammatory diseases. Clin Microbiol Rev. 1996;9(4):532–62.
50. Hanash SM, Pitteri SJ, Faca VM. Mining the plasma proteome for cancer biomarkers. Nature. 2008;452(7187):571–9.
51. Schafer ZT, Brugge JS. IL-6 involvement in epithelial cancers. J Clin Invest. 2007; 117(12):3660–3.
52. Yu H, Kortylewski M, Pardoll D. Crosstalk between cancer and immune cells: role of STAT3 in the tumour microenvironment. Nat Rev Immunol. 2007;7(1):41–51.
53. Butterfield LH, Potter DM, Kirkwood JM. Multiplex serum biomarker assessments: technical and biostatistical issues. J Transl Med. 2011;9:173.
54. Potter DM, et al. Pitfalls in retrospective analyses of biomarkers: a case study with metastatic melanoma patients. J Immunol Methods. 2012;376(1–2):108–12.
55. Whiteside TL. Cytokine assays. Biotechniques (2002);Suppl(4–8), 10, 12-5.
56. Iero M, et al. Tumour-released exosomes and their implications in cancer immunity. Cell Death Differ. 2008;15(1):80–8.
57. Somasundaram R, Herlyn M. Melanoma exosomes: messengers of metastasis. Nat Med. 2012;18(6):853–4.
58. Peinado H, et al. Melanoma exosomes educate bone marrow progenitor cells toward a pro-metastatic phenotype through MET. Nat Med. 2012;18(6):883–91.
59. Szczepanski MJ, et al. Blast-derived microvesicles in sera from patients with acute myeloid leukemia suppress natural killer cell function via membrane-associated transforming growth factor-beta1. Haematologica. 2011;96(9):1302–9.
60. Breiman L, Friedman JH, Olshen RA, Stone CJ. Classification and regression trees. Belmont, CA: Wadsworth Press; 1984.
61. Lotze MT, et al. Workshop on cancer biometrics: identifying biomarkers and surrogates of cancer in patients: a meeting held at the Masur Auditorium. National Institutes of Health. J Immunother. 2005;28(2):79–119.
62. Ascierto ML, et al. An immunologic portrait of cancer. J Transl Med. 2011;9:146.
63. Wang E, Uccellini L, Marincola FM. A genetic inference on cancer immune responsiveness. Oncoimmunology. 2012;1(4):520–5.
64. Calcagni E, Elenkov I. Stress system activity, innate and T helper cytokines, and susceptibility to immune-related diseases. Ann N Y Acad Sci. 2006;1069:62–76.
65. Gajewski TF, Fuertes MB, Woo SR. Innate immune sensing of cancer: clues from an identified role for type I IFNs. Cancer Immunol Immunother. 2012;61(8):1343–7.
66. Manjili MH, Najarian K, Wang XY. Signatures of tumor-immune interactions as biomarkers for breast cancer prognosis. Future Oncol. 2012;8(6):703–11.
67. Gowda M, et al. Distinct signatures of the immune responses in low risk versus high risk neuroblastoma. J Transl Med. 2011;9:170.

Index

J.D. Rosenblatt et al. (eds.), *Advances in Tumor Immunology and Immunotherapy*, Current Cancer Research, DOI 10.1007/978-1-4614-8809-5,
© Springer Science+Business Media New York 2014

MIX
Papier aus verantwortungsvollen Quellen
Paper from responsible sources
FSC® C105338

If you have any concerns about our products,
you can contact us on
ProductSafety@springernature.com

In case Publisher is established outside the EU,
the EU authorized representative is:
Springer Nature Customer Service Center GmbH
Europaplatz 3, 69115 Heidelberg, Germany

Printed by Libri Plureos GmbH
in Hamburg, Germany